THE WORLD BIENNIAL OF PSYCHIATRY AND PSYCHOTHERAPY
Volume I

EDITORIAL BOARD

Editor, Silvano Arieti

BRAZIL	*Horus Brazil*
FRANCE	*Pierre Pichot*
GERMANY	*Gerd Huber*
	Paul Matussek
ISRAEL	*Julius Zellermayer*
ITALY	*Pier Francesco Galli*
	Cornelio Fazio
JAPAN	*Masashi Murakami*
MEXICO	*Alfonso Millan*
PERU	*Carlo Alberto Seguin*
POLAND	*Andrzej Jus*
SOVIET UNION	*A. V. Snezhnevsky*
SPAIN	*Ivan Lopez Ibor*
SWITZERLAND	*Gaetano Benedetti*
	Christian Müller
U. S. A.	*Silvano Arieti*
	Francis J. Braceland
	Paul Friedman
	Jacques S. Gottlieb
	Lothar B. Kalinowsky
	Harold Kelman
	Stanley Lesse
	George Mora
	Jurgen Ruesch

THE WORLD BIENNIAL OF PSYCHIATRY AND PSYCHOTHERAPY

◦§ Volume I §◦

1971

Edited by Silvano Arieti

Basic Books, Inc., *Publishers*

NEW YORK   LONDON

© 1970 by Basic Books, Inc.
Library of Congress Catalog Card Number: 70–116847
SBN 465–09221–7
Manufactured in the United States of America
DESIGNED BY VINCENT TORRE

CONTRIBUTORS

SILVANO ARIETI, M.D.
   Clinical Professor of Psychiatry, New York Medical College; Faculty Member, Comprehensive Course in Psychoanalysis, New York Medical College, New York.

JACOB A. ARLOW, M.D.
   Clinical Professor of Psychiatry, State University of New York; Faculty Member, New York Psychoanalytic Institute, New York.

CARLOS P. BARROS, M.D.
   Chairman, Department of Psychology, Pontificia Universidade Catolica do Rio de Janeiro; Director of Psychoanalytic Research, Instituto de Medicine Psicologica, Rio de Janeiro, Brazil.

PETER G. S. BECKETT, M.D.
   Professor of Psychiatry, Trinity College, Dublin; Consultant Psychiatrist, St. Patrick's Hospital, Dublin, Ireland.

JULES RICHARD BEMPORAD, M.D.
   Chief, Child Psychiatry Division, Wilford Hall Medical Center; Assistant Clinical Professor of Psychiatry, University of Texas Medical School at San Antonio, Texas.

BRUNO BETTELHEIM, Ph.D.
   Director, Sonia Shankman Orthogenic School, Chicago; Rowley Professor of Education, Chicago, Illinois.

PIETRO CASTELNUOVO-TEDESCO, M.D.
   Associate Professor of Psychiatry, University of California, Los Angeles; Chief, Department of Psychiatry, Harbor General Hospital, Los Angeles, California.

PIERRE DENIKER, M.D.
   Professeur Agregé at the Faculty of Medicine of Paris, France.

JACQUES S. GOTTLIEB, M.D.
Director, Lafayette Clinic, Detroit, Michigan; Professor and Chairman, Department of Psychiatry, Wayne State University School of Medicine, Detroit, Michigan.

ROBERT E. GOULD, M.D.
Director of Adolescent Services, Bellevue Psychiatric Hospital; Associate Professor of Psychiatry, N. Y. University School of Medicine, New York.

YOMISHI KASAHARA, M.D.
Associate Professor of Psychiatry, Medical School of Kyoto University; Chief of Division of Mental Health, Student Health Center of Kyoto University, Kyoto, Japan.

EINAR KRINGLEN, M.D.
Professor of Clinical Psychology, University of Bergen; Senior Psychiatrist, Department of Psychiatry, Haukeland Sykehus, Bergen, Norway.

HEINZ E. LEHMANN, M.D.
Professor of Psychiatry, McGill University; Clinical Director, Douglas Hospital, Verdun, Quebec, Canada.

STANLEY LESSE, M.D.
Editor, *American Journal of Psychotherapy*; Consultant, Physicians and Surgeons, American Rehabilitation Committee, New York.

FRANCIS A. MacNAB, Ph.D.
Director of the Cairnmiller Institute, Melbourne, Australia.

PAUL MATUSSEK, M.D.
Director, Research Center for Psychopathology and Psychotherapy in the Max Planck Society; Professor of Psychiatry, University of Munich, West Germany.

LEON ROIZIN, M.D.
Chief of Psychiatric Research (Neuropathology), New York State Psychiatric Institute; Professor of Neuropathology, Columbia University, New York.

KENJI SAKAMOTO, M.D.
Lecturer in Psychiatry, Medical School of Kyoto University; Director of Sakamoto Psychiatric Hospital, Higashi-Osaka, Osaka, Japan.

CONTRIBUTORS

CARLOS ALBERTO SEGUIN, M.D.
Director of Instituto de Psiquiatria Social Universidad National Mayor de San Marcos, Lima, Peru.

MARA SELVINI PALAZZOLI, M.D.
Associate Professor, Institute of Psychology, Catholic University of Milan, Italy; Director, Center for Family Study, Milan, Italy.

A. V. SNEZHNEVSKY, M.D.
Director, Institute of Psychiatry, Academy of Medical Sciences, Moscow, Soviet Union.

ALBERTA B. SZALITA, M.D.
Clinical Professor of Psychiatry, Columbia University, New York; Training and Supervising Analyst, Psychoanalytic Clinic for Training and Research, College of Physicians and Surgeons, Columbia University, New York.

YASUHIKO TAKETOMO, M.D.
Assistant Professor of Psychiatry, Albert Einstein College of Medicine; Chief, Mental Retardation Service, Bronx State Hospital, New York.

J. ROBERTSON UNWIN, M.D.
Director, Adolescent Service, Allan Memorial Institute; Assistant Professor of Psychiatry, McGill University, Montreal, Canada.

D. W. WINNICOTT, M.D., F.R.C.P.
Honorary Cons. Physician, Paddington Green Children's Hospital, London, England.

PREFACE

With the publication of this volume a series is initiated, unique in the history of psychiatry, which every two years will report from the various parts of the world the latest views on man and his psychiatric disorders.

Until a few years ago, psychiatric progress was made in a relatively small number of countries. Today, research is proceeding at an increasingly rapid pace, and many countries have made major contributions to psychiatric knowledge. Moreover, the psychiatric community can anticipate the creative involvement of the several new nations.

The Editorial Board of this project believes that, although an exchange of information now takes place through journals and international meetings, a book published at regular intervals will make more accessible to the psychiatrist, the psychologist, the student, and all people working in related fields the latest contributions, irrespective of where they have been made. Newness and value will be the two major criteria for selection, and no worthy study will be omitted purely for thematic reasons.

The compilation of this book, however, serves more than a practical purpose. It reflects, as does the restive cultural scene, the new spirit that pervades man. Frontiers, political divisions, and separate histories have increasingly less significance, for while we respect our distinctiveness more and more, we feel more and more alike. This book will, hopefully, prove once more that anyone can benefit from whatever psychiatric achievement is made in any part of the world; it will, thus, in its own way, be a humble testimony to that which needs constant reaffirmation—the universality of man. Further, in that it will simultaneously highlight the benefit that all can derive from that which is specific to certain groups of men in particular conditions in different lands, it will reassert the importance of man's diversity within the greater realm of his universality.

In this volume, thirteen countries are represented. The book is divided into four parts: the first deals with theoretical or general issues; the second, with specific clinical problems; the third, with childhood and youth; the fourth, with biological advancements. I have already mentioned that in the selection of the articles newness and importance were given first priority. A few of the chosen topics are not new, but they have been approached from a new angle or in a way which seems definitive.

The nature of this volume can, in part, be defined by the contrasting and yet complementary aspects of the chapters. Several topics, like drug addiction in youth, the hippie alienation, and psychiatric considerations in the heart transplant, are striking in their immediacy. Some chapters, such as those on decreasing the length of psychotherapy, the state of the emotionally isolated woman, anorexia, and consultation in child psychiatry, stand out for their practical value. Still others—for example, Arlow's study on current psychoanalytic thought and Barros's study of thermodynamics and evolutionary concepts of Freud's metapsychology—deal with fundamental theoretical issues.

Along with names of authors well known in psychiatry or related fields, the reader will acknowledge the appearance of new and promising young contributors. Almost all chapters are written in an easy, accessible style. Nevertheless, a few, like those prepared by Barros, Roizin, and Taketomo, may require some efforts from readers not particularly acquainted with their topics. In the future, these few difficult papers may attain a fuller significance; as a matter of fact, they may constitute original landmarks to which the reader will return time and time again in years to come.

In the volumes which are to follow, we will strive for consistency with the principles adopted in the preparation of the present book. However, no principle will be rigidly enforced without taking into consideration changes suggested by the current circumstances. Even in the preparation of this first volume, an exception was made to one of the principles. Though the Editorial Board intended not to publish more than one article by any one author, it happened that Dr. Castelnuovo-Tedesco, who had already prepared a chapter for this book, had the opportunity to see psychiatric complications in a heart transplant patient. We chose not to forgo this timely contribution.

New York SILVANO ARIETI, M.D.
August 1970

CONTENTS

PART ONE
Psychiatric Theory, General Issues, and Reviews

1. *The Structural and Psychodynamic Role of Cognition in the Human Psyche* — 3
   SILVANO ARIETI
2. *Some Problems in Current Psychoanalytic Thought* — 34
   JACOB A. ARLOW
3. *Decreasing the Length of Psychotherapy: Theoretical and Practical Aspects of the Problem* — 55
   PIETRO CASTELNUOVO-TEDESCO
4. *Thermodynamic and Evolutionary Concepts in the Formal Structure of Freud's Metapsychology* — 72
   CARLOS P. BARROS
5. *Levels of Temporality in Psychopathology* — 112
   YASUHIKO TAKETOMO
6. *Symptom, Syndrome, Disease: A Clinical Method in Psychiatry* — 151
   A. V. SNEZHNEVSKY
7. *Folklore Psychiatry* — 165
   CARLOS ALBERTO SEGUIN
8. *Medicine, Psychiatry, and Psychotherapy: A Futurologic Projection* — 178
   STANLEY LESSE

PART TWO
Clinical Contributions

9. *Anorexia Nervosa* — 197
   MARA SELVINI PALAZZOLI

10 New Views on the Psychodynamics of the Depressive
    Character   219
    JULES RICHARD BEMPORAD

11 Psychotherapy of the Emotionally Isolated Woman   244
    FRANCIS A. MACNAB

12 The Marginally Asocial Personality: The Beatnik-Hippie
    Alienation   258
    ROBERT E. GOULD

13 Ereuthophobia and Allied Conditions: A Contribution
    toward the Psychopathological and Crosscultural Study
    of a Borderline State   292
    YOMISHI KASAHARA AND
    KENJI SAKAMOTO

14 Psychotherapy and Family Interviews   312
    ALBERTA B. SZALITA

15 Psychoanalytic Considerations in a Case of Cardiac
    Transplantation   336
    PIETRO CASTELNUOVO-TEDESCO

16 Late Symptomatology among Former Concentration
    Camp Inmates   353
    PAUL MATUSSEK

PART THREE
Psychiatric Studies of Childhood and Youth

17 A Psychotherapeutic Consultation in Child Psychiatry:
    A Comparative Study of the Dynamic Processes   377
    D. W. WINNICOTT

18 Infantile Autism   400
    BRUNO BETTELHEIM

19 Contemporary Misuse of Psychoactive Drugs by Youth   426
    J. ROBERTSON UNWIN

PART FOUR
Biological Studies

20 Psychopharmacology: The Role of Clinical Research   463
    PIERRE DENIKER

21	*New Studies on the Genetics of Schizophrenia* EINAR KRINGLEN	476
22	*Advances in the Biology of Schizophrenia* PETER G. S. BECKETT AND JACQUES S. GOTTLIEB	505
23	*Psychophysiological and Related Approaches to Psychopathology* HEINZ E. LEHMANN	529
24	*Evolution of Fundamental CNS Pathogenic Concepts* LEON ROIZIN	560
	Index	603

PART ONE

Psychiatric Theory, General Issues, and Reviews

THE STRUCTURAL AND PSYCHODYNAMIC ROLE OF COGNITION IN THE HUMAN PSYCHE

Silvano Arieti

INTRODUCTION

A strong desire to emulate chemistry and physics and to strive toward the unity of science has predisposed many researchers in the fields of psychology and psychiatry to adopt a positivistic, operationalistic approach.

Most of these researchers insist in viewing the psyche mainly as a complex apparatus that permits and enhances animal species to adapt to environmental reality. In the human being, this apparatus is viewed as having reached a degree of complexity that leads to an increasing understanding and mastery of the world.

This methodology has led to an accumulation of significant data and is responsible for outstanding progress in our knowledge of certain aspects of the psyche, especially by disclosing how previous external influences affect objective behavior. Nevertheless, if it is not complemented by different types of inquiry, this point of view ignores other parts of the psyche—actually those that matter most within a psychiatric and psychoanalytic frame of reference. To be specific, an exclusively empirical, operationalistic approach first minimizes the role that subjectivity plays in psychological processes; second, it deals almost exclusively with that part of the psyche that makes contact with the surrounding world by perceiving, reacting, and approaching. In infrahumans, this part constitutes almost the whole psyche, but in human beings another important part acquires prominence; in the various terminologies this has been called "inner life," "inner reality," "psychic reality," "intrapsychic self," "intrapsychic life," "endopsychic structure," "proprium," "core of man," and the like.

Inner life, or inner reality, may represent, substitute, distort, enrich, or impoverish the reality of the external world. Although this inner reality too has many exchanges with the environment, it has an enduring life of its own. It becomes the essence of the individual. Its organization is what we call the "inner self."

Inner reality is the result of a constant reelaboration of past and present experiences. Its development is never completed throughout the life of man, although its greatest rate of growth occurs in childhood and adolescence. It is based on the fact that perceptions, thoughts, feelings, actions, and other psychological functions do not cease completely to exist once the neuronal mechanisms that mediated their occurrence have taken place. Although they cannot be retained as they were experienced, their effects are retained as various components of the psyche. Freud wrote that in mental life nothing that has once been formed can perish.

From approximately the ninth month of life the child internalizes: he retains as inner objects mental representations of external objects, events, relations, and the feelings associated with these psychological events. Inner objects acquire a relative independence from the correspondent external stimuli that elicited them. They progressively associate and organize in higher constructs.

This chapter illustrates some major elements of inner reality, giving particular consideration to the role of cognition in its development, structure, and psychodynamics.

PSYCHOANALYTIC VIEWS OF INNER REALITY

Whereas some schools (behavioristic, behavior therapy, conditioned response, aversion therapy, and so forth) are interested in studying and altering man's behavior and capacity for adaptation, most psychoanalytic and psychotherapeutic schools are interested in studying and changing the inner self, even if it is more difficult to do so. The premise of psychoanalysis and psychodynamic psychotherapy is that if you change the inner self, sooner or later a change, and a more reliable one, will occur also in the external behavior and capacity for adaptation.

As Guntrip[18] has pointed out, historically psychoanalysis is the first science to illustrate the existence of a psychic reality that is distinct from the reality of the external world. It is one of Freud's great achievements to have demonstrated the existence of this psychic reality as an entity in its own right, an entity that is alterable, but at the same time highly resistant to change. Other points of view, advanced by Freud, are still open to debate: (1) whether the psyche is nearly formed by the age of four or five; (2) whether its only or most important dynamic components are instinctual forces; (3) whether its only conflicts derive from the desire, on one hand, to satisfy instinctual drives and, on the other hand, to abide with the restrictions imposed by society; (4) whether it can be divided into three parts—id, ego, and superego.

Some neo-Freudian schools of psychoanalysis, as well as the existentialistic school of psychiatry, criticize Freudian theory as being too biological, for minimizing that part of man that transcends or even negates nature by not wanting to adapt to the imposition, limitation, or restriction of nature. We can add to this criticism that man, as he is seen by classic Freudian theory, is not even a full biological man: he is fundamentally a hypothalamic organism. The hypothalamic functions of sex and rage dominate all others. All the structures above the hypothalamus are seen predominantly as restricting or controlling or sublimating the functions of the hypothalamus and related organs.

The cultural and interpersonal schools of psychoanalysis have tried to enlarge this view of man. They have rightly stressed that one becomes a person mainly by virtue of relations with other human beings and not predominantly by virtue of inborn instinctual drives. What they do not indicate, however, is that the sequence of external influences is integrated by intrapsychic mechanisms, so that it becomes personal history and part of the inner self. What these cultural-interpersonal schools fail to point out is that the individual is not passively molded by these environmental influences: he does not just react; he acts autonomously. Whatever is above the hypothalamus meets, assimilates, transforms, expands what comes from the external world as well as from within or below the hypothalamus. The integration of all these intrapersonal and interpersonal factors opens up a new universe, the universe of symbols. Merely from the point of view of survival, symbolic function is not so important as hypothalamic regulation; but from the specific point of view of human psychology and psychopathology, it is much more important.

Some psychoanalytic schools have tried, although not very successfully, to include in their theoretical framework the psychodynamic and psychostructural aspects of high symbolism. Melanie Klein,[20] for instance, recognizes that internalized object relations become permanent features of inner life. For her, however, these mental incorporations correspond to oral incorporation. She sees the formation of the psyche in a theoretical framework that retains Freud's oral, anal, and genital stages. She believes that these stages unfold much earlier in life than Freud had postulated, and therefore even more than Freud she is compelled to neglect cognitive forms that develop after the first year of life. Klein repeatedly refers to unconscious fantasies, but does not indicate the cognitive features or the media that sustain these fantasies. It is difficult to visualize how in the three-month-old baby they can consist of ideas, thoughts, images, feelings of hopelessness, abandonment, and so forth. Although Klein has correctly stressed the importance of man's inner world, she has been quite nebulous in her description of the structure and functioning of this inner world. Fairbairn,[14] too, stressed the importance of the endopsychic structure and its relevance to object relations, but did not examine the cognitive elements of this structure. The classic psychoanalytic school has studied internalization, but with a few recent exceptions has studied them predominantly from the energetic or economic point of view.

SIMPLE FEELINGS AND PRESYMBOLIC ORGANIZATION

Although the main aim of this chapter is to discuss the cognitive forms that enter into the constitution of inner reality, we shall at this point give some consideration to feelings and to presymbolic organizations, which are prerequisite to any form of inner reality. Most of these functions start at birth or in the first few months of life and remain throughout the life of the individual.

Feeling is a characteristic unique to the animal world and is the basis of psychological life. Feeling is unanalyzable in its essential subjective nature and defies any attempt toward a noncircular definition. Synonyms of "feeling," which are often used, are "awareness," "subjectivity," "consciousness," "experience," "felt experience." Although each of these terms stresses a particular aspect, all refer to subjective experience.

Transmission of information from one part of the organism to another exists even without subjective experience. For instance, the important information transmitted through the spinocerebellar tracts never reaches the level of awareness. As long as information is transmitted without awareness, the organism is not too different from an electronic computer or a transmitter or transformer of data. When any change in the organism is accompanied by awareness, a new phenomenon emerges in the cosmos—experience. Awareness and/or experience introduced the factor psyche.

As Freud clarified, and as we shall consider later in this chapter, some psychological functions lose the quality of awareness and become unconscious. However, if in phylogeny some functions had not become endowed with awareness, the psyche would not have emerged and the physiology of the nervous system would consist only of unconscious neurological functions.

The most primitive forms of felt experiences are simple sensations and perceptions, such as pain, temperature perception, hearing, vision, thirst, hunger, olfaction, taste. These sensations and perceptions can be considered in two main ways: (1) as subjective experiences that occur in the presence of particular somatic states, for instance, a specific state of discomfort, which we call pain; (2) as functions mirroring (or producing analogs of) aspects of reality.

We encounter here a basic dichotomy. On one hand is the awareness of a particular state of the body or part of the body: that is, the awareness of an inner status of the organism, the experience as experience. On the other hand is the function of mirroring reality, a function that generally expands into numerous ramifications that deal with cognition. The importance of these two components varies a great deal in the various types of perceptions. The experience of inner status is very important in the perception of pain, hunger, thirst, temperature and less important in other perceptions, such as touch, taste, smell. In auditory and visual perceptions, the experience of a change of inner status plays a minimal role. These perceptions make the animal aware of what happens in the external world and become the foundation of cognition.

Elsewhere[8] I have described the various experiences of inner status (sensations, perceptions, physiosensations, such as hunger, thirst, fatigue, sleepiness, sexual urges, other instinctual experiences) and how from all of them we can abstract feelings of pleasure and unpleasure. Motivation becomes connected with the awareness of what is pleasant (and to be searched for) and what is unpleasant (and to be avoided).*

I have also tried to show how not only the simple experiences of inner status, such as sensations, but all emotions or affects can be included in the category of feeling. They are experienced within the organism. They are felt experiences. From all of them the motivational characteristics of pleasure and unpleasure can be abstracted. It is not without reason that in English the word "feeling" has a connotation so vast as to include simple sensations as well as high-level affects.

Emotions can be divided into several ranks or categories. The simplest (protoemotions or first-order emotions) are of at least five types: (1) tension—a feeling of discomfort caused by different situations, such as excessive stimulation, hindered physiological or instinctual response; (2) appetite—a feeling of expectancy that accompanies a tendency to move toward, contact, grab, or incorporate an almost immediately attainable goal; (3) fear—an unpleasant, subjective state, which follows the perception of danger and elicits a readiness to flee; (4) rage—an emotion that follows the perception of a danger to be overcome by fight, not flight; (5) satisfaction—an emotional state resulting from gratification of physical needs and relief from other emotions.

In a general sense, we can say that protoemotions (1) are experiences of inner status that cannot be sharply localized and that involve the whole or a large part of the organism; (2) either include a set of bodily changes, mostly muscular and humoral, or retain some bodily characteristics; (3) are elicited by the presence or absence of specific stimuli, which are perceived by the subject as related in a positive or negative way to its safety and comfort; (4) become important motivational factors and to a large extent determine the type of the external behavior of the subject; (5) in order to be experienced require a minimum of cognitive work.

---

* For the intricate relation between feeling, causality, and motivation see Chapter 2 of reference 8.

For instance, in fear or rage, a stimulus must be promptly recognized as a sign of danger. The danger is present or imminent.

What we have described under the headings of simple sensations, physiological and instinctual functions, perception, nonsymbolic learning, and protoemotions enable the animal organism (human or infrahuman) to survive and adjust to the environment. The effect of all these functions tends to be immediate or almost immediate. If they unchain a delayed reaction, the delay ranges only from a fraction of a second to a few minutes. Protoemotions are not experienced immediately, as are such simple sensations as pain or thirst. They require some cognitive work. However, this cognitive work is presymbolic or, in some cases, symbolic to a rudimentary degree. Presymbolic cognition includes perception and simple learning that have been intensely investigated by experimental psychologists. It also includes the sensorimotor intelligence, which has been accurately studied by Piaget in the first year and a half of life.

The motivational organization, based on the physiological, instinctual, or elementary emotional states we have mentioned, unchains in man, too, powerful dynamic forces, but it does not include all the psychological factors that affect him favorably or unfavorably. Because of the impact of symbolic cognition, man's needs, desires, purposes, and conflicts go far beyond physiologic-protoemotional motivation.

Most of the functions mentioned in this section do not lead to the formation of inner constructs unless associated with other psychological mechanisms. However, it would be inaccurate to state that they have no role in the making of inner reality. In the human being the memory and recall of these experiences become connected with higher level functions, especially after the acquisition of language. Feelings and protoemotions are also part of inner reality as long as they are experienced.

Protoemotions have even a greater role as potentialities, in that they remain as affective or primary predispositions toward a given type of personality, when they are not well balanced by other emotions. There are some human beings in whom fear (later changed into anxiety) is the predominant emotion. Depending on its interaction with other emotions and on the prevailing type of their interpersonal relations, these people may eventually become either detached (that is, prone to withdraw from frightening stimuli) or compliant (prone to placate the source of fear). People in whom rage prevails tend to become aggressive and hostile.

People in whom appetite is the principal emotion tend to become hedonistic. When tension predominates, the individual is likely to be hypochondriacal and more interested in his body than in the external environment. When satisfaction is the principal protoemotion, the person's predominant outlook is conservative, centered on the status quo.

Presymbolic types of learning and a relating to other members of one's species predispose to specific styles of behavior and of personality. Comparative psychologists have reported that when animals are kept together in a certain environment some assume a dominant and some a submissive role. Presumably this role is determined by a preponderance of a protoemotion and by the learning of a type of behavior that fits the environmental circumstances. Among these environmental circumstances, the type of behavior of the other animals and consequent interplay are very important. The preponderance of a protoemotion and of some kinds of presymbolic learning and ways of relating constitute the temperament.

The characteristics and functions that we have described, unless followed by others, constitute a primordial self. Inner reality is still rudimentary. More mature levels or organization of the self are possible because toward the end of the first year of life the human being acquires symbolic cognition. Symbolic cognition is not simply a system of intellectual mechanisms or a content dynamically neutral or conflict free. It permits emotions and emotional states that could not exist without symbolic functions. It introduces new motivations as powerful as those originated at lower levels and establishes the ground where human conflicts originate. Gratification of the self or the self-image (and not of one's physiological or instinctual needs) will eventually become the main motivation.

For expository reasons, we have so far made no reference to evolvement in time and to interpersonal relations. Actually the presymbolic stage of childhood can be divided into many substages. In the first six to eight weeks of life, the infant is predominantly a bundle of proprioceptive and enteroceptive sensations. Then he becomes more and more involved with sensory perceptions and the simplest forms of learning. First the presence of mother, as the overpowering environmental object, and second, the development of locomotion, help the little child to shift the focus of his awareness from his body to his immediate environment.

THE THREE CATEGORIES OF SYMBOLIC COGNITION

The development of new media—imagery and language—changes enormously the child's relation with his environment. Although at this level of maturation the cortical centers of language are ready to begin to function, it is necessary for the child to be in contact with a human environment to transform his babbling and environmental sounds and noises into meanings. He learns to connect them with things, events, or special states of the organism. That's why children who are deaf or without human contacts cannot learn symbolic processes in normal ways. Consensual validation, that is, the recognition that a given sound has the same or a related effect on the mother and on himself, is an absolute necessity to trigger off verbal symbolization in the child. When the function of language is chiefly denotative, consensual validation is easy; this is "daddi" and this is "mamme." From the very beginning, however, language goes beyond its purely denotative functions. In the course of evolving toward maturity, language and other symbolic functions can be classified as pertaining to three categories of cognition: primary, secondary, and tertiary.

The designations primary and secondary derive, respectively, from Freud's[16] original formulation of the primary and secondary processes, made in Chapter 7 of *The Interpretation of Dreams* (1901). To quote Jones[19]:

Freud's revolutionary contribution to psychology was not so much his demonstrating the existence of an unconscious, and perhaps not even his exploration of its content, as his proposition that there are two fundamentally different kinds of mental processes, which he termed primary and secondary. . . .

Freud gave the first description of these two processes but tried to differentiate the particular laws or principles that rule the primary process only. He called the primary process primary because, according to him, it occurs earlier in the ontogenetic development and not because it is more important than the secondary. Freud elucidated very well two mechanisms by which the primary process operates: namely the mechanisms of displacement and condensation. However, after this original breakthrough, he did not make other significant discoveries in the field of cognition. This arrest of progress is to be attributed to several factors. First, Freud became particularly interested in the primary process as a carrier of unconscious motivation. Second, inasmuch as he interpreted motivation more and more in the function of the libido theory, the primary process came to be studied predominantly as a consumer of energy.

The Freudian school, as a rule, has continued to study the primary process almost exclusively from an economic point of view. Its main characteristic would be the fact that it does not bind the libido firmly, but allows it to shift from one investment to another.[11] Some Freudians, however, for instance, Schur,[26] reassert the preponderantly cognitive role of the primary process.

I am also particularly concerned with the cognitive functions of the primary process; namely what I call "primary cognition." I have described primary cognition in numerous publications, but to maintain the continuity of the exposition, I will repeat briefly some of the main concepts.

Primary cognition prevails for a very short period of time early in life as a normal aspect of development. In most cases, it is almost immediately overlapped by secondary cognition, so that it is difficult to retrieve it in pure forms, even in the young child. Primary cognition also prevails and is easier to detect in those mental mechanisms (1) that are classified in classic psychoanalysis as belonging to the id. The dream work to a large extent follows primary cognition; (2) in the early stages of what Werner[33] called the "microgenetic process"; and (3) in psychopathological conditions. Its most typical forms occur in advanced stages of schizophrenia.[1,2,3,4] Some theorists (especially those belonging to the self-actualization schools, such as Fromm, Rogers, and Maslow) do not include in their system anything pertaining to primary cognition. Their omission is in some respects diametrically opposite to that of the Freudian school. Consequently, their contributions, although offering numerous important insights about some aspects of man and about mild psychopathology, is of much less value in understanding severe psychopathology and dream work.

Secondary cognition consists predominantly of conceptual thinking; most of the time it follows the laws of logic and inductive and deductive processes. Tertiary cognition occurs in the process of creativity and most of the time consists of specific combinations of primary and secondary forms of cognition. The important topic of tertiary cognition cannot be dealt with in this essay, and the reader is referred to other writings of mine.[7,8]

In what follows, I shall describe some developmental aspects of cognition. I shall not follow the usual approaches to cognition, not even Piaget's. The contributions of this Swiss author[22, 23, 24, 25] reveal very well the process of cognitive maturation and adaptation to environmental reality and disclose the various steps by which the child increases his understanding and mastery of the world. Although they are very important, they do not represent intrapsychic life in its structural and psychodynamic aspects.

In what follows, we shall give particular consideration to the formation in childhood of various forms of primary cognition, namely to imagery, endocept, and preconceptual thinking. Although for didactical purposes we may divide early childhood in stages or in a hierarchy of levels, generally these levels occur in combination, with one or the other predominating at a certain time.

THE PHANTASMIC STAGE OF INNER REALITY

At first psychological internalization occurs through images.* An image is a memory trace that assumes the form of a representation. It is an internal quasi-reproduction of a perception that does not require the corresponding external stimulus in order to be evoked. The image is indeed one of the earliest and most important foundations of human symbolism, if by symbol we mean something that stands for something else that is not present. Whereas previous forms of cognition and learning permitted an understanding based on the immediately given or experienced, from now on cognition will rely also on what is absent and inferred. For instance, the child closes his eyes and visualizes his mother. She may not be present, but her image is with him; it stands for her. The image is obviously based on the memory traces of previous perceptions of the mother. The mother then acquires a psychic reality that is not tied to her physical presence.

Image formation is actually the basis for all higher mental processes; it starts in the second half of the first year of life. It introduces the child into that inner world that I have called "phantasmic."[8] It enables the child not only to reevoke what is not present, but to retain an effective disposition for the absent object. For instance, the image of the mother may evoke the feelings that the child experiences toward her.

* See Chapter 5 of reference 8.

The image thus becomes a substitute for the external object. It is actually an inner object, although it is not well organized. It is the most primitive of the inner objects, if, because of their sensorimotor character, we exclude motor engrams from the category of inner objects. When the image's affective associations are pleasant, the evoking of the image reinforces the child's longing or appetite for the corresponding external object. The image thus has a motivational influence in leading the child to search out the actual object, which in its external reality is still more gratifying than the image. The opposite is true when the image's affective associations are unpleasant: the child is motivated not to exchange the unpleasant inner object for the corresponding external one, which is even more unpleasant.

Imagery soon constitutes the foundation of inner psychic reality. It helps the individual not only to understand the world better, but also to create a surrogate for it. Moreover, whatever is known or experienced tends to become a part of the individual who knows and experiences. Thus, cognition can no longer be considered only a hierarchy of mechanisms, but also an enduring psychological content that retains the power to affect its possessor, now and in the future.*

The child who has reached the level of imagery is now capable of experiencing not only such simple emotions as tension, fear, rage, and satisfaction, as he did in the first year of life, but also anxiety, anger, wish, perhaps in a rudimentary form even love and depression, and, finally, security. Anxiety is the emotional reaction to the expectation of danger, which is mediated through cognitive media. The danger is not immediate, nor is it always well defined. Its expectation is not the result of a simple perception or signal. At subsequent ages, the danger is represented by complicated sets of cognitive constructs. At the age level that we are discussing now, it is sustained by images. It generally refers to a danger connected with the important people in the child's life, mother and father, who may punish or withdraw tenderness and affection. Anger, at this age, is also rage sustained by images. Wish is also an emotional disposition, which is evoked by the image of a pleasant object. The image motivates the individual to replace the image with the real object satisfaction. Depression can be felt only at a rudimentary level at this stage, if by depression we mean an experience similar to the one the depressed adult

---

* For a study of the phenomenology of images and the formations of their derivatives—paleosymbols—see Chapter 5 of reference 8.

undergoes. At this level, depression is an unpleasant feeling evoked by the image of the loss of the wished object and by the experience of displeasure caused by the absence of the wished object. Love, at this stage, remains rudimentary. For the important emotion, or emotional tonality, called after Sullivan's security, the author must again refer the reader to another publication.[8]

The child does not remain for a long time at a level of integration characterized exclusively by sensorimotor behavior, images, simple interpersonal relations, and the simple emotions that we have mentioned. Higher levels impinge almost immediately, so that it is impossible to observe the phantasmic level in pure culture. Nevertheless we can recognize and abstract some of its general characteristics.

Images, of course, remain as a psychological phenomenon for the rest of the life of the individual. At a stage, however, during which language does not exist or is very rudimentary, they play a very important role. Unless initiated, checked, or corrected by subsequent levels of integration (secondary process), they follow the rules of the primary process. They are fleeting, hazy, vague, shadowy, cannot be seen in their totality, and tend to equate the part with the whole. For instance, if the subject tries to visualize his kitchen, now he reproduces the breakfast table, now a wall of the room, now the stove. An individual arrested at the phantasmic level of development would have great difficulty in distinguishing images and dreams from external reality. He would have no language and could not tell himself or others, "This is an image, a dream, a fantasy; it does not correspond to external reality." He would tend to confuse psychic with external reality, almost as a normal person does when he dreams. Whatever was experienced would become true for him by virtue of its being experienced. Not only is consensual validation from other people impossible at this level, but even intrapsychic or reflexive validation cannot be achieved. The phantasmic level of young children is characterized by what Baldwin[12] called "adualism," or at least by difficult dualism: lack of the ability to distinguish between the two realities, that of the mind and that of the external world. This condition may correspond to what orthodox analysts, following Federn,[15] call "lack of ego boundary."

Another important aspect that the phantasmic level shares with the sensorimotor level of organization is the lack of appreciation of causality. The individual cannot ask himself why certain things occur. He either naïvely accepts them as just happenings or he expects things to take place in a certain succession, as a sort of habit rather than as a result of causality or of an order of nature. The only phenomenon remotely connected with causation is a subjective or experiential feeling of expectancy, derived from the observation of repeated temporal associations.

THE ENDOCEPT

The endocept is a mental construct representative of a level intermediary between the phantasmic and the verbal. At this level, there is a primitive organization of memory traces, images, and motor engrams (or exocepts). This organization results in a construct that does not tend to reproduce reality, as it appears in perceptions or images: it remains nonrepresentational. The endocept, in a certain way, transcends the image, but inasmuch as it is not representational, it is not easily recognizable. On the other hand, it is not an engram (or exocept) that leads to prompt action. Nor can it be transformed into a verbal expression; it remains at a preverbal level. Although it has an emotional component, most of the time it does not expand into a clearly felt emotion.

The endocept is not, of course, a concept. It cannot be shared. We may consider it a disposition to feel, to act, to think that occurs after simpler mental activity has been inhibited. The awareness of this construct is vague, uncertain, and partial. Relative to the image, the endocept involves considerable cognitive expansion; but this expansion occurs at the expense of the subjective awareness, which is decreased in intensity. The endocept is at times experienced as an "atmosphere," an intention, a holistic experience that cannot be divided into parts or words—something similar to what Freud called "oceanic feeling." At other times, there is no sharp demarcation between endoceptual, subliminal experiences and some vague protoexperiences. On still other occasions, strong but not verbalizable emotions accompany endocepts.

For the evidence of the existence of endocepts and for their importance in adult life, dreams and creativity, the reader is referred elsewhere.[8]* In children, endocepts remain in the forms of vague memories that will affect subsequent periods of life. In adult life, they often evoke memories expressed with mature

* Especially Chapter 6.

language, which was not available to the child when the experiences originally took place.

Endoceptual experiences exist even when the child has already learned some linguistic expressions—expressions, however, that are too simple to represent the complexities of these experiences. To avoid misinterpretations, I wish to repeat at this point that the acquisition of language (that is, the verbal level) overlaps the endoceptual, phantasmic, and, to a small degree, toward the end of the first year of life, even the sensorimotor (or exoceptual) level.[8]

PRECONCEPTUAL LEVELS OF THINKING

It is beyond the purpose of this essay to study the child's acquisition of language and the experience of high-level emotions, which presuppose verbal symbols. I am referring to the mature experience of depression, hate, love, joy, and derivative emotions.*
From the acquisition of language (naming things) to a logical organization of concepts various substages follow one another so rapidly and overlap in so many multiple ways that it is very difficult to retrace and individualize them. These intermediary stages are more pronounced and more easily recognizable in pathological conditions.

Some of the stages, which some authors call "prelogical" and which I call "paleological" (or following ancient logic),[1, 2] use a type of cognition that is irrational according to our usual logical standards. However, paleologic thinking is not haphazard, but susceptible of being interpreted as following an organization or logic of its own. A considerable aspect of paleologic thinking can be understood in accordance with Von Domarus' principle,[31] which (in a formulation I have slightly modified) states: Whereas in mature cognition or secondary cognition identity is accepted only on the basis of identical subjects, in paleologic thinking identity is based on the basis of identical predicates. In other publications[6, 8] I have illustrated the relations among part perception, paleological thinking, and some psychological mechanisms reported by ethologists, for instance, Tinbergen.[28]

Paleologic cognition occurs for a short period of time early in childhood, from the age of one to three. It is difficult to recognize because it is, in most instances, overlapped by secondary cogni-

* See Chapter 7 of reference 8.

tion. Here are a few examples: An eighteen-month-old child is shown pictures of different men. In each instance he says, "Daddy, daddy." It is not enough to interpret this verbal behavior of the child by stating that he is making a mistake or that his mistake is owing to lack of knowledge, inadequate experience of the world, or inadequate vocabulary. Obviously, he makes what we consider a mistake; however, even in the making of the mistake, he follows a mental process. From perceptual stimuli, he proceeds to an act of individualization and recognition. Because the pictures show similarities with the perception of his daddy, he puts all these male representations into one category: they are all daddy or daddies. In other words, the child tends to make generalizations and classifications, which are wrong according to a more mature type of thinking. Obviously, there is in this instance what to the adult mind appears a confusion between similarity and identity. Children tend to give the role of an identifying or essential predicate to a secondary detail, attribute, part, or predicate. This part is the essential one to them either because of its conspicuous perceptual qualities or because of its association with previous very significant experiences. Levin[21] reported that a twenty-five-month-old child was calling "wheel" anything that was made of white rubber, as, for example, the white rubber guard that was supplied with little boys' toilet seats to deflect urine. The child knew the meaning of the word wheel as applied, for example, to the wheel of a toy car. This child has many toy cars whose wheels, when made of rubber, were always of white rubber. It is obvious that an identification had occurred because of the same characteristic, namely, white rubber.*

Young children soon become aware of causality and repeatedly ask why. At first, causality is teleological: events are believed to occur because they are willed or wanted by people or by anthropomorphized forces.

We should not conclude that young children must think paleologically: they only have a propensity to do so. Unless abnormal conditions (either environmental or biological) make difficult either the process or maturation or the process of becoming part of the adult world, this propensity is almost entirely and very rapidly overpowered by the adoption of secondary-process cognition. Moreover, they may still deal more or less realistically

---

* This confusion between identity and similarity reacquires prominence in some psychopathological conditions. It has been studied intensely in schizophrenia by Von Domarus[31] and later by Arieti.[1, 2]

with the environment when they follow the more primitive type of nonsymbolic learning, which permits a simple and immediate understanding. In secondary-process cognition the individual learns to distinguish essential from nonessential predicates and develops more and more the tendency to identify subjects that are indissolubly tied to essential predicates.

THE IMAGE OF MOTHER AND THE SELF-IMAGE

The randomness of experience is more and more superseded by the gradual organization of inner constructs. These constructs continuously exchange some of their components and increase in differentiation, rank, and order. A large number of them, however, retain the enduring mark of their individuality. Although in early childhood they consist of the cognitive forms that we have described (images, endocepts, paleologic thoughts) and of their accompanying feelings (from sensations to emotions), they become more and more complicated and difficult to analyze. Some of them have powerful effects and have an intense life of their own, even if at the stage of our knowledge we cannot give them an anatomic location or a neurophysiological interpretation. They may be considered the very inhabitants of inner reality. The two most important ones in the preschool age, and the only two that we shall describe herein, are the image of mother and the self-image.

Before proceeding, we must warn the reader about a confusion that may result from the two different meanings given to the word "image" in psychological and psychiatric literature. The word "image" is often used, as we did in a previous section of this chapter, in reference to the simple sensory images that tend to reproduce perceptions. This word also refers to those much higher psychological constructs or inner objects that represent whatever is connected with a person: for instance, in this more elaborate sense, the image of the mother would mean a conglomeration of what the child feels and knows about her. From the context, the reader will easily realize which of the two denotations we refer to.

In normal circumstances the mother as an inner object will consist of a group of agreeable images: as the giver, the helper, the assauger of hunger, thirst, cold, loneliness, immobility, and any other discomfort. She becomes the prototype of the good inner object. The negative characteristics of mother play a secondary role that loses significance in the context of the good inner object. In pathological conditions, the mother becomes a malevolent object, and an attempt is made to repress this object from consciousness.[9, 10]

Much more difficult to describe in early childhood is the self-image. This construct will be easier to understand in later developmental stages. At the sensorimotor level, the primordial self probably consists of a bundle of relatively simple relations between feelings, kinesthetic sensations, perceptions, motor activity, and a partial integration of these elements. At the phantasmic level, the child raised in normal circumstances learns to experience himself not exclusively as a cluster of feelings and of self-initiated movements, but also as a body image and as an entity having many kinds of relations with other images, especially those of the parents. Inasmuch as the child cannot see his own face, his own visual image will be faceless—as, indeed, he will tend to see himself in dreams throughout his life. He wishes, however, to be in appearance, gestures, and actions like people toward whom he has a pleasant emotional attitude or by whom he feels protected and gratified. The wish tends to be experienced as reality, and he believes that he is or is about to become like the others or as powerful as the others. Because of the reality value of wishes and images, a feeling results that in psychoanalytic literature has been called a "feeling of omnipotence."

In the subsequent endoceptual and paleologic stages, the self-image will acquire many more elements. However, these elements will continue to be integrated so that the self-image will continue to be experienced as a unity, as an entity separate from the rest of the world. The psychological life of the child will no longer be limited to acting and experiencing, but will include also observing oneself and having an image of oneself.

In a large part of psychological and psychiatric literature, a confusion exists between the concepts of self and of self-image. In this section, we shall focus on the study of the self-image.* Also in a large part of the psychiatric literature the self and the consequent self-image are conceived predominantly in a passive role. For instance, Sullivan has indicated that the preconceptual and first conceptual appraisals of the self are determined by the

* The vaster concept of the self will be more accurately dealt with in the last section of this chapter.

relationships of the child with the significant adults. Sullivan[27] considers the self (and self-image) as consisting of reflected appraisals from the significant adults: the child would see himself and feel about himself as his parents, especially the mother, see him and feel about him. What is not taken into account in this conception is the fact that the self is not merely a passive reflection. The mechanism of the formation of the self cannot be compared to the function of a mirror. If we want to use the metaphor of the mirror, we must specify that we mean an activated mirror that adds to the reflected images its own distortions, especially those distortions that at an early age are caused by primary cognition. The child does not merely respond to the environment. He integrates experiences and transforms them into inner reality, into increasingly complicated structures. He is indeed in a position to make a contribution to the formation of his own self.

The self-image may be conceived as consisting of three parts: body image, self-identity, and self-esteem. The body image consists of the internalized visual, kinesthetic, tactile, and other sensations and perceptions connected with one's body. The body is discovered by degrees and also the actions of the body on the not-self are discovered by degrees. The body image eventually will be connected with belonging to one of the two genders. Self-identity, or personal identity or ego identity, depends on the discovery of oneself not only as continuous and as same, but also as having certain definite characteristics and a role in the group to which the person belongs.

Self-esteem depends on the child's ability to do what he has the urge to do, but is also connected with his capacity to avoid doing what the parents do not want him to do. Later it is connected also with his capacity to do what his parents want him to do. His behavior is explicitly or implicitly classified by the adults as bad or good. Self-identity and self-esteem seem thus to be related, as Sullivan has emphasized, to the evaluation that the child receives from the significant adults. However, again, this self-evaluation is not an exact reproduction of the one made by the adults. The child is impressed more by the appraisals that hurt him the most or please him the most. These partial salient appraisals and the ways they are integrated with other elements will make up the self-image.

For a better understanding of the nature of personal images and other complex mental constructs, we must study how these inner objects are formed. Not only early in childhood but throughout the life of the individual experiences of inner and external origin are processed in two different mechanisms, which for didactical purposes I have called spontaneous or protopathic organization and epicritic organization (or organization that tends toward higher forms of rationality).

Both ways tend to transform experiential conglomerations into structures and syntheses that aim at pseudo or real consistency. In structures formed by spontaneous organization, any experience may add to a construct, either by contiguity, conditioned reflex mechanisms, repetition, and so forth, or because an overpowerful emotion or motivation affects all mental processes. For instance, if a person is experienced by the individual as very frightening, any action of this person, even a benevolent one, will be interpreted or experienced as frightening. Every relation with that person may thus accrue to the original negative image. Similarly, an overpowering sexual or aggressive motivation may be reinforced by any stimulus whatsoever emanating from the source of that motivation.

In epicritical organization, the experiences do not accrue by the simple mechanisms that I have mentioned. First, every experience retains a separate existence, even though associated with others. Second, the symbolic processes that we shall study in the following sections and more complicated ones will lead to various degrees of abstraction and inference and will restructure experiences in accordance with high schemata offered by culture or created by the individual himself. In those ages and conditions in which the primary process prevails, spontaneous organization prevails too. And when secondary process prevails so does epicritic organization.

In the psychoneurotic, but especially in the psychopath and in the person who eventually will develop schizophrenia, specific factors contribute to the prevailing of spontaneous organization in the formation of many complex constructs and especially of the self-image.[8, 9, 10]

SECONDARY COGNITION: THE CONCEPT

It is beyond the scope of this chapter to describe the stages intermediary between early childhood and mature adulthood. We shall consider only the role of concepts. As Vygotsky[32] has illustrated, conceptual thinking starts early in life, but it is in adolescence that it acquires prominence. Conceptual life is a necessary and very important part of mature life. Many authors[24, 13, 35] have made important studies of the mechanisms involved in the formation of concepts and of concepts as psychological forms. In this chapter I shall instead stress their content. This position is a departure from what I have done in reference to less mature forms of cognition.[1, 2] In fact, in psychiatric studies, especially in such conditions as schizophrenia, in which severe pathology is found, it is important to study not only content but also form; it is crucial to understand not only what the individual experiences but how he experiences it. Is he perceiving in terms of parts or wholes? Is he using images, endocepts, or paleologic cognition? How are these cognitive modalities varying during the course of the illness or even during the course of a single therapeutic session? What is the meaning of such variety of forms? On the other hand, the psychiatrist's and analyst's main interest in concepts resides in determining how their content psychodynamically affects human life.

In a large part of psychiatric, psychoanalytic, and psychological literature concepts are considered static, purely intellectual entities, separate from human emotions and unimportant in psychodynamic studies. I cannot adhere to this point of view. Concepts and organized clusters of concepts become depositories of emotions and also originators of new emotions. They have a great deal to do with the conflicts of man, his achievements and his frustrations, his states of happiness or despair, of anxiety or of security.[6] They become the repositories of intangible feelings and values. Not only does every concept have an emotional counterpart, but concepts are necessary for high emotions. In the course of reaching adulthood, emotional and conceptual processes become more and more intimately interconnected. It is impossible to separate the two. They form a circular process. The emotional accompaniment of a cognitive process becomes the propelling drive not only toward action but also toward further cognitive processes. Only emotions can stimulate man to overcome the hardship of some cognitive processes and lead to complicated symbolic, interpersonal, and abstract processes. On the other hand, only cognitive processes can extend indefinitely the realm of emotions. As I have illustrated elsewhere,[8] some very important human emotions could not exist without a conceptual foundation. For instance, depression should not be confused with lower feelings, which require no cognitive counterpart at all or only non-symbolic learning. I am referring to the state of deprivation, discomfort, or anaclitic frustration of lower animal forms or human babies. Depression requires an understanding of the meaning of loss (actual or symbolic) and a state of despair (which follows a belief that what is lost cannot be retrieved). The importance of this understanding is not recognized, because it is based on cognitive processes that often become almost immediately unconscious (see below). The conceptual presuppositions to mature love, to symbolic anxiety, to hate (as distinguished from rage or anger) have been described elsewhere.[8]

Reification of concepts (that is the assumption that concepts faithfully correspond to external reality) is considered by science an invalid procedure. It is obvious that concepts do not correspond to external reality, nor do they most of the time represent reality adequately. Nevertheless, they do have an enduring psychological life or a reality of their own as psychological constructs. Even more criticized and reputed unscientific is the reification of emotions or feelings in general.

Certainly, thoughts and feelings do not easily submit to the rigor and objectivity of a stimulus-response psychology. However, to dismiss all studies of thoughts and feelings as mystical is to dismiss most of man as mystical. Thoughts and feelings make up what is most valuable in man. If this essential part of man requires methods of study that do not correspond to those of standardized science, we must be ready to accept unusual methods of inquiry.

Even what I said about the relative lack of importance of concepts as forms needs clarification. Concepts, too, undergo organization of increasing order, rank, and level and become components or organized conceptual constructs, whose grammar and syntax we do not yet know. Undoubtedly, future studies will reveal the structure of these, so far, obscure organizations and configurations.

From a psychiatric and psychoanalytic point of view, the greatest importance of concepts resides in the fact that to a large extent they come to constitute the self-image.[6] When this development occurs, the previous self-images are not completely obliterated. They remain throughout the life of the individual in the forms of minor components of the adult self-image or as repressed or suppressed forms. In adolescence, however, concepts accrue to constitute the major part of the self-image. Such concepts as inner worth, personal significance, mental outlook, more mature evaluations of appraisals reflected from others, attitudes toward ideals, aspirations, capacity to receive and give acceptance, affection, and love are integral parts of the self and of the self-image, together with the emotions that accompany these concepts. These concepts and emotions, which constitute the self, are generally not consistent with one another, in spite of a prolonged attempt made by the individual to organize them logically.

The motivation of the human being varies according to the various levels of development. When higher levels emerge, motivations originated at lower levels do not cease to exist. At a very elementary sensorimotor level, the motivation consists of obtaining immediate pleasure and avoidance of immediate displeasure by gratification of bodily needs. When imagery emerges, either phylogenetically or ontogenetically, the individual becomes capable of wishing something that is not present and is motivated toward the fulfillment of his wishes. He will continue to be wish-motivated in more advanced stages of primary cognition, such as the paleological stage. As we have already mentioned, although the motivation can always be understood as a search for, or as an attempt to retain, pleasure and avoid unpleasure, gratification of the self becomes the main motivational factor at a conceptual level of development. Certainly, the individual is concerned with danger throughout his life: immediate danger, which elicits fear, and a more distant or symbolic danger, which elicits anxiety. However, whereas at earlier levels of development this danger is experienced as a threat to the physical self, at higher levels it is many times experienced as a threat to an acceptable image of the self.

Many psychologic defenses are devices to protect the self or the self-image. Here are a few examples: A woman leads a promiscuous life; she feels she is unacceptable as a person, but as a sexual partner she feels appreciated. The hypochondriacal protects his self by blaming only his body for his difficulties. The suspicious person and the paranoid attribute to others shortcomings or intentions that they themselves have. These examples could be easily multiplied. They represent cognitive configurations that lead the patient to feelings, ideas, and strategic forms of behavior that make the self-image acceptable or at least less unacceptable. Neurotic behavior is to a large extent based on these particular defensive cognitive configurations, which often become unconscious and are applied automatically. Often the patient has learned to apply these configurations in situations in which they were appropriate. Later, because of his lack of security or ability to discriminate, he has extended their sphere of applicability. In most cases, important cognitive configurations are completely repressed, because ungratifying or inconsistent with one's cherished self-image. Contrary to what is often believed, repression and suppression from awareness do not apply only to primitive strivings and to the contents of primary cognition, but also to the content of high conceptual ideation.

In some psychoneuroses, such as phobic conditions and obsessive-compulsive syndromes, the self is also, in specific situations, protected by some use of primary cognition. In the schizophrenic psychosis, the self is defended by an extensive use of primary cognition, which is not corrected or counterbalanced by the secondary. Various forms of displacement and transformation of a cognitive construct into another that is less disturbing (such as in regression, fixation, paleologic thinking) occur in dreams and in many pathological conditions.

As described elsewhere, no anticipation of the future is possible without symbolic processes.[8] In order to feed his present self-esteem and maintain an adequate self-image, the young individual has, so to say, to borrow from his expectations and hopes for the future. It is when a present vacillating self-esteem cannot be supported by hope and faith in the future that severe psychopathological conditions may develop.[9, 10]

Most concepts that affect the individual are learned from others, either private persons or social and cultural institutions. This point has been stressed in the Whorf-Sapir theory of cognition.[36] Culture, with its system of knowledge, languages, beliefs, and values, bestows on each person a patrimony of concepts that becomes part of the individual. The acknowledgment of this fact should not induce the field of psychiatry and psychoanalysis to equate a cognitive approach to an interpersonal-cultural one. Certainly, a cognitive approach is closer to the cultural than to one based on instinctual theories. However, it does not conceive the individual as molded entirely by culture or by interpersonal relations. First, innate functions and structures vary and affect each individual in different ways. Second, temperament and primary cognition have different shaping influences on the individual. Third, the person's various uses of the different modalities of cognition confer on him a certain individuality that is not derivative from cultural factors.

Nevertheless, it is accurate to say that a given culture predisposes the individual to build some self-images rather than others and special patterns of defenses. This topic is too vast to be discussed here. However, it is relevant to mention that even the need to build and retain a self-image that is gratifying is to a large extent culturally determined. In some medieval cultures, for instance, the prevailing philosophy was that of mortifying the self and of depicting the individual as an insignificant entity, a sinner, an individual who is not "his own." This self-effacing cultural attitude should not be confused with individualistic masochistic traits.

We must acknowledge that learning has a very important role in the organization of inner reality. However, we must specify that the content of a learning experience becomes part of inner reality when it becomes integrated with the rest of the psyche and has an effect that transcends the original experience. Undoubtedly, there are intermediary stages between learning experiences and components of inner reality. Generally, but not in an absolute sense, we can state that:

1. The more emotional the effect of the experience, the more it tends to become part of inner reality. On the contrary, the less emotional the experience, the more it may be viewed as a learning process.

2. The more diffuse the effect of the experience (that is, related to many aspects of the life of the individual, such as the interpersonal relation with a parent), the more related to inner life it becomes. On the contrary, the more specific the effect, the more it remains part of learning.

3. The more the experience is seen as particular (that is, as belonging to a specific member of a category: for instance, how to feel and respond in the presence of the family's dog), the more the experience becomes part of the inner self. On the contrary, the more the experience is from the very beginning categorical or universal (for instance, how to respond or feel in the presence of any member of the whole class of dogs), the more it tends to remain a learning experience. This third point has many exceptions that cannot be discussed here. Thus, although many learning experiences accrue the inner reality, many others remain limited or preponderantly connected with specific behavioral problems and patterns.

Table 1 outlines the cognitive and affective components of inner reality, which we have discussed in this chapter.

TABLE 1

Presymbolic Organization
  A. Simple feelings
  B. Immediate (nonsymbolic) learning
  C. Protoemotions
     1. Tension
     2. Appetite
     3. Fear
     4. Rage
     5. Satisfaction

Symbolic Organization
  A. Primary
     1. Phantasmic stage
        a. Images
        b. Second-order emotions
           i. Anxiety
          ii. Wish
         iii. Anger
          iv. Primitive love
           v. Primitive depression
          vi. Security
     2. Endoceptual stage
        a. Ineffable thoughts
        b. Atmospheric feelings
     3. Preconceptual
        a. Paleologic thinking
        b. Primitive language
        c. Primary generalization
        d. Teleologic causality
        e. Third-order emotions
           i. Depression
          ii. Hate
         iii. Love
          iv. Joy
  B. Secondary
     1. Conceptual
        a. Abstract thinking
        b. Highly connotative language
        c. Deduction and induction
        d. Deterministic causality
        e. High-order emotions
  C. Tertiary
     Creativity

⟶ Progressive formation of inner objects ⟶

GENERAL ASPECTS OF THE SELF AND CONCLUSIONS

The comparative developmental approach I have followed is in many respects similar to the one advocated by Werner.[35] Probably, insights obtained through new approaches, such as the one introduced by Von Bertalanffy's general system theory,[29, 30] will do much to clarify the intricacies of inner reality. I have already referred to the self as an "open system," always related to external reality.

From a general point of view, the self (and in particular, the inner self) can be examined from five different aspects: (1) representational function, (2) subjectivity, (3) potentiality, (4) integration, (5) desubjectivization. These aspects are so interrelated that we cannot understand any of them without taking into consideration the others. For didactical reasons only we shall discuss them separately.

The representational function is the formation of inner constructs that represent objects or events of the external world. These representations are not analogic reproductions of what they stand for. They are mediated by various kinds and ranks of intrapsychic mechanisms and are under the influence of previous experience. Psychologically, they may become more important than external reality.

The second aspect of the self refers to the fact that what is objective or objectivizable becomes subjective, is appropriated by the individual as a subjective experience, acquires a subjective reality, and becomes part of the individual himself. This subjectivization is not adequately accounted for by psychological or psychiatric authors who give exclusive or almost exclusive importance to the environment. This subjectivization is a phenomenon as difficult to understand as the whole mind-body problem. The intensity of a subjective construct does not correspond to the external objective event or stimulus to which it is related. It depends, as we have already mentioned, on the mechanisms triggered off in its formation, on the selections of other constructs with which it is integrated, and on the processes used in such integration. The subjective aspect is particularly evident when we study sensations and emotions, but emotions accompany and transform cognitive constructs and in their turn are transformed by them.

The potentiality of the self can be seen (1) in the way it affects the behavior of the individual in relation to other people, himself, the world in general; (2) it affects itself. In other words, the self feeds on the external world as well as on itself.

The term integration refers to a large number of psychological mechanisms, most of them unknown, by virtue of which all functions of the psyche are related to one another and synthesized into higher ranks of organization.

Desubjectivization is the fifth property and, in a certain way, the opposite of subjectivity. It refers also to a group of phenomena that tend to decrease the private or subjective aspects of the experience. We have seen that in subhuman animals and during the first year and a half of human life the inner self exists only in rudimentary form. In the growing and grown human being, however, it becomes so intense that during the evolution of *Homo sapiens* mechanisms developed that had the purpose of decreasing its intensity and prominence. These various mechanisms have been described, under various terminologies, in psychological, psychiatric, and psychoanalytic literatures. We have already mentioned some of these mechanisms as the adoption of special cognitive configurations or special types of cognition. Others should be considered under the heading of desubjectivization:

1. Decrease of affective or sensuous content, for instance by the mechanisms of denial, reaction-formation, undoing, blunting of affect, depersonalization, alienation, hysterical anesthesia, and so forth.

2. Suppression, or more or less voluntary removal of some psychological content from the focus of attention or of consciousness. This content goes into a state of quiescence, like a language or skill that is not used.

3. Repression or removal of psychological content from consciousness. The study of this mechanism is the main topic of psychoanalysis.

These mechanisms alter and complicate but do not eliminate inner life. Desubjectivization is not necessarily a useful procedure. Although, from the point of view of the whole human race, it may have statistically useful survival effects, it often has undesirable consequences on the individual. As a matter of fact, it is the aim of psychoanalysis to make conscious again what became unconscious. According to me and other writers, this psychoanalytic procedure is not therapeutically sufficient in most instances.

Therapy must also aim at reintegrating harmoniously with the rest of the self what was restored to consciousness.

The respective role of these five aspects or functions of the self can be appreciated particularly in relation to the self-image. The first aspect is easy to understand, as it is obvious that the self-image is a representation of the self to the self. The second aspect is recognized when we consider that the self-image is not a collection of data, but something that is subjectively experienced and evokes in the individual satisfaction or discomfort, security or anxiety. The self-image has the potentiality of changing the behavior of the individual in order to effect a desirable change in itself. The self-image, of course, is the result of the integration of many data and mechanisms. Finally, the self-image may undergo suppression, repression, or distortions of some parts that are disturbing to the rest of the inner self.

This enumeration of the aspects of the self and the separation of the self from the self-image may seem an unwarranted dissection of something that is experienced and therefore by somebody supposed to exist only as a unity. However, all these separate characteristics and their blending together into a subjective unit appear more clearly in the state of dreaming, which is one of the normal states of the self. When an individual dreams, that part of him that makes the dream is the representational function. The part of him that experiences the dream as a felt experience is the subjectivity. The effect of the dream (assuaging, waking up, sexual arousement, enlightenment, and so forth) is related to the potentiality. The integrative aspect consists of all the mechanisms that made the dream possible as a synthesis of many psychological factors. At first impression, desubjectivization does not seem to occur in dreams. As a matter of fact, the main function of the dream seems to make alive and representational again what was in a state of quiescence. However, often compromises occur in dreams, as Freud[16] demonstrated: events take place after they have been made less unacceptable by the dream work.

What about the self-image? It corresponds to the individual himself, as he sees himself in the dream. What in the state of wake is predominantly a cognitive-affective entity becomes a visual image in the dream. Thus, in the dream, the representational function is perfectly fused with the subjectivity. At the same time that the dreamer produces an image of himself, he experiences that image as himself. For instance, if he sees himself threatened by a danger or kissed by his sweetheart, he experiences the horror of the threat or the pleasure of the kiss in himself, not in an object of his observation.

REFERENCES

1. Arieti, S. "Special Logic of Schizophrenic and Other Types of Autistic Thought," *Psychiatry*, **11** (1948), 325–338.
2. Arieti, S. *Interpretation of Schizophrenia*. New York: Brunner, 1955.
3. Arieti, S. "Schizophrenia: The Manifest Symptomatology, the Psychodynamic and Formal Mechanisms," in S. Arieti (ed.), *American Handbook of Psychiatry*. New York: Basic Books, 1959. Vol. 1, pp. 455–484.
4. Arieti, S. "The Microgeny of Thought and Perception," *Archives of General Psychiatry*, **6** (1962), 454–468.
5. Arieti, S. "Contributions to Cognition from Psychoanalytic Theory," in J. H. Masserman (ed.), *Science and Psychoanalysis*. New York: Grune & Stratton, 1965. Vol. 3, pp. 16–37.
6. Arieti, S. "Conceptual and Cognitive Psychiatry," *American Journal of Psychiatry*, **122** (1965), 361–366.
7. Arieti, S. "Creativity and Its Cultivation: Relation to Psychopathology and Mental Health," in S. Arieti (ed.), *American Handbook of Psychiatry*. New York: Basic Books, 1966. Vol. 3, pp. 722–741.
8. Arieti, S. *The Intrapsychic Self: Feeling, Cognition, and Creativity in Health and Mental Illness*. New York: Basic Books, 1967.
9. Arieti, S. "New Views on the Psychodynamics of Schizophrenia," *American Journal of Psychiatry*, **124** (1967), 453–458.
10. Arieti, S. "The Psychodynamics of Schizophrenia: A Reconsideration," *American Journal of Psychotherapy*, **1** (1968), 366–381.
11. Arlow, J. A. "Report on Panel: The Psychoanalytic Theory of Thinking," *Journal of the American Psychoanalytic Association*, **6** (1958), 143.
12. Baldwin, J. M. Quoted in J. Piaget, *The Child's Conception of the World*. New York: Harcourt, Brace, 1929.
13. Bruner, J. S., Goodnow, J. J., and Austin, G. A. *A Study of Thinking*. New York: Wiley, 1956.
14. Fairbairn, W. *Psychoanalytic Studies of the Personality*. New York: Basic Books, 1952.
15. Federn, P. *Ego Psychology and the Psychoses*. New York: Basic Books, 1952.
16. Freud, S. "The Interpretation of Dreams" (1900), in J. Strachey (ed.), *Standard Edition*. London: Hogarth Press. Vol. 4, pp. 1–621; Vol. 5, pp. 687–751. (Also published as *The Interpretation of Dreams*. New York: Basic Books, 1960.)
17. Freud, S. "The Future of an Illusion" (1927), in J. Strachey (ed.), *Standard Edition*. London: Hogarth Press. Vol. 21.
18. Guntrip, H. *Personality Structure and Human Interaction*. New York: International Universities Press, 1961.
19. Jones, E. *The Life and Work of Sigmund Freud*. New York: Basic Books, 1953. Vol. 1.
20. Klein, M. *Contributions to Psychoanalysis*. London: Hogarth Press, 1948.
21. Levin, M. "Misunderstanding of the Pathogenesis of Schizophrenia, Arising from the Concept of 'Splitting,' " *American Journal of Psychiatry*, **94** (1938), 877.
22. Piaget, J. *The Child's Conception of the World*. New York: Harcourt, Brace, 1929.
23. Piaget, J. *The Child's Conception of Physical Causality*. New York: Harcourt, Brace, 1930.
24. Piaget, J. *The Origins of Intelligence in Children*. New York: International Universities Press, 1952.
25. Piaget, J. *Logic and Psychology*. New York: Basic Books, 1957.
26. Schur, M. *The Id and the Regulatory Principles of Mental Functioning*. New York: International Universities Press, 1966.

27. Sullivan, H. S. *Conceptions of Modern Psychiatry*. New York: Norton, 1953.
28. Tinbergen, N. *The Study of Instinct*. Oxford: Clarendon, 1951.
29. Von Bertalanffy, L. "General Systems Theory," in L. von Bertalanffy and A. Rapaport (eds.), *Society for the Advancement of General Systems Theory*. Ann Arbor: University of Michigan Press, 1956.
30. Von Bertalanffy, L. "General System Theory and Psychiatry," in S. Arieti (ed.), *American Handbook of Psychiatry*. New York: Basic Books, 1966. Vol. 3, pp. 705–721.
31. Von Domarus, E. "The Specific Laws of Logic in Schizophrenia," in J. S. Kasamin (ed.), *Language and Thought in Schizophrenia: Collected Papers*. Berkeley: University of California Press, 1944.
32. Vygotsky, L. S. *Thought and Language*. Cambridge, Mass.: M.I.T. Press, 1962.
33. Werner, H. "Microgenesis and Aphasia," *Journal of Abnormal and Social Psychology*, **52** (1956), 347–353.
34. Werner, H. *Comparative Psychology of Mental Development*. New York: International Universities Press, 1957.
35. Werner, H., and Kaplan, B. *Symbol Formation. An Organismic-Developmental Approach to Language and the Expression of Thought*. New York: Wiley, 1963.
36. Whorf, B. L. *Language, Thought and Reality*. New York: Wiley, 1956.

SOME PROBLEMS IN CURRENT PSYCHOANALYTIC THOUGHT

Jacob A. Arlow

The purpose of this chapter is to examine some problems in current psychoanalytic thought from a different perspective. The exigencies of our daily work, the exacting schedules by which we dispose of our hours, and the close proximity we maintain to the data of investigation rarely afford us the opportunity to relax and to reflect in a detached way concerning the trends in psychoanalytic thinking.

I propose in this presentation to consider certain predilections in conceptualization and styles of investigation as they pertain to many unsolved problems in psychoanalysis. Methodological biases of one sort or another are inevitable in any field of investigation, but when they are converted into slogans and become the nucleus for a priori conclusions that are foisted onto data, they may impede new developments and new findings. In the case of psychoanalysis, they may serve to lessen the esteem of the tools that are specifically and peculiarly psychoanalytic. Several authors have recently taken note of the fact that the number of clinical papers appearing in the standard psychoanalytic journals has decreased markedly. Bak[4] has spoken of the paucity of new clinical data. Articles on metapsychology and theory, more often than not based on speculation rather than on empirical findings, seem to be the order of the day.

We should not be surprised that these or other trends of thought and styles of conceptualization should become predominant in psychoanalysis. This happens in every scientific field, and psychoanalysis is no exception. But it may be well for us to pause from time to time to consider why certain methodological approaches are so popular and to study what they indicate about the state of psychoanalysis.

How can one understand the predominance of certain types of conceptualizations? I think the answer to this question may be approached under the following headings: (1) the state of development of psychoanalytic knowledge; (2) the need to correlate psychoanalytic theory with relevant data from associated fields of study; (3) some disappointment or dissatisfaction with the standard method of psychoanalytic investigation, that is, with the data derived from the psychoanalytic situation; and (4) the attachment to certain leading figures, teachers, and authors in the psychoanalytic movement.

As psychoanalysts, we may anticipate that the neat separations we establish between different categories will fail to hold up in actual practice. This is certainly true in this instance, as will become apparent in the course of this presentation. All these factors are closely, in fact inextricably, interrelated. We may also anticipate that we will have to give considerable attention to subjective and affective elements in what on the surface appears to be a very intellectual judgment. Much of this is imbedded in the history of psychoanalysis, how it developed and how it continues to be taught. Above and beyond the rational organization of the psychoanalytic curriculum for training there are certain shared, unconscious fantasies, certain outcroppings of a professional mythology whose impact must be appreciated whenever we pause to consider the rise and the decline in the popularity of certain psychoanalytic concepts.

THE STATE OF DEVELOPMENT OF PSYCHOANALYTIC KNOWLEDGE

Certain preferences in psychoanalytic approaches clearly reflect the state of development of psychoanalytic knowledge. One could trace similar historical developments in medicine as well as in physics. Dominated as the early period of psychoanalysis was by the towering figure of Freud, the pattern of its conceptual evolution is clearer than in most sciences. One could, in fact, delineate in five- to seven-year periods the dominant themes of psychoanalytic literature. In fact, it is almost possible to date most of Freud's papers within a year or two of their publication if one extracts the essential themes—for example, narcissism, quantitative factors, self-directed aggression, dual instinct theory, theory of anxiety. The history of the development of psychoanalytic concepts is a very striking one in this regard. Within the setting of a well-defined, though often shaky, frame of reference, data of observation were collected. These, in turn, challenged the existing frame of reference leading to the necessary modifications in the body of theory. In this way, psychoanalysis remained for a long time a vital and vibrant science, growing and changing with the ingenuity and genius of its founder and his collaborators, who worked consistently with the psychoanalytic situation as their investigative tool.

It is true that from time to time what might be called a "cultural lag" could be observed in the literature of psychoanalysis. It is somewhat ironic from the vantage point of history to observe how from 1923 to 1924, when Karl Abraham was publishing his monumental contribution on the development of the libido, Freud was organizing and publishing a new set of concepts that were to supersede much of what Abraham had written. To be sure, Freud was no easy man to keep up with.

In a similar fashion, although at a somewhat slackened pace, this trend was continued by Anna Freud, Hartmann, Kris, Lowenstein, and many others who took their lead from them. The essence of their contribution, it seems to me, represents an attempt to correlate more precisely the body of analytical data with the body of analytical propositions within the context of the structural theory and ego psychology. Once again, therefore, the problems posed by the data collected under the new rubric and incapable of being fitted neatly within the established propositions call for the elaboration of new theories, for the reexamination of old data, and for new correlations that in themselves constitute fresh data. Let me cite one example of how this process operates in actual experience and how it has served to indicate which path could lead to new data and to fresh observations.

Having placed intrapsychic conflict at the hub of the structure of psychoanalytic theory, the question of how the ego resolves conflicts necessarily takes a commanding position in psychoanalytic thinking. Many things depend on the solution of this question—for example, the difference between health and illness, adaptation and maladaptation, the evolution of character, the selection of sublimations, the development of neurosis. Once the role of anxiety as a signal of impending danger is emphasized, major interest had to shift to the organization of the defenses. How are the defenses adopted? Why are some defenses preferred to others? Are they always related to identification, or are there perhaps biological models that indicate which defenses will prove most effective and, if so, under what circumstances? If identification with objects is so important in building up the ego, how are these identifications made? Why do some object relations eventuate in valuable, that is, adaptive identifications, whereas others eventuate in harmful, that is, maladaptive, identifications? Why do some identifications leave their lasting imprint on the organization of the personality, whereas others seem to have little effect on the developing ego of the young child? And do these effects on the young child persist, or are they altered by subsequent experience, especially by the events of adolescence?

These are rigorous and exacting questions. The answers are not easy to come by, particularly when we bear in mind that psychoanalytic technique is both a method of treatment and a tool for research. I might point out that in outlining the difficulties that have to be faced, I have chosen only one of many areas of psychoanalysis to illustrate my point.

I need hardly point out that not all psychoanalysts have chosen to follow the difficult methodology that current psychoanalytic developments pose for us. In Europe, South America, and some parts of the United States, the followers of Melanie Klein have pursued quite a different course, a course that is easier and less exacting. By projecting the major causes in the individual's conflict back into the first few months of life and by positing a very elaborate system of intricate mental contents, they have spared themselves the arduous task of correlating the data of adult analysis with what is known from child development and direct observation of children. By establishing a firm base in the preverbal period of the individual's life, the followers of Melanie Klein can give free rein to broad and imaginative speculation that is hard to confirm, but at the same time very difficult to invalidate. They are able to generate a certain aura of credibility because the sense of empathy so deeply rooted in our psychological constitution can be extended through imagination into areas to which, on rational reflection, we know it could not possibly pertain. We almost think we can feel what a newborn child experiences. We know that we cannot. The Kleinians have created a mystique of empathy, and on it they have attempted to found a set of propositions that they call psychoanalytic. We should not think that a discussion of the limitations of Kleinian theory and technique is only of historical significance. Quite the contrary. I propose to demonstrate how in a disguised form the appeal of the facile, empathic, and mystic quality of the Kleinian approach reverberates, in a more highly sophisticated manner, in some of the popular concepts that are regarded as in the mainstream of psychoanalytic conceptualization. I hope to demonstrate that in certain areas we are not quite so free as we would like to think we are of the Kleinian pantheon of demonological projections, introjections, and projective identifications.

CORRELATION OF DATA WITH THOSE OF ASSOCIATED FIELDS

The need to bring psychoanalytic hypotheses in line with established findings in other, that is, related fields, influences the nature of which psychoanalytic concepts are singled out for emphasis. Psychoanalytic theories, of course, should not run counter to the findings clearly established by other fields. The other fields, however, ought to return the compliment. Unfortunately, often this is not the case. For example, Harlow studied the reaction of infant monkeys to two types of mother surrogates—terry cloth and wire mesh. The latter was the feeder: it had the bottle. The infant monkey found sustenance in the wire-mesh mother. It sought comfort from the terry-cloth, contact-gratifying mother. These observations, Harlow concluded, disproved psychoanalytic theories about the significance of oral gratification in the early life of the infant. This experiment is based on a naïve concept of orality, but if Harlow had been sufficiently acquainted with psychoanalytic propositions he would have been aware of the fact that this experiment as well as his so-called love-box experiment actually illustrated the usefulness, if not the validity, of the psychoanalytic concept of the primary process operation of the mind, that is, the tendency in states of drive frustration to try to re-experience a set of sensory impressions congruent with memories of earlier gratification. In fact, one could have gone further and made certain predictions on the basis of these experiments. Some years ago, at a symposium at the Albert Einstein Medical School devoted to instinct behavior, I was asked to discuss a presentation by Dr. Harlow in which he described his early experiments. I confessed at that occasion to a lack of certain knowledge of monkey nature. I did admit, however, to some familiarity with human nature. No human infant, I said, raised under the circumstances under which these infant monkeys had been raised, would grow up to exhibit anything even approximating human nature. The pioneer work of Spitz on hospitalism, the work of Bender, Mahler, and others, had demonstrated many years earlier the inevitability of abnormal development under such circumstances of nurture. I was gratified, therefore, to read some two or three years later that what was learned by psychoanalysts about human infants applied accurately to monkey infants. None of Harlow's experimental animals did, in fact, develop into any facsimile of what a well-behaved, self-respecting monkey should be.

I mention this example because there are a number of new and exciting disciplines whose findings are of utmost significance to psychoanalytic investigation. These include ethology, experimental animal psychology, developmental psychology, communications theory, and, more recently, psychophysiological studies of sleep and the dream process. A proper wedding of the findings from these disciplines with psychoanalysis would require respect from the party of the first part as well as from the party of the second part. The match should be based on mutuality of regard. Too often, it seems to me, the particular and unique contribution that psychoanalysts have to make using the data of their special form of investigation is brushed aside, even by analysts, in favor of what seems to be more "scientific," the more experimental data of the other disciplines. It seems to me, for example, that psychoanalysts have a more sophisticated body of knowledge to offer on the subject of imprinting than do the ethologists. In the field of psychophysiological studies of sleep and dreaming, similar trends may be observed. A quick and facile equating of REMing and dreaming has been asserted. Based on this questionable equation, one can observe a tendency to diminish the significance of the dream as a part of the continuity of mental life (altered, it is true, in its appearance under the special circumstances of sleep). The specifically psychological factors of the dream experience are treated as if they ranked second to the physiological findings. Similarly, I doubt if the nightmare can be taken out of the context of dream psychology and related almost exclusively to the physiology of sleep, simply because the nightmare has been found to occur during stages 3 and 4 of the sleep cycle. These are but a few examples of a trend that unwittingly diminishes the significance of the conclusions to be drawn from data gathered within the psychoanalytic situation.

At a recent meeting of the American Psychoanalytic Association, there was presented a panel on the ideological wellsprings of psychoanalysis. It was, I believe, the first time in the history of the association that so many professional scholars equally versed in the history of science as well as in psychoanalysis investigated in depth the relevant data and concepts in neurology, psychiatry, evolutionary theory, hypnosis, and philosophy that Freud had to assimilate in formulating his theories. A surprising conclusion followed inexorably from the total effect of these contributions. The presentations demonstrated with striking uniformity that almost all the concepts that Freud used in his early theory construction were in the air, as it were, at the time, not vaguely but explicitly. They could be quoted almost verbatim from the writings of his teachers. What, then, was the contribution that Freud made? It was a twofold one: first, by reason of his massive intellect, he was able to integrate and correlate the findings and theories of so many fields relating to human behavior. Second, and of overriding significance, he alone of all the workers at the time who were trying to devise a rational objective method for studying the mental life of man was successful in doing so. Through his genius, he fashioned the investigative tool that we now call the "psychoanalytic situation." This was based on the ideas of a dynamic unconscious and the principle of psychic determinism. With this tool, he could turn to collecting data more relevant and significant than those produced by any other method of research. Thus, though we of this generation face a similar task of integrating knowledge from related fields, we are in a much more advantageous position than Freud was. We have a research tool and a methodology that he invented and that has been improved over the years. I am not certain that we have exhausted its usefulness. It is possible that we have not been sufficiently mindful of its methodology and its limitations.

DISAPPOINTMENT WITH THE METHOD OF PSYCHOANALYTIC INVESTIGATION

This brings me to the third heading under which I propose to examine why certain concepts and styles of investigation have been most prominent in psychoanalysis. I refer to the disappointment or dissatisfaction with the psychoanalytic process as a tool of research. Some of this may be traceable to therapeutic frustration following on the widening of the scope of application of psychoanalysis. Several authors have already called for considering the narrowing of the scope of psychoanalysis. Psychoanalysis, as Ernst Kris said, is human nature viewed from the vantage point of conflict. Without the necessary impetus that comes from serious intrapsychic conflict, it is difficult indeed to set in motion the psychoanalytic process—and unless this takes place the data we gather are no more meaningful than what can be learned from a set of anamnestic interviews meticulously conducted by a sensitive psychiatrist. It is valuable, but it is not of the same order of relevance as analytic data, because the methodological criteria of contiguity, similarity, contrast, repetition, convergence, and the other forms of confirmation do not obtain under those circumstances. Without a dynamic process influenced primarily by endogenous forces, the observer must fall back on interpreting surface phenomena rather than derivatives of fixed or repetitive patterns of unconscious fantasy. Such interpretation, often useful and intuitive, is at best a surmise and cannot be submitted to validation in the same manner as constructions formulated within the psychoanalytic process. Interpretation of phenomenology outside of the dynamic context takes the study of mental life back to where it was before psychoanalysis. Many of the methodological errors to be observed in clinical and theoretical papers represent a tendency to interpret data in terms of phenomenological appearance without reference to free associations and the contexts in which the phenomena appeared.

For all the weight we attach to nonverbal communication in psychoanalysis, we cannot disregard the fundamental approach of psychoanalysis. It is a talking cure, but not in the sense that one talks out, that is, discharges his pent-up emotions. It is a talking cure in the sense that the vague hints, the symptomatic acts, the painful symptoms, the perplexing dreams and fantasies are all ultimately recast in the rational language of the secondary process as we are accustomed to referring to it in our psychoanalytic language. Through interpretations based on communication that is ultimately limited to word concepts, primitive fears are exposed, the automatic defenses of the ego are isolated and studied, insight is obtained, and hopefully mastery over conflict ensues. If we despair of the arduous effort entailed in the work, or if we find uncertainty too difficult to sustain, or if we try to push our instrument beyond the inherent limits of its application, then disappointment is certain to follow. Under the circumstances, the gaps can be filled either by a structural mystique such as the Kleinian system or by a set of extrapolations based on empathic identification rather than on observation. Here I am referring to the fascination for reconstructing the events of the first few months of life not on the basis of developmental studies or of direct observation of children, but on the basis of speculation derived from data supplied by the verbal experience of the patient and projected backward in an attempt to reconstruct the events of the preverbal period. This is followed by an extension of the preverbal experiences in order to demonstrate their continuing effects in adult life.

It is to be questioned whether the analytic instrument alone is capable of achieving this goal. It was not devised for such a task. The data of the analytic situation alone are not sufficient to realize it. A proper combination of methods of study that use psychoanalytic propositions in connection with extra-analytic methods of observation is more appropriate in this area. Longitudinal studies and direct observation are two such methods. It is encouraging to note the modest claims of those who work with children in contrast to the more ambitious claims of those who reconstruct the events of the first few months of life on the basis of data obtained in the consultation room.

LEADERS IN THE PSYCHOANALYTIC MOVEMENT

I turn now to the fourth element that I suggest helps determine the popularity of certain concepts in psychoanalysis. This is the attachment to leading teachers and authors in the psychoanalytic movement. Once again it is important to note that there is nothing unique about this phenomenon. One meets it in every field of science, especially in this age of huge laboratories established in the large universities and subsidized by massive grants from the federal government. Hierarchal organization and schools clustering around distinguished, creative, and inspiring teachers have been with us, should be with us, and will surely continue to be part of the scientific scene for a long time. What is different in the case of psychoanalysis is the impact of the apprentice-master model of training on the development and education of future practitioners and investigators. This is rendered all the more significant by the exceptionally close tie that comes into being as a result of the training analysis, which is usually referred to under the heading of transference phenomena.

The problems attendant on these ties are aggravated all the more by the fact that much more is involved than matters of individual transference psychology. The most powerful alliances are strengthened by group processes that are part of the history of psychoanalysis and that are built into the educational and training practices of all the institutes. Large or small, young or old, orthodox or dissident, by whatever name one may refer to it, the process is repeated in one way or another at various training centers. The process of group formation around idealized images may be traced to the operation of several leading unconscious fantasies that are shared in common by the members of the group and thus come to constitute its unofficial mythology.

Because I have discussed this matter elsewhere,[1,2] I will present here only the briefest outline of how the mythology of the institutes operates to influence the style of conceptualization. Favored concepts become fixed or associatively linked with certain societies, groups, or subgroups in psychoanalysis. Most often they are identified with one particular leader. The particular leader is almost always a training analyst of repute in the particular institute to which he belongs.

The training analyst in general and the particular outstanding teacher is the culture hero of psychoanalysis. He is the victorious end product of the psychoanalytic odyssey, a route of training fraught with more trials, tests, examinations, and transition experiences than almost any other profession.

In every culture, the hero of the myth becomes at some point the external representation of the collective ego ideal. Through a common relationship to the collective ideal, as Freud pointed out, a group may be formed. The members of the group are bound to one another through ties of mutual identification, and the group thereby becomes stable and coherent. The organizational dynamism is furnished by the affective forces associated with an unconscious fantasy that is shared in common by members of the group. The myth represents a more sophisticated and better integrated version of the fantasy. Through its mythology, each group sets about creating a climate that will foster the establishment of appropriate identifications, appropriate in the sense that such identifications lead to the realization of the character structure of the individual members of certain ideal qualities and attitudes. This is an important, unspoken, unconscious element of every educational system.[6] Organized groups that have a history, a continuity of ideology, and a developing body of knowledge for transmission to generations of newcomers utilize some form of mythology whether they are aware of it or not. Mythology is built into the social or educational institutions, and it is formalized in ceremony and ritual. The form that the educational experiences take, that is, the total curriculum or ritual through which we cause students to pass, evolves slowly in keeping with the conscious goals of the educators and the unconscious methodology of the discipline. In any discipline there is more to training than the transmission of knowledge. The professional attitude and with it the leading concepts and points of view have to be inculcated; identification is the prime psychological mechanism by which this is accomplished. Consciously or intuitively, the educational experience is structured in such a way as to favor such identifications.

There are two myths that give coherence to the psychoanalytic training experiences. The first is the myth of Prometheus. The second is the family romance. The two are, of course, intimately connected. There is a little bit of the Promethean fire thief in every scientific investigator. Somewhere in the recesses of his fantasy life he pictures his work as the equivalent of stealing at least an odd, glowing coal of omniscience from the altar of the gods. In the analytic mythology, Freud, of course, is the archetypal Prometheus, and the splendor of his achievement is universally acknowledged. But endless disputes have taken place over who is the legitimate heir, the confirmed possessor and protector of the magical knowledge. The myth of Prometheus is, of course, a socialized version of the private fantasy of stealing the omnipotent phallus from the father. In any training experience that accentuates the master-apprentice model, the emergence and activation of this universal fantasy must sooner or later be anticipated. To become the true heir and the possessor of the magical omniscience is confirmed by the initiation experiences and eventuates in an identification with the master.

The second leading fantasy of psychoanalysts is the family romance. The force of this universal fantasy is enhanced, in fact, it is intensified, by certain sociological, economic, and cultural factors. Most psychoanalytic candidates are recruited from the ranks of the liberated, intellectually enlightened middle class. They belong to that group that the sociologists have designated as upwardly mobile. Their education and liberal political tradition have weakened the ties of organized religion, the significance of patriotism, and any strong intellectual commitment to the economic system under which they live. For people who feel cut off from their own historical past, the existential dilemma calls for new allegiances. These are found in psychoanalysis. Candidates frequently express the thought that in analysis they have found an outlook that supersedes all other outlooks and a set of teachers who can be taken as models because of their rational, objective approach, their dedication to truth, and so forth. It is hard within the transference situation to counter, to tease out the irrational fantasy-based derivatives of the family romance, especially because it is true that analysis does offer a view of man that is objective, rationally different and, as we believe, superior to other approaches. Nonetheless, in every training analysis this derivative of the family romance must be analyzed if we are to achieve our educational goal—a free, independent, inquiring spirit not bound to a particular outlook by irrational, emotional concepts that see the analyst as a superior, parental imago superseding the denigrated parents of one's childhood years.

The unanalyzed residua of the phallus-stealing fantasies as exemplified by the Prometheus myth and of the family romance fantasies as exemplified by a whole series of complementary myths reinforce the graduate's espousing of his analyst's point of view. Anna Freud, Waelder, and others have given rich illustrations of the principles involved. The total effect of these fantasies, organized into a psychoanalytic mythology, is to foster a group process that serves to perpetuate the particular approach and outlook of the central figure, the ego ideal of the organized subgroup in psychoanalysis.

REASSESSMENT OF INFANTILE STATE

It should now be clear which trends in analysis I wish to consider most of all. I refer to the tendency to place the critical, decisive events that serve as the traumatic kernel for neurosis and character disorders earlier and earlier in the individual's life. It seems almost as if one's fate were sealed somewhere in the first few months of life, during the preverbal period dominated conceptually by the vicissitudes of the mother-child relationship.

I would like to emphasize at the very beginning of this discussion that that there can be no overestimating the significance of the early events of life. I propose to consider two questions. Just how do these early events influence the significant conflicts that form the bases of neurosis? And, second, how does one decide the nature of their impact and on the basis of what data? It should be clearly understood from the outset that the patterns of drive discharge, the predisposition to anxiety, and the shaping of the ego's function of defense in particular are probably influenced more strongly by the events of the earliest years of life than by all other subsequent events. The problem I am discussing is a methodological one. How can one establish from the data of the psychoanalytic situation which are the decisive, critical traumatic events behind the conflicts at the basis of the neuroses and the neurotic character disorders?

There are many methodological problems involved. It is very hard to comprehend the mental experience of the neonate and the young infant in terms of data from the verbal period. The rate of mental development in the neonate must at least equal the rate of physical development. Probably it is much greater. The mental functioning of a two-month-old child must be enormously different from that of an eight-month-old child. Everything that we have learned from developmental psychology and direct observation of children points to that conclusion. Furthermore, a revolutionary turning must take place with the acquisition of symbolic communication, at first nonverbal and soon afterward verbal as well.

How can we really conceptualize such ideas as wish, drive, danger, and fusion in the experience of the neonate or the recent neonate? Do these wishes, which we ascribe to this period on the basis of derivatives that we observe in analysis, actually stem from the experiences of this phase? It is doubtful. At best it is hard to know. As we know, every oral wish does not necessarily have to begin only in the early oral phase. Many oedipal wishes may be expressed in oral terminology. A little boy who wishes to eat so that he can become big and strong like his father and thereby win the love and admiration of the mother is actually expressing an oedipal wish in oral terms.

Lewin,[9] for example, described the triad of oral wishes supposedly operating in the mind of the nursling. These are the wish to eat, the wish to sleep, and the wish to be devoured, that is, to be fused with the mother. These concepts found wide circulation in psychoanalytic circles. Several authors tried to link a major portion of psychopathology to the sleep-wakefulness cycle, as a variant of the cycle of hunger and satiety. Every symptom represents to them a partial falling asleep, a miniscule fusing with the mother. For others the nursing situation becomes the model for psychic functioning in general and for the organization of psychic structure. And for still others, the nursing situation is repeated not only in the experience of the patient in the analytic situation but in the response of the analyst to the material produced by the analysand. This latter concept comes very close to the idea of projective identification so popularly held among Kleinian psychoanalysts, especially in South America.[5]

More recently Lewin[10] felt it necessary to clarify his earlier statements concerning the oral triad. He felt that he could not assert that these wishes actually obtained in the case of the nursling. They are, he said, the three-to-four-year-old child's fantasy of what is the mental state of the little rival whom he observes at his mother's breast, in his mother's arms. I think we should all welcome such clarification. How, indeed, is it possible to entertain the notion of fusing with another object prior to the development of individuation, prior to the distinct sense of separation between the self and the object world? Most evidence seems to indicate that this process of individuation and separation does not seem to take place until well into the second year. Furthermore, why should fusion as such be regarded as a danger? Sleep is a prized, wished-for, heaven-sent gift. It could be regarded as dangerous, however, by a three- or four-year-old child entertaining a fantasy of being devoured and incorporated into the mother's body.

A variant of the same theme can be seen in the writings of other authors. For example, Greenson,[7] in a study of phobias, felt that in each case the primal anxiety over separation from the mother in the earliest months of life was repeated in the phobic situation. It was essential, he said, for the individual to reproduce and master this trauma during treatment in order to get well. The same objections that applied to certain applications of the oral triad mentioned in the paragraph above apply in this case. Furthermore, the essential requirement in treatment that every patient reexperience the terror of separation from the mother in a preverbal type of experience does not conform with the observations of most practitioners. I have not seen it in my own cases or in cases I have supervised, except in connection with deep problems of depression.

In order to demonstrate how this methodological bias operates, I would like to illustrate with an experience from a discussion of a clinical paper I presented recently. This paper was based on a study of the relationship of certain character traits to antecedent perversions, perversions that had been practiced during early adolescence. In this contribution I made the analogy to character neurosis, that is, a situation in which a conflict at one stage in life gave rise to symptoms, but later, following alteration in the life experience, maturity, and so forth, gave rise instead to neurotic character traits. Pursuing the analogy, I advanced the concept of character perversion. I referred to unusual character traits that appeared during late adolescence and that replaced earlier perversions or tendencies toward perversion. The striking fact was that the unconscious reassuring fantasy and the defense mechanisms were the same in the perversion as in the character trait based on it. I discussed several types of character perversions—the unrealistic character, the petty liar, the practical joker. More recently I have added another type, the petty swindler.

The unrealistic character represents a transformation of fetishism, to be observed in individuals who make the unconscious equation of the female genital and reality.[8] These individuals cannot look at the heart of the matter, must beat around the bush and find reassurance by focusing their attention on some peripheral, tangential perception that serves to deny the unpleasant reality perceived in the form of the female genital without a phallus. In the analytic situation, such patients are glancers rather than lookers. When they are forced to confront an unpleasant reality during sessions, they tend to shield their eyes, to rub their eyes, to blink, or to turn their gaze away, literally and figuratively. The second type of character perversion described was that of the petty liar who resembles the first one, the unrealistic character just described. There is an important variant. This type of character perversion is based on a special requirement characteristic of the fetish. The fetish had to be in earlier years an object that could be looked through but through which one could not actually see, for example, some black lingerie, silk stockings. Such patients tell petty lies, adorn and embellish the truth. They prefer to treat reality, as one patient said, as if it were a bad dream. The petty lie is like the fetish that is interposed between the observer and reality. If the patient is able to convince other people of his lies, he achieves reassurance by proxy.[13] The third type of character perversion described is that of the practical joker, or hoaxer. This character trait is a transformation of what had once been the transvestite perversion. In his perversion, the transvestite creates the external facsimile of a woman, but has the reassuring knowledge that if one could only look underneath and examine the real truth one would see a percept that would be alleviating of anxiety, namely, the presence of the phallus. The practical joker loves to stimulate anxiety in others and gets the pleasure of exposing the hoax. This has the unconscious significance of stating, "There was nothing really to worry about from the very beginning. You might think that the situation looked terrifying but if you got to know the real truth you would see that there was never anything to worry about." These patients in childhood characteristically would play at being blind or being crippled. The joy in the game came not from the exercise thereof, but from the sense of mastery and pleasure that came with the reassuring ending of the game and the restoring to oneself of one's capacity for sight and locomotion. As children, such patients characteristically used to play in front of the mirror, pressing back the phallus between the thighs in order to simulate the appearance of the female genital and achieving the reassuring pleasure of releasing the thighs and watching the penis reappear to vision. The petty swindler is based on the type of homosexuality described by Nunberg.[11] He refers to the type of individual who assumes the passive, submissive, ingratiating, so-called feminine attitude in sexual experiences with another male. While doing so, however, he unconsciously entertains a fantasy of identifying with the more powerful male partner by seizing and possessing during the act of intercourse the powerful phallus of the dominant male partner. The petty swindler whom I have observed entraps his victims through ingratiation, submission, and even a feminine adoring attitude toward the male who is dominant. In the end, however, the situation is dramatically reversed as the swindler comes away with the money and the advantage, and the so-called dominant male finds himself bereft of his possessions.

In reviewing the essence of this contribution, one can see that this was primarily a study of the transformation of an established perversion or tendency to perversion into a character trait. The origin of the perversion was not really germane to the clinical problem nor essential to the theoretical constructs deriving therefrom. In presenting these contributions, however, a certain trend could be observed in discussions. The discussions represent a concrete illustration of the methodological biases I have discussed earlier. The main points of the discussions centered around the following:

1. It is impossible to discuss perversion without considering preoedipal factors, because perversion is clearly a preoedipal problem dealing with the mother-child relationship.

2. The essence of transvestism is the wish to fuse and become one with the mother, to become the mother, in order to offset the danger of losing her, the danger of separation. In other words, if you cannot have the mother, you become her. The situation, it was argued, was self-evident: because the transvestite dresses up as his mother, he therefore becomes the mother.

3. Fetishism represents an attempt to cling to the mother, if not to all of her at least to a part of her. The fetishist object is derived from the transitional object, that is, something that is at one time part self and part external object. The danger of separation is negated or mastered through clinging, if not to the entire object, at least to a part of her.

4. Fetishism is a recapitulation of the wish to continue the passive, dependent pleasures of the mother-child relationship. Proof of the fact can be seen in the evidence that the fetishistic objects are precisely those involved in the mother's nursing, protecting, feeding, and rearing the infant.

I wish to make the following observations about the points raised in the discussions. There is no doubt that preoedipal experiences do influence the outcome of intrapsychic conflict when perversion is the result, but the conflict itself is phase specific (Hartmann). Without the castration anxiety of the oedipal phase there is no fetishism or probably no other male perversion. In other words, though preoedipal traumata are relevant to the problem of fetishism, they are neither sufficient nor decisive in themselves to account for this phenomenon.

Clinical evidence suggests no definite relationship between undue attachment to the transitional object and to the subsequent development of fetishism. Once again following Hartmann, one could observe that emphasis on such a relationship is an example of the genetic fallacy in psychoanalysis. The early clinging to an object resembles but is not identical with the later clinging to the fetish. The clinging experience undergoes a change of function. In a new context, it has a different meaning and serves an entirely different purpose.

This latter point illustrates a fundamental problem in current psychoanalytic thinking. The approach that identifies the clinging experience with the origin of fetishism is an approach based on phenomenology rather than on empirical findings in the analytic situation. A man who dresses up in a woman's clothing may have many different unconscious fantasies about the activity while he is practicing it. One can no more deduce the meaning of the perverse behavior and the purpose it serves from the manifest behavior of the pervert than one can interpret the meaning of a dream from its manifest content.

Finally, it is not true that the items chosen by the fetishist are especially related to the child care situation; thus one cannot conclude that the fetishist expresses in his choice the wish to re-create the passive, protected, dependent, nurturing mother-child relationship. I have yet to hear of a fetishist who concentrated on a milk bottle, a teething ring, or a can of ZBT baby powder. The fetish is more often than not an exotic object, chosen in a very specific context and rather late in life, much later than infancy.

It is perhaps in the treatment setting that one can observe biases operating most forcefully. The analytic situation and the transference have come to be regarded as replicas of the infantile state, because the analysand restricts his activity and is in that sense passive, because he turns to the analyst for help, because he bares his secrets to the analyst who reveals nothing of himself. Several authors in a symposium on the subject[12] concluded that the effectiveness of the analytic situation and the origin of the transference must be related to the early mother-child situation. Anna Freud, on the other hand, felt that many other conditions, especially the experiences of having turned to someone for help, influence the development of trust in general and the ability to enter into the analytic situation and to effect a transference in particular.

In connection with the working alliance or the therapeutic alliance, that is, the nontransference analytic compact that operates in the treatment situation, several authors have stated rather categorically that those patients who did not enjoy a good mother-child relationship cannot enter into the therapeutic alliance. For them treatment is impossible. Discussions of this sort led one outstanding practitioner to protest that because of his own strong sense of masculine identity he did not find it easy to be a mother in the treatment situation. Nevertheless he felt that he had been rather effective in working with his patients. Others[3] have pointed out that cases have been reported in which a good working alliance was effected between analysand and analyst on the basis of an earlier relationship with the father and in the face of an extremely bad relationship with the mother during the earliest phase of life. Though there is no doubt that the basic patterns of turning in a trusting way to adults are laid down in childhood, one must be careful nonetheless to prevent this observation from becoming a fixed and immutable principle in discussing problems of treatment and technique.

TERMINATION OF ANALYSIS

A final point may be made about considerations concerning termination of analysis. In keeping with the bias discussed above, termination of analysis has been regarded as necessarily recapitulating the trauma of early childhood separation from the mother. Each patient, accordingly, is expected to go through a mourning reaction in the closing phases of treatment. This is certainly true in many cases; it is not true in all cases. The fantasies and conflicts involved in the experience of termination cover a wide range that not only recapitulates separation from the mother in early childhood but also activates fantasies about completion vs. incompletion, castrated vs. phallic, life vs. death, and disappointment over the fact that the analysis has failed to fulfill all those unconscious childhood fantastic wishes that the patient brings in to the analysis under the guise of the wish to get well. It is worth repeating that in all the elements concerned with the treatment situation in which the bias in favor of the early mother-child relationship is emphasized, namely, the significance of the analytic situation and the origin of the transference, the effectiveness of the therapeutic alliance, and the experience of termination; in all these, the methodological error consists of interpreting the surface phenomena from the manifest experience rather than utilizing the analytic situation to elicit the nature of the concomitant unconscious fantasy of which these phenomena are the observable derivatives.

Another aspect of the problem should be mentioned here, unfortunately only in passing. It deserves fuller treatment in a separate communication. There is another corollary of the methodological bias concerning the traumatic impact of the earliest childhood experiences. Those who emphasize the early phases of childhood but who do not project speculative guesses about the content of these experiences tend to fall back on a concept of trauma that makes it identical with noxious biological experiences, for example, physical illness or speculations about the nature of psychosomatic distress. Accordingly, a contentless anxiety is described in biological terms, or organismic distress comes to replace the more palpable types of danger situation that can be conceptualized only by an older child. Derivative expressions of anxiety that actually reflect the patient's reaction to the danger situation are treated as primary causes in themselves. Thus one deals seriously with such situations as fear of dissolution, fear of loss of ego boundaries, or fear of loss of ego functions. It is hard to establish that a patient unconsciously experiences such highly structured psychological concepts as constituting dangers and that these provoke anxiety.

CONCLUSION

In this communication I examined some elements contributing to the general emphasis in current psychoanalytic thought on the traumatic effect of the events of the first few months of life and of their lasting influence on later psychic structuring and neurotic conflict and character formation.

Some consideration was given to the methodological problems involved in reconstructing the events of the preverbal period. The analytic situation can hardly define in great detail the precise speculative reconstructions that have been offered.

One of the effects of this tendency has been to diminish the significance of the analytic situation as a research tool. Data obtained through its use are given less weight than they should get. Instead, one observes unconfirmed speculations about the first few months of life put forward as if they were established fact.

I have suggested that the study of psychoanalytic methodology has to be refined and deepened to utilize more fully the data obtainable from direct observation and longitudinal studies, group dynamics, and the like.

Contributions to the literature based on speculations concerning the first few months of life seem to have crowded out, to have discouraged clinical contributions based on empirical findings using psychoanalytic data. This is a trend that is a cause for concern, and every effort should be made to revive interest in clinical studies.

REFERENCES

1. Arlow, J. "Ego Psychology and the Study of Mythology," *Journal of the American Psychoanalytic Association*, 9 (1961), 371–393.
2. Arlow, J. "Myth and Ritual in Psychoanalytic Education," in C. Babcock, *Training Analysis*. 1969.
3. Arlow, J., and Brenner, C. "The Psychoanalytic Situation," R. E. Litman (ed.), *Psychoanalysis in the Americas*. New York: International Universities Press, 1966. Pp. 23–43.
4. Bak, R. Paper presented at the American Psychoanalytic Association, Miami, Florida, May 4, 1969.
5. Baranger, M., and Baranger, W. "Insight in the Psychoanalytic Situation," in R. E. Litman (ed.), *Psychonanalysis in the Americas*. New York: International Universities Press, 1966. Pp. 56–72.
6. Freud, A. "Psychoanalysis and the Training of the Young Child," *Psychoanalytic Quarterly*, 4 (1935), 15–24.
7. Greenson, R. "Phobia, Anxiety, Depression," *Journal of the American Psychoanalytic Association*, 7 (1959), 663–674.
8. Lewin, B. D. "The Nature of Reality, the Meaning of Nothing, with an Addendum on Concentration," *Psychoanalytic Quarterly*, 17 (1948), 524–526.
9. Lewin, B. D. *The Psychoanalysis of Elation*. New York: Norton, 1950.
10. Lewin, B. D. *The Image and the Past*. New York: International Universities Press, 1968.
11. Nunberg, H. "Homosexuality, Magic, and Aggression," *International Journal of Psycho-Analysis*, 19 (1938), 1–16.
12. Waelder, R., Zetzel, E. R., Hoffer, W., Spitz, R. A., Winnicott, D. W. "Symposium on Transference," *International Journal of Psycho-Analysis*, 37 (1956), 367–388.
13. Wangh, M. "The Evocation of a Proxy," in P. Greenacre (ed.), *Psychoanalytic Study of the Child*. New York: International Universities Press, 1962. Vol. 17, pp. 451–469.

DECREASING THE LENGTH OF PSYCHOTHERAPY: THEORETICAL AND PRACTICAL ASPECTS OF THE PROBLEM

Pietro Castelnuovo-Tedesco

In 1937 Freud[10] said:

Experience has taught us that psychoanalytic therapy—the liberation of a human being from his neurotic symptoms, inhibitions and abnormalities of character—is a lengthy business. Hence, from the very beginning attempts have been made to shorten the course of analysis. Such endeavors required no justification: they could claim to be prompted by the strongest considerations alike of reason and expedience.

Of the questions that are asked today about psychotherapy, one that still receives much attention is how the length of treatment can be limited. In fact, during the past ten years—under the rubrics of brief, short-term, or crisis psychotherapy and similar headings—much emphasis has been given to this problem.

The impetus to shorten treatment has been enormous and has derived from many sources, which we shall have occasion to consider. A result of this concern has been an outpouring of books and articles; their number is such that only a few will be specifically mentioned here. A quick scanning of the psychotherapeutic scene reveals a tendency still to regard brief treatment as quite new and as a replacement for the longer and more intensive forms of psychotherapy rather than as an approach with definable and reasonably specific indications (and also reasonably predictable limitations). There is also a trend to consider it in isolation without reference to other known psychotherapeutic modalities, glossing over differences in goals and in characteristic methods. Finally, although much of the brief psychotherapy that is done in this country is analytically inspired or, at least, dynamically oriented, it is also looked on as favoring, in fact requiring, eclecticism of technique. Thus, on the issue of technique as well as on that of duration, brief treatment often is viewed not as an approach sui generis, but as somehow opposed to long-term treatment and, in particular, psychoanalysis. Brief treatment then becomes a rallying point for those who plead for special causes, among them "flexibility of technique" and nonintensiveness of contact.

Of course, nothing intrinsic places these treatment methods (the long and the short, the more intensive and the less intensive) in opposition to each other. This opposition, when it occurs, is more an expression of individual outlook than of inherent contradiction in the subject matter. In this connection, it is important to remind ourselves that the early history of analysis and of brief psychotherapy is jointly shared. Breuer's[3] cathartic method was really an example of brief psychotherapy. Dora,[8] from whom Freud learned so much about the workings of transference, was in treatment only three months. Freud employed what later was to be regarded as an important technical device of brief psychotherapy when he introduced a limit into the treatment of the Wolf-man.[9] Even after he was established as an analyst, Freud treated some patients for only a few sessions, when this was indicated, as in the case of Gustav Mahler,[13] the composer, and that of Bruno Walter,[23] the conductor.

The enormous interest in short-term treatment apparent in the last decade derives from at least several important sources. Primary, probably, is the newly acquired significance—social as well as medical—of brief treatment. Increasingly, the need has been felt to make psychotherapeutic help accessible to broad segments of the population, and the hope has grown that brief psychotherapy, often combined with drugs, could provide the needed vehicle for this "psychiatry for everyman."[25] Also, over the years our knowledge of the workings of brief psychotherapy has increased considerably. Our greater understanding of transference, ego mechanisms, and crisis has taken brief treatment out of the realm of the personal virtuosity of the individual practitioner, as tended to be true in its early days, and shaped it into a discipline that can be described, taught, and tested. With this has come greater confidence in its effectiveness. Although there are still important differences of opinion about the true reach of brief psychotherapy—what it can do, what it cannot do, and what realistically it can be expected to provide—there is fairly general agreement that its potential as a therapeutic tool is noteworthy and that probably it has much to contribute to the practical solutions that currently are sought. However, we should also not forget that at times an outspoken interest in brief treatment results, paradoxically, from the progressive disenchantment with *all* psychotherapy and with its long forms in particular. Here the wish, really, is to reduce contact with the patient down to the vanishing point. The attitude is not new and Freud,[10] in fact, had occasion to remark on it:

There probably lurked in them some trace of the contempt with which the medical profession of an earlier day regarded the neuroses, seeing in them the unnecessary results of invisible lesions. If it had now become necessary to deal with them, they should at least be got rid of with the utmost dispatch.

WHAT IS BRIEF PSYCHOTHERAPY?

Although "brief" and "short-term psychotherapy" are labels that are often used interchangeably, they do perhaps imply recognition that even limited treatment covers variable time spans. Possibly, "brief psychotherapy" might be used to refer to the briefest interventions and "short-term psychotherapy" to those lasting several weeks or a few months. In a similar vein, Gill[11] has suggested that there are not only brief but also intermediate forms of psychotherapy. The names, however, are not significant. What is important is that they refer to a range of time alternatives and not to a single prescription. Moreover, often both are distinguished from "long-term psychotherapy," but here, too, the dividing line is arbitrary. Empirical considerations have led most writers in this field to consider as brief any treatment involving not more than ten to twenty-five sessions, spread out over a period of three or four months, but others allow as many as forty or more sessions or permit the span of treatment to be six months or even a year if the sessions are spaced far apart and their total number is small.[1, 16] It is clear, therefore, that the concept of brief treatment involves questions of depth and intensity and, as we shall see later, also of goals and methods, as well as of duration. (The common denominator between treatment that lasts four weeks and treatment that lasts a year but where the sessions occur infrequently is that in both instances intense transference reactions [certainly a full-fledged transference neurosis] are not given a chance to develop. More will be said about this later.)

Where appropriate, treatment frequently consists of only several sessions, five or so, or even fewer,[1, 14, 20] and occasionally a pre-established time limit is used.[6, 7] The empirical considerations referred to above have to do with the observation that as treatment is extended beyond ten to twenty-five sessions, the focus inevitably broadens to include, in addition to the current predicament, examination of the patient's fundamental and long-standing ways of reacting—that is, of his personality and character.

In brief treatment, the frequency of the visits usually is once (or twice) a week, although, if initially the patient is highly distressed and symptomatic, the first few sessions may need to be closer together. The duration of each visit generally is the standard fifty-minute hour, but recently there has been also experimentation with sessions of lesser duration.[6, 7, 15, 17] An example of the latter is the "Twenty-Minute Hour,"[6, 7] which was introduced as a model for supportive work by the nonpsychiatric physician. Clearly the length of the psychotherapeutic session should be geared to the goals of the therapy and to the technical devices by which it tries to achieve these. Fifty-minute periods are appropriate (and needed) when the aim is the interpretive analysis and working through of conflicts, whereas shorter visits may be quite sufficient where the time is given primarily to catharsis, clarification, and simple reassurance. Again, this, too, is a variable matter because, occasionally, significant amounts of interpretive work can be accomplished during briefer periods.

Reference should be made also to a type of brief treatment, which perhaps might be called "truncated psychotherapy," where the length of treatment is chosen arbitrarily out of deference to factors that are extrinsic to the patient and may have nothing to do with his particular problem. A common example is the practice in certain clinics of seeing patients only for a standard, fixed number of sessions to distribute available professional time as widely as possible. Many patients manage reasonably well even with an arbitrarily set time limit, although some do not, and then special arrangements have to be made to deal with the complications. Obviously, it is preferable if the time limit can be used selectively and adjusted to the patient's particular situation rather than applied across the board to all comers.

FUNDAMENTAL ISSUES OF BRIEF PSYCHOTHERAPY

"Brief" or "short-term psychotherapy," then, is not a one-dimensional process, to be accounted for mainly in terms of its duration. Other crucial issues must be considered inasmuch as they define its essential nature and help to establish a rational basis for its indications. Time does more than measure the length of treatment; it also influences its scope, shapes its goals and methods, and creates priorities.

Always, the primary purpose of brief psychotherapy is to relieve the patient's suffering and, in particular, his most pressing symptoms, as promptly and as expeditiously as possible. When more is achieved, this is to be regarded as a special bonus not counted on or even actively sought. Brief treatment is particularly indicated where the patient's distress is not the expression of a long-standing neurotic struggle, but rather of an unfortunate predicament that has noticeably taxed his endurance and social effectiveness and has rekindled an internal conflict, previously dormant or, at least, adequately managed. No attempt is made to modify and reorganize the patient's basic personality or to disturb well-established defensive patterns. Rather, the emphasis, always a highly practical one, is on taking care of first things first. The psychotherapeutic effort is directed in the main not at "changing" the patient, that is, bringing about a new level of organization, but at restoring him to the one that existed before his acute difficulties began.*

These remarks, however, must be qualified. Brief psychotherapy

---

* "Crisis therapy," or "crisis intervention,"[5, 19] recently has re-emphasized the considerable clinical usefulness in brief psychotherapy of focusing sharply on the present, especially on the disruption of significant current relationships. Also, it has given special recognition to the finding that patients often are more accessible to psychotherapy during states of emergency than at other times. However, as a theoretical concept, the notion of crisis, which attempts to straddle intrapsychic and environmental events, is less successful and tends to blur the important distinction between what happens inside the patient and what happens around him, between internal conflict and external stress. Emotional disturbance occurs not only in apparent response to new circumstances (positive as well as negative) but also endogenously (that is, without striking or manifest environmental participation).

is not limited to the removal of troublesome symptoms and alleviation of general distress, nor is more fundamental and lasting change the exclusive province of long-term, intensive psychotherapy. Depending on the presenting symptoms, on the vigor and effectiveness of the patient's personality, on the favorableness of his social circumstances, and on the skill of the therapist, important reorganizations of sectors of the personality can take place; these changes may well go beyond a temporary improvement of the homeostatic balance. Actually, the spectrum of results is very wide, and from time to time one is impressed by an outcome that is truly remarkable for its unexpected breadth and sturdiness. Nonetheless, such results, when seen, are a comment less on the scope of brief treatment than on the strength and resourcefulness of certain personalities who can respond to a little help with a great spurt of growth and rapid progress. These cases are the counterpart of instances, not infrequent in everyday life, of persons who with minimal assistance have lifted themselves from extremely restricted circumstances to achieve notable careers in one or another field.

Brief treatment achieves its primary goal of maximal possible effectiveness in the context of brevity and economy of time through the workings of several fundamental and interrelated processes. Time, within limits, decides what is feasible and what is not.

1. Emphasis is deliberately on the present and on the reactions that are shaping it, inasmuch as these are most fluid and readily accessible. Attention is given to the patient's major current conflict(s) and to the main object relationship(s) involved in the current upset. This is in keeping with the usual psychoanalytic procedure of approaching material from the surface. Although the contributions of the past are not totally neglected, the focus primarily is on the present (What ails him now?) rather than on the past (How did he become what he is?) or the future (Where is he going? Is his life fulfilling its basic goals?).

2. Analysis of resistance is restricted, in the main, to those more superficial defenses that are, again, readily accessible and closely related to current material. Defenses of long standing, especially those frozen into the character, cannot be usefully approached and should, in fact, be circumvented.

3. Transference reactions may be recognized and dealt with, especially if they are negative but fairly superficial (for example,

expressions of doubt, disappointment, mild resentment). On the other hand, negative manifestations that appear related to deep-seated paranoid and depressive anxieties are usually left untouched for fear of stirring up issues that cannot be settled in the limited time available. Also untouched (and deliberately unresolved) are the positive transference reactions: they are the glue that binds the cure. A full transference neurosis is not desirable and does not develop, in part because time is insufficient and in part because of specific steps taken to prevent it: the regressive state which a full-fledged transference brings about is not in keeping with the aim of promoting a rapid recompensation.

4. The patient's ability to work through the issues touched on during the limited period of treatment determines to a large degree what is accomplished in brief psychotherapy. This depends on the ego's synthetic capacity, which is variable, and on the fact that working through is greatly foreshortened for want of time. Actually, much of this process is left to the patient to complete on his own after treatment has stopped. Consequently, an adequate interval should be allowed, and a follow-up is particularly important to evaluate the final result.

THE TECHNIQUES OF BRIEF PSYCHOTHERAPY

The therapeutic techniques commonly used in brief treatment are multiple and varied. In fact, although there are major points of agreement about the proper conduct of brief psychotherapy, there has also been a general feeling that a "standard technique" belongs less here than in the longer forms of psychotherapy and, in particular, psychoanalysis. There has been a tendency to see the situation in brief treatment as highly idiosyncratic, unique, and unpredictable and therefore rather unsuited to a systematic and methodical approach. Indeed, it has been felt to favor, at times even to require, bold improvisation and an individualistic style. Both analytic and nonanalytic therapists have contributed to this viewpoint. Whether reliance was placed on a "deep" Stekelian interpretation that would unlock the unconscious secret or on a timely piece of directive prodding for the patient who seemed to need it, the notion has been that a single therapeutic act, shrewdly chosen and well applied, quickly would resolve a complex neurotic impasse. The problem with this view has been that though it fails to account for the usual course of events, occasionally things happen just as hearsay would have them. Every busy therapist can recall encounters of this sort, and notable examples have been reported in the literature.* The notion that the therapeutic approach should be eclectic in orientation and flexibly applied has arisen not only from the uniqueness and heterogeneity of the problems treated, but also from the very fact that the treatment is expected to be short. For some the task of brief treatment—doing a big job fast—has meant that the therapist should bring to it every possible means at his disposal. As a result, there has been a tendency to maintain or resurrect manipulative techniques of exhortation, advice-giving, and direct pedagogy to a degree well beyond their probable usefulness. At any rate, in the longer forms of treatment these devices have not been found especially helpful. There has also been the view that as brief treatment often deals with emergent situations and pressing problems, special means are called for: as one fights fire with fire, one treats conversion with suggestion, compulsion or inhibition with direct injunction. The question raised here is whether these techniques, useful though they are on occasion, have not been oversold and whether the case for eclecticism has not been overstated.

The technical devices currently used (and advocated in the general psychiatric literature) as applicable to brief psychotherapy cover the widest range, and this seems to be in keeping with the idea, already referred to, that here, as in love and war, all is fair play. One might list:

1. Establishing (and maintaining) a positive transference. Of relevance here are a variety of devices that are known to affect the quality of the transference, for example, a time limit, the frequency of sessions, the "role" adopted by the therapist, his degree of activity, focusing on the healthy aspects of the patient, and so forth.
2. Ventilation and emotional catharsis.

---

* One about whom many such tales are told was the late N. Lionel Blitzsten, of Chicago. As Douglass Orr[18] recalls, "Then there is the story of the diva with acute aphonia, quickly cured when Lionel thrust a wiener at her mouth and made her scream. ... One woman tells this of herself: She went to Lionel extremely upset in a marital crisis and dramatically announced that she would throw herself out of the window. Lionel drew aside and said, 'Well, there is the window,' after which they got down to the business at hand." Stekel's[22] writings are full of examples, whether real or slightly fictitious, of the successful "one-punch" intervention.

3. Reassurance and suggestion. Occasionally the latter may take the form of hypnosis.
4. Exhortation, counseling, advice, and environmental manipulation.
5. Explanations and pedagogic remarks.
6. Drug-giving.
7. Desensitization by counterconditioning techniques,[27] especially for phobias and other focal anxiety responses.
8. Interpretive techniques. These include clarifications (of feelings, thoughts, attitudes), confrontations, and interpretations proper. Occasionally, a dream may prove a useful starting point for the analysis of a crucial current conflict.

The choice of techniques depends not only on the requirements of the particular case, but also on the special preference of the individual therapist and on his level of training. It is important to note here that at least *some* brief psychotherapy can be carried off—just because time is limited and it is possible to stay close to the surface—with simple methods, a rudimentary theoretical orientation, and relatively untrained therapists. For example, one of the purposes of the "Twenty-Minute Hour"[6, 7] was to define certain conditions in which treatment could be managed safely and effectively by the occasional psychotherapist. On the other hand, in some situations brief treatment can become unexpectedly complex and demanding of skills, and this, of course, makes the task a variable and highly uneven one. Many psychotherapists achieve quite satisfactory results by relying on the two mainstays of brief treatment, namely, the benefits of a positive relationship and adequate catharsis. Others add in varying proportions suggestion, exhortation, explanation, manipulation, drug-giving, or, perhaps, desensitization. Finally, still others employ primarily interpretive techniques which, despite modifications, are used similarly as in the more intensive forms of long-term treatment. They emphasize insight and self-understanding and try to go as far in this direction as time and the opportunity for working through of conflicts allow. The work accomplished depends, among other things, on the accessibility of the conflict, on the patient's ability to ally himself with the therapist and his interpretive efforts, and on the time available for working through. Of course, there is great variation even among analytic therapists, because in addition to the inevitable differences of personal style, there is also, as has been noted, hardly anything that even approximates a standard technique. As Stone[24] has observed,

One [therapist] actively engages the patient's attention to himself and the therapeutic relationship by leading questions and by prompt interpretations of the transference; another proceeds very much as in analysis; another proceeds vigorously with id interpretations with or without transference emphasis; a third gives a great deal of advice about the conduct of life, but minimal interpretation except of a general didactic nature; and so forth.

Of significance is whether predominantly interpretive or predominantly manipulative techniques are used. There is general agreement that manipulative devices have a necessary and sometimes critical role in brief treatment. Here the important question refers to the degree to which they are employed by the individual therapist. A statement by Gill[11] is applicable to this discussion, even though it was made in the context of trying to separate classical analysis from analytic psychotherapy. He said, "There is a vast difference between attempting to maintain a position of neutrality . . . and deciding that since perfect neutrality cannot be maintained anyhow, we might as well plunge into emotional participation with the patient." The point is that in brief treatment reliance can be placed, as much as the clinical situation permits, on interpretation, which is the therapist's most dependable tool, and that manipulative maneuvers can be employed in a planned way with careful dosage of the ingredients rather than as expression of some general viewpoint, such as that it is good to be oneself and do what comes naturally. Gill,[11] too, says, "I believe we have failed to carry over into our psychotherapy enough of the nondirective spirit of our analyses. I do not refer to the emergency situations where active intervention seems unavoidable and where the essential goal is supportive, but to the less urgent problems seen over longer periods of time with more ambitious goals." In other words, one should distinguish between the extent to which such devices may be needed to stabilize an otherwise uncertain treatment situation and the extent to which they are indulged in, because of the therapist's predilection, for their own sake. In writings on brief psychotherapy, it has become almost a cliche to emphasize the need for activity, responsiveness, and enthusiasm by the therapist. These characterizations cover a great deal of ground, which cannot be examined here in detail. However, it may sharpen the point to say that in brief therapy there is perhaps an even greater need than elsewhere to catch accurately the drift of the patient's feelings and to represent them to him in a lively, dramatically emphatic way.

INDICATIONS AND LIMITATIONS OF BRIEF PSYCHOTHERAPY

In considering the scope of brief psychotherapy, we must include not only its range of goals (as we have already done) but also the types of conditions to which it is applicable. Brief treatment has much to offer to a variety of patients, and for some it is specifically the treatment of choice. However, it is not suitable for all patients or all conditions, and there are some for which it is quite unsuitable. It would be attractive if decisions about the appropriateness of brief psychotherapy could be made on clinical grounds alone, that is, on the specific features of the patient's disturbance, but in practice consideration often must be given to extraneous factors, the patient's financial resources, and the therapist's available time. Frequently, also, the therapist's personal preference definitely tips the scales for one or another mode of treatment. Yet, as Gillman[12] correctly (but somewhat idealistically) points out, "Selection must not be based merely on the absence of some criterion for psychoanalysis, or because a particular therapist needs to feel the power of directive therapy and quick cure, or because the predilection is for more limited goals rather than getting to the bottom of things."

The question of the indications for brief psychotherapy is a complicated one because it immediately involves issues of treatment goals and the therapist's orientation toward these. In speaking here about the indications and limitations of brief psychotherapy, we are referring to those conditions and situations where this mode of treatment can be expected to provide reasonably stable and definitive results. On the other hand, the range of indications can be broadened considerably beyond what will be discussed in the following paragraphs, and in practice a wide variety of patients are treated with brief psychotherapy, including many that by more stringent criteria would be regarded as unsuitable. My purpose here is not to attempt a list of "treatable" (and "untreatable") conditions, which would be unrealistic and arbitrary, but to survey the factors that make patients more or less accessible to brief treatment, emphasizing as space permits the rationale for the decisions that must be made in the individual clinical instances.

Brief psychotherapy probably is best limited to patients of reasonably mature personality and adequate motivation whose emotional disturbance is focal, acute (rather than chronic), of less than extreme intensity, and associated with fairly apparent situational factors.*

It is highly desirable that the patient, despite his distress (which in some instances may be very great), still be able to function in his accustomed social role. We are talking, therefore, about the ego's relative competence, in particular about its synthetic, integrative, and adaptive capabilities. We include, then, mainly neurotic patients, not grossly incapacitated, who see their previous functioning as reasonably satisfactory or at least not troublesome enough to warrant a more extended therapeutic commitment. However, brief treatment may also be indicated initially as a first-stage procedure for sicker patients in an acute turmoil before a more intensive approach with more ambitious goals is even considered.

The presenting symptoms bear some relationship (but not an overly close one) to the suitability for brief treatment. Those who suffer mainly from the simpler symptomatic manifestations —anxiety, moderate depression, or minor hysterical conversions— usually respond especially well,[7] although those with mild obsessive manifestations not infrequently also show surprisingly good results.[21, 26] Yet, more significant than any one particular symptom or diagnosis is the patient's accessibility and his capacity and readiness for rapid involvement with the therapist. This is a function not only of the patient's psychopathology, but also of his motivation, which in turn relates to the typical transference attitude he brings to the treatment situation. Patients who often do very well and are able to make the most of the opportunity are those who show a "latency type transference," that is, who present themselves as father's (or mother's) helpers; they identify strongly with the therapist's efforts and get busy tidying up the neurotic struggle. They are similar to certain couples who consult a marriage counselor when they have already decided that they are going to save their marriage. By the same token, there are also patients who bring with them transference attitudes that are less adaptive. For example, some want help but also need to score

---

* We might pause briefly to consider what we are describing when we say that a particular patient's conflict is situational and acute. We mean that when he comes for treatment he has already chosen some key person in his environment, often a spouse, a boss or a co-worker, to serve as the transference object onto whom he tries to displace some aspects of his infantile struggles. In these acute cases, the neurotic conflict is already full blown and the transference very much there, except that it is being elaborated and worked out in the context of a real relationship rather than in the treatment. Thus, it presents itself to the doctor as already developed and ready to be interpreted within the metaphor of the displacement.

points against the therapist, and others need to prove that the treatment is really for *him* and at *his* request. These patients are not necessarily sicker or more incapacitated than those in the adaptive group, but they are less suited (sometimes quite unsuited) for brief psychotherapy. Berliner's[2] observations also follow along this path. He says:

> The quick removal of a symptom . . . is best achieved under a state of positive mother transference to which persons with an oral disposition are particularly inclined. . . . They absorb friendly transference influences readily. . . . They are easy to guide, in contradistinction to people of an anal disposition. However, the result of this guidance remains superficial. The old ambivalence pattern is always ready to get the upper hand . . . [S]ymptoms of oral origin . . . require great caution, and their quick disappearance must be judged with reservation.

Brief psychotherapy is of limited value when, because of ego impairment, the patient is no longer able to function in his accustomed social role. It is worth emphasizing again that brief treatment places especially great demands on the ego's power to rally and particularly on its synthetic and integrative functions; when these are badly compromised, the patient's responsiveness is also substantially diminished. In the category of patients who are likely to respond unimpressively, one specifically wishes to include psychotic patients, those with massive character disorders of long standing (for example, alcoholics, drug addicts, and the severely unstable and self-destructive), and those with chronic, complex, and disabling psychosomatic illnesses (for example, ulcerative colitis, rheumatoid arthritis, and the like). With the latter group, brief psychotherapy may help to make periods of hospitalization significantly less stressful. Yet, mainly, it tends to highlight the need for more prolonged treatment. Often, in fact, it serves as an entrée into, and preparation for, more definitive long-term treatment.

Special care must be taken with some depressed patients who are a suicidal risk; brief treatment frequently offers them neither enough protection nor enough time to resolve their difficulties. Schizoid patients who are bland, detached, and disenchanted have trouble becoming involved in brief treatment and often show a very limited response. The problem of patients with difficult transference attitudes has already been mentioned. Prominent here are markedly dependent patients who often need the continuing support of an extended relationship. Closely related are those who derive strong secondary gains and neurotic satisfaction from their symptoms. Finally, long-term intensive treatment (perhaps psychoanalysis) is called for whenever there is clear and patent need for personality reconstruction.

Not all authors would concur with the foregoing statement of indications. Burdon,[4] for instance, says, "I am convinced that almost all patients can profit from brief psychotherapy . . . [and that] a therapeutic trial . . . [is] indicated in most cases . . ," although later he allows that the optimal indications for brief psychotherapy are in the range of those given above. Similarly, Wolberg[26] says, "The best strategy, in my opinion, is to assume that every patient, irrespective of diagnosis, will respond to short-term treatment unless he proves himself to be refractory to it," but then he, too, acknowledges that certain conditions (for example, presence of pronounced dependency and immaturity, major character disorders with persistent acting-out, near psychotic states with massive anxiety, and so forth) sharply prejudice the outcome. He adds, however, that he has used short-term methods in treating patients with chronic disorders, including obsessive-compulsive neurosis and borderline schizophrenia, and has "observed in many gratifying results." Koegler and Brill[15] also report a favorable response in some severe cases, including, again, instances of borderline schizophrenia. Malan[16] has expressed the belief that patients with disturbances of moderate severity may actually do better than mildly ill patients, especially if they are highly motivated and if they show an ability to work in interpretive therapy. Nonetheless, from his evidence it appears that the poorest therapeutic results were obtained with the sickest patients. One is reminded here of Berliner's[2] observation that "the feasibility of short treatment does not depend on the acuteness and duration of the illness but on the depth of the neurotic disposition."

Approaches vary also when an adequate response to short-term treatment is not obtained. Provisions may be made for long-term treatment, unless the patient is seen again for one or more courses of brief psychotherapy. This involves not only some judgment of how the patient will manage the regressive trends that, in varying degrees, accompany long-term treatment, but also reflects the therapist's preference. Repeated courses of brief treatment often are the approach of choice with many poorly compensated patients who should not be exposed to the risks of a serious regression and of a prolonged dependent transference. On the other hand, such courses also are preferred by therapists who are skeptical about long-term treatment and who believe that the main contribution of psychotherapy is to provide support to the patient who is in a crisis.

BRIEF PSYCHOTHERAPY: IMPLICATIONS FOR THE PRESENT

Although there are notable exceptions, the current literature on brief treatment is often handicapped by what appears to be a limited historical perspective, which tends to be more enthusiastic than critical and frequently conveys the implication that brief treatment represents a new discovery rather than something that has long been part of the psychiatric experience. It seems at times as if each generation of psychiatrists must come to terms over and over again with certain issues and that some topics are particularly prone to repeated rediscovery (brief psychotherapy is one, hypnosis is another, the role of social and environmental forces is a third).

It is much easier to say something about what brief psychotherapy is or what it is not and how it accomplishes certain specifically clinical goals than to make a statement about its place in contemporary psychiatric practice. The latter depends not only on technical characteristics, but also on questions of values and personal preference that have much greater difficulty reaching consensus. What makes brief psychotherapy so important is that it touches on philosophical as well as purely clinical issues. One simply skirts the controversy if one makes the sound but obvious point that brief psychotherapy is one of a range of therapeutic approaches and that it should be employed according to its clinical indications.

Among the basic questions that are still asked is whether psychotherapy is truly curative (that is, able to alter and reverse fundamental psychopathology) or primarily palliative (that is, able to console and support). In other words, do we have a psychotherapy of character or do we have only a psychotherapy of crisis? Is there a difference between surmounting a crisis and resolving or, at least, alleviating a neurosis? For a psychoanalyst (and for many other therapists), the answer is clear, but then it is not one that is uniformly accepted. And what is adult neurosis? Is it the internalized legacy of the maldevelopments of childhood, or is it mainly a reflection of current social conditions? And what should young therapists be trained to do? The place assigned to brief treatment techniques will affect not only what the patient receives, but also what the doctor becomes and what skills he has an opportunity to develop. Paradoxically, though brief treatment at times presumes the most complex psychotherapeutic skills that are slowly garnered through intensive work with patients, it can also be practiced with reasonable safety and often noticeable effectiveness by the relative beginner. This, in turn, has implications for the goals of training programs, the level of practice, and the future of psychotherapy as a science and an art. It is difficult to predict how (and whether) these questions can be answered. It is clear, however, that the issue of decreasing the length of psychotherapy encompasses much more than simply how much time needs to be devoted to the cure.

REFERENCES

1. Alexander, F., and French, T. M. *Psychoanalytic Therapy*. New York: Ronald, 1946.
2. Berliner, B. "Short Psychoanalytic Psychotherapy: Its Possibilities and Its Limitations," *Bulletin of the Menninger Clinic*, 5 (1941), 204–213.
3. Breuer, J., and Freud, S. *Studies on Hysteria* (1895). New York: Basic Books, 1957.
4. Burdon, A. P. "Principles of Brief Psychotherapy," *Journal of the Louisiana Medical Society*, 115 (1963), 374.
5. Caplan, G. *Principles of Preventive Psychiatry*. New York: Basic Books, 1964.
6. Castelnuovo-Tedesco, P. "The Twenty-Minute 'Hour': An Experiment in Medical Education," *New England Journal of Medicine*, 266 (1962), 283.
7. Castelnuovo-Tedesco, P. *The Twenty-Minute Hour: A Guide to Brief Psychotherapy for the Physician*. Boston: Little, Brown, 1965.
8. Freud, S. "Fragment of an Analysis of a Case of Hysteria" (1901), in J. Strachey (ed.), *Standard Edition*. London: Hogarth. Vol. 7, pp. 7–122. (Also in *Collected Papers of Sigmund Freud*. New York: Basic Books, 1959. Vol. 3, pp. 13–146.)
9. Freud, S. "From the History of an Infantile Neurosis" (1918), in J. Strachey (ed.), *Standard Edition*. London: Hogarth. Vol. 17, pp. 7–122. (Also in *Collected Papers of Sigmund Freud*. New York: Basic Books, 1959. Vol. 3, pp. 473–605.)
10. Freud, S. "Analysis Terminable and Interminable" (1937), in J. Strachey (ed.), *Standard Edition*. London: Hogarth. Vol. 23. (Also in *Collected Papers of Sigmund Freud*. New York: Basic Books, 1959. Vol. 5, pp. 316–357.)
11. Gill, M. "Psychoanalysis and Exploratory Psychotherapy," *Journal of the American Psychoanalytic Association*, 2 (1954), 771.
12. Gillman, R. D. "Psychotherapy: A Psychoanalytic View," *American Journal of Psychiatry*, 122 (1965), 601.
13. Jones, E. *The Life and Work of Sigmund Freud*. New York: Basic Books, 1955. 2 vols.
14. Knight, R. P. "Application of Psychoanalytic Concepts in Psychotherapy: Report of Clinical Trials in a Mental Hygiene Service," *Bulletin of the Menninger Clinic*, 1 (1937), 99.
15. Koegler, R. R., and Brill, N. Q. *Treatment of Psychiatric Outpatients*. New York: Appleton-Century-Crofts, 1967.
16. Malan, D. H. *A Study of Brief Psychotherapy*. London: Tavistock, 1963.

17. Mandell, A. G. "The Fifteen-Minute Hour," *Diseases of the Nervous System*, **22** (1961), 1.
18. Orr, D. W. "Lionel Blitzsten, the Teacher," in *N. Lionel Blitzsten, M.D., Psychoanalyst, Teacher, Friend, 1893–1952*. New York: International Universities Press, 1961.
19. Parad, H. G. (ed.). *Crisis Intervention: Selected Readings*. New York: Family Service Association of America, 1965.
20. Saul, L. "On the Value of One or Two Interviews," *Psychoanalytic Quarterly*, **20** (1951), 613.
21. Sifneos, P. E. "Psychoanalytically Oriented Short-Term Dynamic or Anxiety-Provoking Psychotherapy for Mild Obsessional Neuroses," *Psychiatric Quarterly*, **40** (1966), 271.
22. Stekel, W. *Conditions of Nervous Anxiety*. New York: Liveright, 1950.
23. Sterba, R. "A Case of Brief Psychotherapy by Sigmund Freud," *Psychoanalytic Review*, **38** (1951), 75.
24. Stone, L. "Psychoanalysis and Brief Psychotherapy," *Psychoanalytic Quarterly*, **20** (1951), 215.
25. Wagner, P. S. "Psychiatry for Everyman," *Psychiatry*, **30** (1967), 79.
26. Wolberg, L. R. *Short-Term Psychotherapy*. New York: Grune and Stratton, 1965.
27. Wolpe, J., and Lazarus, A. A. *Behavior Therapy Techniques*. Oxford: Pergamon, 1966.

THERMODYNAMIC AND EVOLUTIONARY CONCEPTS IN THE FORMAL STRUCTURE OF FREUD'S METAPSYCHOLOGY

Carlos P. Barros

To provide a frame of reference for a critical examination of the thermodynamic and evolutionary foundations of psychoanalytic metapsychology it is useful to reexamine the historical development of Freud's theories, not as the traditional chronology of a number of crucial shifts in his scientific interests and methodology, but as the unfolding of the coordinated steps of a comprehensive, systematically elaborated problem-solving enterprise.

As my investigation proceeded, the historical sequence of psychoanalytic formulations emerged clearly as an ordered series of intermediate solutions, skillfully worked out by Freud for the series of intermediate clinical and theoretical problems subsidiary to his main scientific undertaking, namely, the physiopathological explanation of the neuroses. In such a context it has not been difficult to detect the formal structure of Freud's system, clearly shaped in the molds of the metascientific presuppositions and the dynamic-evolutionary concepts that oriented his researches in pathological physiology. But this formal organization of the psychoanalytic theories only became articulated when I decided to scrutinize Freud's own writings[15, 22, 25] with no obligation to retain any of the persistently held misunderstandings of psychoanalytic vocabulary and methodology—even those that happen to be cherished as the distinctive features of a true depth-psychological type of scientific knowledge.

This chapter is an effort in the direction of theory clarification, and in the first section I will summarize my attempt at a reconstruction of theoretical psychoanalysis, viewed as an interconnected system of psychological, bioevolutionary, and physicochemical propositions formulated to explain the entire range of psychoanalytic empirical findings. The subsequent three sections discuss those topics that appear to represent the most relevant issues in current psychoanalytic theorizing, namely (1) the metascientific assumptions, (2) the physicalistic basic concepts borrowed from thermodynamics, and (3) the biological explanatory constructs ("equal in dignity" to the physiocochemical ones) borrowed from evolutionary theories. In the course of this discussion I will acknowledge, in the form of a critical review, my main sources of stimulation and qualified guidance:

1. Rubinstein's essay on the ambiguity of psychoanalytic theory with regard to the mind-body problem,[92] which conducted my inquiry into related metatheoretical questions;

2. Holt's study on the vitalistic nature of Freud's concept of psychic energy,[65] which suggested my extensive investigations into the thermodynamic roots of psychoanalysis; and

3. Guntrip's paper on the concept of psychodynamic science and on the psychodynamic-psychobiologic dichotomy in psychoanalytic theories,[57] which stimulated my researches into the evolutionary and learning-theoretical foundations of Freud's most important psychodynamic concept—the secondary wishful impulse (*Triebregung*). Freud's use of *Trieb* for *Triebregung* has permitted serious conceptual misunderstandings—made worse by the erroneous English translations ("instinct," "instinctual impulse").

THE STEPS IN THEORY CONSTRUCTION—A PROPOSED SYSTEMATIZATION

The following account of Freud's steps in theory-building has been prepared with a view to disclosing the main lines of his articulated system, thus providing a workable framework, hitherto unavailable, for an adequate assessment of the scientific status of psychoanalytic theory and, eventually, for the reintegration of metapsychology into the realm of the regular scientific disciplines, where it belongs.

The Nosographic Account and the Physiopathological Formula

Dissatisfied with Charcot's purely nosographic (atheoretical) approach, and trained in the tradition of the physiological method of the German school of medicine, Freud considered it the task of neuropathology to discover the physiopathological formula for the diseases of the nervous system: "So far as we know, there is not as yet any theory of hysterical attacks, but only a description of them, coming from Charcot."[49] "While the description of clinical pictures is the subject-matter of nosography, the task of clinical medicine is to follow out the individual form taken by cases and the combination of their symptoms . . . a tendency to make a physiological interpretation of the clinical conditions; . . . the French method . . . the German method . . . "[26]

In the case of the purely functional nervous diseases, or neuroses, neuropathological interpretation would be identical with the finding of the still unknown physiopathological formula: "Hysteria is a neurosis in the strictest sense of the word . . . based wholly and entirely on physiological modifications of the nervous system and its essence should be expressed in a . . . physiopathological formula . . . not yet . . . discovered . . . "[23] "I have heard Charcot say: 'Je fais la morphologie pathologique, je fais même un peu l'anatomie pathologique; mais je ne fais pas la physiologie pathologique, j'attend que quelqu'un autre la fasse.' "[26]

In his contribution to Villaret's encyclopedia[23] Freud had already outlined the physiopathological formula for hysteria, somewhat as follows: (1) a surplus of excitation in the nervous system (the hereditary hysterical status), and (2) an abnormal distribution of excitation in the different parts of the nervous system, provoked by physical or by psychic factors (the *agents provocateurs*).

But impressed with Breuer's case of Anna O, and with Charcot's demonstrations of artificial hysterical paralyses, Freud became predominantly interested in the mechanism of the psychic factors.

The Psychological Mechanisms in Hysteria

Extending Charcot's explanation of the artificial imitation of the hysterotraumatic paralyses, and based on the data obtained by the cathartic method, Freud (and Breuer) admitted that in the pathogenesis of common nontraumatic hysteria, the part played by the psychic traumas, that is by the memories of experiences whose quota of affect had not been eliminated (by association or motor reaction), could be demonstrated.[12, 27, 49]

In psychically provoked hysteria, the psychological lesion consists in the associative inaccessibility of those groups of ideas that have become involved with the memory of the trauma.[12, 27] The psychic mechanism, therefore, consists in a "dissociation—a splitting of the content of consciousness"[49] resulting from the occurrence of retention, defense, or hypnoid states.[28]

The Techniques of Psychic Analysis

The entirely functional lesion of hysteria could not, by definition, be revealed even by the most delicate methods of anatomical analysis.[27] And because the pathogenic psychic traumas usually eluded analysis by simple anamnesis, it was necessary to develop special techniques of clinicopsychological analysis—Breuer's hypnotic analysis and Freud's psychoanalysis.[12, 28]

Thus, based on Charcot's explanation of traumatic hysteria, and improving on Breuer's cathartic method, Freud was able to comply with John Stuart Mill's methodological dictum, expressed by John Hughlings Jackson in the words: "We are to rid ourselves as much as possible of psychological bias in what is an anatomical and physiological inquiry. I do not mean that we have no concern at all with psychology. On the contrary, it is perfectly obvious that it is impossible for us to begin to study the anatomical substrata of mind without prior psychological analysis."[67]

The Physiopathology of the Psychic Mechanisms

Proceeding with his physiopathological program, Freud explained the operation of the psychic mechanisms as follows:

whereas the hereditary foundation of the hysterical disposition corresponds to a surplus of excitation in the nervous system, the psychological traumas correspond to an accretion of excitation in the cerebral cortex (the organ of mind), thus altering the conditions of stable equilibrium and of excitability within the nervous system.[23, 49]

The Basic Neurophysiological Hypothesis

Scientific physiopathologists (from Claude Bernard and John Hughlings Jackson to the German school, represented in Vienna by Stricker and Brücke) always conceived abnormal processes as departures from normal functioning, and not as qualitatively new, irreducible phenomena. The physiopathological formula for the neuroses, therefore, ought to be expressed in terms of alterations of the normal physiology of the nervous system, that is, alterations of a physiological quality, such as nervous excitability.[27]

Following the prevailing natural-scientific paradigm,* Freud, from the beginning, endeavored to formulate the alterations of excitability in terms of a physiological quantity—neuronic excitation.[49, 53]

The elaboration of the physiopathological formula, accordingly, was in strict dependence of previous neurophysiological knowledge, and we know that Freud's earliest contributions were intended to fill the gaps in the physiological theory of neuronic excitation.[12, 49, 52] And in this search for the basic postulates about the normal functioning of the nervous system (including the organ of mind), Freud proposed a series of formulations—true to his reductionistic ideal[107]—from the purely physiological propositions[27] to the quasiphysical and physical principles.[28-54]

1. The qualitative (physiological normal) formulation. In his studies on the functional aphasias (1891),[25] Freud had adopted Bastian's three levels of reduced excitability as the physiological modification that occurs in the intact speech apparatus. Two

---

* See, for instance, Duhem: "Franklin, Oepinus, Coulomb, Leplace, Poisson—all the creators of the science of electricity thought that qualities could not be admitted into the constitution of a physical theory and that only quantities have the right of entry. Hence, underneath this quality of electric charge manifest to their senses, their reason sought a quantity, 'the quantity of electricity' . . . due to the presence within the charged body of a certain 'electrical fluid' . . ." (p. 119).[16]

years later, discussing the nature of the dynamic lesion responsible for the hysterical paralyses, Freud suggested a diminution of excitability as the probable physiological alteration in the nervous system of the hysterical patients.[27]

On the other hand, in the "Studies on Hysteria" (1895),[12] Freud (and Breuer) admitted that certain hysterical phenomena correspond to Oppenheim's "abnormal expression of the emotions," hence to increased excitability in particular nervous pathways.

To account for those physiopathological states as departures from healthy conditions, Freud had to establish the physiological laws of nervous excitability. In view of the lack of experimental data, he postulated the principle that nervous "excitability ... normally remains constant or varies within fixed limits."[27] This is the hypothetical principle of constancy of nervous excitability, structurally identical (isomorphic) with Claude Bernard's theory of the constancy of the internal environment.

2. *The quantitative ("stationary state") formulations.** Oppenheim attributed the abnormal nervous excitability of hysterics to the instability of the molecules, and Jackson, before him, had attributed the increased nervous excitability of epileptics to the increased instability of nerve tissue. Probably influenced by Fechner's ideas, however, Freud's explanation of abnormal excitability was based on a more encompassing investigation of the conditions of equilibrium of the amounts of excitation within the nervous system.

In his contribution to Villaret's encyclopedia in 1888, Freud had already suggested that the psychic disturbances of hysterics correspond to alterations of the normally stable distribution of excitation in the nervous system.[23] This distribution, he added in 1894, "turns out to be an unstable one."[28] The "mechanism of the neuroses" could therefore be interpreted as "disturbances of equilibrium owing to increased difficulty in discharge."[50]

From his encyclopedia article (1888) to his metapsychological considerations about the quantitative factor, in "Analysis Terminable and Interminable" (1937),[47] Freud proposed a series of slightly different quantitative formulations of the basic hypothesis, but they all fall within three distinct formal categories: the

---

* A detailed and more rigorous treatment of the physicochemical concepts and propositions essential for an adequate understanding of the basic structure of Freud's metapsychology is developed by the present writer in a monograph form, expanded version of this chapter (in preparation).

stoichiometric, the quasienergetic, and the true energetic formulations.*

The stoichiometric formulation: The normal distribution of the amounts of excitation (*Erregungsgrösse*) in the nervous system corresponds to the conditions of stable equilibrium ($V=0$; $P=constant$).[23, 28] Or, to be more accurate, we should reformulate Freud's statement thus: the normal distribution of the amounts of excitation in the nervous system corresponds to the conditions of stable stationary state ($P=$constant), or, still more generally, to the conditions of displacement of equilibrium (P varies, but its initial and end values always correspond to configurations of stationarity).

The quasienergetic formulation: the normal distribution of the amounts of excitation (*Erregungsgrösse*) in the nervous system is such that a certain quantitative factor is either kept at a constant level (below threshold value) or brought back to that level whenever the threshold is crossed.[28, 30, 37, 41, 44, 47, 49] This quantitative factor has the characteristics of a parameter of state, related to the evolution of the amounts of excitation (that is, of the masses of excitation).†

Another formulation of the quasienergetic statement: the normal distribution of the masses of excitation in the nervous system is such that a certain parameter described as the sum of excitation (*Erregungssumme*) is always kept at (or restored to) a constant value. This precondition of health is put into effect because the nervous system is capable of disposing of every sensible accretion of the masses of excitation, either associatively or by appropriate motor reaction, thus keeping the sum of excitation constant.[49]

The concept "sum of excitation"[28, 49] is only another name for the quantitative factor (*quantitativ Faktor*)[30] and should not be

---

* Stoichiometry concerns itself with the material transformations of systems in evolution. Its main subdivisions are: (1) kinetics, which deals with the velocities of transformation (V) and with the changes of P, the parameters of state; (2) statics, which deals with systems in true equilibrium (where $V = 0$ and $P = $ constant); stationary states (where V is not zero, but P is kept constant); and those cases of displacement of equilibrium where the changes depend only on the initial and final values of P, independent of the intermediate steps.

Quasi energetics: In cases of displacement of equilibrium it is customary to consider the structural correspondence (homology) between the state parameters P and the intensity and the capacity factors of an energy and to apply Le Chatelier's principle. The result is a sort of quasienergetics, only structurally related to the true energetics.

True energetics corresponds to the energetics, in the strict sense, of any system, that is, with real energy transformations.[80]

† See the formal correspondence with Le Chatelier's principle (p. 80, footnote).

confused with the concept "amount of excitation."[39] Whereas the sum of excitation is a parameter of state, the amount of excitation is a materialized energetic concept, like the electric fluid of early physicists. The confusion between these two concepts has led Jones,[73] among others, to believe that Freud's principle of constancy "was evidently derived from Helmholtz's principle of conservation of energy" (p. 434).

The quantitative factor has been interchangeably designated by Freud as the "sum of excitation,"[28, 49] "quota of affect,"[28] "level of stimuli,"[37] and "quantity of excitation."[41] It corresponds unequivocally to Breuer's intracerebral tonic excitation.[12] Incidentally, Breuer's concept of tonic excitation is not equivalent to Freud's concept of cathexis, as Holt supposed (p. 482).[63] Tonic excitation corresponds to the intensity factor of cathectic energy—the level of cathexis.

Freud's definition of the quantitative factor has consistently been given in terms of a ratio between economic and structural concepts, such as load/capacity,[30] quota of libido/ego's ability,[35] amount of cathexis/structures,[42] strength of the instinct/strength of the ego,[47] and so on. The quantitative factor is therefore isomorphic with the electric potential U, of a conductor, defined as the ratio between the electric charge Q and the electric capacity C. Thus, $U=Q/C$. Freud, of course, was always unaware of the correct physical analogies and related his quantitative factor now to the electric charge (p. 60),[28] now to the electric current (the flowing electric fluid) (p. 61).[28] He left to Breuer the adequate homology with the electric potential (p. 194n).[12]

The true energetic formulation: the libidinal tension of the psychic apparatus is normally kept at (or restored to) a constant level.[29, 33, 53] This constant level corresponds to a zero point, that is, the minimum value of the tension compatible with the structure of the apparatus. Freud was not aware of the fact that the constant is a minimum characteristic of a given apparatus that may conventionally be equated to zero. Hence his indecision:[41] "The pleasure principle, then, is a tendency operating in the service of a function whose business it is to free the mental apparatus entirely [zero] from excitation or to keep the amount of excitation in it constant [constant] or to keep it as low as possible [minimum]. We cannot yet decide with certainty in favour of any of these ways of putting it . . ." (p. 62).[41]

Another formulation of the true energetic statement: whenever energetic inputs (stimuli and drives) raise the libidinal tension above the minimum value (equilibrium state), there appears an urge to bring the tension back to the original level (stable equilibrium); or, more generally, an urge to bring the tension to a new value, compatible with an equilibrium state (displacement of equilibrium).

Whereas the quasienergetic hypotheses bear only a formal relationship to the physicochemical principle of Le Chatelier, the true energetic formulations represent the same principle applied to the psychic apparatus as a real thermodynamic system.*

Some of the energetic formulations represent essentially the enunciation of the Helm-Ostwald intensity law. Take, for instance, the one we find in the third part of the "Project"[63]: "If the level of cathexis in the ego-nucleus rises, the extent of the ego will be able to expand its range; if it sinks, the ego will narrow concentrically" (p. 427).[53] Here, of course, the level of cathexis (g_i-g_e) and the extent of the ego (G) correspond, respectively, to the intensity and the capacity factors of the total energy of the psi neuronic system.

Neurophysiology as an Evolutionary Neuroenergetics

Trained in the tradition of the German physicalistic physiology,[7, 73] to which Brücke had added an evolutionary (Darwinian) orientation, Freud was ready to adopt Jackson's views (with which he became acquainted while studying the problem of the aphasias): (1) the definition of neurophysiology as the "physics of the nervous system"[68] and the tripartite explanation of nervous diseases in terms of disturbances of anatomy, physiology, and nutrition of the nervous system[66] that inspired the metapsychological conceptions and (2) the application of Spencer's hypotheses of evolution and dissolution as the bases for the construc-

---

* "Every system in chemical equilibrium, under the influence of a change of any single one of the factors of equilibrium, undergoes a transformation in such direction that, if this transformation took place alone, it would produce a change in the opposite direction of the factor in question.

The factors of equilibrium are temperature, pressure, and electromotive force [that is, the intensity factors], corresponding to three forms of energy—heat, electricity and mechanical energy" (*Recherches sur les équilibres chimiques*, 1888, quoted, in English, by Lotka[80]).

Le Chatelier's principle may be expressed by the relation $\frac{dG}{dt} \gtreqless 0$, where $g_i \gtreqless g_e$, and G and g stand for the capacity and the intensity factors of an energy (Helm-Ostwald intensity law).

tion of a scientific neuropathology[70] that oriented the psychoanalytic developmental ideas.

Freud's theory of development deals with the evolution of the nervous system (and of the erogenous sources of excitation) through the following stages:[32-41, 53]

1. The uncathected phi neuronic system (and the primary neuronic function). The most primitive, phi neuronic system only transmits the energy it receives from exogenous stimuli. The energies transmitted by these phi neurones—quantities in a state of flow (or flowing Q)—constitute the hypothetical current in the neuronic paths of conduction.

The phi neuronic system, pressed by the tendency to divest itself of Q and regulated by the principle of inertia, is the scene of action of the primary neuronic function (discharge, or flight) (p. 357).[53]

The phi neurones are neither filled with cathexis (energy stored in the psi system) nor supplied with psychic energy (energy of the psychic apparatus). But they do contain an appreciable amount of flowing Q, in the form of a steady state current, maintained by a continuous input of exogenous stimuli, that compensates for the continuous striving to divest themselves of quantities. We agree with Glick's statement that the phi neurones are uncathected,[56] but this does not in any way mean that they are anergic or empty, as Glick maintains, except, of course, in the abnormal conditions of afferent isolation. Freud's complete model is quite in keeping with the most recent data on sensory deprivation, exploratory behavior, and craving for stimulation. The isolated phi neurones, when abstracted from their theoretical context, cannot retain their explanatory value (like any other limiting models).

2. The cathected psi neuronic system (and the secondary neuronic function). As the phylogenetic development proceeds, under the pressure of the exigencies of life, there comes into being the psi neuronic system, less permeable in the contact barriers. Connected with the somatic sources of drives (endogenous stimuli), the psi neurones do not transmit energy, because they have learned (phylogenetically) to store up the quantities coming from the somatic cells. These energies, retained by the psi neurones, are grouped together to make up what Freud designated as the "stored Q," or "cathexis" (*Besetzung*). The concept of cathexis, therefore, corresponds to the total energy of the psi neuronic system (see the concept of total energy, p. 97).

Whereas the phi neurones are homologous with energy conductors, the psi neurones are homologous with thermodynamic systems capable of storing up the energetic inputs. The opposition between cathexis (in psi) and current (in phi) is not equivalent to the opposition between delay and discharge, as stated by Pribram.[87] Cathecting processes are thermodynamic transformations, whereas the phi currents are pure propagation processes. Therefore, when the cathexes are eventually discharged to perform the specific action, we are not thereby entitled to say that they have been converted into a current.

Holt's daring attempt to disentangle the concepts of bound and free cathexis[63] would certainly have been successful if only he had a workable definition of cathexis to start with. The lack of an adequate understanding of the Freudian concepts of cathexis and other thermodynamic constructs has caused the failure of other equally brilliant theoretical endeavors.[1, 3, 9, 14, 55, 60, 64, 65, 72, 73, 77, 78, 97, 98, 105, 106]

Further phylogenetic development brings up the differentiation of the psi neurones into two classes: (1) the psi neurones of the nucleus, cathected from the endogenous sources, and (2) the newly developed psi neurones of the pallium, cathected both from the soma (through the nuclear psi) and from the exogenous sources (through phi). The nuclear psi neurones, when cathected from the erogenous sources, manifest an urge (*Drang*) to discharge the accretion of excitation along preformed motor paths.

The nuclear psi neuronic system, pressed by the urge to discharge the accretion of excitation, and regulated by the principle of constancy, is the scene of action of the secondary neuronic function (adequate reflexes).[53]

Under the pressure of internal development trends and the influence of external factors, the nuclear psi system in each individual evolves through the phases of libidinal development, becoming successively connected with appropriate erogenous zones* (oral, anal, phallic), on one hand, and with the corresponding functional motor pathways on the other.[33] Further ontogenetic development of the nuclear psi system toward the genital organization depends on parallel development of the pallium psi system and the ego.[32–47, 53]

3. The newly developed pallium psi neuronic system (and the primary psychic processes). In addition to the secondary neuronic

---

* See the theory of the somatic drives, p. 86.

function that it has in common with the nuclear neurones, the pallium psi system is capable of memory and of associative learning, of wishful impulse, and of affective repulsion.

With regard to the pallium, therefore, we may say that (1) it keeps the mnemic images of the external objects perceived by phi; (2) it keeps the kinesthetic images of the reflex movements; (3) it establishes associative links between those two images and the state of libidinal tension in the nucleus by means of facilitations left behind after an experience of satisfaction; (4) it evokes the memories of the objects of satisfaction, whenever the nuclear neurones are recathected from the soma; (5) it manifests an emergent wish, that is, an impulse (*Regung*), to reestablish the perception of those objects of satisfaction as soon as their memories are evoked (an impulse, that is, to achieve perceptual identity); (6) it establishes associative links between the memories of hostile objects and the secretory neurones after an experience of pain; (7) it excites the secretory neurones (releasing an unpleasurable affect) whenever the mnemic image of the hostile object is recathected (perceptually or associatively); (8) it manifests an emergent repulsion toward the hostile object, that is, a tendency to decathect its mnemic image (primary defense or repression).

This summary, abstracted from "A Project for a Scientific Psychology"[53] and from the "Interpretation of Dreams"[32] (section C of Chapter 7), shows us that the concept of wish—as a psychic impulse to reestablish the perception of the object—is a truly Object Relations construct (in Guntrip's sense),[57] equivalent to Fairbairn's object-seeking libido.[17] Although it deserves a place among Freud's other basic postulates (inertia, constancy-pleasure, and reality principles), the concept of wish has been usually neglected and often confused with the concepts of urge and drive. The wishful impulse (*Wunschregung*), or instinctual impulse (*Triebregung*), or psychical motive power (*psychische Triebkraft*) is an emergent psychodynamic concept and should be carefully distinguished from the concept of the nuclear neurone's urge to discharge (*Drang*) and from the concept of the somatic drives (*Triebe*).

The concept of affect has not been elaborated by Freud except in the first part of the "Project." As a consequence, (1) he met with serious difficulties when trying to explain anxiety dreams with the sole concept of wish fulfillment,[32] and (2) he has felt the need to develop the discursive constructs of the threat of unpleasure (*Unlustdrohung*), in Part 3 of the "Project," and of threat of castration (*Kastrationsdrohung*), in the "Dissolution of the Oedipus Complex,"[46] to explain the origin of the ego and of the ego ideal, respectively, in dynamic (conflictual) terms.

The pallium psi neuronic system, pressed by the wishful impulses and by the tendency to primary defense, and regulated by what might be called the "principle of object relations," is the scene of action of the primary psychic processes (wish fulfillment and primary defense).[32, 53]

The pallium neuronic system, therefore, corresponds to the id of post-1920 formulations. It is an extremely complex, structured system, rich in inborn (instinctive) and learned harnessing devices. It is far from being "a chaos, a cauldron full of seething excitations," except in the literary parlance of the "New Introductory Lectures,"[46] where Freud intended to emphasize the richer organization of the ego. The concepts employed in the explanation of the psychic primary processes, contrary to common belief, are already personal-theoretical, psychodynamic constructs, irreducible to psychobiological ones.[57]

4. The emergence of the binding ego (and the secondary psychic processes). In order to avoid the biologically damaging situations, the neuronic system, pressed by the threat of unpleasure, learns (phylogenetically) to inhibit the primary psychic processes, thus permitting the indications of reality. Ontogenetic experiences only actualize the maturational trends of the inherited, potential structure of the ego.

This inhibition (binding) of the free cathexes is operated by the ego, that is, by the whole cathectic mass, kept in equilibrium within the structured (differentially facilitated) psi neuronic system.

The ego-inhibited pallium psi neuronic system, pressed by the secondary wishful impulses and regulated by the principle of reality, is the scene of action of the secondary psychic processes (that lead to the specific action and to the satisfaction of the needs).[32, 34, 37, 53]

The pallium system plus the ego constitute Freud's psychic apparatus. The secondary wishful impulses, in turn, constitute the subject matter of the so-called psychoanalytic theory of drives (or instinct theory). These ego-inhibited impulses are, no doubt, "the derivatives of the drives" (instincts), but this does not mean that they should be called drives, let alone the designations instincts and instinctual drives.[59, 95, 103] In the famous *Triebe und Triebschicksale*[22] (vol. 10) Freud uses twice the correct term

Triebregung (p. 223), translated as "instinctual impulse" (p. 131).[37] Unfortunately, in the rest of the paper, although it is clear that he is always referring to *Triebregungen* ("instinctual impulses"), he uses the shorter term *Triebe* ("instincts"). *Triebregung* means "drive-energized impulse," or an impulse that is a derivative of the drives. Freud's paper on "Repression"[38] begins with the phrase: "One of the vicissitudes of an instinctual impulse . . ." (. . . *das Schicksal einer Triebregung*), thus giving further evidence that he is studying the vicissitudes of the *Triebregung*, only out of carelessness designated as *Trieb*. And in "The Interpretation of Dreams,"[32] on pages 548, 568, and 603–604 (corresponding to pages 554, 574, and 609 in volumes 2–3 of the *Gesammelte Werke*), we can see the meanings of the concepts "wishful impulse" (*Wunschregung*) and psychic motive force (*psychische Triebkraft*) to be equivalent to the instinctual impulse (*Triebregung*), but certainly different from the motive force (*Triebkraft*) and the drive or instinct (*Trieb*).

Freud's Theory of the Somatic Drives

As his researches proceeded, in addition to the neurophysiopathological formula (and its energetic-evolutionary reduction), Freud was soon confronted with another pathological problem—the etiological equation for the neuroses and the physiology of the sexual life.[29, 30, 31, 33]

As he revised Charcot's doctrine of the *famille névropathique* and the exclusively hereditary theory for the neuroses, Freud admitted (1894) the existence of purely acquired neuroses,[28] hence the need for an inquiry into their etiological formulas.[29, 30, 31]

THE ETIOLOGICAL EQUATION

The occurrence of a neurotic illness depends on the satisfaction of the etiological equation: (1) quantitatively, when the quantitative factor (cf. the quasienergetic formulation above) crosses the threshold value, irreversibly, and (2) qualitatively, by the presence, in the equation, of the specific etiological factor that cannot be replaced by other (predisposing, concurrent, or precipitating) causes.

The specific factor was found to be always a disturbance in the patient's *vita sexualis*, either in contemporary sexual life (actual neuroses) or in the past sexual life (psychoneuroses).

THE THEORY OF THE SOMATIC DRIVES (SEXUAL EXCITATIONS)

When, led by clinical and theoretical considerations, Freud had to elevate the sexual factors to the rank of specific causes of the neuroses, he recognized the need for an investigation of the physiological problem of the sexual life.[31] The study of the sexual excitations (*somatische Sexualerregungen*),[29] that is, the sexual motive forces (*sexuelle Triebkräfte*),[32] or sexual drives (*Sexualtriebe*),[51] thenceforth became an integral part of the physiopathological formula and consequently of theoretical psychoanalysis.

The etiology of the fundamental disturbance of hysteria—the surplus of excitation in the nervous system—was no longer to be looked for in heredity, but in the peculiarities of the *vita sexualis*.

The chemical energy of the somatic cells (particularly of the sex glands),[33] therefore, constitutes the ultimate driving force[53] (*Triebfeder*) of the psychic mechanism.

Helmholtz's principle of conservation of energy (or of the excluded perpetual motion)[62, 85, 89] forbids any natural system—including the psychic apparatus—to be set in motion by itself. Freud had to look for the source of the moving power (or driving energy) of the psychic apparatus and proposed the sex glands as the main source of the energetic input to the psychic system. The workings of the psychic apparatus were no longer in contradiction with the conservation principle. The apparatus had inputs and outputs of amounts of excitation (*Erregungsgrösse*), whose vicissitudes (transformations and redistributions) could, at least in principle, be followed out and quantitatively estimated (p. 181).[39]

We have already pointed out that the subject matter of Freud's instinct theory (*Triebtheorie*)[37] are the secondary wishful impulses that are "a derivative of the drives"[53] (*Abkömmling der Triebe*),[52] but are not drives (*Triebe*).

Freud's Theory of Development

The energetic-evolutionary approach has been utilized by Freud to explain the origin and the development of the psychic apparatus, of the psychic energetics, and of the psychic impulses (forces) under the headings:

1. The development of the (topographic) *delaying structures:* (a) the contact barriers that inhibit the primary neuronic function; (b) the facilitations between the nuclear psi and the two memory images retained by pallium psi that divert the original

energetic flow, thus inhibiting the secondary neuronic function; (c) the lateral cathexes of the ego that inhibit the primary psychic processes, leading to the emergence of the most developed, secondary psychic processes.

2. The development of the hierarchically superimposed agencies, or (topographic) *systems*, that is, the subdivisions of the psychic apparatus: (a) the first psi system, that is, the pallium psi system with all the delaying structures, except the lateral cathexes of the ego, and (b) the second psi system, inhibited (bound) by the ego (p. 599).[32]

In his metapsychological paper on "The Unconscious,"[39] Freud introduced the terms "system Ucs" and "system Pcs (Cs)" to designate the first and the second systems, respectively. He was thus abandoning the purely evolutionary criterion (according to early or late emergence of the system) and adopting a new criterion to divide the psychic apparatus—that of the accessibility to consciousness.

Eight years later, in "The Ego and the Id,"[43] Freud proposes a third criterion for the distinction of the psychic subdivisions or systems, namely, the structural criterion—the presence or the absence of the delaying structures of the binding ego (and of the corresponding dynamic structures discussed below). The id and the ego (superego) are, therefore, two topographic systems obtained in accordance with a structural criterion. It is customary —though erroneous—to designate the Ucs/Pcs (Cs) division as the topographic point of view and the id/ego (superego) division as the structural point of view.[4, 90, 91] Gill has recently revised his own position on the subject (p. 54).[55]

3. The development of the *impulses*, that is, the (dynamic) harnessing structures that convert the cathectic energies into bodily movements, by releasing, and channeling these energies appropriately: (a) the urge (*Drang*), that is, the preformed reflex contrivances of the nuclear neurones capable of releasing the cathexes whose level of tension is raised above constant and channeling them into the neural patterns of the adequate reflex; (b) the wish (*Wunsch*), that is, the complex set of innate and learned facilitations and inhibitions of the pallium neurones, capable of releasing the pallium (and nuclear) cathexes when perceptual identity is achieved and channeling them into the neural patterns of the adequate reflex; and (c) the ego-inhibited wishful impulse (preconscious wish), that is, the complex set of inhibitions and facilitations of the ego, capable of releasing the bound

cathexes when the indications of the presence of the real object are signaled by the omega neurones[54] and of channeling them into the appropriate motor pathways of the specific action that will lead to the satisfaction of the biological needs.

In physicochemical terminology, the dynamic harnessing devices correspond to generalized forces capable of overcoming the topographic resistances.

4. The development of the (economic) *regulative principles* of the neuroenergetic processes: (a) principle of inertia; (b) principle of constancy (or pleasure principle); (c) principle of wish fulfillment, or principle of object relations (never enunciated by Freud as such); and (d) principle of reality.

5. The development of the (economic) erogenous *sources* of sexual drives (input)—(a) oral, (b) anal, (c) phallic, and (d) genital phases—that runs parallel with the development of the corresponding types of specific actions (output).

Freud's Metapsychological Theory

The subject matter of metapsychology is the study of the fully developed psychic apparatus and its functioning. Metapsychology, therefore, consists of:

1. The topographic point of view—the study of the fully developed psychic apparatus with its delaying structures and its systems. Topography, therefore, is not restricted to the study of the Ucs vs. Pcs (Cs) antithesis, as it has been erroneously supposed.[4, 90]
2. The dynamic point of view—the study of the fully developed harnessing structures, that is, of the most developed generalized forces, capable of overcoming the topographic delaying structures and of releasing the cathexis along certain directions—the specific motor pathways. The fully developed forces are the ego-inhibited wishful impulses, erroneously designated as instincts.
3. The economic point of view—the study of the most organized energetic processes, comprising the most developed thermodynamic regulative principle, that is, the principle of constancy* and the thermodynamic conservation principle, which holds in the energy transformations and redistributions that occur when the most developed psychic apparatus receives energetic inputs from the most

---

* We have already seen that the principle of wish fulfillment and the reality principles are not strictly thermodynamic. They contain (dynamic as well as topographic) structural components.

developed somatic sources and discharges them in the efferent pathways onto the external world (outputs).

In Freud's own words, "In the theory of psychoanalysis . . . the course taken by mental events is automatically regulated by the pleasure principle. . . . In taking that course into account . . . we are introducing the 'economic' point of view . . ." (p. 7).[41] And, "Besides the dynamic and the topographical points of view, we have adopted the economic one. This endeavours to follow out the vicissitudes of amounts of excitation [*Erregungsgrösse*] and to arrive at least at some relative estimate of their magnitude (p. 181).[40]

In physicochemical terms, the economic point of view studies a *principle of stability* of stationary state (constancy principle) and a *principle of equivalence* between the somatic drives, the neuronic cathexes, and the efferent discharges (usually misunderstood as a principle of conservation of libido).

Whereas Freud's economic point of view studies the conservation causality relations, the dynamic point of view deals with the instigation causality relations, if we adopt Von Bertalanffy's illuminating distinction.[100]

It is clear that Freud's dynamics, anticipating Colby's[14] and Fairbairn's[17] contributions, has always been inseparable from structure, that is, the harnessing structures that release, along certain pathways, the energies that are kept in equilibrium by the topographic, delaying structures. The alleged "divorce of energy from structure"[17] in Freud's system, therefore, only reflects the divorce of reinterpreted Freudian theory from the original formulations laid down by Freud.

The Additional Points of View in Current Metapsychology

The genetic and the adaptive points of view, proposed by Rapaport and Gill,[91] belong to Freud's theory of development and are not metapsychological principles. The alleged structural point of view,[4, 90, 91] as we have seen, is only one aspect (or criterion) of the topographic theory. The four additional points of view proposed by Rapaport (empirical, organismic, Gestalt, psychosocial)[90] either belong to the metascientific assumptions of psychoanalysis or are already included in one of the classic metapsychological points of view. Needless to say, Freud's metapsychology is not a metatheory, but a well-defined part of psychoanalytic theory. (See the section on metascientific problems, and the concluding remarks.)

Freud's Theory of Involution (The Reverse of Development)

In addition to the explanation of the development and the functioning of the mature psychic apparatus, the energetic-evolutionary approach has also permitted the investigation of the involutional processes (related to Spencer's concept of dissolution).

The explanatory value of the concept of regression, both in normal psychology (dreams, parapraxes, jokes) and in psychopathological interpretation (neurotic and psychotic syndromes), is too well known to need further elaboration. It is, undoubtedly, one of the most important contributions of psychoanalysis to modern scientific psychiatry. On the other hand, another derivative of the involutional phase of the energetic-evolutionary theory—the postulate of a death instinct—is only a scientific curiosity and deserves examination as a social psychological phenomenon.

Usually misinterpreted, now as a philosophical speculation, now as one of the most profound of Freud's psychological insights, the concept of *Todestrieb* is nothing but the result of an understandable parapraxis, a *Fehlleistung*, or "faulty action," in the task of theory construction.

It will be demonstrated below (in the section discussing thermodynamic concepts) that the postulate of a death drive is the end result of a series of distortions and condensations of meanings of some thermodynamic concepts (p. 101). The scientific curiosity consists in the fact that such a postulate, a misconstruction of a scientific genius, has gained the status of a psychological (or biological) truth and has been maintained for almost two decades as a scientific proposition by no less a man than Sigmund Freud. And the social-psychological phenomenon consists in the failure to recognize the clear-cut nonsensical character of the famous postulate, demonstrated by a legion of extremely able research workers, only because they knew that they were dealing with a statement that happened to have associative bonds with a high-valued source. We refer to the laboriously worked out, but disconcertingly naïve, contributions of first-rate psychoanalysts and brilliant scholars, such as Alexander,[2] Bernfeld and Feitelberg,[8]

Bibring,[10] Choisy,[13] Fletcher,[19] Flugel,[20] Foxe,[21] Heimann,[61] Jones,[72, 73] Kapp,[74] Klein,[76] Money-Kyrle,[83] Orr,[84] Penrose,[86] Segal,[94] Sterba,[96] Szasz,[99] Waelder,[103] and Walker.[104]

METASCIENTIFIC PROBLEMS

Against the background of the theoretical framework developed in our investigation—and summarized in this chapter—some of the most relevant metascientific assumptions of psychoanalysis have been clearly delineated.

The Mind-Body Problem

On the metaphysical problem of the mind-body relationship we have found that Freud consistently adopted a sort of materialistic monism, related to Jackson's doctrine of concomitance[71] and to Haeckel's evolutionary physicalism.[58]

The passages quoted below are apt to reveal Jackson's methodological materialism (consistent with his metaphysical parallelistic dualism) and Freud's methodological empirical parallelism (consistent with his metaphysical materialism—a materialistic-oriented epiphenomenalism).*

1. Jackson's metaphysical parallelism:

I am not competent to discuss the metaphysical question of the nature of the relation of mind to nervous activities. There are three doctrines: (1) that mind acts through the nervous system (through highest centres first); here an immaterial agency is supposed to produce physical effects [interactionistic dualism]; (2) that activities of the highest centres and mental states are one and the same thing [identity theory], or are different sides of one thing [double-aspect theory]. A third doctrine, (3) one I have adopted, is that (a) states of consciousness (or synonymously states of mind) are utterly different from nervous states of the highest centres; (b) the two things occur together, for every mental state there being a correlative nervous state; (c) although the two things occur in parallelism, there is no interference of one with

* The traditional philosophical positions concerning the mind-body problem are usually characterized as (1) dualism, admitting two substances, and adopting either an interactionistic or a parallelistic interpretation of the mind-body relationship, and (2) monism, admitting only one substance, matter (materialistic monism), mind (spiritualistic monism), or a neutral reality (neutral monism, roughly equivalent to identity theory). For an authoritative survey of the problem, see Feigl.[18]

the other [parallelistic dualism]. Hence we do not say that psychical states are functions of the brain . . . but simply that they occur during the functioning of the brain. . . . A critic of my Croonian Lectures . . . says that the doctrine of concomitance is Leibniz's "two clock theory" . . . (p. 84).[71]

2. Jackson's methodological materialism:

The reader must never forget that an absolute distinction is made in this paper between mental states and their corresponding physical states, and that no attempt is made to explain the former by the latter . . . whilst admitting, as of course, that prior psychological analysis is necessary, we are directly concerned [methodologically] not with psychology, but with certain questions in the anatomy and physiology of the nervous system (p. 41).[68]

Scientific materialism is quite a different thing from crude popular materialism. Scientific materialism distinguishes betwixt mind and nervous system in order to study each thoroughly. . . . Scientific materialism is only materialistic as to what is material, the nervous system (p. 325 n.). [69]

3. Freud's metaphysical materialism (epiphenomenalism):

We possess no criterion which enables us to distinguish exactly between a psychical process and a physiological one, between an act occurring in the cerebral cortex and one occurring in the subcortical substance . . . (p. 84).[24]

Perhaps it would be more correct to say that these processes are not of a psychical nature at all, that they are physical processes whose psychical consequences [psychic epiphenomena] present themselves as if . . . [they] had really taken place ["as if" reality of the mental] (p. 53).[28]

4. Freud's methodological empirical parallelism:

The relationship between the chain of physiological events in the nervous system and the mental processes is probably not one of cause and effect. The former do not cease when the latter set in. . . . The psychic is, therefore, a process parallel to the physiological, a dependent concomitant (p. 55).[25]

Freud expresses here the empirical parallelism between the two chains of phenomenal events—the physiological and the psychological. But the expression "dependent concomitant" already implies his metaphysical epiphenomenalism.

The passages quoted above also reveal that Freud's materialistically oriented epiphenomenalism is patterned after an evolutionary type of biological materialism that ought to be distinguished from the classic French mechanistic materialism and from German physicialism. The material reality, in Freud's system, includes the highly organized, biologically developed nervous structures, in addition to the purely mechanical or physicochemical components of the pre-Darwinian materialistic models. The same is true of Jackson's doctrine, of Haeckel's cosmology, and of other dynamic-evolutionary theories.

The Postulational Concepts

In his endeavor to arrive at an explanation of the psychoanalytic empirical findings, Freud elaborated his theoretical concepts now on the psychological level, now on the metapsychological (neurophysiological) level.

In a letter to Fliess of March 10, 1898, Freud wrote: "It seems to me as if the wish-fulfilment theory gives only the psychological and not the biological, or rather metapsychological explanation. . . . Biologically, dream-life seems to me . . ."[11]

In spite of his unambiguous commitment to a materialistic position, Freud did not shy away from psychological formulations whenever they were considered methodologically useful: "I only ask permission to move on to psychological ground—which can scarcely be avoided in dealing with hysteria" (p. 170).[27]

Or, again, in "The Interpretation of Dreams":[32] I shall entirely disregard [methodologically] the fact that the mental apparatus . . . is also known to us in the form of an anatomical preparation, and I shall carefully avoid the temptation to determine psychical locality in any anatomical fashion. I shall remain upon psychological ground, . . ." (p. 536). But, he added: "And since at our first approach to something unknown all that we need is the assistance of provisional ideas, I shall give preference in the first instance to hypotheses of the crudest and most concrete description [psychological intervening variables discussed below]" (p. 536).

But Freud really meant it; the psychological provisional ideas should eventually be replaced by real neurophysiological (metapsychological) constructions[35]: "we must recollect that all our provisional ideas in psychology will presumably some day be based on an organic substructure . . . special substances and chemical processes . . . " (p. 78).

In contemporary (Russellian) metatheoretical terminology, we may say that Freud developed two types of postulational concepts: (1) the psychological constructs, with no existential commitment apart from systemic existence, and (2) the metapsychological inferred entities, with actual or hypothetically real existence.

Constructs and Inferred Entities

Following Russell's distinction between "constructions" and "inferences,"[93] the terms "construct" and "inferred entity" have been explicitly defined by Beck:[6]

An inferred entity is the supposed real existent whose existence is inferred if and only if a given substantive hypothetical proposition about it is confirmed. . . . A substantive hypothesis is an hypothesis to be tested. . . . A construct is that entity whose systemic existence is affirmed by the confirmation of the relevant hypothesis. . . . Systemic existence is the mode of existence of an entity all descriptions of which are analytic within a system of propositions. Real existence is the mode of existence attributed to an entity if there is any true synthetic proposition that can be made about it . . . (pp. 369–370).

Hypothetical Constructs and Intervening Variables

If, instead of Beck's, we follow MacCorquodale and Meehl's distinction of postulational concepts,[81] we may say that Freud developed two types of concepts: (1) the psychological intervening variables, abstracted from the empirical relationships, and (2) the metapsychological hypothetical constructs, involving supposition of entities or processes not among the observed.

According to MacCorquodale and Meehl,[81]

the phrase "intervening variable" . . . will involve no hypothesis as to existence of nonobserved entities or the occurrence of nonobserved processes; it will contain . . . no words which are not definable . . . in terms of the empirical variables. . . . As a second linguistic convention, we propose that the term "hypothetical construct" be used to designate theoretical concepts which . . . involve terms which are not wholly reducible to empirical terms; they refer to processes or entities that are not directly observed (although they need not be in principle unobservable); . . . The validity of intervening variables . . . cannot be called into question except by an actual denial of the empirical facts. . . . Since hypothetical constructs assert the existence of entities and the occurrence of events not reducible to the observable, it would seem to us that it is the business of a hypothetical construct to be "true" . . . (pp. 605–607).

Incidentally, when MacCorquodale and Meehl[81] try to examine an example of one psychoanalytic intervening variable (pp. 608ff.), they select, erroneously, the concept of libido—a true hypothetical construct. In addition to this, they get involved in pointless discussion about the (irrelevant) hydraulic analogue of the libido concept, thus failing to examine, metatheoretically, the concept itself, a sound neurobiochemical hypothetical construct.

The Rules of Correspondence (or Epistemic Correlations)

The postulated, unobserved relations between the empirical data and the inferred entities (hypothetical constructs) "has been called by Northrop the 'epistemic correlation' and by Margenau a 'rule of correspondence' " (p. 375).[6]

When we examine the "rules of correspondence" that have been established between the psychoanalytic empirical data and the metapsychological hypothetical constructs, we have to distinguish the intermediate types of "epistemic correlations," namely, the correlation between the empirical data and the psychological intervening variables and the correlation between the provisional (and fictional) intervening variables and the potentially real, metapsychological hypothetical constructs.

Freud's assertions about moving onto psychological ground, and staying in psychological ground (quoted above), therefore, always refer to the psychological intervening variables (*Hilfsvorstellungen*) and not to real psychological entities. The neurophysiological bases of psychoanalysis have never been ostensibly dropped (or replaced by psychological concepts), as Strachey and Jones[73] gladly assumed.

Rubinstein's Critical Comments on the Mind-Body Problem

In a brilliant and challenging metatheoretical analysis Rubinstein[92] inadvertently failed to distinguish the assumptions connected with the mind-body relationship from the statements concerning the epistemic correlations in psychoanalytic literature. Whereas the mind-body relationship refers to metaphysical entities, the epistemic correlations refer to the empirical data, on one hand, and to the theoretical concepts on the other; the latter, we have seen, may have real (metaphysical) or systemic (epistemological) existence.

Though it is true that Freud's metaphysical position corresponds to a materialistic monism, described by Rubinstein[92] as the *empiricist* view, it is unjustifiable to suppose that "psychoanalytic theoreticians have vacillated uneasily between . . . dualism, pseudodualism, and empiricism . . . [a] dilemma that accounts for the ambiguity of psychoanalytic theory . . . in regard to the mind-body problem" (pp. 47–48).

The epistemic correlations between the real existent neurophysiological hypothetical constructs and the systemic existent psychological intervening variables may be referred to as an as-if dualism (or *pseudodualism*), but because this pseudodualism is not a metaphysical position, psychoanalysis may accept both empiricism and pseudodualism simultaneously, without ambiguity or vacillation.

Some of Freud's metapsychological concepts (neurophysiological hypothetical constructs) have been given psychological names (psychic energy, ego, psychic apparatus, system Cs, wish, and so forth). Such nomenclature has misled Rubinstein[92] into the conclusion that those terms "have as referents purely psychological entities" (p. 45), thus admitting that a *dualistic theory* has been espoused by psychoanalysts. As the psychologically named entities are actually neurophysiological ones, psychoanalytic dualism only reflects a common misinterpretation of metapsychological nomenclature.

THERMODYNAMIC CONCEPTS AND THERMODYNAMIC HOMOLOGIES

In addition to those metascientific questions, it has been the purpose of our investigation to attempt a clarification of the meanings of some of the most important psychoanalytic concepts that are related to physical or biological theoretical entities. Through a careful examination of the types of correspondence[100, 102] that exist between the metapsychological and the physicobiological models, we have separated (1) the superficial analogies from (2) the logical homologies and (3) the reductionistic identities. A logical homology, or isomorphism, is said to hold between the concepts of two different fields of science when we can find a formal identity, or a structural correspondence, between those concepts. Reductionistic identity is said to exist when the events of one science are explained in terms of the concepts of the reducing science. Because the concept of psychic energy refers to a physical entity, we have here an example of reductionistic identity. On the other hand, the principle of constancy of the sums of excitation is only formally identical with Le Chatelier's principle, and hence is an example of logical homology. And the postulate of a death instinct is only a poor analogue of the second law of thermodynamics.

This preliminary work provided the frame of reference in which it has been possible to ascertain the logical status and the heuristic value of the psychoanalytic principles that have their roots in thermodynamics and in evolutionary biology.

In this section we will summarize the results of our systematization of the most controversial questions related to the energetic (or quasienergetic) nature of some metapsychological concepts—and it is hoped that they will become sufficiently clarified to invite further, and more enlightening, critical inquiries.

Psychic Energy

Freud's concept of psychic energy has no correspondence whatever (identical, homological, or analogical) with the physical concept of the interconvertible *forms of energy*, such as heat, chemical, electrical, mechanical, or radiant energy. Psychic energy, therefore, is not a form of physical energy. The alleged homology with vital force[64, 92] is still less justifiable (see below).

Freud's concept of psychic energy is unmistakably identical with the physical concept of *total energy* of a thermodynamic system, Adrian's[1] and Holt's[65] opinions notwithstanding. The total energy of a system is usually made up of several terms, the sum of the different forms of physical energy, internal to, or stored in, the system under consideration.

Psychic energy, therefore, designates the total energy* of a well-defined thermodynamic system—the psychic apparatus (see below). It corresponds to the sum of several forms (or alleged forms) of physical energies (libidinal energy, aggressive energy, neutral energy, and so forth) that happen to be stored in the

---

* In psychoanalysis, as in physicochemical problems, we only deal with changes in the total energy, although we may theoretically assume the existence of the absolute value of the total energy.

psychic apparatus. As the concept of cathexis (p. 81) corresponds to the total energy of the psi system, the psychic energy corresponds to the total energy of the psychic apparatus (pallium psi system, plus the binding ego).

Bernfeld and Feitelberg's Contributions

In a long and elaborate paper, *"Über psychische Energie, Libido und deren Messbarkeit,"*[9] Bernfeld and Feitelberg developed the concept of *personierte Energie*, defined as the total energy of the central nervous system (*Zentralapparat*), plus the potential difference between the CNS and the soma. They would have come closer to their aim of clarifying Freud's concept of psychic energy had they defined their *personierte Energie* as the total energy of the psychic apparatus (a detail of the CNS) in equilibrium plus the difference in the total energy that occurs when the apparatus is driven from the equilibrium condition (minimum potential) to a nonequilibrium state of libidinal tension.

The proposed technique for the measurement of *personierte Energie*, if feasible, would apply to the concept of their definition and not to the Freudian psychic energy.

The Psychic Apparatus

Freud's concept of psychic apparatus is identical with the physical concept of a thermodynamic system. Although not yet anatomically well defined, the psychic apparatus (like its forerunner, the speech apparatus[25]) is a physically existent, functionally represented, topographic region situated in the body. In Freud's own words:[25] "Our concept of the organization of the central apparatus of speech is that of a continuous cortical region occupying the space between the terminations of the optic and acoustic nerves and of the areas of the cranial and some peripheral motor nerves . . ." (p. 67). And,[32] "we will picture the mental apparatus as a compound instrument. . . . we shall ascribe a sensory and a motor end to the apparatus" (pp. 536–539).

"We have refused to localize the psychic elements of the speech process in specified areas within this region . . . " (p. 67).[25] "Mental activity is bound up with the function of the brain. . . . But every attempt to go on from there to discover a localization of mental processes . . . has miscarried completely. . . . Our psychical topography has for the present nothing to do with anatomy; it has reference not to anatomical localities, but to regions in the mental apparatus, wherever they may be situated in the body" (pp. 174–175).[39]

The psychic apparatus, therefore, corresponds to a provisionally hypothetical (supposedly real) thermodynamic system made up of several subsystems, the so-called psi systems, that may not be "arranged in a *spatial* order" (p. 537),[32] but have the characteristics of being "extended in space, expediently put together, developed by the exigencies of life . . . " (p. 196).[48] The "bodily organ and scene of action" of our mental life is "the brain (or nervous system)," even though we have no knowledge of the "exact localization of the processes of consciousness" (p. 144).[48]

Libidinal Energy

Among the various *forms* of physicochemical energy that are grouped together to make up the *total* psychic energy, Freud distinguished (and investigated carefully) one particular form—libidinal energy, or libido,[33] characterized by its origin in the special chemistry of the sex glands and by its function of energizing the "group of sexual ideas which is present in the psyche" (p. 108).[29] In the period between the papers on metapsychology and the publication of "Beyond the Pleasure Principle," it is true, Freud identified libidinal energy with the total psychic energy, admitting no other forms of energy within the psychic apparatus.[36, 37, 38, 39, 40]

The Psychic Apparatus—A Closed (but Nonisolated) System

Though the psychic apparatus may ideally be conceived as a closed system (which exchanges energy, but no matter, through its boundaries), it has never been considered by Freud as an isolated system (which can exchange neither energy nor matter with the environment)—if we use those terms in accordance with standard thermodynamic nomenclature.[88, 89, 101] Hence, the fact that there are inputs and outputs of energy in the psychic apparatus is quite in keeping with the assumption of a closed system, Holt's assertion[65] to the contrary notwithstanding: "Of course, Freud always realized that there are inputs (principally from the instinctual drives) and outputs (which he called discharge); what he did not realize was that this state of affairs destroyed the assumption of a closed system, and that only within a closed system did his *economic* conceptions make sense" (p. 34).[65]

If we adhere to the correct thermodynamic definitions of closed and open systems, however, it becomes clear that Freud's economic conceptions (principle of equivalence and principle of constancy) do make sense in any nonisolated system (closed or open). On the other hand, the economic conceptions are superfluous or inapplicable when we deal with isolated systems (Holt's closed system).

Thermodynamic-Isomorphic and Thermodynamic-Identical Principles

The energetic processes in the psychic apparatus are regulated by principles and limiting conditions [27–44, 49, 53] that are either isomorphic with or identically equivalent to thermodynamic laws and constraints.[15, 62, 79, 80, 82, 88, 89, 100, 101]

Some examples: (1) the principle of constancy (corresponding to Le Chatelier's principle); (2) the impulse to wish fulfillment (corresponding to the generalized forces called "affinities"); (3) the reality principle (corresponding to the constraints determined by the outside world); (4) the binding function of the ego (corresponding to the phenomenological coupling of irreversible processes, leading to stationary states).

Libidinal Tension—A Thermodynamic Potential

Freud's statement[29] that when "the group of sexual ideas which is present in the psyche becomes supplied with energy ... there comes into being the psychical state of libidinal tension" (p. 108) is a true thermodynamic proposition that can be rephrased thus: when the psychic apparatus, a nonisolated, stable, stationary system, receives drive energies (*Triebkräfte*) from the somatic sources, there comes into being a thermodynamic state of increased (above minimum) thermodynamic potential.

Urgency, Urge, or Pressure (Drang)—A Generalized Force*

Freud's statement[29] that the "psychical state of libidinal tension . . . brings with it an urge to remove that tension (p. 108) is, again, a true thermodynamic proposition that can be rephrased thus: the increase (above minimum) of the thermodynamic potential brings with it a generalized force that gives the direction of the spontaneous transformation that will remove the difference in thermodynamic potential.

A Note on the Death Instinct

The removal of the libidinal tension from the psychic apparatus (by means of association or discharge) rigorously corresponds to a displacement of equilibrium (Le Chatelier's principle) and not to a simple reattainment of equilibrium (owing to stability of stationary state).

If we decide to use those concepts loosely, failing to distinguish the displacement of equilibrium (that actually takes place) from the reattainment of equilibrium (of easier conceptualization), then we may admit that the end states are always identical with the initial states. And we may agree with Freud[29] that the psychic apparatus—a stable system—when acted on by external forces (somatic drives) undergoes an increase in its thermodynamic potential that brings with it "an urge to remove that tension" (p. 108), that is, *"an urge . . . to restore an earlier state of things . . . a compulsion to repeat"* (p. 36).[41]

Now, if we further confuse the concepts of drive (*Trieb*—the external work done on the system) and urge (*Drang*—the force that performs work on the environment), we may admit that the living thing has an urge (*Drang*) to restore the earlier inanimate condition, and call this urge the "death drive."

Finally, if we adopt the erroneous translation of *Trieb* as "instinct," then we may be able to accept the postulate of a death instinct as a scientific (or philosophical) assumption.

---

* Freud's concept of *Drang*[22, 52] has been, alternatively, translated as urgency,[53] urge,[29] and pressure[37] in the *Standard Edition*. Freud, occasionally, confuses the terms *Drang* ("urge") and *Wunsch* ("wish"),[52] but it was the confusion of the terms *Drang* and *Trieb* ("urge" and "drive," or "instinct"[41] that ended up in the *Todestrieb* jumble.

The Directional (Entropic) Character of Freud's "Urge"

Freud's concept of psychic energy is not directional and, on this ground, not a vitalistic concept. On the other hand, Freud's concept of urge is directional, because it corresponds to the physical concept of a generalized force—a directional concept. All generalized forces (including Freud's "urge") are directional but not vitalistic concepts.

The Directional (Enthalpic) Character of Freud's "Wish"*

Whereas Freud's "urge" is directional because it strives for equilibrium, for discharge (and for pleasure), Freud's concept of wish is directional in another sense—it is teleological and object-seeking. This new kind of generalized force (homologous with chemical affinity) appears in the psi neurones of the pallium as residues of the "experiences of satisfaction,"[32, 53] and it is teleological and object-seeking in the sense that it has the purpose of producing the perceptual identity with the mnemic image of the object of satisfaction. A thermostat also seeks to establish the set temperature, as if it were a goal.[5] Freud's "wish," "chemical affinity," "error controlled devices," the enthalpy component of Gibbs free energy, all are examples of directional, goal-seeking concepts that are not vitalistic.

Fairbairn's "Libido" and Freud's "Wish"

It is my belief that Fairbairn would have withdrawn his criticism of Freud's "libido" and his proposal for the introduction of the supposedly original concepts of object-seeking libido and dynamic structure,[17] if he had been given the opportunity to reevaluate Freud's theories in the light of the posthumously published "Project"[52, 53] and of the German text of *Die Traumdeutung*.[22] The concepts of object-seeking libido (wish) and dynamic structure (ego-inhibited wishful impulse) had already been exhaustively elaborated by Freud in his theories of wishes

---

* The thermodynamic state function Gibbs free energy G is given by the relation $G = H - TS$, where T is the temperature, H, the enthalpy, and S, the entropy of the system.

(and affects)[53] and in his dynamic concepts of *Wunschregung* ("wishful impulse"), *Triebregung* ("instinctual impulse"), and *psychische Triebkraft* ("psychic motive force"),[22] unfortunately obscured in the English translations[32, 33, 37] and usually misinterpreted as synonyms of "libido," of "libidinal tension," of "urge," or even of the "somatic drives" ("instincts").

Holt's Analysis of Freud's Energetic Concepts

In a recent paper[65] Holt presents a series of arguments to demonstrate "that psychic energy is a vitalistic concept in the sense of being similar to and influenced by vital force, and being to a large extent functionally equivalent to it. They are at least historically and methodologically homologous—buds from the same branch" (p. 24).

The main arguments put forward by Holt are (1) Freud's alleged dualistic theory, as demonstrated by Rubinstein[92] (similar to the vitalist's dualism); (2) Freud's nonspatial psychic apparatus (similar to the nonspatial entelechy's "seat"); (3) the nonphysical character of Freud's psychic energy (in the same sense that vital force is nonphysical); and (4) the directional and teleological character of psychic energy (in the same way as vitalistic forces are directional and teleological).

We have seen above (1) that Freud's position is consistently monistic, (2) that the psychic apparatus is extended in space, (3) that psychic energy is an aggregate of physical energies, and (4) that psychic energy is neither directional nor teleological and should not be confused with the concept of urge.

In this brilliant and enlightening paper Holt's argumentation has been led astray by the following reasons:

1. The mentalistic misconstruction of Freud's momentous decision to abandon any attempt to discover the anatomical localization of the psychic apparatus, restricting his researches to the elaboration of a neurophysiological model, inferred from clinical data. Actually, Freud was candidly stating his intention of proceeding with his neurologizing program, only avoiding the pitfalls of premature localization in the same vein of his previous position in regard to the nonlocalizatory (but neurophysiological) interpretation of the speech apparatus.[25]

2. The nonexistential misinterpretation of Freud's statement about the psi systems that need not be arranged in a spatial order;

we have seen that the lack of spatial ordering does not imply lack of spatiality of the psi systems.

3. The influence of Rubinstein's scholarly demonstration of the (presumed) dualism that was behind Freud's psychological theories.[92]

4. Finally, the uncritical utilization of very inadequate thermodynamic concepts, those oversimplified and grossly distorted notions that, unfortunately, have become an undisputed part of the theoretical equipment of contemporary psychology.

THE EVOLUTIONARY "EMERGENCE" OF FREUD'S PSYCHODYNAMIC CONCEPTS

Closely related to the thermodynamic constructs examined in the last section are the developmental and the learning theoretical concepts that Freud had explicitly superimposed on his quantitative psychology.[53]

Under the heading of "biological acquisition" (not reducible to mechanical principles) Freud elaborated, in great detail, the concepts of phylogenetic (Darwinian) and ontogenetic (roughly recapitulationist) development of (1) the neuronic system and (2) the somatic sources of excitation.

In ontogenetic processes Freud distinguished (1) the maturational factors, that is, the "phylogenetically prescribed programme,"[40] and (2) the effects of environmental pressure and adaptive learning.

We have seen, in the first section, the combination of the energetic and the evolutionary concepts to explain the development of the structure and functions of the psychic apparatus, from primary neuronic function to secondary psychic processes. In these secondary psychic processes, the dynamic factors correspond to the ego-inhibited wishful impulses, that is, the ego-inhibited instinctual impulses, inadequately designated as drives or instincts, the result of Freud's adoption of the term *Triebe*, when he was referring to *Triebregungen* in the classic paper "Triebe und Triebschicksale,"[22] translated as "Instincts and Their Vicissitudes."[37] In this paper Freud developed the following concepts:

1. Source—a physiological, physicochemical entity, needed to explain the origin of the somatic drives. These somatic energies on entering the psychic apparatus constitute the so-called psychic

energy. The secondary wishful impulses, in turn, are the generalized forces that correspond to psychic energy harnessed by pallium and ego structures.

2. Pressure (or urge)—a thermodynamic entity, that is, a generalized force related to the functioning of the nuclear psi system, under the principle of constancy. The secondary wishful impulse is, therefore, another generalized force, corresponding to a modification of the pressure, under the influence of pallium and ego structures.

3. Aim—a psychodynamic concept that consists of both inherited (instinctive) and learned patterns of adequate motor reactions. The secondary wishful impulse is the generalized force that releases the specific action, whose ultimate aim is the satisfaction of the biological needs.

4. Object—a mixture of psychobiological entity and psychodynamic construct. It corresponds to a part of the real external world (a physicochemical, psychobiological entity) capable of removing the state of stimulation at the source. It is also a mnemic image in the pallium, whose perceptual cathexis functions as a cue for the ego to release the consummatory phase of the specific action; this perceptual identity, in turn, is obtained by means of the appetitive phase of the specific action—a cybernetic-modeled programmed behavior. The secondary wishful impulse, therefore, is a generalized force that sustains the appetitive (object-seeking) behavior—as long as there is dissimilarity between the wishful cathexis and the perceptual cathexis of a memory—and releases the consummatory action when perceptual identity is obtained.

GUNTRIP'S CRITIQUE OF FREUD'S PSYCHOBIOLOGY

Guntrip's criticism of the psychobiological type of personality theory is unquestionably correct, but it does not apply to Freud's models, even to those of the pre-1920 biological stage.[57] If, as Guntrip maintains, the theory of the superego is a psychodynamic concept, the same is true of the theories of wishes and affects (1895), the rules of attention and defense (1895), the theory of the wishful impulses (1900), the theory of the (secondary) wishful impulses (1915), and so on. They all have psychobiological and psychodynamic aspects.

Contrary to Guntrip's opinion, Freud's *Triebtheorie* is not a biological theory, even when presented under the misnomer "instinct theory." It is a true psychodynamic theory, and its subject matter is the *Triebregungen*, unfortunately designated, as we have seen, as *Triebe*, thus bringing unnecessary confusion with the somatic drives.

CONCLUDING REMARKS

If we now review the different meanings of the term "psychoanalysis," in Freud's writings,[22] we may distinguish:

1. Psychoanalysis as a technique, both as a special psychological investigative procedure and as a new psychotherapeutic method.

2. Psychoanalysis as a wealthy collection of special psychological data, obtained with the help of psychoanalytic techniques.

3. Psychoanalysis as a new scientific discipline, the science of the unconscious mental processes, or depth-psychology, that is, the system of psychoanalytic basic concepts and postulates proposed to account for the psychoanalytic empirical data. This new science—theoretical psychoanalysis—consists of (a) the metascientific presuppositions, and (b) the scientific sets of propositions—psychological, metapsychological, developmental, and the physicochemical theory of the biological or somatic drives.

4. Psychoanalysis as an ideologic "movement"—dogmatic Freudianism or any of its current ramifications—originally, a healthy reaction against the resistances to psychoanalysis, but now the most awkward obstacle to the scientific and technical advances so badly needed in psychoanalytic psychology and psychotherapy.

Ten years ago we would probably close this chapter with George Kelly's ominous words that revealed his preoccupation with the harm that had been done to psychoanalytic theories and techniques by the outmoded but still influential psychoanalytic movement:

As the years go by, Freudianism, which deserves to be remembered as a brave outpost on the early frontier of psychological thought, is condemned to end its days as a crumbling stockade of proprietary dogmatism. Thus, as with other farseeing claims to absolute truth, history will have a difficult time deciding whether Freudianism did more to accelerate psychological progress during the first half of the twentieth century than it did to impede progress during the last half (1958).[75]

It is our belief, however, that the growing concern of many psychologists and psychoanalysts, with the need for an over-all clarification and systematization of psychoanalytic theory and for a radical rebuilding of certain theoretical models, will inevitably reintegrate psychoanalysis into the community of the truly investigative sciences and into its position of a brave outpost on the frontier of psychological thought.

NOTE: The preparation of this chapter was supported (in part) by a grant from the *Instituto de Medicina Psicológica*, a private post-graduate training institution in psychiatry and intensive psychotherapy.

REFERENCES

1. Adrian, E. D. "The Mental and the Physical Origins of Behavior," *International Journal of Psychoanalysis*, 27 (1946), 1–6.
2. Alexander F. *Fundamentals of Psychoanalysis*. New York: Norton, 1948.
3. Apfelbaum, B. "Ego Psychology, Psychic Energy, and the Hazards of Quantitative Explanation in Psychoanalytic Theory," *International Journal of Psychoanalysis*, 46 (1965), 168–182.
4. Arlow, J. A., and Brenner, C. *Psychoanalytic Concepts and the Structural Theory*. New York: International Universities Press, 1964.
5. Ashby, W. R. *Design for a Brain*. London: Chapman & Hall, 1954.
6. Beck, L. W. "Constructions and Inferred Entities," in H. Feigl and M. Brodbeck (eds.), *Readings in the Philosophy of Science*. New York: Appleton-Century-Crofts, 1953.
7. Bernfeld, S. "Freud's Earliest Theories and the School of Helmholtz," *Psychoanalytic Quarterly*, 13 (1944), 341–362.
8. Bernfeld, S., and Feitelberg, S. "Der Entropiesatz und der Todestrieb," *Imago*, 16 (1930), 187–206.
9. Bernfeld, S., and Feitelberg, S. "Über psychische Energie, Libido und deern Messbarkeit," *Imago*, 16 (1930), 66–118.
10. Bibring, E. "Zur Entwiclung und Problematik der Triebtheorie," *Imago*, 22 (1935), 147–176.
11. Bonaparte, M., Freud, A., and Kris, E. (eds.). *The Origins of Psycho-Analysis: Letters to Wilhelm Fliess, Drafts and Notes, by Sigmund Freud (1887–1902)*. New York: Basic Books, 1954.
12. Breuer, J., and Freud, S. "Studies on Hysteria" (1895), in J. Strachey (ed.), *Standard Edition*. London: Hogarth, 1955. (Also in *Collected Papers of Sigmund Freud*. New York: Basic Books, 1924–1950.)
13. Choisy, M. *Sigmund Freud: A New Appraisal*. London: Owen, 1963.
14. Colby, K. M. *Energy and Structure in Psychoanalysis*. New York: Ronald Press, 1955.
15. D'Abro, A. *The Rise of the New Physics*. New York: Dover, 1951.
16. Duhem, P. *The Aim and Structure of Physical Theory*. New York: Atheneum, 1962.
17. Fairbairn, W. R. D. *Psychoanalytic Studies of the Personality*. London: Tavistock, 1952.
18. Feigl, H. "The 'Mental' and the 'Physical,'" in H. Feigl, M. Scriven, and G. Maxwell (eds.), *Minnesota Studies in the Philosophy of Science*. Minneapolis: University of Minnesota Press, 1958.

19. Fletcher, R. *Instinct in Man.* New York: International Universities Press, 1957.
20. Flugel, J. C. "The Death Instinct, Homeostasis and Allied Concepts," *International Journal of Psychoanalysis*, Supplement, **34** (1953), 43–73.
21. Foxe, A. N. "Critique of Freud's Concept of a Death Instinct," *Psychoanalytic Review*, **30** (1943), 417–427.
22. Freud, A. et al. (eds.). *Sigmund Freud: Gesammelte Werke.* London: Imago, 1952.
23. Freud, S. "Hysteria" (1888), in J. Strachey (ed.), *Standard Edition.* London: Hogarth, 1966. Vol. 1.
24. Freud, S. "Hypnotism and Suggestion" (1880–1889), in *Collected Papers of Sigmund Freud.* New York: Basic Books, 1959. Vol. 5, pp. 11–24.
25. Freud, S. *On Aphasia* (1891). New York: International Universities Press, 1953.
26. Freud, S. "Preface and Footnotes to the Translation of Charcot's *Tuesday Lectures*" (1892–1893), in J. Strachey (ed.), *Standard Edition.* London: Hogarth. Vol. 1.
27. Freud, S. "Some Points in a Comparative Study of Organic and Hysterical Motor Paralyses" (1893), in J. Strachey (ed.), *Standard Edition.* London: Hogarth. Vol. 1. (Also in J. Strachey (ed.), *Collected Papers of Sigmund Freud.* New York: Basic Books, 1959. Vol. 1, pp. 42–58.)
28. Freud, S. "The Neuro-Psychoses of Defence" (1894), in J. Strachey (ed.), *Standard Edition.* London: Hogarth. Vol. 3. (Also published as "The Defence Neuro-Psychoses," *Collected Papers of Sigmund Freud.* New York: Basic Books, 1959. Vol. 1, pp. 59–75.)
29. Freud, S. "On the Grounds for Detaching a Particular Syndrome from Neurasthenia under the Description 'Anxiety Neurosis'" (1895), in J. Strachey (ed.), *Standard Edition.* London: Hogarth. Vol. 3.
30. Freud, S. "A Reply to Criticisms of My Paper on Anxiety Neurosis" (1895), in J. Strachey (ed.), *Standard Edition.* London: Hogarth. Vol. 3. (Also published as "A Reply to Criticisms on the Anxiety-Neurosis," *Collected Papers of Sigmund Freud.* New York: Basic Books, 1959. Vol. 1, pp. 107–127.)
31. Freud, S. "Heredity and the Aetiology of the Neuroses" (1896), in J. Strachey (ed.), *Standard Edition.* London: Hogarth. Vol. 3. (Also in *Collected Papers of Sigmund Freud.* New York: Basic Books, 1959. Vol. 5, pp. 288–294.)
32. Freud, S. "The Interpretation of Dreams" (1900), in J. Strachey (ed.), *Standard Edition.* London: Hogarth. Vols. 4–5. (Also published as *The Interpretation of Dreams.* New York: Basic Books, 1955.)
33. Freud, S. "Three Essays on the Theory of Sexuality" (1905), in J. Strachey (ed.), *Standard Edition.* London: Hogarth. Vol. 7, pp. 123–243. (Also published as *Three Essays on the Theory of Sexuality.* New York: Basic Books, 1962.)
34. Freud, S. "Formulations on the Two Principles of Mental Functioning" (1911), in J. Strachey (ed.), *Standard Edition.* London: Hogarth. Vol. 12. (Also published as "Formulations Regarding the Two Principles in Mental Functioning," *Collected Papers of Sigmund Freud.* New York: Basic Books, 1959. Vol. 4, pp. 13–21.)
35. Freud, S. "Types of Onset of Neurosis" (1912), in J. Strachey (ed.), *Standard Edition.* London: Hogarth. Vol. 12. (Also published as "Types of Neurotic Nosogenesis," *Collected Papers of Sigmund Freud.* New York: Basic Books, 1959. Vol. 2, pp. 113–121.)
36. Freud, S. "On Narcissism: An Introduction" (1914), in J. Strachey (ed.), *Standard Edition.* London: Hogarth. Vol. 14. (Also in *Collected Papers of Sigmund Freud.* New York: Basic Books, 1959. Vol. 4, pp. 30–59.)
37. Freud, S. "Instincts and Their Vicissitudes" (1915), in J. Strachey (ed.), *Standard Edition.* London, Hogarth. Vol. 14. (Also in *Collected Papers of Sigmund Freud.* New York: Basic Books, 1959. Vol. 4, pp. 60–83.)
38. Freud, S. "Repression" (1915), in J. Strachey (ed.), *Standard Edition.* London: Hogarth. Vol. 14. (Also in *Collected Papers of Sigmund Freud.* New York: Basic Books, 1959. Vol. 4, pp. 84–97.)
39. Freud, S. "The Unconscious" (1915), in J. Strachey (ed.), *Standard Edition.* London: Hogarth. Vol. 14. (Also in *Collected Papers of Sigmund Freud.* New York: Basic Books, 1959. Vol. 4, pp. 98–136.)
40. Freud, S. "Introductory Lectures on Psycho-Analysis" (1916–1917), in J. Strachey (ed.), *Standard Edition.* London: Hogarth. Vols. 15–16.

41. Freud, S. "Beyond the Pleasure Principle" (1920), in J. Strachey (ed.), *Standard Edition*. London: Hogarth. Vol. 18, pp. 1–64.
42. Freud, S. "Certain Neurotic Mechanisms in Jealousy, Paranoia and Homosexuality" (1922), in J. Strachey (ed.), *Standard Edition*. London: Hogarth. Vol. 18, pp. 223–232. (Also in *Collected Papers of Sigmund Freud*. New York: Basic Books, 1959. Vol. 2, pp. 223–243.)
43. Freud, S. "The Ego and the Id" (1923), in J. Strachey (ed.), *Standard Edition*. London: Hogarth. Vol. 19.
44. Freud, S. "The Economic Problem of Masochism" (1924), in J. Strachey (ed.), *Standard Edition*. London: Hogarth. Vol. 19. (Also published as "The Economic Problem in Masochism," *Collected Papers of Sigmund Freud*. New York: Basic Books, 1959. Vol. 2, pp. 255–268.)
45. Freud, S. "The Dissolution of the Oedipus Complex" (1924), in J. Strachey (ed.), *Standard Edition*. London: Hogarth. Vol. 19. (Also in *Collected Papers of Sigmund Freud*. New York: Basic Books, 1959. Vol. 2, pp. 269–276.)
46. Freud, S. "New Introductory Lectures on Psycho-Analysis" (1933), in J. Strachey (ed.), *Standard Edition*. London: Hogarth. Vol. 22.
47. Freud, S. "Analysis Terminable and Interminable" (1937), in J. Strachey (ed.), *Standard Edition*. London: Hogarth. Vol. 23. (Also in *Collected Papers of Sigmund Freud*. New York: Basic Books, 1959. Vol. 5, pp. 316–357.)
48. Freud, S. "An Outline of Psychoanalysis" (1940), in J. Strachey (ed.), *Standard Edition*. London: Hogarth. Vol. 23.
49. Freud, S., and Breuer, J. "On the Theory of Hysterical Attacks" (written with Josef Breuer in 1892) (1940), in J. Strachey (ed.), *Standard Edition*. London: Hogarth. Vol. 1. (Also in *Collected Papers of Sigmund Freud*. New York: Basic Books, 1959. Vol. 5, pp. 27–30.)
50. Freud, S. "Draft D" (1954), in J. Strachey (ed.), *Standard Edition*. London: Hogarth. Vol. 1.
51. Freud, S. "Draft E" (1954), in J. Strachey (ed.), *Standard Edition*. London: Hogarth. Vol. 1.
52. Freud, S. "Entwurf einer Psychologie" (1950), in M. Bonaparte, A. Freud, and E. Kris (eds.), Sigmund Freud: *Aus den Anfängen der Psychoanalyse—Briefe am Wilhelm Fliess, Abhandlungen und Notizen (1887–1902)*. London: Imago, 1950.
53. Freud, S. "A Project for a Scientific Psychology" (1954), in Marie Bonaparte et al. (eds.), *The Origins of Psycho-Analysis*. New York: Basic Books, 1954.
54. Freud, S. "Letter to Fliess of January 1, 1896" (1954), in J. Strachey (ed.), *Standard Edition*. London: Hogarth.
55. Gill, M. M. "Topography and Systems in Psychoanalytic Theory," in G. S. Klein (ed.), *Psychological Issues*. Monograph 10. New York: International Universities Press, 1963.
56. Glick, B. S. "A Note on Freud's 'Empty' Neuron," *British Journal of Medical Psychology*, 40 (1967), 159–162.
57. Guntrip, H. "The Concept of Psychodynamic Science," *International Journal of Psychoanalysis*, 48 (1967), 32–43.
58. Haeckel, E. *Die Welträthsel*. Bonn: Strauss, 1903.
59. Hartmann, H. "Comments on the Psychoanalytic Theory of Instinctual Drives" (1948), in *Essays on Ego Psychology*. London: Hogarth, 1964.
60. Hartmann, H. "The Mutual Influences in the Development of Ego and Id" (1952), in *Essays on Ego Psychology*. London: Hogarth, 1964.
61. Heimann, P. "Notes on the Theory of Life and Death Instincts," in M. Klein et al. (eds.), *Developments in Psychoanalysis*. London: Hogarth, 1952.
62. Helmholtz, H. L. F. von. *Wissenschaftliche Abhandlungen*. Leipzig: Barth, 1882–1885.
63. Holt, R. R. "A Critical Examination of Freud's Concept of Bound vs. Free Cathexis," *Journal of American Psychoanalytic Association*, 10 (1962), 475–525.
64. Holt, R. R. "A Review of Some of Freud's Biological Assumptions and Their Influence on His Theories," in N. S. Greenfield and W. C. Lewis (eds.), *Psychoanalysis and Current Biological Thought*. Madison: University of Wisconsin Press, 1965.
65. Holt, R. R. "Beyond Vitalism and Mechanism: Freud's Concept of Psychic

Energy," in J. H. Masserman (ed.), *Science and Psychoanalysis*. Vol. 11. *The Ego*. New York: Grune & Stratton, 1967.
66. Jackson, J. H. "On the Anatomical, Physiological and Pathological Investigation of Epilepsies" (1873), in J. Taylor (ed.), *Selected Writings of John Hughlings Jackson*. New York: Basic Books, 1958. Vol. 1, pp. 90–111.
67. Jackson, J. H. "On the Scientific and Empirical Investigation of Epilepsies," (1874–1876), in J. Taylor (ed.), *Selected Writings of John Hughlings Jackson*. New York: Basic Books, 1958. Vol. 1, pp. 162–273.
68. Jackson, J. H. "On the Anatomical and Physiological Localisation of Movements in the Brain" (1875), in J. Taylor (ed.), *Selected Writings of John Hughlings Jackson*. New York: Basic Books, 1958. Vol. 1, pp. 37–76.
69. Jackson, J. H. "On Temporary Paralysis after Epileptiform and Epileptic Seizures: A Contribution to the Study of Dissolution of the Nervous System" (1880–1881), in J. Taylor (ed.), *Selected Writings of John Hughlings Jackson*. New York: Basic Books, 1958. Vol. 1, pp. 318–329.
70. Jackson, J. H. "Remarks on Dissolution of the Nervous System as Exemplified by Certain Post-Epileptic Conditions" (1881), in J. Taylor (ed.), *Selected Writings of John Hughlings Jackson*. New York: Basic Books, 1958. Vol. 2, pp. 3–28.
71. Jackson, J. H. "Remarks on Evolution and Dissolution of the Nervous System" (1887), in J. Taylor (ed.), *Selected Writings of John Hughlings Jackson*. New York: Basic Books, 1958. Vol. 2, pp. 76–91.
72. Jones, E. "Psychoanalysis and the Instincts," *British Journal of Psychology*, **26** (1936), 273–288.
73. Jones, E. *Sigmund Freud: Life and Work*. London: Hogarth, 1956–1958. New York: Basic Books, 1953–1957.
74. Kapp, R. O. "Comments on Bernfeld and Feitelberg's 'The Principle of Entropy and the Death Instinct,'" *International Journal of Psycho-Analysis*, **12** (1931), 82–86.
75. Kelly, G. A. "Man's Construction of His Alternatives," in G. Lindzey (ed.), *Assessment of Human Motives*. New York: Evergreen, 1960.
76. Klein, M. *Contributions to Psycho-Analysis*. London: Hogarth, 1948.
77. Kubie, L. S. "The Fallacious Use of Quantitative Concepts in Dynamic Psychology," *Psychoanalytic Quarterly*, **16** (1947), 507–518.
78. Laplanche, J., and Pontalis, J.-B. *Vocabulaire de la Psychanalyse*. Paris: Presses Universitaires de France, 1967.
79. Lindsay, R. B., and Margenau, H. *Foundations of Physics*. New York: Dover, 1957.
80. Lotka, A. J. *Elements of Mathematical Biology*. New York: Dover, 1956.
81. MacCorquodale, K., and Meehl, P. E. "Hypothetical Constructs and Intervening Variables," in H. Feigl and M. Brodbeck (eds.), *Readings in the Philosophy of Science*. New York: Appleton-Century-Crofts, 1953.
82. Maron, S. H., and Prutton, C. F. *Principles of Physical Chemistry*. New York: Macmillan, 1965.
83. Money-Kyrle, R. E. "An Inconclusive Contribution to the Theory of the Death Instinct," in M. Klein et al. (eds.), *New Directions in Psychoanalysis*. New York: Basic Books, 1955.
84. Orr, D. W. "Is There a Homeostatic Instinct?" *Psychoanalytic Quarterly*, **11** (1942), 322–335.
85. Ostwald, W. *Vorlesungen über Naturphilophie*. Leipzig: von Veit, 1905.
86. Penrose, L. S. "Freud's Theory of Instinct and Other Psychobiological Theories," *International Journal of Psycho-Analysis*, **12** (1931), 87–97.
87. Pribram, K. "Freud's Project: An Open, Biologically Based Model for Psychoanalysis," in N. S. Greenfield and W. C. Lewis (eds.), *Psychoanalysis and Current Biological Thought*. Madison: University of Wisconsin Press, 1965.
88. Prigogine, I. *Étude Thermodynamique des Phénomènes Irréversibles*. Paris: Dunod, 1947.
89. Prigogine, I. *Introduction to Thermodynamics of Irreversible Processes*. New York: Wiley, 1965.
90. Rapaport, David. "The Structure of Psychoanalytic Theory. A Systematizing Attempt," in G. S. Klein (ed.), *Psychological Issues*. Monograph 6. New York: International Universities Press, 1960.
91. Rapaport, D., and Gill, M. M. "The Points of View and Assumptions of Meta-

psychology," *International Journal of Psychoanalysis,* **40** (1959), 153–162.
92. Rubinstein, B. B. "Psychoanalytic Theory and the Mind-Body Problem," in N. S. Greenfield and W. C. Lewis (eds.), *Psychoanalysis and Current Biological Thought.* Madison: University of Wisconsin Press, 1965.
93. Russell, B. *Mysticism and Logic* (1918). London: Penguin, 1953.
94. Segal, H. *Introduction to the Work of Melanie Klein.* London: Heinemann, 1964.
95. Spitz, R. A. *The First Year of Life.* New York: International Universities Press, 1965.
96. Sterba, R. "The Cosmological Aspect of Freud's Theory of Instincts," *American Imago,* **6** (1949), 157–161.
97. Strachey, J. "The Emergence of Freud's Fundamental Hypotheses," in J. Strachey (ed.), *Standard Edition.* London: Hogarth. Vol. 3.
98. Strachey, J. "The Nature of Q," in J. Strachey (ed.), *Standard Edition.* London: Hogarth. Vol. 1.
99. Szasz, T. S. "On the Psychoanalytic Theory of Instincts," *Psychoanalytic Quarterly,* **21** (1952), 25–48.
100. Von Bertalanffy, L. "An Outline of General System Theory," *British Journal for the Philosophy of Science,* **1** (1950), 134–165.
101. Von Bertalanffy, L. "The Theory of Open Systems in Physics and Biology," *Science,* **111** (1950), 23–29.
102. Von Bertalanffy, L. *Problems of Life.* London: Watts, 1952.
103. Waelder, R. *Basic Theory of Psychoanalysis.* New York: International Universities Press, 1960.
104. Walker, N. "Freud and Homeostasis," *British Journal for the Philosophy of Science,* **7** (1956), 61–72.
105. Weiss, E. *Principles of Psychodynamics.* New York: Grune & Stratton, 1950.
106. White, R. W. "Ego and Reality in Psychoanalytic Theory," in G. S. Klein (ed.), *Psychological Issues,* Monograph 11. New York: International Universities Press, 1963.
107. Wolman, B. B. "Principles of Monistic Transitionism," in Benjamin B. Wolman (ed.), *Scientific Psychology.* New York: Basic Books, 1965.

LEVELS OF TEMPORALITY IN PSYCHOPATHOLOGY

Yasuhiko Taketomo

INTRODUCTION

"Temporality," in this chapter, will refer to time as immanent in experience. It dovetails such concepts as psychological time, subjective time, internal time, personal time, experiential time, and lived time—all concepts used by researchers on the subject. Aside from avoiding the risks of confusion that emerge with the use of these alternative terms, "temporality" has the additional advantage of brevity.

The specific aspect of temporality explored here is that of the temporal awareness involved in the integration of ongoing experience, that is, the temporal-integrative field of experience. The concept of such an integrative field is operational, akin to such constructs as that of "temporal perspective,"[31] "field at a given time,"[64] and "ordination."[76]

The present discussion deals with the hierarchical status of the temporal-integrative field as well as with its relevance to the psychopathology of temporality. It is suggested that a given unit of experience can be studied as integrated in a field that is at one or another of the hierarchic levels of the time orders. This conceptual tool will then be tested on some questions about temporality in psychopathology.

The totality of a behavior—that is, of a behavioral process—from its inception to its termination can be viewed as being integrated. The model for such integration, which steers the movement of the ongoing phases toward a goal, has already been presented by ethologists[101] and neuropsychologists[58, 74] within the observational frame of reference.

If we shift the frame of reference, however, to the introspective one, the same behavioral process can be studied as a course of experience. We experience our own behavioral processes either as currently going on or as thoughts of such a process, embedded in memory, prospect, plan, or, possibly, in fantasy and dream. Our experience includes all those elements of any given phase of a behavioral process that can be delineated in relation to the totality of that process. If one adopts the analogy with road markers, which relate the various positions of the traveler to the course of his travels, it is also conceivable to consider an analogue to the scale (or yardstick) that constitutes the underlying measure. Such an analogue—that is, the underlying medium of temporal experience that relates any one phase of a behavioral process to its total course—is provided by the time orders.

The scale-reading in the medium of road markers can be extended to either side of any particular segment of the road. Can a time order (or, more specifically, the time order of one particular experiential-integrative field) be similarly extended when the behavioral process in question is a constituent of a larger integrated behavior (or experience)? This is the central point of discussion in this chapter.

Levy,[62] in discussing the psychodynamic significance of the study of sequential structure in purposive behavior, has pointed to a hierarchy of behavioral processes, from the elementary to the complex. His work has inspired me to study the temporality (in the experiential sense) involved in the sequential (in the observational sense) structure of purposive behavior. In a preliminary presentation,[99] the possibility was put forward of matching a hierarchy of the levels of time order with the corresponding levels of the behavioral processes. This suggestion is here summarized, with some modifications, as Table 1.

In spite of the profound relevance of temporality to psychopathology, research in the field encounters a number of difficulties. Aside from the more familiar problems, which arise out of attempts to cross the conceptual barriers between different theoretical systems, there is one serious problem that stems from inadequate delineation of the particular aspect of temporality under discussion. It is hoped that this presentation will clarify the conception of time orders and their relevance to psychopathology and contribute thereby to future research on temporality.

TABLE 1

Behavioral Context of Temporality		Hierarchy of Time Orders
LEVELS	EXPLANATION	LEVELS
(Functional unit)	A fraction of the stream of experience segmented by the experimental procedure; not directly comparable to the spontaneous structure of the process of experience	
act	the elementary unit of purposive behavior	practical order
simple act	the act as divided into appetitive phase consummatory phase	
complex act	emergence of conflicting goals during the appetitive phase	
performance		
simple performance	a series of acts integrated toward a goal	subjective order
complex performance	interruption during the course of a planned performance	objective order
performance in reference to life trajectory	experience integrated in terms of one's own life trajectory or major stages (epochs) thereof	representative order (life trajectory)
performance in reference to historical perspective	experience integrated in terms of one's historical perspective	representative order (historical perspective)

THE EARLY EPIGENESIS OF THE TEMPORAL FIELD

Time Orders in the Sensorimotor Period

Piaget's[79] study of the development of the temporal field between ages 0:0 and 2:0 (the sensorimotor period) is of unique relevance here. Because verbal communication is not available, the observer must infer the essential aspects of the child's temporality, along with the cognitive features of his experiences, from observed behavior patterns.

As understood by Piaget, temporal organization includes five constituent elements—duration, consciousness of before and after, seriation, memory, and concepts regarding time. Of these, seriation and memory, which together comprise his temporal field, most clearly reveal the epigenetic development that differentiates his six substages. In each substage, behavior patterns are viewed in correlation with four areas of the child's cognitive world—object, causality, time, and space.

It should be noted that, though memory is, for Piaget, a major constituent element, he does not speak of any anticipatory constituent. This is despite what we know of anticipatory behavior in early life.[3, 68] The rigorous exclusion of an anticipatory constituent from Piaget's discussion would seem to be his way of emphasizing that futurity is not a simple extension "on the other side" of that "pastness" in which memory rests.

The development of the cognition of causality plays the primary role in preparing the organization of the experiential modalities of futurity of intention and futurity of anticipation. Although "anticipation" and "expectation" are generally (except for Arieti[3]) used interchangeably in the literature, Piaget uses the former term to refer to the cognition of spatial causality and the latter to refer to the cognition of intentional causality.

It should further be noted that Piaget deals with the rhythm of the infant's repetitive movement as essentially spatial in character, based on the return to the initial position. Grasp of the temporal rhythm involved lies within the capacity of the observer; what is questionable, however, is whether such a temporal medium is also available for experiencing by the observed, the infant.

Nevertheless, it is striking how closely the various stages of sequence postulated by Piaget fit the time orders that have been here (see Table 1) postulated for some levels of behavior—so much so that Piaget's work can be taken as having established the preverbal developmental prototypes of these time orders. Thus, the time order for "act," postulated in Table 1 as the elementary unit of purposive behavior is designated as "practical order," in keeping with Piaget's prototypical "practical sequence."

Similarly with "objective order" and Piaget's "subjective series," as well as "objective order" and his "objective series." In the case of the former, the focus is "simple performance," as a series of acts directed toward a goal; in the latter, it is "complex performance," in which there is the beginning of active handling of the social time scale. The infant is brought to see the time order as placed outside and above his own activity and, in that sense, objective.

By the time the infant has reached the level of "representative order," he is already departing from the preverbal period and entering the verbal one. Nevertheless, his attainment of a new time order does not mean that the time orders previously attained now pass out of existence for him. At the close of the six substages, neither the practical, subjective, nor objective series has been rendered obsolete. When the child enters the world of verbal learning, it is with all these earlier time orders still available to him as modalities of experience.

In view of the significance for our psychodynamic inquiry of Piaget's contribution, it is of interest to recall that the earliest psychoanalytic study on time experience as such by Spielrein[94] was stimulated by Piaget's current research.

In regard to the temporality during the early developmental period under discussion, Gifford[42] attempted to integrate the neurophysiological findings of Kleitman and Engelmann[57] with the psychoanalytic issues of orality-sleep-temporality. The latter issue, in part discussed in the following, was also suggested by Sacks.[47] It seems that the need for the differentiation of the time of the observer (therefore the biological time) and the temporality of the child is particularly germane to a discussion in this area.

Time Orders in Children's Verbalized Experiences

It is clear that the prototypes of the hierarchy of time orders make their appearance during the preverbal period. Psychopathological methodology, however, approaches temporality from the standpoint not only of observed behavior but of verbalized content as well. Time orders involved in experiences that can be verbalized are therefore no less relevant than those inferred from the infant's behavior during the sensorimotor period.

In their "Ontogenesis of Time Experience," Werner and Kaplan have summarized what is now known about verbal expressions of time.[106] Their four steps are differentiated as follows: (1) The temporal aspect is implied in monoremic (purely referential) expressions, with temporality being imbedded, as it were, in the total event, comprising inextricably both the subjective and objective aspects. (2) Temporal aspects are more and more carried by action words, now increasingly differentiated from thing words. (This does not mean, however, that these temporal aspects are any less fused than previously with particular events and affects.) (3) Temporal aspects as such begin to be articulated as variable characteristics of a relatively self-contained action. That is to say, action words begin to be modulated, although the modulated forms still express temporality in terms of a present event. (4) The mastery of temporality qua tense occurs, a process facilitated by the emergence of adverbs and other words of tense. At this stage, the child at length becomes able to codify activity at specific positions on a time line.

Study of this same ontogenetic scheme from the standpoint of time orders leads to the following considerations. In Step 1, the child is still unable to express, in verbal form, a temporality that has been detached from the sum total of events. The range of temporality includes only the immediate future and the immediate past, both clearly connected with the ongoing present. The only experiences that can be verbalized in this step are therefore those integrated by the practical and subjective orders. In Step 2, as noted, action words provide the vehicle for expressions of temporality, and futurity is expressed in the form of imperatives. This is in line with the extent to which preverbal development of a sense of futurity has leaned on development of the cognition of causality. The experiences that can be expressed in this step, therefore, are those that are integrated by the subjective order; this can be seen from the way in which the child's own affective involvement determines how he refers to the disappearance of the object. In Step 3, with the appearance of tense-like modulations of action words, the expression of the time order begins to be independent of the expression of behavior. Yet, objectification is not yet firmly established, so that the time order expressed in the verbalizations of this period constitutes a transition from the subjective to the objective order. Finally, in Step 4, although it is still an affectively toned situation—including the speaker's attitude—that is being referred to, the child is now, for the first time, able to refer verbally to the objective series, independently of his own action. Expressions in this step, therefore, refer to the objective order.

Thus, despite the fact that the child enters, at roughly the same time, on both verbal acquisition and the development of representative order, it is not possible for him, at the start, to avail himself of all the time orders for verbal expression. It is only by steps—

beginning with the practical-subjective orders—that the child attains the verbal skill to express his experiences, as these have been integrated by the higher time orders.

On this question, some highly relevant findings emerged in a study by Cromer of the development of temporal reference in the language of children.[15] In his studies of children's spontaneous speech, he found that, following the emergence of structured utterances, there was a slight increase with increasing age, in the ability to refer to past time. On the other hand, the ability to refer to needs, desires, or wishes or to some other kind of immediate future makes its appearance with the start of two-word utterances. At 4:0–4:6 there merges a certain cognitive ability that enables children to utilize their newly acquired linguistic devices for such specific modes of temporal references as viewpoints (a viewpoint in the future), unactual (possibility that can or cannot happen) and so on. These devices are discussed by Cromer as design features of temporal references. On the strength of these findings, Cromer hypothesized that the child has acquired, during the first half of the fourth year, a new ability to "decentrize in time" (analogous to Piaget's[80] concept of "decentrizing in space"). This meant that he was now able to free himself linguistically from the immediate situation and from the actual order of events.

Tests designed to validate this hypothesis, however, revealed that it was only after age five that the child was actually able to decentrize. Throughout the previous period, when the child was being exposed to the entire range of linguistic devices employed in his environment for temporal reference, his own ability to employ any such device correctly would still have had to wait till a later age. Initially, he would be able to use that device in a limited way, and one that did not necessarily correspond to its generally accepted meaning. What emerges during the fourth year is not the ability to decentrize in time, but rather the cognitive ability prerequisite to it—what Bruner has called "deactionizing."[8]

For Bruner, with the very young child, "the tempo and metric of time is given . . . by the tempo and segmentation of the actions occurring within it." Because what is decisive for the child of that age is "the activity itself and its inherent temporal order," he is unable to treat time independently. Nevertheless, the point at which time and action do become separated is arrived at, and neither any longer has to borrow the other's terms in order to be expressed by the child.

Taken together, these findings confirm the position stated above with regard to temporal-integrative fields in the various time orders available to children, both preverbally and after the attainment of verbalization. Up to the point at which deactionizing has been achieved, the only temporal fields in which the child's behavior can be integrated verbally by him are those of the practical and subjective orders. (These previously had been available to him for preverbal integration, of course, along with both the objective and the representative order.) With deactionizing, the objective order becomes for the first time available for verbal integration, insofar as the time order is now independent of the behavior itself; with decentrizing, later on, the child begins to be able to integrate verbally in the representative order in that his conceptual ability now includes a temporal field that extends beyond the field of direct perception.

The unique experiments by Werner and Kaplan on time expression in nonverbal media[106] have shown that these various levels of time order are all latently functional for the integration of experiences by a "normal" adult. Subjects were required to express temporal references, as set forth in groups of sentences, by way of either linear patterns or verbally expressed visual images. Several different modes of representing temporal references by way of these nonverbal media were then delineated. In the medium of "expressive lines," these included representation in terms of "affective reaction" or "agent characteristics" (posture or attitude), or of characteristics of one phase of a temporally extended event; they also included representation in terms of spatial-vectorial relations of action to object or goal, as well as in terms of such generic aspects of action as "anticipation," "ongoingness" or "cessation." In the medium of visual imagery there also appeared such modes of representation as situational elements, spatial relation of agent's action to situational context, and qualities inherent in the medium.

Viewed from the standpoint of the hierarchy of time orders, these results are highly relevant. Ordinarily, when the adult resorts to verbal representation, his temporal-integrative field is at the representative order—even though latently he still has access to all four levels. Temporarily deprived in these tests, however, of the opportunity to represent temporal integration by verbal means, he is obliged to find substitute means of expression for temporal integration and resorts to other levels of time order for this purpose.

Only in reference via generic aspects of action (in the "expressive line" medium) does he employ the representative time order. In all other instances, what he does, in effect, is to transpose the given public meaning, such as he would otherwise verbalize in the representative order, into any one of the lower time orders—practical, subjective, or objective—or to the intermediate level transitional from subjective to objective order. Which lower order the transposition is made to depends on the personal meaning he attaches to the ongoing temporal integration of experience.

When such transpositions take place, it must be noted, there is a concurrent detachment of the relevant integration from the temporal context of all time orders in the hierarchy that are above the order to which the transposition is effected. Thus, for example, in an r-s transposition—from *r*epresentative to *s*ubjective time order—neither the temporal-integrative field of the representative order (life trajectory) nor that of the objective orders (the planning of a complex performance) is available; the highest behavioral context of the temporal field is the one that takes in a series of acts leading toward a goal. Similarly with the r-o (*r*epresentative to *o*bjective) transition: though the temporal-integrative fields of both the practical and the subjective order are still available, that of the representative order is no longer. Figure 1 represents a diagram of the processes of transposition and detachment at issue.

LEVELS OF TIME ORDER IN DYNAMIC PSYCHOPATHOLOGY

Dynamic psychology, as motivational psychology, can be divided into two major areas—one dealing with a longer (enduring) temporal process, the other with shorter (transient) ones.[9] Both these, however, when considered from the standpoint of experiential time, or temporality, are germane to the levels of time orders. The longer process is the temporal field of life trajectory, whereas the shorter ones are those temporal fields that integrate experiences on the lower levels of temporal orders.

Considered from the standpoint of someone other than the experiencing subject (for example, a psychiatrist), the shorter processes are relevant to the time span of behavioral contexts at the lower levels (see Table 1), whereas the longer process is relevant to the patient's personal history. It is in reference to the latter

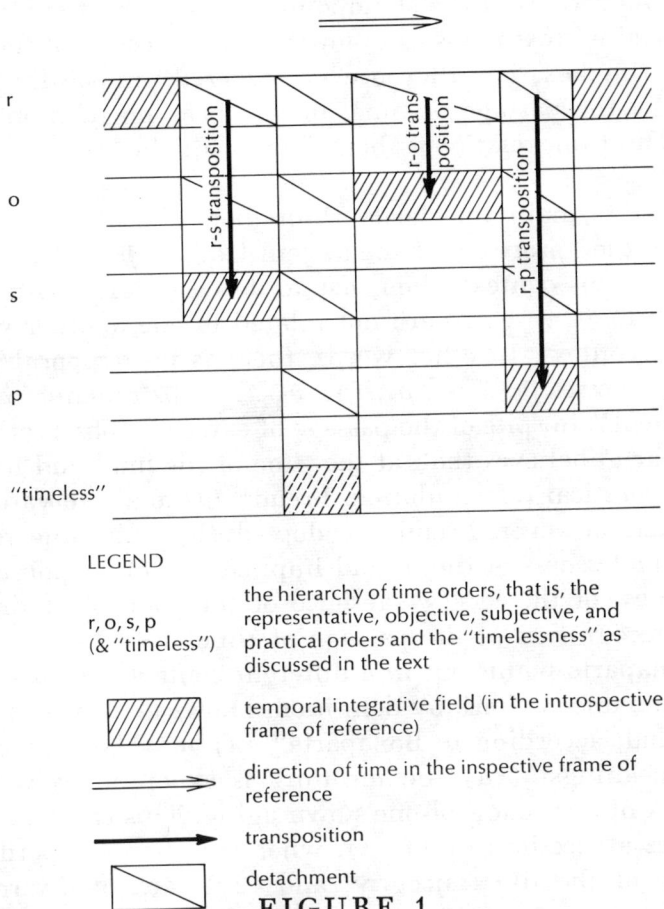

FIGURE 1

that Levenson has reminded us of the change that took place in the fundamental concept of time—from Newtonian to Gibbsian—as dynamic psychopathology developed from the Freudian to the post-Freudian period.[61] Lewis discussed time from the psychoanalytic structural point of view.[65]

The Timelessness of the Unconscious Process and the Discontinuity of the Awareness of Time

Of greater relevance to the subject of this chapter, however, is the fact that both longer and shorter time processes are involved in Freud's well-known premise about "the timelessness of Ucs."[36]

As an initial step in the exploration of levels of temporality in dynamic psychopathology, I would like to attempt an explication of this premise, from the standpoint of our present study.

The original text reads as follows: "The processes of the system Ucs are timeless: i.e., they are not ordered temporally, are not altered by the passage of time, in fact bear no relation to time at all. The time relation is bound up with the work of the system Cs."

In order to maintain clarity throughout the discussion, let us designate the "processes of the system Ucs" as $\bar{p}_1, \ldots, \bar{p}_n$. Timelessness in this context, then, has to do essentially with the following: (1) $\bar{p}_1, \ldots, \bar{p}_n$ are not related to one another within a temporal context. In other words, there is no temporal integration of processes $\bar{p}_1, \ldots, \bar{p}_n$; (2) $\bar{p}_1, \ldots, \bar{p}_n$ remains unaltered (permanent), in spite of the passage of external (observer's) time.

Bonaparte[6] believes that, at the time of his final and most dramatic theoretical reformulation, Freud[38] made a reservation as to (2). Later, however, Freud[39] readopted (2), this time referring to the timelessness of the id and implied two other points in the timelessness of the id: (3) absence of the concept of time; (4) lack of recognition of the passage of time.

As Bonaparte points out in a different context, (3) is a truism, in that the unconscious, by definition, knows no concepts. On the other hand, according to Bonaparte,[7] (4) may have several different meanings: (4a) the meaning is synonymous with (1); (4b) lack of awareness of one's own aging. This can be regarded simply as a specific case of (1), where the temporal order is at the level of the life trajectory; and (4c) lack of awareness of passage of time during the course of ongoing processes $\bar{p}_1, \ldots, \bar{p}_n$ themselves. Among these, the only real addition is (4c). Though the temporal nature of $\bar{p}_1, \ldots, \bar{p}_n$ has already been suggested in the term "processes," experience of the processes themselves is now explicitly claimed not to accompany awareness of the passage of time while they are taking place.

In order to prevent the apparent redundancy involved in denying awareness of unconscious processes, the statement may be rephrased as follows: though the unconscious processes $\bar{p}_1, \ldots, \bar{p}_n$ are to be taken as equivalent of conscious processes (designated respectively as $p_1, \ldots, p_n$—as extrapolated in the nonreporting range of the working mind[81]—), their conscious counterparts $p_1, \ldots, p_n$ are behavior processes (or processes of experience) in which the subject does not have any awareness of the passage of time.

But what are these processes ($p_1, \ldots, p_n$) that are lacking in awareness of the passage of time? Freud's theory of dream interpretation,[33] in particular his discussion of wish fulfillment, indicates that they are phases of the gratification of motivational behavior, induced by (infantile) need tension. That is to say, the timelessness of $\bar{p}_1, \ldots, \bar{p}_n$ is equivalent to the experiential aspect of the consummatory phase of the act (the latter in the sense of Table 1).

This interpretation of timelessness in psychoanalytic theory is supported by the lucid exposition of related issues by Arlow.[4] In it, he explains timelessness as being "the diminution of self-consciousness [that is] characteristic of the ego [when it is] immersed in gratifying experience." Along with B. D. Lewin,[63] Arlow points to the specific relevance here of the satiation of oral needs as "the earliest experience of satiety as timeless," this being the essential meaning of "eternity," as sought by suicidal individuals, mystics, and drug addicts. (See also Rado.[81])

What follows immediately from this premise is that the unpleasurable experiences of frustration, anxiety, and the like awaken the motivational phase (that is, appetitive phase).* Both self-awareness and the awareness of the passage of time are then simultaneously prodded into existence.

But what about those appetitive-phase behaviors that lead to the consummatory phase $p_1, \ldots, p_n$? Do they not, following their repression, constitute the significant part of those unconscious processes that are seeking immediate gratification? Further, being integrated in the practical time order (see Table 1), are they not thereby detached from the higher context of the temporal field?

As we have seen, the experience cannot be regarded as timeless, because integration on the practical order accompanies it, as the result of which it is intermingled with the feelings of need, impatience, anticipation, and so forth. One could speak of the repressed behavior of the appetitive phase as timeless unconscious processes, but only if one chose to neglect the specific temporality

---

* The division of a motivational behavior pattern into appetitive and consummatory phases has been a useful concept in ethology. Tinbergen[101] credits the concept to Craig.[16] The counterpart of this ethological concept is to be found in Mead's study of the temporal organization of human behavior.[70] Some aspects of Mead's ideas were incorporated into Levy's handling of the "act as a unit" in psychodynamics,[62] which will be referred to later. Such division of motivational behavior is now found to be quite relevant to the levels of temporality.

inherent in practical-order integration. Therefore, if one considers the meaning of "timeless" more strictly, the timeless unconscious process can apply only to the final phase of the repressed acts, that is, to their consummatory phase. This also seems to be the meaning of the term as used by Freud,[33] Arlow,[4] and B. D. Lewin.[63] To summarize our interpretation of this premise: The repressed motivational process, under the dictate of the primary process, is the repressed act (integrated on the practical order)— both its appetitive phase and its consummatory phase. It is the latter that is the timeless unconscious process.

From the standpoint of the time order, therefore, psychoanalytic investigation divides the act into two phases of different nature: the appetitive phase as temporally integrated (awareness of the passage of time intermingling with the feeling of need, effort, and so on) and the consummatory phase as lacking temporal integration (that is, taking place without awareness of the passage of time).

The time sense (more specifically, awareness of the passage of time) is, according to Arlow,[4] switched on and off, depending on the level of self-awareness. One clinical example he offers is an interesting pattern of the sequence of the patient's verbalization during the analytic treatment. Perhaps this can be taken as a magnified demonstration, akin to a high-speed film presentation of a fast process, of what is happening in a more elusive fashion in the stream of consciousness.

Arlow's discussion of this question may be summarized as follows:

1. It is an illusion that self-awareness operates constantly and always at the same level. It is, in fact, a highly intermittent function, being sometimes stimulated to intense activity by situations of frustration, unpleasure, pain, and anxiety.
2. A series of apparently successive instances of self-awareness, organized into a continuity by our inner perceptual activity and correlated with memory, furnish the data in terms of which we conceptualize the individual as an entity operating in extended time.
3. It is the illusory conception of a succession of moments of self-awareness, all equal in duration, that forms the subjective basis for the concept of a continuous time of equal units. Projected and materialized in terms of the motions of concrete objects, this basically egocentric concept gives rise to practical and poetical representations of the passage of time, such as "a river of time flowing."

I believe that there is a fundamental disruption of continuity in the awareness of time as well as an essential heterogeneity of such awareness, depending on the ongoing field of integration. Nevertheless, it seems that the idea of a continuous and homogeneous flow of experiential time is more likely to be adopted in psychopathology. This is in spite of the fact that James's[52] concepts of the stream of consciousness and of time awareness were not actually that oversimplified. The process by which time sense is evolved through successive instances of self-awareness may be depicted in our transpositional scheme as shown in Figure 1.

Symbolism of Time

While the course of consciousness proceeds by way of fluctuating levels of self-awareness, the time sense is switched on and off intermittently. Arlow[4] does not explicate the plurality of levels of self-awareness; nor does he mention whether or not there are levels of time sense when it is functioning. It is possible that Arlow's discussion of the symbolism of time might have some bearing on levels of temporality.

Symbolism of time has been a central theme in the discussion of temporality in psychoanalytic literature.[4, 5, 7, 14, 21, 47, 51, 71, 72, 89]

The symbolic use of time revolves importantly around "time-as-father" (for example, Kronos*)—that is, time as the "frustrator of anal and oedipal wishes"—and "time-as-mother" (Horae)—that is, as the "frustrator of the oral wish." "Time-as-mother" is thus to be taken as referring to the integrative field of the appetitive phase (on the practical order), its prototype being the experience of a hungry infant.

Erikson has suggested that the infant's achievement of basic confidence, which accrues from the integrative experience of this particular temporal field, is closely tied to the genesis of basic trust, as the attitude toward futurity that lies at the core of the healthy personality.[21] His epigenetic chart indicates that this basic trust is the primordial form of temporality (that of the practical order, in our concept); it later develops into the temporal perspective (of the order of historical perspective, in our concept) as a constituent of ego identity.

Though the baby remains, during the period of growth under discussion, a passive participant in the integration of the appeti-

* The equation of Kronos and Chronos is, however, not altogether supported philologically.[11, 47]

tive phase, active participation in or control of that integration emerges when the "frustration of anal wishes" is at issue. Such active participation is to be found either in so-called sphincter control or in a variety of acts of primordial self-assertion that emerge during this period. Parental frustration here consists of interfering with the infant's own temporal integration in the name of an externally imposed schedule, which demands compliance from what would otherwise be the infant's own schedule. The course of events involves the integration of (or the refusal to integrate) the act, within the context of a segment of social time; the relevant time order is the transitional level between the subjective and the objective orders.[1, 47, 53]

The temporal field of integration during the frustration (that is, appetitive phase) of the oedipal wish is that of the time order of life trajectory. Though the child is not old enough to marry his mother, neither will she remain unaging up to the time the child is old enough to be eligible to do so. Reinforcing the symbolization at this level is time as the symbol of death (or castration)—that is, as the ultimate point in the primordial life trajectory, due punishment for the death wish raised against the father.

Regardless of the fact that higher level orders integrated the situations of "anal and oedipal frustration," repressed ideation with regard to both must be understood as being integrated at the practical order. That is to say, the ideation is detached from its higher context and represented by the terminal chain of constituent acts (both appetitive and consummatory phases).

Distortion of Speed of Passage of Time—Various Meanings of That Speed

One question discussed with great frequency in relation to psychopathology is that of awareness of change in the speed of the passage of time. Whatever hypothesis may be put forward about the underlying processes, there are no grounds for assuming that the time that is passing in these different experiences is identical with a hypothetical flow of time that is continuous and homogeneous.

It is often suggested that comparison between awareness of the passage of experienced time and awareness of the passage of public (external world) time is at the heart of such an experience. If so, this psychic process of comparing would hold for the temporal-integrative field only at the level of objective order or at that of representative order (especially life trajectory). The reason for this is that external time, as a referent for psychic correlation (whether it take the form of comparison, interference, juxtaposition, or compliance), is available only in these particular integrative fields.

At the level of the practical and subjective orders, where such a correlation is not feasible, a sense of slowness in the passage of time cannot be anything other than a feeling of impatience about the progress of the event in which the person is involved. The feeling can have no genuine reference to speed per se. Because, at this level, there is no distinction among the temporalities of actor, action, object, and world, there cannot be any comparison between public time and personal time.

Boredom is a phenomenon closely related to impatience. It is known to be linked with the experience of having the subjective feeling of time lengthened—without, and sometimes against, one's own wishes in the matter. Fenichel in his classical paper suggested that

> boredom is characterized by the coexistence of a need for activity and activity-inhibition, as well as by stimulus-hunger and dissatisfaction with the available stimuli. The central problem here is the inhibition of the drive to activity and the inhibition of the readiness to accept the craved-for stimuli.[26]

The meaning of this theoretical position becomes clarified when Fenichel rephrases it through the hypothetical thinking of a child who is crying out of boredom:

> I am excited. If I allow this excitement to continue, then I shall get anxious. Therefore, I tell myself, I am not at all excited; I don't really want to do anything. Simultaneously, however, I feel I do want to do something; but I have forgotten my original goal and do not know what I want to do. The external world must do something to relieve me of my tension without making me anxious. It must make me do something, but so that I shall not be responsible for it. It must divert me, distract me, so that what I do will be sufficiently remote from my original goal. It should accomplish the impossible, afford a discharge without drive-action.[26]

If subjective conditions prevent external stimuli from being experienced as tension-releasing, Fenichel points out, time passes slowly. The time disturbance can thus be either secondary to boredom—that is to say, its consequence—or else it can be primary and dispose the person to boredom. The latter is the case with those who sexualize their time experience; this is found in certain anal characters.[47] The meaning of inhibition in boredom was further clarified by Bieber.[6] In this respect, boredom is like impatience, primarily an issue of temporal integration at the level of the practical-subjective time orders.

What emerges, within our context, as a salient difference between the mode of temporal integration at the practical-subjective orders and that at the higher time orders was set forth by Freud.[35] He pointed to the ability to delay—that is, drive control—as the crucial aspect differentiating temporal integration under the dictates of the reality principle from that under the dictates of the pleasure principle. As Rappaport[84] has suggested, inability to delay is closely connected with boredom and other related disturbances in time experience. It is felt, however, that the two modes of temporal integration with regard to the issue of delay are not in themselves sufficient to explore the character of the time experiences.

At the level of the subjective order, as has been noted, it is not yet possible to speak of temporality as independent of the sequence of acts in progression. Clock time, therefore, and calendar time constitute public time as integrated, respectively, at the level of the objective order and at that of the representative order. This means that there is a basic difference in the meaning of these two public time scales, experientially speaking, even though clock time and calendar time do not represent any essential differences in the time reckoning of a scientist (or when used as the time scale in the observational frame of reference). The experience of time passing (or having passed) quickly, for example, while one has been absorbed in interesting work or in entertaining a charming visitor, is different in meaning from time's fast passage as experienced by Arlow's patient, who said that "the summer passed in the blink of an eye."[4] The former represents an experience integrated at the level of objective order, whereas the latter experience is integrated at the level of the life trajectory.

On the other hand, the historical perspective of temporality is not a field in which we can compare the passing of public and experiential time—with the exception of one's own life trajectory, for which the historical perspective may provide the context. Such an experience as "Society changes so fast" (the experience of a man living in that history, rather than that of a man studying it) has to do with a sense of the discontinuity of the social ethos within the context of that person's life trajectory rather than with his internal experience of the speed of historical time per se.

Death as the eventuality of the life trajectory has already been mentioned. The meaning of "eventuality," in terms of temporality (or experiential time), however, naturally depends on the subject's conception of his own life. His life trajectory may extend, in his eyes, beyond his actual life, so that the field of integration on the order of life trajectory will therefore include the posthumous phase. Such an integration often becomes the carrier of intense emotional motivation, particularly by way of repression. The extended life trajectory becomes represented by an unconscious act, which corresponds to the terminal chain of integration in the life trajectory.

Clinical reports indicate that the experience of unconscious temporal integration, when it takes place in this fashion in the practical order, sometimes distorts the experienced speed of time. For instance, slowing down may correspond to the experience of impatience. An obsessive woman patient of Scott's complained that she was living "so slowly" and that time dragged.[90] Analysis revealed her "unconscious desires to reach her deathbed, to be with her dead sister so that she could undo the harm she had done to this sister." The slowness of time, as integrated on the practical order, slowly disappeared as the patient became conscious of the need for expiation. In thus becoming conscious, the integration is regarded as being placed back in the extended life trajectory.

Scott reported on a man of forty, who had become depressed after having had an anesthetic during which he thought he might die and thus be with a woman, now dead, whom he had once loved.[90] The unconscious meaning of living on was that of approaching death, at which point he would come face to face with the woman he had deserted, as well as his mother, whom he also felt he had deserted. According to Scott, the conflict in this patient between omnipotent fantasies of rolling time back (or of reversing what had happened) and the passage of real time produced the experience of quickening time—through, that is, the comparison of experienced and public time.

Fearful anticipation as the primordial temporal experience of integration in the practical order might have been the basic meaning of the supposed "quickening," in this case, in a way analogous to impatience being converted into slowing. Such fearful anticipation is inherent in the act of flight (back to the past), which is unconsciously integrated at the level of the practical order as the terminal chain of the extended life trajectory. But extended life trajectory can also induce the experience of living forever. Eternity, then, means not an endless flow of time, but rather timelessness of gratification. In the latter instance, the extended life trajectory is represented, in the unconscious practical order, by the consummatory phase of the act of the terminal chain.

Disintegration of the Hierarchy—Sustained Detachment from the Higher Context

Rado maintained that the primary constituent of the motivational organization of depression is "regressive yearning for the alimentary security of the infant."[82] There are, in his formulation, two other constituents: alteration of mood to that of sustained gloomy repentance and a struggle among excessive emotions, in which submissive fear finally defeats coercive rage. This points to a prevailing integration at the level of the practical order (the search for so-called oral gratification). In terms of levels of temporality, one can then guess at (1) the experience of impatience as the primordial temporal feeling, which is expressed as the slowing of time; (2) some manifestation of the detachment of the integrative field at the practical level from such fields at the higher levels.

Some basic questions of the distorted experience of time in the depressive state were enumerated and discussed by Erwin Straus in his classical phenomenological contributions.[96, 97] "Within the developing whole of our life history, we experience our existence in each moment as growing or shrinking, advancing or standing still." This "standstill of becoming" is regarded as inducing the maximum discordance between personal time and clock time and that discordance as serving to explain, in the main, the distorted experience of time.

Expressions of alienation from one's personal past (for example, "I cannot remember yesterday morning," as meaning "It no longer belongs to my life" or "Everything seems ages ago") or from a personal future (for example, "The future to me is remote. I feel hopeless. Before, I could look for the future, but I can't now. There's something that won't let me.") are indicative of the standstill of becoming. The latter is then quite close to our concept of the detachment of the lower integrative fields, especially the one at the practical order level, from the context of integration on the life trajectory.

"Time doesn't seem to move at all" can be taken as an expression both of alienation from the time of personal becoming (that is, the detachment) and of the ensuing alienation from world time, inasmuch as the latter has lost its integration into personal time. Levy's discussion of his patient, a woman subject to depressive episodes most of her life, sheds important light on the problem of loosening and of eventual detachment from the higher temporal-integrative field.

There might be full interest and enjoyment in the theatre, during a visit to an art museum, listening to a concert, purchasing a gift and during any number of social events. There were also positive feelings on receiving letters of appreciation, a response fairly frequent in her work for social agencies. As soon as any one of these particular episodes was over, however, she lapsed back into her depressive state. Her pessimistic attitude returned, as well as her feelings of worthlessness and obsessional thoughts about suicide, an act she attempted several times.[62]

Levy explains this way of experiencing gratifications (which is also to be found in presumably normal persons), from his standpoint of the act as an operational concept in psychodynamics, as follows:

The feeling that arises in each episode, however gratifying at the time, is almost completely transitory. I wish to bring to your attention *a kind of weakness in the cumulative value of feelings that arise in acts of the same relevance. They do not mesh; they are disparate events bound only by a cognitive thread* (italics mine—Y. T.).

Each of the gratifying social experiences enumerated above was temporally integrated, in the main, at the level of objective order; it was certainly not integrated at that of the practical order. What is, however, the "weakness in the cumulative value of feelings" to which Levy refers above? Our interpretation is that this indicates that the integrative field of life trajectory is losing its ability to serve as the context of integrations at the lower time orders. We also suggest that that loss presents an intermediary stage, leading to the sustained detachment of the integrative field of practical order from that of the life trajectory.

Another mode of detachment of lower temporal fields from that of the life trajectory is indicated in the adaptive pattern of a juvenile delinquent, as discussed by Kardiner: "He does everything for the moment; every activity is disconnected from everything else. 'Having a good time' seems an end in itself."[55] This boy, however, is sufficiently capable of integrating his experience on the objective order to be able to participate in the social life of a local gang. A corollary of this detachment is impoverishment with regard to those meanings and values of living that can be integrated into one's life only within the integrative field of the life trajectory. This boy

> can give meaning to, and relate in a very primitive way to, only a small segment of the stimuli [in the sense of cues for an adaptive challenge] and situations that reach him. The rest remain meaningless and unstructured. Hence, the constant complaint of boredom, which reflects a good deal of unengaged potential interest.

What differentiates the detachment of a depressed person from that of a juvenile delinquent? Why is the slowdown of time experienced in certain cases of depression and not in others? Such factors as the different routes by which detachment is reached and the impact of the prevailing mode of emotional integration, such as coercive rage or guilty fear, may be among the relevant ones. But our knowledge of the hierarchy under discussion is so far too meager for us to be able to answer these questions about nosological specificity.

A more pressing problem, perhaps, is arriving at an understanding of the hierarchy of temporality in relation to the patterns of human adaptation. According to Erikson, a crisis in human developmental adaptation introduces an element of time diffusion.[25] To surmount this, a historical perspective becomes available as the subject's newly acquired temporal-integrative field. Erikson's epigenetic concepts suggest how germane the temporal-integrative field may be to the changing tasks of human adaptation. Temporal integration is, after all, the integration of experience and behavior in the social milieu. The hierarchy of time orders, as a determinant of adaptive patterns rather than of nosological entities, seems also to be in keeping with a contemporary trend in psychopathology.[55]

In order to apply the concept of hierarchy directly to the study of the distortion of temporality in schizophrenia, as so dramatically presented in Fischer's pioneering work,[27] the special function of interpretation—ability to penetrate the schizophrenic language and thought—is required. This is perhaps what was implied by Schilder, when he said:

One cannot help but feel that many of these protocols of Fischer's have a more or less artificial character. They are not merely descriptions of experience the patients had, but they express in a symbolic way the feelings of the patients that their libido has withdrawn from the changing experiences concerning the outside and inside world. These time-disturbances are further away from the immediate experiences than the time-disturbances observed in depressive cases and in depersonalization cases. But it is important that the patients use a time symbolism.[89]

A schizophrenic experience of time reported by Bergler and Róheim[5] suggests the existence of a symbolic relationship between time and oral trust, such as we touch on elsewhere in this chapter. A schizophrenic patient of Dooley's once complained that everything happened "so fast she didn't know where she was."[19] The patient explained that her powers of synthesis were inadequate and that the time units therefore needed both to be made smaller and to come in slower succession. The patient fragmented the temporal experience, withholding her attention from large parts of both past and present experience, that is, evincing detachment.

An ingenious, statistically designed study by Melges and Fougerousse also found fragmentation of temporal perspective among schizophrenics and severely delusional patients.[73] The inventory used, however (a modification of the one devised by Hoffer and Osmond),[50] does not permit us to obtain an unambiguous picture of the meaning of the time perspective in terms of the time order levels.

Dooley has also commented on the meaning of "turning time back," or "turning the world back," as these expressions are used by many psychotics.[19] The patient mentioned above needed to turn time back in order to be able to synthesize the rapidly flowing stream of external events with the strongly stimulated flow of internal desires and thus to feel herself master of both—that is, overwhelmed by neither. Dooley thinks that to "turn time back" means not only to return to that point in the patient's life at which the catastrophe had not yet occurred, but also, in some cases, to re-establish a synchronism that has been lost in the rush of succeeding events. The former, one might say, constitutes flight within the temporal-integrative field of the life trajectory, whereas the latter may be no more than an effort to restore a lost synchronism on the objective order.

In early infantile autism, the "as if" attitude that is discussed in the following section is lacking.[54] The schizophrenic child, according to Goldfarb,[43] is committed to an existence in which he does not concern himself either with delays in gratification or with boundaries of time and space. (Time here means the temporality of the objective and representative orders, as Goldforb's report refers to the schizophrenic child's inability to accept such institutional subdivisions of time as school time or meal time.) Basically, this stems from the child's primordial anxiety, which in turn is the consequence of his inability to give form and meaning and, more importantly, predictability to his experience. Such primary perceptual-conceptual incompetence, and the ensuing impairment in organizing meaning in the world and in communication, is reflected in the delayed auditory feedback experiment.[44] One aspect of the tremendous challenge for the therapist who is treating a schizophrenic child, as discussed by Goldfarb,[43] is the task of stimulating and guiding the child to learn an adaptive pattern that is then to be integrated into the field of the objective and representative time orders. (See also Ekstein.)[23]

In his contribution to the conjoining of psychoanalysis and historical science, Erikson[25] has pointed to the importance of historical perspective in the adaptive patterns of an individual and to the pioneering concepts, in this regard, of Mannheim.[69]

Lifton's methodology for the study of historical perspective in the individual is to approach youth who have been trapped in cultural discontinuities during an ongoing historical phase of a foreign culture—Japan.[67] The types of historical perspective that have emerged in his study are highly reminiscent of the types enumerated by Mannheim as having prevailed in the successive phases of Western thought. Differentiation of life trajectory and historical perspective, however, might have made the discussions in this unusual contribution more cogent than they are.

Eissler[22] refers to Spengler's[92] typology of temporality that characterizes three epochs in Western history: Apollonian, Magian, and Faustian. These three, to a certain extent, have the features of practical-subjective, objective, and representative time orders, respectively.

As Werner,[106] Whorf,[107] Meerloo,[71, 72] Smith,[91] Bergler and Róheim,[5] and Spiegel,[93] among others, reminded us, the comparative linguistic or cultural anthropological dimensions are basically relevant to the meaning of temporality in psychopathology. These areas are, however, beyond the scope of this chapter.

Quantitative and Qualitative Differences among the Time Orders

In an early contribution, Arieti discussed the need for establishing a conceptual differentiation between "anticipation" and "expectation" in psychopathology.[3] The differentiation suggested here is not in terms of Piaget's distinction between "intentional" and "spatial" causalities. Arieti's was rather the difference between "immediate expectancy" (or the ability to foresee certain events while an external stimulus is present) and "distant anticipation" (or the ability to predict future events, in the absence of external stimuli that are directly or indirectly related to them). "Expectancy of danger" is reacted to with fright, whereas "anticipation of danger," which is "not yet an act," is reacted to with anxiety.[38]

According to Arieti: (1) Developmentally, expectation is present during the first year of life, as inferred from the "as-if" attitude of an infant (see von Domarus).[102] Anticipation appears during the anal period. During the genital and latency periods,

> the ability to anticipate the future will develop enormously, and in the early part of adolescence, will expand to include all its implications. . . . In adult life, this future anticipation occupies the greatest part of men's thoughts, and consequently determines the greatest number of men's actions.

The aging individual becomes less and less concerned about the future, and, when senescence arrives, his concerns are practically confined to the present time—the state known as "restriction of the psychotemporal field." (2) Nosologically, senile psychosis and arteriosclerosis are characterized by an intensification of the picture of senescence. Chronic psychoneurotics, who think mostly about the past and little about the future, are described as examples of an "apparent psychotemporal inversion," determined by an escape mechanism. Schizophrenia produces considerable restriction of the psychotemporal field: temporal orientation becomes "more and more similar to that of the narcissistic period—that is, as related to the present time." A delusion, however, particularly that of the early paranoid type, does require the process of anticipation.

Arieti's concept of "psychotemporal field" has much in common with that of the temporal-integrative fields—that is, time orders—discussed in this chapter. Nevertheless, the sketch of Arieti's discussion presented above should suffice to indicate the basic difference between his concept and ours.

His discussion, which is couched in such terms as "immediate" or "distant," "expansion" or "restriction," is focused primarily on variations in the stretch of one single psychotemporal field that holds true in both development and pathology. In addition to postulating different levels, however, and seeking their primordial forms in the epigenesis of the cognitive experience of sequence, our discussion also postulates qualitative differences among the several temporal-integrative fields, as far as the introspective experience of temporality is concerned.

Arieti's discussion is, by contrast, directed primarily toward the quantitative aspect of the psychotemporal field. There are, in his discussion, suggestions as to the qualitative aspects, but these are not made the major criteria of the differences among the variations in the psychotemporal field. Our schema began by first delineating the levels of behavioral context, which hinge very much on the stretch of the temporal integrative field. In spite of the overlap, the difference, or rather the complementarity, still remains.

Restriction of the psychotemporal field to the present does not mean an absolute obliteration of futurity, even though it may mean that futurity in the context of life trajectory is hardly available. It can be seen rather as a mode of detachment from the life trajectory. The patient's psychotemporal field is not only short, but also changed qualitatively, in terms of the predominant level of time order—a qualitative difference that is already suggested in the epigenetic considerations.

Data that in part lend support to the concept of a qualitative change resulting from quantitative change are derived also from a series of experiments by Cohen, Hansel, and Sylvester.[12] They asked the subject to mark off, on a given line, a length that would correspond either to the period of time that had elapsed since certain portions of the subject's past history or to the span that he expected to intervene up to a given point in the future. Both in the rate of increase of the experienced interval and in the difference in scope between the experienced past interval and the anticipated future interval, the lengths beyond one year followed trends different from those of less than one year.

Because the time stretch has to do with the subject's own course of experience, cannot this result be evaluated in the light of the shift of his temporal-integrative field from that of the lower time order (objective order) to that of his life trajectory? In this experiment, the subject had agreed to represent, on a straight line, his image of the course of his time and of the proportion between relevant portions of it. Cohen himself cautions that this is not always an easy thing to do naturally.[11] Taketomo has discussed the helical course of time as a mode of the symbolization of time order at the level of life trajectory.[99]

Nature of the Disintegration of the Levels

In what has preceded, some examples of the distortion of temporality, as one aspect of the disordered adaptive patterns, have been discussed in terms of the hierarchy of time orders. The functional nature of the relationship among the levels, as these are differentiated both quantitatively and qualitatively, was expressed in such terms as "transposition" and "detachment."

Our attempt to describe distortion in temporality by way of a hierarchy of time orders quite closely approaches the concept of pathological "primitivization of the notion of time" as proposed by Werner:

However different in clinical cause and appearance the pathological degenerated ideas of temporality may be, all the regressive changes exhibited have certain formal characteristics in common. The basic factor behind these structural changes is a dedifferentiation of the acting subject and the objective world against him. Through this shrinking of the gap between object and subject, the individual is plunged into a swift stream of events; he more or less loses *the ability to enmesh this flux of activity within a temporal schema*, and thus to fix and order it (italics mine—Y. T.).[105]

There are two major points, however, that differentiate our concept of the hierarchy of time orders from Werner's proposals. First, personal time and world time are regarded by Werner as a fundamental conceptual polarity. On the contrary, my belief is that the interrelation of the two concepts, as well as the many varieties of personal time, requires explanation.

World time—whether it be in the daily range of clock time,

calendar time, or time in the historian's chronology; or in such technical times as astronomical time or the "ultramicro" time involved in submolecular phenomena—is derived from the representative time order. This time order, which is as personal as any other level of temporality, constitutes the substratum of world time, the segmentation of which is made by public timepieces. If public time and personal time had no such common denominator, then the very possibility of comparison or integration of the two would not exist.

On the representative order, a person not only commands his life trajectory and historical perspective as his personal time, but also, whenever necessary, adopts (or reintegrates) world time. This enables him to function in a general way as a member of the social milieu and also as a specialist, utilizing the time axis of the various ranges of world time. Of the total scope of world time, it is only for a limited range that any one person can directly grasp the meaning; in a way, this is analogous to the range of visibility as compared with the total spectral scope of the wavelength. Astronomical time and ultramicro time, such as 10^{-4} sec,* belong to that portion of world time outside the range of the directly apprehendable.

The public segmentation of the substratum that is derived from personal time (hence also the possibility of the interaction of world time and personal time) actually emerges, as the reader will recall, at the level of objective order. "Objectification of time" meant, in Piaget's sense, cognition of sequence as completely independent of the subject's behavior process. But it should be noted that such objectification opens up the possibility that the time order becomes amenable to segmentation by a public timepiece. It was also part of the definition of the objective order that, although the time order has become independent of ongoing behavior, the actual stretch of personal time relevant to the objective order does not go beyond that of the field, as determined by the sequence of ongoing integration of behavior. What differentiates importantly the representative order quantitatively from the objective order is that the relevant range of personal

---

* Dr. Carroll Alley calculated the effects on the Apollo astronauts of two phenomena described by Einstein's relativity equations: (1) time actually runs slower for an object as its speed increases; (2) time speeds up for an object as it moves away from a body (such as the earth) exerting a gravitational force.

The result: during all their missions in space, Lovell and Borman respectively spent 200 and 100 microseconds less time than was recorded on earth—which means that they were paid for more time than they actually worked.[2]

time in the former extends far beyond that of the direct integrative field of ongoing behavior.

When the duration of what is experienced as 1 sec is compared with the duration of 1 sec as segmented by a chronometer, to what order of temporality does the former (that is, the 1 sec of personal time) belong? We try to answer this question by examining to what personal meaning of behavioral integration we can possibly relate the reintegrated 1 sec. It may be related to tapping on a piano,[48] or perhaps to blinking the eyes. Such actions as these, however, when taken in isolation, can hardly be regarded as units of behavior that have been purposely integrated in the subject's interaction with the social milieu. This is despite the fact that they may constitute elements of a significant action, directed toward aesthetic expression, or of a reflex component in a dangerous situation. If we follow the epigenesis and hierarchy of time order in the context of behavior, as we do here, the duration of 1 sec, as personal time, has to be placed outside the hierarchy of the time orders. In Table 1, a category of "functional unit" was given for this aspect of personal time, as segmented without direct relation to the integration of purposive behavior.

In the light of the concepts here presented—namely, that there are several levels of temporality (personal time), that the relation between personal time and world time differs depending on the particular levels, and that world time is itself derived from (personal) temporality, as the substratum to be segmented by a public timepiece—the polarity of world time and personal time appears to be only the conceptual beginning of the issue.

Second, primitivization or regression can be applied only within limits to what we discussed as transposition in the hierarchy. The prevailing temporal integration at a lower time order per se is not synonymous with a disturbance in adaptation. Higher level integration is organized by means of lower level constituents. When the normal subject is involved with lower level constituents, the higher level integration retreats into the background, even though it remains available wherever adaptively necessary. "Disintegration," on the other hand, refers to a condition in which there is a break in the otherwise elastic functional correlation between the levels of the hierarchy; a state of sustained difficulty in adopting one (or more) particular level(s) of the order, even though such adoption is necessitated by the adaptive task.

"Detachment," in our usage, is the loss of availability of the higher contexts of temporal integration, at a time when the ongoing temporal integration is taking place at the level of a lower time order. "Transposition," on the other hand, is the placement of experiential content that had originally been integrated at a higher time order into the temporal-integrative field of a lower time order. Transposition, therefore, rests on detachment from the higher context, which has now been rendered unavailable.

From the psychodynamic standpoint, what do we know of the underlying processes that may produce transposition, detachment and, through either or both, disintegration?

1. Regression. As Dooley said,[19] "yet the almost universal craving to be free of it [time] and to be cut off from objects shows how powerful is the *backward pull into the great reservoir from which the ego emerged—into the id*" (italics mine—Y. T.). The italicized portion depicts transposition to the unconscious practical time order.
2. Repression. Temporal disorientation and amnesia—that is, partial detachments from the context of the life trajectory—are induced in cases of hysteria by repression.
3. Isolation. Freud defined isolation as follows: "When something unpleasant has happened to the subject, or when he himself has done something which has a significance for his neurosis, he interpolates an interval during which nothing further must happen, . . . during which he must perceive nothing and do nothing" (p. 120).[38] (See also Freud, p. 256.)[35] Though an experience that takes place during that interval is not forgotten, it is stripped of its affect, and its associative connections are either suppressed or interrupted. The experience therefore fails to be integrated into the larger context of the sequence of behavior, and to be reproduced during the course of one's mental activity. Such a psychic process is obviously detrimental to the ongoing hierarchic organization of the time orders.

Eissler's discussion of one of his patients elucidates the clinical picture of the outcome of isolation.[22] The patient, a twenty-year-old woman, "lacked the capacity to experience any contents of the present and the past as being connected with each other. Her biography was to her an aggregate of anecdotes." (She experienced partial but severe detachment from the life trajectory.) "It became evident that she had no feeling of a stream of time, but that the process of subjective life was for her an accumulation of disparate time units, of strictly separated and isolated moments." (The "feeling of a stream of time" depends, of course, on temporal integration, and particularly at the life trajectory.)

Isolation was in her instance "not something of which she complained, but was a formal principle of her personality and well-integrated into the structure of her ego. . . . She claimed to be amnesic for the greater part of her life, except for a few events.

Subsequently it became evident that she actually had no such defect but could recall, on the spur of the moment and in detail, the events of the past, even though they had happened many years ago. . . . The past was not represented as an organic whole, which continued to grow or which formed a unit, but consisted of simple experiences, scattered, independent and disconnected. When asked about her past, she faced a collection of disjointed contents."

(The partial detachment may perhaps have been extending to the level of the objective order.)

This patient, a very punctual and intelligent person, had a horror of time; it was only very late that she had learned how to read time. Related symptoms included isolation and "inverted" isolation of emotions; depersonalization and periodic (at the time of ovulation) impulsiveness.

4. Undoing. In compulsive neurosis, or in the traumatic neurosis of wartime, undoing involves repetition—but detached from the context of the life trajectory.
5. Depersonalization and related phenomena. Schilder discussed disturbance in the experience of time, concurrently with his discussion of depersonalization.[88, 89] One important dynamic factor that Schilder found in these cases was fear of death. One example is that of an obsessional neurotic who was fearful that his death might come before he had satisfied his aggressiveness. The patient said,

> I had the feeling that time was flying. I was here one minute and gone the next. I feel like I am talking to you one minute and talking to someone else the next. I have the feeling that time is flying away. I figure how short time is. We die soon. The pictures in front of me never stay; they are always moving. I cannot concentrate on my work. I feel depressed. The thought of time flying depresses me. I know that we all will die in forty or fifty years, yet the idea depresses me.

Death as the ultimate point in the temporal field of life trajectory must have a great bearing on the personal meaning of identity. This is another example of reference to the changed speed of time concurrent with distortion of the temporal field.

Oberndorf's patient virtually replaced his own life trajectory with that his mother had worked out and imposed on him.[78] This all-encompassing, yet nevertheless borrowed, life trajectory was adaptively inadequate as the highest context for the temporal integration of the patient's behavior. His temporal integration at the level of the objective order was, as may well be imagined, full of obsessional features.

Arlow[4] has pointed to the defensive use of déjà vu (with regard to anxiety evoked by a new situation), as well as premonition (with regard to the guilty fear evoked by recognition of having harbored a death wish). The latter has been studied by Stein.[95] Freud's experience of derealization at the Acropolis was similarly a defensive encroachment on the temporal field at the life trajectory.[40]

6. Inhibition. The psychic mechanism that can be responsible for the disturbance in the aspects of temporal integration of an act such as its initiation or completion[6, 62] (see also the discussion on boredom).

Defensive reinforcement of the hierarchy of time orders—Dooley also reminded us that the hierarchy of time orders may be kept intact precisely by the defensive need of the patient.[19] With instructive clinical examples, she has shown that "keeping track of" time—that is, maintaining the integrity of the life trajectory as well as of the objective time order—may be motivated by the desire to avoid the following danger situations: loss of the world of objects; loss of a portion of the mind (and/or the body, especially the penis); loss of identity and/or of the entire body (death); loss of superego approval through failure to perform a task imposed on one; being overwhelmed by sadistic, masochistic, and erotic drives; being drawn back into the mother—that is, into the timeless existence, without identity, of prenatal life. The last two items are the dangers that appear in the regression mentioned under point 1. Intellectualization about time during puberty can be seen as modality of time within the context of defense.

Studies of Temporality in Introspective and Inspective Frames of Reference

This chapter has dealt with the problem of temporality, as studied within the introspective frame of reference, and particularly with such temporality as emerges in the essentially dyadic commiunciation between the patient and the psychiatrist.

The significance of the rapprochement of the dynamic school with the phenomenological school for the study of psychopathology within the introspective frame of reference has been discussed by Ellenberger[24] and Weigert,[104] among others. It was the phenomenological school that made the classical contribution to the psychopathology of temporality, as in the works of Minkowski,[75] Von Gebsattel,[103] Straus,[96] and Fischer.[27] One major problem in the way of this rapprochement lies in the conceptual differences that exist between the two schools, the phenomenology of temporality being closely tied to the philosophical concepts of Husserl, Bergson, Scheler, Heidegger, and Merleau-Ponty, among others.

Though the present work cannot aspire to cover this important field, it is hoped that the hierarchy of time orders, here presented as being inherent in the meaning(s) of temporality, may also have relevance to the meaning(s) of temporality in phenomenological psychiatry. The same applies to temporality as explored by hypnosis.[15] It is also hoped that such relevance will contribute to the rapprochement of these viewpoints, to the extent that they explore temporality in the introspective frame of reference.

The position presented here constitutes an attempt to re-examine temporality from the standpoint of "the ego's need to be aware of itself as experiencing and acting."[19] For this purpose, "the libidinous situation" as the determinant of experiences of time[89] has been considered within the context of the total hierarchy of time orders, as these have developed.

Various hypotheses about the introspective experience of temporality have been proposed in the inspective (or observational) frame of reference, in which some aspects of temporality are treated as the intervening variables, or the psychic correlates, of the observed phenomena. More recent contributions involve such areas as the biological clock, or periodicity; estimates of brief duration, the microstructure of time; temporal distortion, induced by psychotomimetic drugs; and the neuropsychological correlates of temporal integration. Such contributions as those by Fraisse,[30] Goldstone,[46] Fisher[28] Hoagland,[49] Lehmann,[60] and Talland[100] have included a review of the relevant literature.

From the vantage point of psychopathology, what is required of these findings is some stipulation as to the specific aspect of temporality to which they are relevant. Lehmann's attempt does elucidate some significant differences among aspects (i.e., basic modes of experiencing the flow of time), that is, external time calculation, internal time estimation, internal time awareness, and internal time perspective. Even when such differentiation as this is made, however, a single psychopathological time scale is assumed, which is supposedly applicable to all the different modes of experiencing the flow of time. When one adopts this viewpoint it inevitably becomes an unexpected discovery that anxiety, depersonalization, derealization is capable of influencing a person's subjective awareness of time, while still leaving quite intact his objective estimation of time intervals.[10, 13, 60, 73]

In some research, temporality has been studied in relation to a predetermined length of time, which has no direct connection with the spontaneous motivational state of the subject.

For instance, Lhamon, Goldstone, and Goldfarb found, after systematic study of extensive data, that the estimation by schizophrenic patients of 1 sec auditory duration is shorter than that of normal persons.[66] This is a significant contribution to the psychophysical characterization of the nosological group. But in order for this differentiation and the inferred internal tempo to become correlates of the temporality that is involved in a schizophrenic patient's adaptive pattern, the context of temporality itself needs to be worked out far beyond where it has been. The compartment, in Table 1, for the functional unit is thus reflective of the current state, methodologically speaking, of the study of temporality.

Lehmann[59, 60] presented a model of psychological time based on the quantum* of consciousness which he called oligon. This is, to my knowledge, the first attempt by a psychopathologist to present a model of psychological time with the conceptual tools of information theory, an approach also taken by Fogel.[29] Such tools for the study of the formal aspect of communication have proven effective in the experimental exploration of the issues of functional unit (see for a review of the area, Efron[20]). Until Lehmann's model is developed to explain the hierarchy of temporality as discussed in this chapter, relevance of the model to psychopathology also appears to be confined to the functional unit.

Some methods of approach to the contents of communication, on the other hand, have been found instrumental in exploration of the hierarchy, as evinced by the linguistic-cognitive studies discussed earlier. An inventory of temporality taken in this chapter may help to make psychopathology more amenable to communicational research.

Psychological researchers[11, 17, 45, 85, 100] have offered experimental methods for the study of some of the basic issues relevant to temporal integration. The significance of these contributions for psychopathology depends, to a great extent, on the context of temporality available for introspective psychopathology.

A reconsideration of the context of temporality, we believe, is also relevant to such therapeutic issues as have been discussed by Freud[41]—to give only one notable example—Kelman,[56] French and Wheeler,[32] and Novey.[77]

---

* Regarding the quantal concept, see also Bonaparte[7] and Schaltenbrand.[87]

SUMMARY

1. This chapter deals with temporality: time considered within the introspective frame of reference and as a methodological issue in psychopathology.
2. A hierarchy is discussed of four levels of the substratum (called time orders) of the field of temporal integration of experience. The hierarchy is conceptualized in connection with the epigenesis of the behavior patterns.
3. Some recent contributions to the psychology of development and to the study of symbolic communication support this hierarchy of time orders.
4. In order to describe the functional relations within the hierarchy, the terms "transposition" and "detachment" are adopted.
5. Some questions of temporality in dynamic psychopathology are discussed in the light of the hierarchy and its disintegration through transposition and detachment.
6. The meaning of levels of time orders is discussed by delineating the present approach from related contributions in the field.

NOTE: The author wishes gratefully to acknowledge the support of Career Scientist's Award of the Health Research Council, the City of New York.

The author also acknowledges the kind offices of Dr. Jacob Arlow and Dr. Roger Brown, through whom the author could avail himself of two yet unpublished papers: in the first case, Dr. Arlow's own unpublished paper, and in the second case, the doctoral dissertation of Dr. Richard Cromer, his student. The author wishes to express his gratitude for the interested discussions with Drs. Arlow and Brown, as well as Drs. Silvano Arieti, Henry Lennard, David Levy, Warren McCulloch, John Millet, Charles Muses, Edwin Straus, Joseph Schachter, Daniel Schapiro, and Michiko Takaki.

REFERENCES

1. Abraham, K. "Contributions to the Theory of the Anal Character," *International Journal of Psycho-Analysis*, 4 (1923), 400–418. Also in D. Bryan and A. Strachey, trans., *Selected Papers of Karl Abraham*. New York: Basic Books, 1953. Pp. 370–392.
2. Alley, C. In "Relativity: A Matter of Overtime," *Time*, 93 (March 7, 1969), 42.

3. Arieti, S. "The Processes of Expectation and Anticipation: Their Genetic Development, Neural Basis, and Role in Psychopathology," *Journal of Nervous and Mental Diseases*, **106** (1947), 471–481.
4. Arlow, J. A. "A Contribution to the Problem of the Psychology of Time." Unpublished.
5. Bergler, E., and Róheim, G. "Psychology of Time Perception," *Psychoanalytic Quarterly*, **15** (1946), 190–206.
6. Bieber, I. "Pathological Boredom and Inertia," *American Journal of Psychotherapy*, **5** (1951), 215–225.
7. Bonaparte, M. "Time and the Unconscious," *International Journal of Psycho-Analysis*, **21** (1940), 427–468.
8. Bruner, J. S. Personal communication, cited in R. F. Cromer, "The Development of Temporal Reference during the Acquisition of Language," doctoral dissertation, Harvard University, 1968.
9. Brunswik, E. "The Conceptual Framework of Psychology," in O. Neurath, R. Carnap, and C. Morris (eds.), *International Encyclopedia of Unified Science*. Chicago: The University of Chicago Press, 1938. Vol. 1, no. 10. (Combined edition published in 1955.)
10. Cappon, D., and Banks, R. "Experiments in Time Perception," *Canadian Psychiatric Association Journal*, **9** (1964), 396–410.
11. Cohen, J. "Subjective Time," in J. T. Fraser (ed.), *The Voices of Time*. New York: Braziller, 1966. Pp. 257–275.
12. Cohen, J., Hansel, C. E. M., and Sylvester, J. D. "An Experimental Study of Comparative Judgements of Time," *British Journal of Psychology*, **55** (1954), 108–114.
13. Cohen, S., and Mazey, A. "The Effect of Anxiety in Time Judgment and Time Experience in Normal Persons," *Journal of Neurology, Neurosurgery, and Psychiatry*, **24** (1961), 266–268.
14. Cohn, F. "Time and the Ego," *Psychoanalytic Quarterly*, **26** (1957), 168–189.
15. Cooper, L. P., and Erickson, M. H. *Time Distortion in Hypnosis*. Baltimore: Williams & Wilkins, 1959.
16. Craig, W. "Appetites and Aversions as Constituents of Instincts," *Biological Bulletin*, **34** (1918), 91–107.
17. Craik, K. H. "Of Time and Personality," Contribution to the Symposium "Human Time Structure" at the Annual Meetings of the American Psychological Association, Chicago, 1965.
18. Cromer, R. F. "The Development of Temporal Reference during the Acquisition of Language," doctoral dissertation, Harvard University, 1968.
19. Dooley, L. "The Concept of Time in Defense of Ego Integrity," *Psychiatry*, **4** (1941), 13–23.
20. Efron, R. "The Duration of the Present," *Annals of the N.Y. Academy of Sciences*, **138** (1967), 713–729. Art. 2. (Interdisciplinary Perspective of Time.)
21. Eisenbud, J. "Time and the Oedipus," *Psychoanalytic Quarterly*, **25** (1956) 363–384.
22. Eissler, K. R. "Time Experience and the Mechanism of Isolation," *Psychoanalytic Review*, **39** (1952), 21–22.
23. Ekstein, R. "The Space Child's Time Machine: On 'Reconstruction' in the Psychotherapeutic Treatment of a Schizophrenic Child," *American Journal of Orthopsychiatry*, **24** (1954), 492–506.
24. Ellenberger, H. F. "A Clinical Introduction to Psychiatric Phenomenology and Existential Analysis," in R. May, E. Angel, and H. F. Ellenberger (eds.), *Existence: A New Dimension in Psychiatry and Psychology*. New York: Basic Books, 1958. Pp. 92–124.
25. Erikson, E. H. "The Problem of Ego Identity," *Journal of the American Psychoanalytic Association*, **4** (1956), 56–121.
26. Fenichel, O. "On the Psychology of Boredom," (1934), in *Collected Papers of Otto Fenichel*. New York: Norton, 1953–1954. Vol. 1, pp. 292–302.
27. Fischer, F. "Zeitstruktur und Schizophrenie," *Zeitschrift für der gesamte Neurologie und Psychiatrie*, **121** (1929), 544–576.

28. Fisher, R. "The Biological Fabric of Time," *Annals of the N.Y. Academy of Sciences,* **138** (1967), 440–488.
29. Fogel, L. J. "A Note on the Fourth Dimension," *Proceedings of the Institute of Radio Engineers,* **42** (1954), 1699.
30. Fraisse, P. *The Psychology of Time* (1957), trans. J. Leith. New York: Harper & Row, 1963.
31. Frank, L. K. "Time Perspective," *Journal of Social Philosophy,* **4** (1939), 293–312.
32. French, T. M., and Wheeler, D. R. "Hope and Repudiation of Hope in Psychoanalytic Therapy," *International Journal of Psycho-Analysis,* **44** (1963),304–316.
33. Freud, S. "The Interpretation of Dreams" (1900), in J. Strachey (ed.), *Standard Edition.* London: Hogarth Press. Vols. 4–5. (Also published as *The Interpretation of Dreams.* New York: Basic Books, 1955.)
34. Freud, S. "Notes upon a Case of Obsessional Neurosis" (1909), in J. Strachey (ed.), *Standard Edition.* London: Hogarth Press. Vol. 10, pp. 151–249. (Also in *Collected Papers of Sigmund Freud.* New York: Basic Books, 1959. Vol. 3, pp. 293–383.)
35. Freud, S. "Formulations on the Two Principles of Mental Functioning" (1911), in J. Strachey (ed.), *Standard Edition.* London: Hogarth Press. Vol. 12, pp. 213–226. (Also published as "Formulations Regarding the Two Principles in Mental Functioning," *Collected Papers of Sigmund Freud.* New York: Basic Books, 1959. Vol. 4, pp. 13–21.)
36. Freud, S. "The Unconscious" (1915), in J. Strachey (ed.), *Standard Edition.* London: Hogarth Press. Vol. 14, pp. 159–215. (Also in *Collected Papers of Sigmund Freud.* New York: Basic Books, 1959. Vol. 4, pp. 98–136.)
37. Freud, S. "A Note upon the 'Mystic Writing Pad'" (1925), in J. Strachey (ed.), *Standard Edition.* London: Hogarth Press. Vol. 19, pp. 225–232. (Also in *Collected Papers of Sigmund Freud.* New York: Basic Books, 1959. Vol. 5, pp. 175–180.)
38. Freud, S. "Inhibitions, Symptoms and Anxiety" (1926), in J. Strachey (ed.), *Standard Edition.* London: Hogarth Press. Vol. 20, pp. 75–175.
39. Freud, S. "New Introductory Lectures on Psycho-Analysis" (1933), in J. Strachey (ed.), *Standard Edition.* London: Hogarth Press. Vol. 22, pp. 1–182.
40. Freud, S. "A Disturbance of Memory on the Acropolis: Open Letter to Romain Rolland on Occasion of His Seventieth Birthday" (1936), in J. Strachey (ed.), *Standard Edition.* London: Hogarth Press. Vol. 22, pp. 227–248. (Also in *Collected Papers of Sigmund Freud.* New York: Basic Books, 1959. Vol. 5, pp. 302–312.)
41. Freud, S. "Analysis Terminable and Interminable" (1937), in J. Strachey (ed.), *Standard Edition.* London: Hogarth Press. Vol. 23, pp. 209–253. (Also in *Collected Papers of Sigmund Freud.* New York: Basic Books, 1959. Vol. 5, pp. 316–357.)
42. Gifford, S. "Sleep, Time and the Early Ego: Comments on the Development of the Twenty-Four-Hour Sleep-Wakefulness Pattern as a Precursor of Ego Functioning," *Journal of the American Psychoanalytic Association,* **8** (1958), 5–42.
43. Goldfarb, W. "Anxiety and Conflict in Schizophrenic Children," in J. H. Masserman (ed.), *Childhood and Adolescence.* New York: Grune & Stratton, 1969. Pp. 151–162.
44. Goldfarb, W., and Braunstein, P. "Reactions to Delayed Auditory Feedback among a Group of Schizophrenic Children," in P. Hoch and J. Zubin (eds.), *Psychopathology of Communication.* New York: Grune & Stratton, 1958. Pp. 49–63.
45. Goldstone, S. "The Human Clock: A Framework for the Study of Healthy and Deviant Time Perception." *Annals of the N. Y. Academy of Sciences,* **138** (1967), 767–783. Art. 2. (Interdisciplinary Perspective of Time.)
46. Goldstone, S. "The Perception of Time by Children," in A. H. Kidd and J. L. Rivoire (eds.), *The Perceptual Development in Children.* New York: International Universities Press, 1967. Pp. 445–486.
47. Hárnik, J. "Die triebhaft-affektiven Momente in Zeitgefühl," *Imago,* **2** (1925), 32–57.
48. Hoagland, H. "The Physiologic Control of Judgment of Duration: Evidence for a Chemical Clock," *Journal of General Psychology,* **9** (1933), 267–287.

49. Hoagland, H. "Some Biochemical Considerations of Time," in J. T. Fraser (ed.), *The Voices of Time*. New York: Braziller, 1966. Pp. 312–329.
50. Hoffer, A., and Osmond, H. "The Relationship between Mood and Time Perception," *Psychiatric Quarterly*, **36** (1962), Supp. 87–92.
51. Hollós, S. "Über das Zeitgefühl," *Internationale Zeitschrift für Psychoanalyse*, **8** (1931), 421–439.
52. James, W. *The Principles of Psychology*, Vol. 1. London: Macmillan, 1891. Esp. Chs. 9 & 15.
53. Jones, E. "Anal-Erotic Character Traits," in E. Jones, *Papers on Psycho-analysis*. London: Bailliere, Tindall & Cox, 1918. Pp. 664–688.
54. Kanner, L. "Autistic Disturbances of Affective Contact," *Nervous Child*, **2** (1943), 217–250.
55. Kardiner, A. "The Relation between Frame of Reference and Nosology" (1959), in G. E. Daniels (ed.), *New Perspectives in Psychoanalysis: Sándor Rado Lectures, 1957–1963*. New York: Grune & Stratton, 1964. Pp. 108–123.
56. Kelman, H. "Life History as Therapy," *American Journal of Psychoanalysis*, **15** (1955), 144–162, **16** (1956), 68–78, 145–166.
57. Kleitman, N., and Engelmann, T. G. "Sleep Characteristics of Infants," *Journal of Applied Physiology*, **6** (1953), 269–282.
58. Lashley, K. "The Problem of Serial Order in Behavior," in L. Jeffress (ed.), *Cerebral Mechanisms in Behavior. The Hixon Symposium*. New York: Wiley, 1951. Pp. 121–122.
59. Lehmann, H. "Discussions," in P. Hoch and J. Zubin (eds.), *Psychopathology of Perception*. New York: Grune & Stratton, 1965. Pp. 104–110.
60. Lehmann, H. E. "Time and Psychopathology," *Annals of the N.Y. Academy of Sciences*, **138** (1967), 798–821.
61. Levenson, E. A. "Changing Time Concepts in Psychoanalysis," *American Journal of Psychotherapy*, **12** (1958), 64–78.
62. Levy, D. M. "The 'Act' as an Operational Concept in Psychodynamics," *Psychosomatic Medicine*, **24** (1962), 49–57.
63. Lewin, B. D. *The Psychoanalysis of Elation*. New York: Norton, 1950.
64. Lewin, K. "Defining the 'Field at a Given Time,'" *Psychological Review*, **50** (1943), 292–310.
65. Lewis, W. C. "Structural Aspects of the Psychoanalytic Theory of Instinctual Drives, Affects, and Time," in N. S. Greenfield and W. C. Lewis (eds.), *Psychoanalysis and Current Biological Thought*. Madison: The University of Wisconsin Press, 1965. Pp. 151–180.
66. Lhamon, W. O., Goldstone, S., and Goldfarb, J. "Psychopathology and Time Judgment," in P. Hoch and J. Zubin (eds.), *Psychopathology of Perception*. New York: Grune & Stratton, 1965. Pp. 164–188.
67. Lifton, R. "Individual Patterns in Historical Change: Imagery of Japanese Youth," in *Disorders of Communication*. Baltimore: Williams & Wilkins, 1964. Pp. 291–306.
68. Lipsitt, L. P. "Learning in the First Year of Life," in L. P. Lipsitt and C. C. Spiker (eds.), *Advances in Child Development and Behavior*. New York: Academic Press, 1963. Vol. 1, pp. 147–195.
69. Mannheim, K. "Ideology and Utopia" (1929), in K. Mannheim, *Ideology and Utopia: An Introduction to the Sociology of Knowledge*, trans. L. Wirth and E. A. Shils. New York: Harcourt, Brace & World, 1936. Ch. 4.
70. Mead, G. H. *Mind, Self and Society*. Chicago: The University of Chicago Press, 1934.
71. Meerloo, J. A. M. *The Two Faces of Man: Two Studies on the Sense of Time and on Ambivalence*. New York: International Universities Press, 1954.
72. Meerloo, J. A. M. "The Time Sense in Psychiatry," in J. T. Fraser (ed.), *The Voices of Time*. New York: Braziller, 1966. Pp. 235–252.
73. Melges, F. T., and Fougerousse, C. E., Jr. "Time Sense, Emotion and Acute Mental Illness," *Journal of Psychiatric Research*, **4** (1966), 127–139.
74. Miller, G. A., Galanter, E., and Pribram, K. H. *Plans and the Structure of Behavior*. New York: Holt, 1960.

75. Minkowski, E. *Le Temps vécu*. Paris: d'Artrey, 1933.
76. Murray, H. A. "Drive, Time, Strategy, Measurement, and Our Way of Life," in G. Lindzey (ed.), *Assessment of Human Motives*. New York: Rinehart, 1958. Pp. 183–196.
77. Novey, S. *The Second Look: The Reconstruction of Personal History in Psychiatry and Psychoanalysis*. Baltimore: The Johns Hopkins Press, 1968.
78. Oberndorf, C. P. "Time, Its Relation to Reality and Purpose," *Psychoanalytic Review*, **28** (1941), 139–155.
79. Piaget, J. *The Construction of Reality in the Child*, trans. M. Cook. New York: Basic Books, 1954.
80. Piaget, J., and Inhelder, B. *The Child's Conception of Space*. London: Routledge & Kegan Paul, 1956
81. Rado, S. "The Psychoanalysis of Pharmacothymia (Drug Addiction)," *Psychoanalytic Quarterly*, **2** (1933), 1–23.
82. Rado, S. "Psychodynamics of Depression from the Etiologic Point of View," *Psychosomatic Medicine*, **13** (1951), 51–55.
83. Rado, S. "Hedonic Control, Action-Self, and the Depressive Spell," in P. Hoch and J. Zubin (eds.), *Depression*. New York: Grune & Stratton, 1954.
84. Rappaport, D. *Organization and Pathology of Thought*. New York: Columbia University Press, 1951.
85. Renner, K. E. "Temporal Integration: An Incentive Approach to Conflict Resolution," *Progress in Experimental Personality Research*, **4** (1967), 127–177.
86. Schachtel, E. "On Memory and Childhood Amnesia," *Psychiatry*, **10** (1947), 1–26.
87. Schaltenbrand, G. "Consciousness and Time," *Annals of the N.Y. Academy of Sciences*, **138** (1967) Art. 2 (Interdisciplinary Perspective of Time), 632–645.
88. Schilder, P. *Selbstbewusstsein und Personlichkeitsbewusstsein*. Berlin: Springer, 1914.
89. Schilder, P. "Psychopathology of Time," *Journal of Nervous and Mental Diseases*, **83** (1936), 530–545.
90. Scott, W. C. M. "Some Psychodynamic Aspects of Disturbed Perception of Time," *British Journal of Medical Psychology*, **21** (1948), 111–120.
91. Smith, M. W. "Different Cultural Concepts of Past, Present and Future: A Study of Ego Extension," *Psychiatry*, **15** (1952), 395–400.
92. Spengler, O. *The Decline of the West*, Vol. 1. *Form and Actuality* (1918), Vol. 2. *Perspectives of World History* (1922), trans. C. F. Atkinson. New York: Knopf, 1926 and 1928.
93. Spiegel, J. P. "Conflicting Formal and Informal Roles in Newly Acculturated Families," in *Disorders of Communication*. Baltimore: Williams & Wilkins, 1964. ARNMD Proceedings. Pp. 307–316.
94. Spielrein, S. "Die Zeit im Unterschwelligen Seelenleben," *Imago*, **9** (1923), 300–317.
95. Stein, M. H. "Premonition as a Defense," *Psychoanalytic Quarterly*, **22** (1953), 69–74.
96. Straus, E. "Das Zeiterlebnis in den endogenen Depression und in der Psychopathischen Verstimmung," *Monatschrift für Psychiatrie und Neurologie*, **68** (1928), 640–656.
97. Straus, E. "Disorders of Personal Time in Depressive States," *Southern Medical Journal*, **40** (1947), 254–259.
98. Taketomo, Y. "Psychological Time," *Proceedings of the Fourth World Congress of Psychiatry*, Madrid, 1966. Amsterdam: The Excerpta Medica Foundation, 1968. Pp. 1528–1531.
99. Taketomo, Y. "An Exploration into Psychodynamics of Time Experience: Helical Structure of Experienced Temporal Dimension at the Level of Life-Trajectory," *Journal for the Study of Consciousness*, **2** (1969), 37–54.
100. Talland, G. A. *Deranged Memory: A Psychonomic Study of the Amnesic Syndrome*. New York: Academic Press, 1965.
101. Tinbergen, N. *The Study of Instinct*. London: Oxford University Press, 1951.
102. Von Domarus, E. "The Specific Laws of Logic in Schizophrenia," in J. S. Kasanin

(ed.), *Language and Thought in Schizophrenia*. 2d ed. New York: Norton, 1964. Pp. 104–114.
103. Von Gebsattel, W. E. "Zeitbezogenes Zwangsdenken in der Melancholie," *Nervenarzt*, 1 (1928), 275–287.
104. Weigert, E. "Goals in Psychoanalysis" (1957) in G. E. Daniels (ed.), *New Perspectives in Psychoanalysis: Sándor Rado Lectures 1957–1963*. New York: Grune & Stratton, 1965. Pp. 253–281.
105. Werner, H. *Comparative Psychology of Mental Development* (1948). rev. ed. New York: International Universities Press, 1957.
106. Werner, H., and Kaplan, B. *Symbol Formation: An Organismic-Developmental Approach to Language and the Expression of Thought*. New York: Wiley, 1967.
107. Whorf, B. L. "The Relation of Habitual Thought and Behavior to Language," in L. Sapir (ed.), *Language, Culture and Personality: Essays in Memory of Edward Sapir*. Menasha, Wisc.: Sapir Memorial Publication Fund, 1941. Pp. 75–93.

[[[6]]]

SYMPTOM, SYNDROME, DISEASE:
A CLINICAL METHOD IN PSYCHIATRY

A. V. Snezhnevsky

If the United States may rightly be called the second motherland of Freudism, then the Soviet Union with full justice may be considered the second motherland of traditional clinical psychiatry. A synthesis and a further development of classical French, German, English, and Russian psychiatry is being carried out by Soviet psychiatry.

The American psychiatrists usually call clinical psychiatry phenomenological. This is so only partially and only in relation to one stage of the development of clinical psychiatry. They have in view the studies of Karl Jaspers and his followers—psychopathologists and pathopsychologists. In recent times, the studies in question are of an existential character. Previously, dynamic theories prevailed in psychiatry.

Phenomenological theories in science are those that limit themselves to the description of external aspects of phenomena and do not attempt to investigate the internal reasons conditioning the different properties of these phenomena. Dynamic theories, on the contrary, do not limit themselves to the description of external sides of phenomena, but attempt to disclose internal causes, conditioning the corresponding properties of phenomena. In any scientific discipline, depending on the complex conditions, phenomenological theories may prevail on one level and dynamic ones on another level.[1]

In psychiatry, dynamic theories were prevalent. But, in the past as well as at present, they were not all identical; the psychoanalytical theory of Freud and the psychobiological theory of Adolf Mayer are dynamic theories. Dynamic theories are being developed in Soviet psychiatry, and in particular the clinicopathogenetic theory, which is rather widespread. This theory consists in interpreting the manifestation of diseases—the clinical picture —as an external expression (a peculiar code) of pathogenetic and pathokinetic mechanisms of the disease. Refined descriptions and studies reveal the nature and development of symptoms and syndromes.

The theoretical basis of contemporary clinicopathogenetic approaches in Soviet psychiatry are the principles of general human pathology. Contemporary original concepts of Soviet pathologists I. V. Davidovsky[3, 4] and S. N. Davidenkov[2] may be presented in the following concise way:

Diseases are special forms of reactions to the environment. They are the same products of evolution as the whole organism, its physiological systems and biological and social potentials. Adaptive variability includes the existence of different forms of disease. Any cause of a disease brings on different manifestations (clinical pictures) only through the evolutionarily formed, or historically predetermined, physiological mechanisms. As a result of infinite reiterations and by a fixation in the posterity, they form stereotypes. Schizophrenia and epilepsy, for instance, possess a very variable inherited development that occurred in mankind long ago, possibly even in prehistoric man.

The human being is a social being, and the etiology of his diseases is always socially conditioned. But the social etiology of human diseases does not coincide with its essence. The etiology of human starvation is social. The essence of the process of starvation is biological. Any external noxious factor sooner or later loses significance in the development of the disease. Causa externa inevitably becomes causa interna. The influence of high temperature in burns usually lasts only several fractions of a second. The subsequent phenomena are a very complicated disseminated chain of physiological, morphological, and other acts that form a stereotype picture of a disease—the clinical picture of burns. Noxious factors cannot begin in the organism nor bring on anything more than it contains in the form of historically developed potentials. Pathogenetic mechanisms of diseases are evolutionarily strictly programmed, as are all biological phenomena. Such programs were formed historically, reflecting the century-old experience of human adaptation to environmental factors. Noxious factors may produce different stereotypes, that is, clinical pictures, of diseases, but moderated through the historically predetermined physiological mechanisms. The clinical picture of any disease reflects the historically trained different functional systems, conditioned by a durative action on the organism of corresponding factors. Whatever the noxious factors may be, they may bring on only a corresponding, in other words, adequate, change in the organism. The organism itself should have internal bases for such changes, that is, a functional readiness, determining the possibility of developing different processes.

In each individual life, the reason for diseases may be absolutely accidental: trauma, infections, carcenogenesis. Contrary to this, the pathogenetic mechanisms of diseases are the priority of a species. They are regular, stable, conservative. The pathogenesis determines the appearance of a process, its cycle and completion. The existence in the organism of definitely constructed and definitely functioning mechanisms condition the possibility or impossibility of developing corresponding pathologic processes. This possibility, as any other biological predisposition, becomes a reality as a result of the action of corresponding external factors.

The relation of causes and sequences is not linear, but always multilateral, structurally complicated processes. The form of causal relations in the organic world is extremely complex. Causes are inseparable from action.

Thus, the action of noxious factors is moderated by the organism by its adaptive mechanisms, formed in the evolutionary process. The clinical picture of disease, the successiveness of its modifications, externally express the chain reactions of the organism. At the basis of pathogenesis lie the profoundly automatized chain mechanisms, acting according to the principle of self-development and self-movement, as do all physiological mechanisms. The chain character of processes is the fundamental principle of pathogenesis. Pathogenesis actually includes two aspects: genesis, that is, the occurrence of pathological phenomena, and kinesis (pathokinesis), that is, the development of the appearing phenomena in the direction of some (general pathological or nosological) stereotype. A dynamic, in relation to chain reactions, development of physiological, morphologic, biochemical reactions, reflecting the functional state of the organism at the moment of illness is related to the closest and oldest anamnesis of mankind, his ontogenesis.

PSYCHIATRIC NOSOLOGY

Along with an individually conditioned manifestation and development of a disease, the community of biological, social, nutritional, and metabolic factors to a certain extent erase the individual variability, giving the disease human traits, those stereotypical mechanisms of development that permit individual diseases to unite into nosological forms.

The nosological independence of a disease is based on the unity of its etiology and pathogenesis. Nosology integrates separate cases and knows only general forms, the stereotype of development. It reflects the objective difficulties of individual and species adaptation. Nosology is not a scholastic simplification of facts. Nosological forms of diseases illustrate the most essential factors, the formation of causal relations. It is impossible to treat an individual patient not having a general concept of the disease as a nosological unit, not knowing general regularities engendering the disease (for example, social, professional, domestic, and geographical factors).

The complexity and ramification of pathogenetic mechanisms condition the most important prerequisite of the extremely variable forms of nosologically independent diseases. Individually and hereditarily conditioned refraction of the influence of the environment on the organism is a most important biological basis of the diverse forms of diseases.

The specificity of nosologically independent diseases is rather relative. Specificity has a relation only to integrative reactions and processes, and not to particular phenomena. Inflammation as an integrative reaction is specific and differs from atrophic, degenerative processes and new growths. Particular processes—tubercular, leprous, syphilitic, brucellous granulomas—quite often cannot be differentiated historically, nor even cytologically. The elimination of infectious from other (noninfectious diseases) is accomplished rather voluntarily, ignoring the principle of relativity. There is not one single symptom or syndrome that would be absolutely infectious. Depending on the economic utilization of adoptive measures (pathogenetic mechanisms) of the organism, in some cases, the action of different noxious factors responds in identical ways, that is, equifinally.

SYMPTOM AND SYNDROME

A disease is a group of pathologic disorders. Any disease, including mental ones, is not expressed in separate, uncoordinated signs or symptoms, but in the form of a syndrome, that is, a typical complex of internally connected symptoms. A syndrome is a system of interconnected typical disturbances of symptoms (elements), which are subordinated to a special regularity.

A symptom beyond this system has no sense.

A syndrome from the point of view of the given moment is static (*status praesens*). From the point of view of the time dynamic, any process, including a pathologic one, is always directed into the future. The development of a disease is accompanied by an increase of symptoms with a change in their interrelationship, as well as in an appearance of new symptoms. This may lead to a modification of the clinical picture of the disease and a transition of one syndrome into another. The cognition of a disease should not be limited to the knowledge of its cause. It is no less important to know the connection of different states (shifts of syndromes) in the disease, the regularities according to which one state is substituted by another.

The cause of the disease and the successive shift of syndromes reflect the pathologic process. The pathologic process determines the character of connections and, vice versa, the character of connections in the state of any pathologic process assumes certain cause and effect relations.

The syndromes and their transformation reflect externally the features of the pathologic changes in the brain activity ("internal origin of diseases"—Maudsley[9]) and regularities of their development ("the logic of the brain process"—Schüle[10]), the pathokinesis of the disease.

The syndromes and their regular shifts shape the clinical picture of the disease in its development. In other words, a disease is expressed in a continuous shift of syndromes, which is an external manifestation of pathogenetic chain reactions. A clinical manifestation of each nosologically independent mental disorder is characterized by a prevalence of some syndromes over others and regularities of their transformation, that is, a stereotypical mechanism in the development of the disease. All diseases, and mental disorders in particular, are characterized by diverse individual deviations. Nevertheless, despite these deviations, the typical prevalence of some syndromes over others, the reiteration of their successive appearance inherent to each separate mental disease is firmly preserved. The latter circumstance permits clinical elimination of separate mental diseases (nosological units).

GENERAL PATHOLOGIC REGULARITIES

A stereotype of a disease may be demonstrated as a general pathologic process, inherent to all diseases. It may also be a nosological stereotype, inherent to separate diseases. Each mental disease, proceeding from the features of its development and consequently irrespective of its nosological position, may be expressed in different disturbances. Consequently, it is necessary to display common regularities for all psychoses. In the past, such regularities were studied by the representatives of the concept of a common psychosis,[5,10] who established that each mental disorder begins with a depression. As the diseases become more profound, depressions are substituted by manic states, then they are transformed into delusional states, and finally they terminate in dementia. The study of general regularities by the followers of the concept of a common psychosis was limited by historical conditions. These investigations were exhausted by studies of only the most serious patients, who were in psychiatric custodial care at that time. Further investigations, in mental outpatient clinics, displayed that all mental diseases in the initial stages of their development have asthenic, affective, neurotic, and subsequently paranoial and hallucinatory disorders, clouded consciousness, and crude organic symptoms. Any pathologic process, once it appears, develops as a chain reaction, preserving at the same time the phases and periods of its development. From modern theories of reliability of technical and living systems, it ensues that in all refusals of work, the system refusing totally will without fail go through all phases of partial refusal. Processes, related to refusals, are continuous in time.[12]

Figure 1 demonstrates the typical syndromes occurring in the course of all mental diseases. They are a scale of gravity of disease, a generalization of mental disturbances; their successive change reflects the general pathologic pathokinesis. In their typical form, the above-mentioned mental disorders should not be identified with the direct expression of the causal action nor with the independent classes of nosological classification of mental disorders. In the development of separate diseases, we usually see regularities common for all diseases. This pertains to the complication of the clinical picture as the disease develops, to the successive transformation of minor, simple, syndromes into more complicated, major, ones.

The concept of minor and major syndromes assumes a different degree of generalization of the pathologic process, an involvement in the disorder of one organ, one system of organs, or several organs and systems. This finds expression in the homogeneity or complexity of the clinical picture.

The clinical picture of any progressive psychic disease, irrespective of the way it proceeds—continuously, in the form of attacks, or periodically, but with the deteriorating quality of remission—will always become more complex as the disease develops. The initially homogeneous clinical state (asthenic, depressive, obsessive, hysterical, paranoial, and so forth) becomes more complex with the development of the disease. A typical example of such a complicating course may serve the systematized hallucinatory-paranoid insanity of Magnan (the contemporary paranoid schizophrenia). As the disease progresses, the homgeneous paranoial state is stereotypically substituted by a more complex hallucinatory-paranoid condition with diverse symptoms of the Kandinsky-Clerambault syndrome. Further on, these states are transformed into paraphrenia. The clinical picture is then composed of delusions of persecution, physical influence, diverse symptoms of psychic automatisms, dreamlike megalomanic delusions, and different degrees of emotional disorders.

A complication of the clinical picture in psychotic states, as an expression of a progressive disturbance of mental activity, is based as well on the confrontation of the clinical picture of depressive and manic phases of a circular psychosis and attacks of schizoaffective psychosis. The clinical picture of attacks in schizoaffective psychosis, unlike the homogeneous picture of manic-depressive psychosis, is, as a rule, a major syndrome. It is usually composed of affective disturbances, dreamlike fantasical delusions, and oneiroid-catatonic disorders.

The existence of complex syndromes is confirmed as well by the effectiveness of therapy by some psychotropic drugs. Chlorpromazine treatment of depressive-paranoid attacks of the schizoaffective psychosis leads to a disappearance or reduction of delusions and hallucinations while the depressions remain untouched or at any rate almost untouched. A prescription in such cases of tofranil will reduce or eliminate the depression, but leaves intact and sometimes even increases the delusions and hallucinations. In both cases, there is a splitting of the complex syndrome into more simple ones as a result of the influence on the separate links of the pathogenesis.

The exacerbation of simple syndromes* (minor or homogeneous) shows that each may become complicated at the expense of any other. For instance, a depression may become paranoid or hallucinatory-paranoid. At the crucial stage of a depressive-paranoid state, oneiroid changed consciousness or stuporous states may appear. Depressive-amnestic states have also been described. The manic syndrome in the course of different diseases is sometimes complicated by the adjoinment of catatonic-oneiroid disorders, confabulosis, expansive-fantastic delusions, delusions of physical influence, phenomena of psychic automatisms. The clinical picture of delirious states changes, becomes complex, if amentive disorders ensue. In asthenic states, depressions and obsessions may occur as well.

As the clinical picture of a psychosis in its development becomes more complicated, another principle of common development appears. A simple phenomena is an outcome in the process of development; it is less developed and is on a lower level compared to more complex phenomena. Complex phenomena are terminal in the same process of development, but more developed on a higher level.

The clinical picture of a psychosis seen at a given moment in a patient is always a product of a previous development of the disease and at the same time contains prerequisites of a further development. The clinical picture of a psychosis that manifests itself in the combination of affective disorders, catatonic-oneiroido features, and fantastic delusions indicates, as a rule, a remittent or intermittent course of the disease. And vice versa, systematized delusions, ideas of physical influence accompanied by symptoms of psychic automatisms, testify to a tendency of a continuous chronic course of the disease. If a recovery or remission sets in, the transformation of the clinical picture takes place in a di-

---

* The simple homogeneous syndromes are the asthenic, depressive, manic, hysterical, obsessive, paranoial, verbal hallucinogenic, syndromes of clouded consciousness, and amnestic ones.

rection opposite to its development. Complex (major) syndromes gradually become more and more simple (minor).

The shift of simple syndromes into more complex ones does not occur chaotically. However complex be the syndrome, it nevertheless continues to preserve the so-called genus belonging. Delusions, oneiroid stupor states, and phenomena of psychic automatisms that complicate the depression possess another quality, differing from those disorders that occur as complicating factors in other states, for example, in paranoial states. The depression in this example remains till the end as a prevalent disorder. The same pertains to the complication of other simple syndromes. But the prevalent disorder, depending on the concrete conditions of the disease development, may for a certain period of time be shadowed by complicating symptoms. For instance, in general paralysis, the depression during the initial period may be so dominant in the clinical picture as to obscure the organic symptoms.

The above-mentioned syndromes were referred to according to their pathological productive structures. But each syndrome, besides the pathologically productive (positive) structures, contains negative elements (destruction, defect, disintegration). Both occur in unity; there is an organic connection between them; they form the peculiar structure of separate syndromes. The idea of an interdependency of the positive and negative disturbances was first proposed and developed by Don D. Jackson.

A clinical study of psychopathologic syndromes shows a correspondence of definite positive disturbances to definite negative ones. Asthenic, affective, neurotic, paranoial positive manifestations correspond to negative disorders in the form of temporary or stable personality disharmony. Hallucinatory-paranoid, fantasiophrenia, catatonic disturbances correspond to phenomena of regression and convulsive and psychoorganic ones, to dementia. (See Figure 1.) However, the negative and positive disturbances are not identical. Negative disturbances may be depicted without or almost without positive ones. The positive symptoms are extremely variable: they depend on the age, sex, mental development, and outcome state of mental activity. The negative symptoms are rather stable.

These data may only be considered as a continuation in the search of general regularities of disturbed mental activity, which was begun by the followers of the concept of a common psychosis

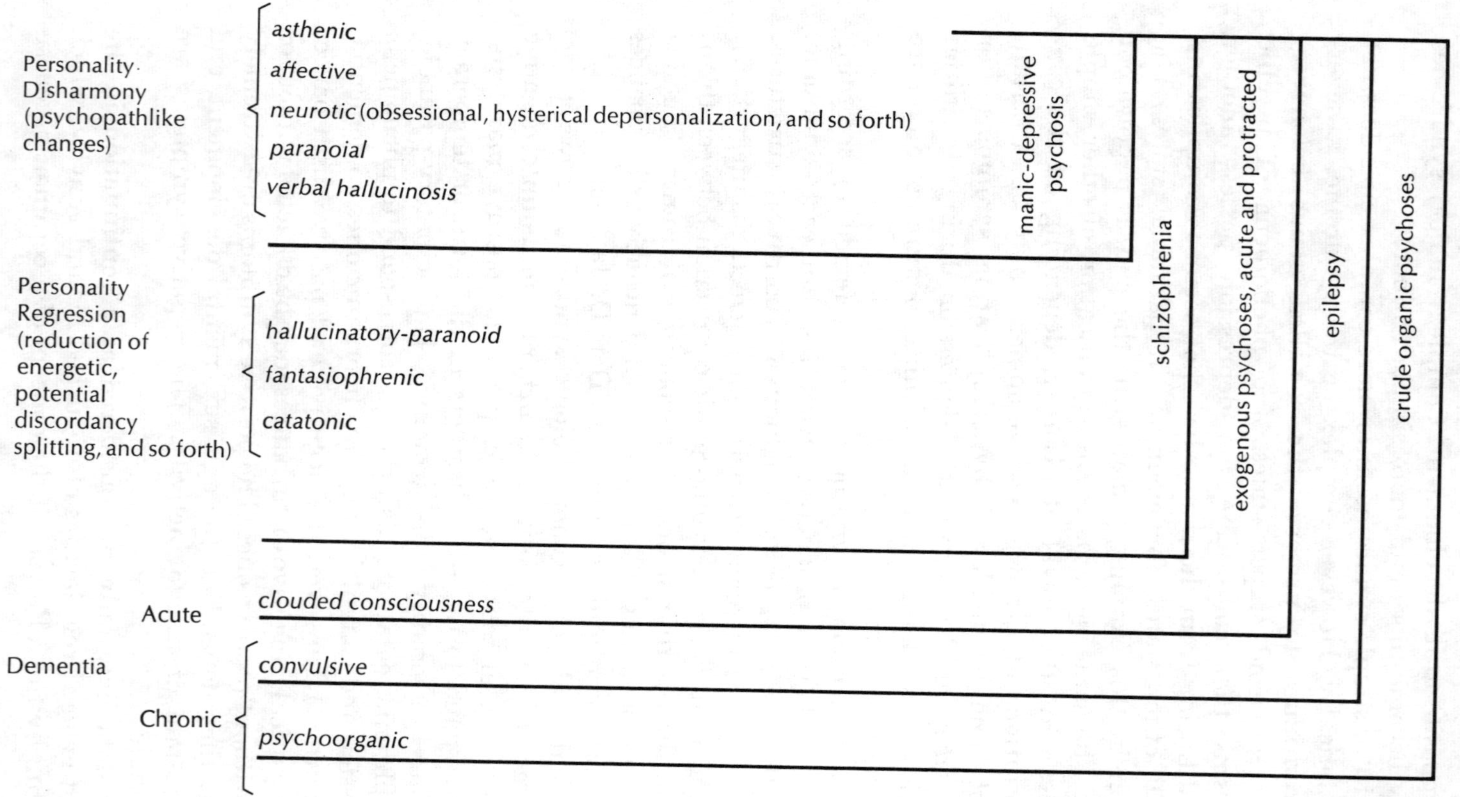

```
                                              ┌─ crude organic psychoses
                                        ┌─ epilepsy
                                  ┌─ exogenous psychoses, acute and protracted
                            ┌─ schizophrenia
                      ┌─ manic-depressive psychosis

Personality          ⎧ asthenic
Disharmony           ⎪ affective
(psychopathlike      ⎨ neurotic (obsessional, hysterical depersonalization, and so forth)
changes)             ⎪ paranoial
                     ⎩ verbal hallucinosis

Personality          ⎧ hallucinatory-paranoid
Regression           ⎨ fantasiophrenic
(reduction of        ⎩ catatonic
energetic,
potential
discordancy
splitting, and so forth)

                     Acute  { clouded consciousness

                     Chronic ⎧ convulsive
Dementia                     ⎩ psychoorganic
```

FIGURE 1

and continued by Emil Kraepelin[8] and Jackson, and is now being developed by Henri Ey.

An attempt to abstract from the immense diversity of nosological and individual forms of mental disturbances has the purpose of depicting disorders common for all diseases, conditioned by internal features of the brain structure and its activity. Human general pathology of diseases has outlined the concept of fever, inflammation, new growths, and so forth. In general psychiatry, such sections in the study of mental pathology do not as yet exist. But the success of such studies depends on the progress in research studies of the pathogenesis of separate psychic diseases. This determines the necessity of investigating the correlations in the pathology of mental diseases of general (general pathological), exceptional (nosological), and singular (individual)—"a universal is that which incarnates the wealth of exceptional, individual, separate . . ."[6]

NOSOLOGICAL REGULARITIES

The general pathologic stereotype of development does not contradict nor cancel nosology. It equips it. In general practice, the psychiatrist does not depict the general regularities of mental pathology, but regularities inherent to the given disease in its actuality; not asthenia in general, but neurasthenia, arteriosclerotia, paralytic asthenia, and so forth; not dementia in general, but epileptic, senile, or oligophrenic dementia.

Each nosologically independent disease has a typical range of syndromes in which it is being exposed (Figure 1). The clinical picture of manic-depressive psychosis is exhausted by affective, asthenic, and obsessive disturbances. In schizophrenia, the range of syndromes is wider. In the course of schizophrenia, there are not only asthenic, affective, obsessive, and hysterical disorders, but paranoial, hallucinatory-paranoid disturbances, psychic automatisms, and paraphrenic and catatonic syndromes as well. The range of syndromes in symptomatic psychoses is even wider (in acute and especially protracted psychoses). Excepting the named syndromes, the clinical picture of symptomatic psychoses is characterized by states of changed consciousness. Even more diverse clinical pictures can be seen in epileptic psychoses, in the course of which, along with convulsive fits and other paroxysms, such syndromes as hallucinatory-paranoid, stuporous, and affective disorders can appear. And finally, the most polymorphic clinical pictures are usually seen in crude organic psychoses. In the course of such diseases, any of the known syndromes can be depicted.

An attempt to display the essence of nosological specificity on a more profound level of vital activity was futile. "The specificity withdraws further and further from us as we absorb ourselves into the cytological details, into the field of electronic microscopy."[3, 4] The morphological brain changes in schizophrenia, for instance, are not only nonspecific, but display an extreme similarity to changes appearing in patients affected by X-rays and radiation.[11]

The studies convened by M. E. Vartanyan and his collaborators[13] have established that patients with malignant forms of schizophrenia as well as patients with Picks disease and those exposed to radiation show similar pathological metabolites in the blood. The pathologic metabolites of all three groups of patients evince (1) marked arrest of development in experimental animals; (2) an antimitotic action; (3) a disarrangement of the normal stress reactions; (4) antoimmune reactions; (5) free radical compounds.

On grounds of the depicted nosological nonspecific disturbances seen on a profound level of vital activity ensue the following conclusions:

1. The nosological specificity of pathology seems to level out on a profound level of vital activity. The questions in mind in such cases are the features of functioning in elementary mechanisms of reliability in living systems.

2. The nosological specificity of a disease is demonstrated not in elementary processes, but in the peculiar disorders of the entire organism.

3. Identical disorders, established in patients with such different diseases, testifies to the fact that general regularities of pathology exist not only for nosologically different psychoses, but for all diseases of man, including mental diseases.

4. It is almost impossible to divide the different diseases (including mental) into functional and organic. Recent morphological studies, done on a subcellular and molecular level, have established that structural changes precede functional disorders, that is, purely functional changes do not exist. The division of mental

disorders into fully reversible and unreversible is also relative. From the general human pathology of diseases, it is known that, after a full recovery from any disease, a complete restitution of the organism to the previously existing physiological state does not occur. The most elementary example of this may be the development of immunity as a result of some infectious disease.

THE INDIVIDUAL REALIZATION OF A DISEASE

From general pathology, it is known that in biological processes even the most insignificant shifts in the complex of causal relationships may give absolutely new results. Individuality, as a qualitative category, is most significant here. It makes the causal connections unique. The individual refraction of pathogenetic factors makes abstract nosological categories absolutely concrete phenomena with a wide range of deviations. In the symptomatology of mental diseases, the features of the pathologic changes in the personality are being fully exposed. The quality of the symptoms in the disease depend on the features of the patient's personality, his individual traits preceding the onset of the disease, and his age. The latter is of special importance and was justly pointed out even by Maudsley.[9] In early childhood, mental disorders, irrespective of their nature, are expressed in the form of motor excitation. Hallucinations and delusions do not occur at this period. In those of preschool age, along with excitation, hallucinations may appear, and in adolescence, delusions are also possible. All psychiatrists are aware that in presenility the clinical picture of all psychoses is characterized by a prevalence of anxiety-depressive symptoms, whereas in senescence by amnestic-confabulatory ones.

Diseases of the past also modify the clinical picture of an appearing mental disorder. The whole personality of the patient, his constitutional qualities and those acquired during life modify the expression of the disease and the outcome of mental activity.

Establishing the individual traits of mental disorders, the investigator penetrates into the general regularities. After that, he returns to the individual traits, their modification and concrete expression in the given patient. This method of investigating is then realized in the diagnosis of the disease.

THE CLINICAL METHOD AND LABORATORY INVESTIGATIONS

Contemporary studies of the nature of any disease on all levels of vital activity (a multidisciplinary study) may be achieved on conditions of evaluating clinically comparable cases. The biggest mistake in the estimation of any laboratory study arises in those cases when the investigations are not preceded by detailed and comprehensive studies of clinical phenomena, by an observation of the natural development of the disease. A clinical study cannot be in a contraposition to a laboratory or experimental study. Any experimental study will be futile if there is no previous study of the phenomena, as it were, at the bedside of the patient. Laboratory investigations should be premised by observations and selections of comparable cases. Clinical studies should precede and subordinate all the laboratory and experimental studies. Observations should occur first, then generalizations ensuing from the observations, then laboratory investigations, and only then modelizing.

REFERENCES

1. Aronov, R. A. *Voprosy Fiilosofii*. N. 1, 1969.
2. Davidenkov, S. N. *Evoluzionno—Genitichkye Problemy V Nevropatologii*. Leningrad, 1947.
3. Davidovsky, I. V. *Obshaya Patologya Cheloveka*. Moscow, 1961.
4. Davidovsky, I. V. *Problema Prichiinosty V. Medizine/Etiologya*. Moscow, 1962.
5. Griesinger, V. *Duschernye Bolezni*. Petersburg, 1867.
6. Hegel. *Sochinenia. Moscow*, 1937. Tom V, Str. 38.
7. Kannabich, U. *Istoriya Psychiatrii*. Moscow, 1928.
8. Kraepelin, E. *Zeitschrift f.d.g. Neurologie u Psychiatrie*. Bd. 62, 1923.
9. Maudsley, G. *Fizyologya y Patologya, Dushi*. Petersburg, 1871.
10. Schüle, G. *Rookovodstvo K. Dushevnim Boleznyem*. Kharkov, 1880.
11. Snesarev, P. E. *Teorytecheskie Osnovy-Patologicheskoi Anatomii Pschitscheskich Bolezney*. Moscow, 1950.
12. Ushakov, I. A. *Voprosy Filosofii*. N. 6, 1967.
13. Vartanyan, M. E. *Vistniik Akademii Medizinskich Naook*. No. 4, 1969.

[[[7]]]

FOLKLORE PSYCHIATRY

Carlos Alberto Seguin

INTRODUCTION

If we try to understand the evolution of psychiatry by comparing the representative publications of successive decades, we may be able to see the change of emphasis and broadening of scope. We may say that, from almost purely individualistic considerations, psychiatry has been moving toward the study of man's pathology in relationship to his world in a more general, more comprehensive perspective. This trend is not exclusively for psychiatry, of course. All the sciences of man have followed the same evolution. The individualistic considerations of the Renaissance have been replaced by an emphasis on the consideration of man as a part of humanity. I can only point to the modern emphasis of such sciences as sociology and anthropology and, in the philosophical field, to the importance given to existential theories in which man is considered, ontologically, as a being-in-the-world. One aspect of this trend has been the collaboration of psychiatry with the related behavioral sciences. Witness the ever increasing cooperation of psychiatrists with psychologists, sociologists, anthropologists, ecologists, and the like.

Two fields of modern psychiatry have been of special interest to the scholars and the researchers: social psychiatry—the understanding of the very complex net of interrelationships of the human group, from family to society—and trans-cultural psychiatry, the relating of the phenomena of each culture to the psychological and psychopathological pictures and their comparison intra-culturally and cross-culturally.

There is, of course, a wealth of work done in these fields, but, curiously enough, one obvious aspect has been neglected—folklore psychiatry.

We might define "folklore psychiatry" as the study of the ideas, beliefs, and practices concerning psychiatric conditions and their treatment and cure as maintained in each culture by popular tradition.

We must very clearly distinguish folklore psychiatry from ethnopsychiatry. Ellenberger[7] defines ethnopsychiatry as "the study of mental illness as a function of ethnic of cultural groups to which the diseased person belongs." Ellenberger differentiates ethnopsychiatry from

1. "*The psychology of populations* which, as Mirollo (1958) has shown, is one of the branches of the descriptive sociology;
2. *Cultural anthropology;* which could be considered as a branch of ethnology.
3. *Social psychiatry,* i. e., the study of mental illness in function of the social (nonethnic) group, to which the sick people belong."

Ethnopsychiatry deals, therefore, with the ethnic or cultural groups in their own cultural environment, whereas folklore psychiatry concerns itself with the part of folklore practices and beliefs maintained in any culture—even the most Occidental one—in relation to psychiatric conditions.

Folklore psychiatry must also be differentiated from the wide world of the "quack," the "fake," the "charlatan," and so forth. This distinction is not, however, clearly cut. Folklore psychiatry, historically linked to the cultural traditions of each society, maintains very definite relations with the ways of the quack, because even the most Westernized of them has, in underdeveloped countries, some connection with the folklore psychiatry of his people and his cultural region.

Folklore psychiatry, it must be emphasized, exists in the present. It participates in the traditions of the culture in which it acts and grows, but only through the different influences that such traditions have imparted during the culture's history. This gives it its particular flavor and unique characteristics.

As we shall see, folklore psychiatry is of particular usefulness in understanding underdeveloped countries. In Lima, at the Institute of Social Psychiatry,* we have been working on different research

---

* The former Institute of Social Psychiatry has been replaced by the Peruvian Institute for Socio-Psychiatric Studies (Instituto Peruano de Estudios Socio-Psiquiátricos). Its address is Av. Angamos 387, 2nd piso, of. 3, Lima, Peru.

projects connected with folklore psychiatry, and it is my conviction, re-confirmed each day, that this rich material is a source of incomparable data. This chapter is a sketch of our preliminary program of work and some of the early findings.

HISTORY OF FOLKLORE PSYCHIATRY

The history of folklore psychiatry is seen from two aspects: (1) what has been accomplished in the general history of the field, defined, as we did, apart from ethnopsychiatry, transcultural psychiatry, and cross-cultural psychiatry; (2) the history of folklore psychiatry in each cultural setting, that is, the evolution of ideas, beliefs, and practices concerning psychiatric conditions in a definite society.

At the institute we have begun a bibliographic research of folklore psychiatry in Peru, from the pre-Inca period to the present. This research has started with the Spanish *cronistas*, the first written reports about pre-Hispanic Peruvian folklore, and it is giving us a very rich, broad view, not only of psychiatry itself, but—as could be expected—of many related cultural and social problems.

FOLKLORE PSYCHIATRY FROM THE ANTHROPOLOGICAL POINT OF VIEW

The relationship between folklore psychiatry and anthropology does not need to be emphasized. To understand the meaning of different aspects of folklore psychiatry in a culture we have to know about the culture itself.

Our country affords ideal conditions for such research. Peru extends through three geographical regions—the Pacific coast, the Andean region, and the Amazon jungle. Along the coast lie the modern, Westernized cities. Going inland, we enter the Andean region, the *sierra*. Inhabited by Indian and *mestizo* populations, it offers a completely different cultural picture, because its inhabitants maintain many Inca and pre-Inca traditions mixed with Spanish influences. Farther east, we go into the Amazon jungle, with Brazil our eastern limit. There the situation is totally different. Primitive tribes, living in small villages among the rivers and maintaining their own individuality, are quite apart from the civilization of the coast and the general life of the country.

Given these conditions, the area offers great possibilities for anthropological research. There is an enormous amount of data concerning folklore psychiatry, not only related to psychiatry itself, but the historical evolution of the culture and the influences of the different forces acting on it as well.

We have been working on several projects at the institute. One of them concerns very interesting findings in a village on the *sierra* of northeast Peru in which we discovered the, for us fruitful, fact that almost one of every five inhabitants is a native healer. One anthropologist studied the characteristics of the native healers, and her work has been published in Spanish and English and read to different scientific societies.[3, 4, 5, 6]

Another project, already in the evaluation phase, is concerned with the use of ayahuasca, a psychedelic plant, by a tribe in the village of Marcos in the Amazon jungle.[12] A psychiatrist and anthropologist team is making a one-year study at the Amazon jungle city of Iquitos, in northeast Peru of certain phenomena of folklore psychiatry related to the magical use of another psychedelic plant.[11]

Yet another research team is studying the magical basis of the practice of the *curanderos* ("native healers") in Lima.

SOCIOLOGY AND FOLKLORE PSYCHIATRY

Any attempt to understand folklore psychiatry has also to consider the sociological factors related to it. The native healer, witchdoctor, or *curandero* is, of course, a social institution. He fulfills a role in his society, and the description of his role and his ways of influencing the community, as well as the reaction of such a society, are a real challenge for the investigators.

Our first steps in Peru have offered us a wealth of findings, opening wide horizons in the interpretation, not only of sociological issues, but also of the foundations of some healing techniques of psychiatry itself. For instance, a project—conducted by a team of behavioral scientists in a village in northern Peru—investigated the ability of some native healers to cure chronic alcoholics.

The native healer and his community are also being studied in relationship to the sociological evolution of his role. Retracing the path of the Indian civilizations from the Amazon jungle to the Peruvian coast, along the Inca highways, we have been able to follow the evolution of the conceptions, ideas, and practices of the native healers and to appreciate their close relationship to the changing sociological conditions.*

One interesting example is that, in the Peruvian *sierra*, the etiology of diseases is connected by the people with the natural forces. The soul is "stolen" by the mountains or the rivers, and such stealing is the cause of the disease. On the coast, the disease is not produced by nature, but by men, who produce the *daño* ("harm"). This contrast shows the relationship of these beliefs to the different emphasis in the struggle for life. In the Amazon jungle, man has to fight for his life against nature; therefore, nature is the enemy, the one who will cause disease. On the coast, nature is no longer the main enemy; it is man. It is he who causes the disease. Another feature is the mixture of magic, "primitive" thinking with Western ways, a mixture whose proportions and characteristics change along the same lines. Of course, these are only hints that have been useful for the elaboration of research projects that we are developing presently.

PATHOGENESIS AND ETIOLOGY FROM THE POINT OF VIEW OF FOLKLORE PSYCHIATRY

I have already said something in connection with this theme, and I shall elaborate on it later. The ideas the native healers in different parts of Peru (of course, that would apply to any other part of the world) have about the etiology of disease are also worthy of investigation. In my country, where we are beginning such investigation, we can say that they have very definite concepts and that the study of them is instructive.

The pathogenesis of the different psychiatric pictures we observe from the point of view of folklore psychiatry is interesting, too. I cannot go into details here, but it goes without saying that this also offers many fruitful research possibilities.

---

* One of the members of the institute, Dr. Mario Chiappe, is presently studying this aspect of the problem.

FOLKLORE PSYCHIATRY NOSOGRAPHY

Folklore classification of psychiatric clinical pictures is also fascinating. The native healers and the population at large have precise ideas on the matter. In Peru, they classify diseases in two clearly differentiated groups: *enfermedades de Dios* ("God diseases") and *enfermedades de daño* ("harm diseases"). God diseases are supposed to be caused by natural forces: these are the ones the doctors of the hospital are able to cure. When one of the native healers diagnoses these diseases, he will not treat them, but will send the patient to the hospital doctors. Harm diseases, on the contrary, are supposed to result from some kind of *daño*, done by means of different forms of supernatural, magic forces. Doctors at the hospital don't understand them and, of course, are unable to cure them. They are the province of the native healer.

There are many other features in the folklore psychiatric nosography we are studying in Peru, and we are trying to understand their theoretical basis.

A few words are perhaps necessary here (though only as an anticipation of a future study on the matter) about the classification of folklore clinical pictures. There have been many attempts to force their inclusion into different schemes closely related to Occidental nosographies. Such attempts are bound to fail because they are basically unsound. They treat these "exotic" clinical pictures as diseases, that is, as something that can be isolated and compared to the other "civilized" diseases already classified, forgetting the essential fact that they cannot be understood or even conceived except relatively to their own cultural background. Any attempt at classification or nosographic ordination must be grounded on an understanding of the cultural and social roots and characteristics. In other words, I do not believe that we can study them (much less classify them) from the Western point of view, disregarding all their anthropological significance.

FOLKLORE PSYCHIATRIC THERAPY

Two different aspects of the native healers' therapy must be taken into consideration: the therapeutic act itself and the drugs used to perform it.

Native healers in Peru follow different types of treatment according to the region in which they live and, of course, to the cultural background of that region. Witch doctors and shamans from the Amazon jungle have quite different ways of curing than do the native healers, or *curanderos*, of the coast.

It is interesting, as stated before, to note the evolution of the native healers' practices from the jungle to the coast along the Inca road according to the changes imposed by history and culture.

Another feature being studied is the influence of Catholic beliefs and practices on the native healers in Peru. As we know, Catholicism is the most influencing religious force in this country. The native healers have adopted many elements of the Catholic ritual —images of saints, prayers, songs, and so forth—and they use them during their rites, creating a true syncretism. The similarities between the symbolisms of the ritual followed by the native healers and the different rites of Western religions are quite suggestive and will be studied thoroughly in the future.

The patron saint of most native healers in the *sierra* and coast of Peru is San Cipriano. As the legend goes, this man was a magician who was converted to Catholicism and, later on, became a martyr. They pray to San Cipriano and have his image in their "chapels."

PLANTS AND DRUGS USED IN FOLKLORE PSYCHIATRY

The use of plants and drugs by healers is one of the most important aspects of the study of folklore psychiatry. The witch doctors and native healers use different plants autochthonous of Peru in their procedures. Some have been studied, but most are unknown to the medical profession. One known example is ayahuasca (*Banisteria caapi*), a well-known liana, containing harmine and alkaloid similar to mescaline and producing psychedelic effects. Another is San Pedro (*Trichocereus pachanoi*), containing mescaline, which is used in northern Peru.

We know more than forty different plants used by native healers, and it is our task to see whether these can be employed scientifically and fruitfully.

TRANSCULTURAL OR COMPARATIVE FOLKLORE PSYCHIATRY

Another field of study is the comparison of folklore psychiatric practices. In Peru, there are several regions, and, in a given region, the ways of thinking and acting of the native healers differ widely. Comparing the different ways of facing the same problem will give us the opportunity to understand many features, not only of the healing process itself, but of the cultural and sociological background of the population.

Transcultural studies of the folklore psychiatry of Peru and the other Latin American countries afford another area of study. The practices and beliefs of Peruvian folklore psychiatry are very similar to those of nearby countries—Bolivia, Ecuador, northern Argentina—but not to those of Brazil or Mexico, because the latter have completely different racial and cultural backgrounds.

AN EXAMPLE

To illustrate, very briefly, what has been learned, I am going to relate some features of a project we have been working on at the institute.*

In northern Peru there is a small village that has become renowned because of the conviction that the native healers are able to cure chronic alcoholism. During 1967, a team of anthropologists, psychologists, and psychiatrists went to this village to study some aspects of the treatment. The statistical data of the research are still being processed, but some features are worthy of consideration.

Diagnosis and Prognosis

The healer studies his patients very carefully. He will not act without a previous careful and detailed anamnestic interview. He will ask about details of family relationships, work, status,

---

* This research has been done, under the direction of Dr. Arnold Meadow, by Miss Marlene Dobkin, Drs. Mario Chiappe and Luis Dragunsky, and psychologists Miguel Boado and Delia Matos. A communication has been read at the meeting of the A.P.A., Hawaii, May 1970.

and difficulties of social life. He is interested in hereditary background and previous episodes of alcoholism and intents of cure. He will ask about the kind of liquor the patient takes, the quantities, and the circumstances in which it is drunk.

Some "patients" are immediately rejected. "They came drunk from the womb of their mothers." Those accepted after this first *rastreo** have to pass through a trial period. The native healer tells them that they are very weak and rundown and could not stand the treatment. Therefore, they have to strengthen themselves. To do that, they must abstain from drinking any alcohol for at least one month. At the same time, they have to take a tonic beverage that the healer prescribes. If they are not able to abstain, the healer will not take care of them. He is very strict on this issue and will not admit exceptions. If the patient is able to pass through this period, he is taken for treatment.

Treatment Itself

The patient is submitted to different procedures, among them to therapeutic sessions in which he has to join other patients in meetings with the native healer. These meetings are held during the night in the forest and have very interesting characteristics. I will not describe them in detail here. This has been done by some of my associates.[2] Suffice it to say that they consist of group intoxication with a concoction of "San Pedro," community singing, and the native healer acting in order to cure the patient.

The performance has different aspects worth considering. The whole atmosphere is one of mysticism and strong suggestive influence. Monotonous and prolonged singing (until the first hours of the next day) and the attitudes of the healer contribute to influence the patient. The plant concoction will produce, at the beginning, gastrointestinal symptoms, with vomiting and intestinal expulsion, which are interpreted as "getting rid of the harm." Later on, a psychedelic reaction occurs with the known characteristics of mescaline intoxication. The healer will approach the patients, talk to them, and perform magic gestures in order to free them from *daño*.

The ceremony is not, however, the only way in which the native healer acts. The healer submits some patients to a kind of conditioned adversion. He will give them liquor mixed with a

* *Rastreo* could be translated as "tracing," a diagnostic procedure.

beverage producing vomiting and diarrhea and repeat this therapy until "he won't even like to smell the stuff."

What is more interesting, the healer will give advice to the patient concerning his social life and relationships. He will tell him the one or the ones who "did harm to him" and whom he must avoid in the future. These could be his wife, his mother-in-law, his mistress, or some of his friends, relatives, or working companions. The healer will forbid him to associate with them, because "they will keep doing harm" to him and prevent him from being cured.

This rearranging of the social world of the patient appears to me as the main feature of the treatment. The native healer will really change the whole social environment and, in this way, the whole life of the patient.

Results

Although we are processing the data and cannot offer definite statistical figures, I can anticipate that these native healers are able to cure more than 30 per cent of chronic alcoholics, quite a success considering that there have been cases of twenty or more years of chronic alcoholism among them.

THE IMPORTANCE OF FOLKLORE PSYCHIATRY

Folklore psychiatry is a neglected chapter in the field of modern psychiatry. The ever growing emphasis of our specialty on being scientific has led to an attitude of contempt toward research that is not carried out in the laboratory or that lends itself to the statistical handling of data and the experiment. The treatments used and the ideas of "uncivilized" people were believed unworthy of consideration, being only remains of a primitive and unscientific past that ought to be forgotten as soon as possible.

If we look at this matter from a different point of view, we will be able to realize that folklore psychiatry, as well as all the manifestations of folk art or folk medicine, is the product of deep cultural patterns and carries with it a wealth of meanings that cannot be neglected.

As a matter of fact, folklore psychiatry today is a synthesis, let us say, of cultural anthropology and social psychiatry, both, as we have seen, in the limelight of modern trends in our specialty. If our interests have been going from individual problems to group problems, and from these to social ones, folklore psychiatry enables us to study them in a cultural anthropological context.

On the other hand, the common trend of close collaboration between psychiatry and such disciplines as sociology, anthropology, or psychology finds folklore psychiatry a very fruitful field.

From the point of view of our specialty, I can say now, after some years of experience, that we have a lot to learn from our colleagues, the native healers, witch doctors, and medicine men. We have a lot to learn, not only in the field of new plants and drugs to be used pharmacologically, but in something that we are discovering just now: the handling of family problems, the groups —our group dynamics, group therapy, and family therapy—as well as the management of social and community problems, which we approach as novelties, and they handle traditionally and skillfully.

It is therefore necessary, as I have insisted many times, to include in the psychiatric textbooks a very extensive chapter on folklore psychiatry.* If this is important in the developed countries (even in the most developed ones folklore psychiatry extends itself from the small villages to the big cities),[1, 8, 10, 13] it is really urgent in the underdeveloped areas, where a young psychiatrist, who will know everything about the latest theories on schizophrenia, will be at a loss in many of his daily activities. We see our residents, well instructed in modern psychiatry, up to date in procedures of diagnosis and therapy, but completely ignorant about what they are going to meet daily in their own country, much more so when they have to go inland to practice their specialty.

This reality is shocking in such countries as the Latin American ones, in which there is a terrible contrast between the human resources and the needs of psychiatric assistance. As an example, let us consider the situation in Peru. There are about 100 psychiatrists in practice, ninety of them in Lima, the capital. Of the total of 2,010 psychiatric beds, 95 per cent are in Lima and the rest of the country, which has 83.45 per cent of the population of Peru, has only ninety-three psychiatric beds.

Similar conditions are present in all our subcontinent. In

* This has already been done to some extent in an article by Ari Kiev[9] in the *American Handbook of Psychiatry*.

Mexico, there are 250 psychiatrists for almost 15 million inhabitants, and most are in the principal cities. In Colombia, for a population of almost 20 million inhabitants, there are 162 psychiatrists, which means that there is one psychiatrist per 140,000 inhabitants. Not to mention Haiti, where, for a population of almost 5 million inhabitants, there are four psychiatrists and nineteen psychiatric beds! I have no doubt that in other continents, such as Asia or Africa, the reality will be the same, if not worse.

Under these conditions, our psychiatrists know nothing about folklore psychiatry and are not prepared at all to face the needs of their daily practice. It is, then, time to study folklore psychiatry seriously in all its aspects and to include in the textbooks chapters dedicated to that knowledge. Such chapters will be very instructive for the developed countries and especially important for the underdeveloped areas.

CONCLUSION

In psychiatry, as well as in any other field of human endeavor, there is no one and only way to learn. Human behavior must be studied in all possible ways. Real human wisdom lies perhaps in the old traditions of mankind that have to be rediscovered in a kind of Renaissance that will revitalize the Western world and give it new perspectives.

REFERENCES

1. Borgolts. "La Psychiatrie en pratique rurale" (abstract), *Transcultural Research,* 8 (1960), 46–47.
2. Chiappe, M. "El Curanderismo en la Costa Norte del Peru," paper presented at the Fifth Latin American Congress of Psychiatry, Bogota, November 25–30, 1968.
3. Dobkin, M. "Folk Healing with a Psychedelic Cactus in North Coastal Peru," *International Journal of Social Psychiatry,* xv (1969), 1.
4. Dobkin, M. "Fortune's Malice: Or Divination, Psychotherapy, and Folk Medicine in Peru," *Revista del Instituto de Psiquiatría,* in press.
5. Dobkin, M. "The Religious Significance of Folk Healing with a Psychedelic Cactus in North Coastal Peru," presented at the Third Annual Meeting of the R. Bucke Society, McGill University, Montreal, Canada.
6. Dobkin, M. "*Trichocereus Pachanoi*—A Mescaline Cactus Used in Folk Healing in Peru," *Economic Botany,* in press.
7. Ellenberger, H. F. "Ethnopsychiatrie," in *Enciclopédie Médico-Chirurguali.* Vol. 3. *Psychiatrie.*

8. Garbe, E. "La Psychiatrie en clientele rural," *Concours Medical* (1960), 1489–1498.
9. Kiev, A. "Prescientific Psychiatry," in S. Arieti (ed.), *The American Handbook of Psychiatry*, Vol. 3. New York: Basic Books, 1966. Pp. 166–179.
10. Leighton, A. "Mental Illness and Acculturation," in Iago Galdston (ed.), *Medicine and Anthropology*. New York: International Universities Press, 1959.
11. Rios, O., and Dobkin, M. "Psychotherapy with Ayahuasca (a Harmine Drink) in Northern Peru: Research Report and Proposal," *Transcultural Psychiatric Research*, 4.
12. Siskind, J. "Informe Preliminar de una Investigación sobre el uso de Ayahuasca en una Tribu de la Selva Peruana," presented at the Peruvian Congress of Psychiatry, Lima, October 1968.
13. Tanzi, E. "II. Folk-lore nella patologia mentale," *Revista di Filosofia Scientifica*, 9 (1890), 385–419.

[[[8]]]

MEDICINE, PSYCHIATRY, AND PSYCHOTHERAPY: A FUTUROLOGIC PROJECTION

Stanley Lesse

During the past decade, the terms "futurology" and "futuristic" have been used with increasing frequency in the literature. The term "futurology" was coined by Ossip Flechtheim during the 1940's. As conceived now, it is not a universal science, but it does embrace such diverse phenomena as types of prognoses, projections, linear programming, planning procedures in the social sciences, education, assessments of goals, norms, and values. Therefore, those interested in futurologic research must use a broad spectrum of methods.[1]

Futurology, under different designations in different eras, has preoccupied man throughout the ages. The theologic projections of heaven, hell, nirvana, and the like carry with them implications of man's preoccupation with tomorrow and his attempts to formulate a pragmatic method by means of which he might guarantee for himself the "good" future.

From a philosophic standpoint, there is a small but very stimulating literature that may be divided roughly into utopian and counterutopian projections. The utopian concept can be witnessed in Plato's *Republic* and in Thomas More's *Utopia*. Counterutopian conceptualization can be viewed in such works as Jack London's *The Iron Heel*, Jevgenyi Samiatin's *We*, Aldous Huxley's *Brave New World*, and George Orwell's *1984*. Utopian concepts are based on values of love, hope, and faith designed to establish a new world of goodness and beauty. The counterutopian philosophic model of civilization carries with it a concept of absolute tyranny in which positive human values are degraded. Though, at first glance, some of the utopian conceptualizations may appear naïve, hopefully man always will be nagged by desires for a utopia with his efforts in some measure being in the service of a self-fulfilling prophecy.

The futurologic movement has thus far been bypassed by the medicopsychologic sciences. It is dominated by men from the physical and social sciences. In many ways, the general lack of interest in and awareness of the racing future is an indication of the lack of broad psychosocial awareness that characterizes the medicopsychologic sciences, a type of scotoma that has rendered many of our theories, techniques, and physical establishments anachronistic.

This chapter is an encapsulation of general ideas with regard to the future of medicine, psychiatry, and psychotherapy that have evolved during the past ten years. My first tentative probings were published in a brief vignette in 1964.[3] With all respect to the reader, I would like to suggest that whenever one reads an article or listens to a paper dealing with an aspect of the future, he should attempt to detach himself from his current prejudices and value judgments and view tomorrow as it is likely to be rather than the way he would like it to be. At times these views may coincide; more often than not, they do not.

At the outset I would like to emphasize that the conceptualizations described in this chapter are not presented with any sense of dogmatic certainty; rather, they represent tentative probings that will be subject to modification, revision, or radical alterations when dictated by the events of the emerging future. Though the world is always in a state of revolution, the rate of change that has occurred technologically, socioeconomically, sociopolitically, and sociophilosophically since the end of World War II has accelerated to a degree that has never before been experienced. Institutions that were relatively stable for decades or even centuries are now drastically altered or must alter if they are to survive. In the not too distant future, our civilization is likely to show developmental patterns radically different from those we recognize today. In this chapter I attempt to characterize the world of tomorrow, focusing on three elements and drawing on certain basic assumptions and deductions that seem to emerge with Western civilization as it is likely to be in the coming generations. The three elements are socioeconomic and sociopolitical changes; overpopulation with limitation of available space; and automation.

Most of these conceptualizations are the result of the combined studies of the author and William Wolf. Part of what follows is an encapsulation of material that was jointly published for the first time in 1966.[8] Based on projected trends, an attempt will be made to outline the nature of man's illnesses and his expectations with regard to medical treatment.

SOCIOECONOMIC AND SOCIOPOLITICAL FORCES

There appears to be little doubt that our society will become increasingly group oriented and more highly organized. The force of the mass increase in population, which will be discussed later, is likely to accelerate the process. As our society becomes more complex, social organizations will not only tend to become unified, but also more specialized. Man will incline largely to group goals, and expectations emphasizing personal preferences will be much less appreciated. Indeed, great individual expectations are likely to be looked on as odd, reactionary, and antigroup. Unanimity of thinking will be the normal pattern.

In this new, tightly organized society, individual competition must also be greatly reduced. The individual, rather than being preoccupied with his personal self, will find it necessary to orient himself as part of an integrated group in order to be accepted by his society, indeed, to survive. He very likely will strive to become an integral part, a dependent member, of the interdependent structure. In turn, he very likely will perform, as a matter of course, specific functions and tasks. In this process, certain of his capacities, functions, and even his body structure will change, with some areas undergoing atrophy and others hypertrophy.

A man raised in an organized world, such as has been projected above, is likely to develop expectations different from those considered commonplace today. He probably will have been taught to subordinate himself to the purposes of the group; he most likely will not consider himself as an important factor for his own sake, but important only so far as he is part and parcel of a successful group structure. As such, he will hardly expect individually oriented medical care. Rather, he will anticipate being treated on a group-oriented basis, with therapy being directed, in the main, to returning him to the group with optimal speed. He is likely to experience illness as being detached from the group and health as being well integrated into the group. One of his great concerns may well be the threat of physical and psychologic separation from the group. An individualist in all likelihood will be a maverick with expressions of individualism being considered as an ailment, and, as a corollary, rejection by the group may lead to illness.

POPULATION CHANGES AND LIMITATIONS OF AVAILABLE SPACE

Despite current efforts to retard the population increase, it is estimated by many demographers that the world population by the year 2000 will be 6 billion people, or approximately 3 billion more than now. This means that, in fewer than thirty-five years, the number of living persons will have doubled.

One crucial factor that probably will shape our future society will evolve around the fact that land space available for living and working is fixed and limited. This, together with the accelerating trend toward urbanization, will make horizontal expansion difficult, if not impossible, with the result that expansion will have to be upward. Thus, organized megalopolises will be formed. For example, very likely one such megalopolis in the United States will extend from New England to Washington and will contain 80 million people.

Population expansion and the massive trend toward further urbanization will likely necessitate increased structuralization of society, for when individuals are integrated into an organized group, the space necessary to permit effective functioning is reduced. Because it would appear that the group ego will predominate, increased organization of our society is likely to be requested and readily accepted. Though careful specialization in all probability will be stressed, it very likely may be in a context of indivisible relationships.

AUTOMATION

A great misunderstanding exists with respect to the concept of automation. All too often it is confused with very sophisticated mechanization. Indeed, the two are often used interchangeably.

Actually, the most sophisticated mechanical system, no matter how great the number of its components, is an open system that cannot operate unless the controlled loop is closed by a human being. In contrast, a fully automated system is closed, the human component being supplanted by a computing machine.

The new world of the closed, automated system most likely will necessitate a radical change in political, technologic, and social thinking. During the agricultural and industrial revolutions, man developed increasingly complex tools and systems that extended his sense perception and increased his skill and strength. In these systems, however, man was the inevitable factor that could direct and guide these tools. Hence, he was the unavoidable link in providing for his own well-being.

The cybercultural revolution is changing all this. It differs radically from previous innovations, because now man has devices that will largely supplant his labor and certain activities of his mind. As a result, he will have to find new tasks to occupy his time, because he will no longer find it necessary to use it for toiling in the fields or manufacturing his goods. In the age of cyberculture, enormous segments of the population will live in leisure. Only a few will "labor" in the sense of drudgery.

Cyberneticists have written that, in the new development of cyberculture, man must learn to live in leisure and abundance.[8] However, leisure must not be confused with idleness nor abundance with waste. Although computing machines and automation are in their infancy, they have already made far-reaching indelible changes in our current world. Before long our industrial capacity will be of a magnitude that will dwarf the most generous predictions. At the same time, fewer and fewer men will be required to produce more and more. Heretofore, unemployment as the result of automation was considered as affecting principally unskilled labor; automation also will replace those whom we now consider to be highly skilled technicians. This very likely will have the effect of equalizing men, so that automation in itself will have a profound impact on both the economic and philosophic aspects of this new revolution.

One cannot stress too strongly that automation, social and economic change, and the population increase must be viewed as an indivisible, interreacting group of forces. It would lead to serious error if one were to consider the progress of automation without simultaneously taking into account the other factors.

THE NATURE OF ILLNESS IN THE FUTURE

All indications point to the likelihood that we probably will encounter relatively few instances of so-called acute conditions, mostly infectious diseases, with their complications and sequelae, of which we have had such a plethora until recently. They are likely to be rare not only because we will be able to treat them effectively with broad-spectrum therapies, but also because the very transmission of infection will be greatly diminished. Preventive medical techniques will immunize most persons from sources of infection. The problem of resistant organisms will probably be conquered in the coming decades.

The principal acute processes that will be encountered are likely to be the results of traumata, hemorrhage, burns, radiation, and the like. In addition, we very likely will encounter acute phases or exacerbations of chronic illnesses, which will be managed primarily by preventive measures or by treating the more chronic underlying matrix. Acute processes will also include acute psychic problems, some representing exacerbations of congenital defects and some that are precipitated by various psychosocial traumata.

Chronic ailments probably will constitute the bulk of medical practice, partly owing to the fact that life expectancy will continue to increase. There possibly will be problems related to genetic mutations, many secondary to increased radiation fallout. In addition, there may be the effects of toxic materials ingested over a prolonged period of time in the form of preservatives, air pollution, artificial treatment of drinking water, and the like.

Increasingly crowded urban conditions coupled with a possible downgrading of the importance of the family as the basic social unit may be a source of considerable emotional stress for some time to come. In addition, of course, entirely new causes and types of somatopsychosociologic problems are likely to arise.

The sources of psychosocial stresses very likely will differ considerably from those of today. As indicated, they will probably be determined in great measure by the fact that the group ego most likely will supersede the individual ego in importance. Stresses are also likely to result from a probable deemphasizing of the family as the primary teacher of the child. Moreover, as such changes occur, the degree to which the parents no longer will be the prime sources of early instruction may considerably revise our concepts of psychodynamic development. Then, too, the child's relationships with other persons in the community are likely to be markedly different from those that we consider par for today.

The most significant psychosocial difficulties will most likely be traceable to group maladaptation and rejection by the group. Thus, quite new concepts of human relationship leading to other psychosocial stresses are likely to show up. Preoccupation with romantic love may well become diluted, and many interactions between men and women may change considerably. Stress on sexual gratification, which is so intimately incorporated into our present culture, may play a lesser role as a source of psychic disturbance, so that our future society might be far less sexualized than our current one.

PSYCHIATRY AND PSYCHOTHERAPY IN OUR FUTURE SOCIETY

The role of the psychiatrist and psychotherapist, as we currently understand it, is likely to be altered dramatically. Diagnoses probably will be made by means of a closed, automated system in which the psychiatrist or psychologist will be replaced by a programmed computing machine that by means of "computest language" will take most definitive histories. These histories very likely will be coupled with physiologic and biochemical data that will be obtained simultaneously. Though this concept may seem outlandish to some readers, I would like to point out that currently computers are being programmed to take histories, to act as therapists, to act as patients, to make differential diagnoses.

It is not unlikely that many of the psychoses—including the schizophrenias, manic-depressive psychoses, many depressive syndromes, and some hereditocongenital processes—will be managed primarily through biochemical means, either in the form of replacement therapy or by eliminating a biochemical excess.

The theories and techniques of psychotherapy will likely be changed or modified to be compatible to the needs of the day. New techniques probably will be dictated by the shift in the prime sources of psychic stress from real or apparent intrafamilial deprivation to maladaptation to a rapidly changing, increasingly organized, ever more crowded and automated society. Most men, as always, will be able to adapt to the altered scene. The greatest difficulties are likely to arise during the last decade of this century and the first few decades of the next century, for though the rate of change may not be so great during these periods as it will be later in the twenty-first century, the qualitative shifts will be most pronounced.

Psychotherapy will probably find its most important role as a prophylactic tool. Psychotherapists are likely to find their major functions as psychosociologists, as analysts and advisers to government agencies in an attempt to build compensatory factors into the politicoeconomicotechnologic system in order to make it optimally compatible to men and vice versa.[5]

For example, in order to help our society adjust to the forces of automation and its attendant social changes, an entirely new orientation to education is in order. No longer should education be directed mainly toward enabling the individual to earn a livelihood, for this eventually will be produced by machines and provided to all, as a matter of course, by the society. Psychotherapists will likely be involved in the formulation of this new educational framework. Psychotherapists, as psychosociologists, should logically be preoccupied with the question as to exactly what the sources of pride and pleasure will be for the man of the future, when labor will no longer be the prime motivation for his existence. There will likely be a basic concern in the not too distant future with the development of man's inner resources both within himself and within his group constellation. These problems will necessitate a penetrating awareness of the relationship between man's group ego and man's individual ego in an era when the individual ego may be deprecated as being unworthy and as being synonymous with selfishness, while the group ego likely will be extolled.

As noted before, the techniques of psychotherapy optimally should be adapted to the needs of the culture. Because patients are likely to be group oriented in a way and to a degree that would be alien to our current society, psychotherapy will be aimed at reinforcing the group ego, while subduing the threat of the demands of the individual ego. This will necessitate a type of group therapy, because a one-to-one patient-psychotherapist relationship would probably nourish the patient's individual ego.[6]

I believe it not unlikely for a type of group therapy based on learning theory conducted by programmed computerized systems to be one of the main psychotherapeutic techniques. Its main function would be to correct the patient's maladaptation to the group. The therapeutic process probably would deal primarily with conscious factors. However, aspects of the group unconscious would also be a focus of investigation and reinforcement. New conceptualizations of psychodynamics of necessity would evolve that would view individual psychodynamics in an indivisible relationship with sociodynamics, with the latter being weighed as the more important process and individual psychodynamics viewed as an extension of sociodynamics.

It is possible that psychotherapy will include the use of somato-psychic relaxation exercises, with patients attaining states of psychic detachment akin to that described by the Zen Buddhists as satori. Beginning with this relaxed state in which the initial level of anxiety is low, the group therapy social reconditioning processes possibly will proceed with repeated reaffirmations of the need by the patient to readapt to the group and reaffirmations of the dominance of the group ego over the individual ego.

Individual psychotherapy may be preserved and utilized in combination with group therapy. It would be applied to the elite class who will most likely be the programmers of the automated systems. These programmers probably will have highly developed individual ego structures, this being the prime source of their psychic difficulties in a society that probably will depreciate the individual. It is from these discontented, conflict-ridden programmers that future progress is likely to come with ideas generated by frustration.

MEDICINE AND THE FUTURE

I have discussed the social structure of the future (as it appears at the moment), for in order to understand the practice and nature of medicine of the future, one must comprehend the order of the society in which medicine will be an integral part. All too often, we physicians forget that it is society that molds medicine as one of its essential institutions. It is true that medicine does exert an influence on society, but it does not significantly shape its nature. In this connection, it may be well to appreciate that in an automated, heavily populated, group-oriented society, the nature of illnesses, their diagnosis and treatment, is likely to be far different from those we understand and recognize today.

The Need for Two Types of Medical Professionals

In a society structured and integrated in the manner described, with most services being automated, it would appear that two general types of professionally trained individuals will be needed to care for medical needs. Tentatively, they may be called medical academicians (M.A.) and medical technical experts (M.T.E.). Each will fulfill specific roles and will have a working knowledge of the other.

Medical Academician

The medical academician will be trained, primarily in the comprehension, expansion, and pragmatic application of the dynamic interrelationships between physiodynamics-psychodynamics and sociodynamics. This concept ideally will assume increasing importance whereby the mutual interrelationships and interdependencies of all human functions are stressed. These various terms may be defined as follows:

1. "Physiodynamics" refers to the state or changing state of the individual's anatomic structures, physiologic and biochemical functions, their mutual interdependence in relationship to one another and in relationship to psychodynamic and sociodynamic factors.
2. "Psychodynamics" refers to the state, or changing state, of the individual with regard to all psychic functions (conscious and unconscious) and their mutual interdependence in relation to physiodynamic and sociodynamic factors.
3. "Sociodynamics" refers to the state or changing state of an individual's total external environment and its mutual interdependence in relation to physiodynamic and psychodynamic factors.

The central theme to be stressed here is that whenever there is an alteration in one area of human function, there is inevitably an alteration in other areas or aspects of the same function and all other functions, both internal and external, until a state of relative equilibrium is reached. These changes operate and affect every aspect of the individual's life and in turn that of society in an indivisible feedback fashion, whereby a dynamically changing equilibrium is maintained. The equilibrium being dynamic is ever momentary, and when the factor of progressing time is added, the picture of constant flux is evoked.

Historic adaptability is another fresh concept that should be built into the education of the medical academician. This must be stressed, because the concept of intentionally conditioning students to anticipate automatically the necessity for change in response to internal and external stimuli has very little precedence in medical or, for that matter, most other types of education. It means that the medical academician and even the students will be encouraged to scan, as a matter of course, the knowledge and stimuli that they perceive in terms of the passing of time or becoming. In other words, greater emphasis will be placed on process rather than achievement of fixed ends. The real goal will lie in seeking rather than reaching a static end. The medical academician will also be proficient in two basic subsciences: the study of the interrelationships of normal functions and the study of interrelationships of abnormal functions, both in terms of the individual as well as the individual's relationship to society as a whole.

Medical Technical Expert

The medical technical expert working with many sophisticated, automated devices will be trained to take over many of the tasks of today's highly skilled physicians. Most routine diagnoses and therapies will undoubtedly be performed by the medical technical expert-computer combination. It appears likely that automated devices will take histories, perform specialized biochemical, physiologic, and psychologic recordings and examinations, and even indicate correlations. In all likelihood, these studies will be performed much more intensively and accurately and be correlated in a far superior manner than is now possible by skilled diagnosticians. The machines probably will not only correlate and arrive at specific or broad-spectrum diagnostic categories, but may conceivably indicate general and even specific courses of therapy. Other special devices very likely will actually administer some of the therapies. Because therapies in all likelihood will be increasingly broad spectrum in nature, most patients will probably be managed by the M.T.E.-automated device team at the level of a district general medical clinic or regional specialty center.*

Above all, the medical technical expert will be highly trained for very specific, very limited jobs. Even though he probably will be far more knowledgeable than the physician of today as to the details and technique of a special task, because his field of operation will likely be so limited, his education may require far less

* These will be defined later in the chapter.

time than that required to train the present-day medical specialist. Thus, the old saying that "men will know more and more about less and less" will become an ever more cogent truism.

The medical technical expert will find his role greatly narrowed, but at the same time markedly deepened in scope because of the nature of the marked advances in technology. The pragmatically oriented training of the medical technical expert very likely will be much briefer than that required for the medical academician. The former also should be trained to think in terms of interrelationships, but in a relatively superficial fashion. The medical technical expert ideally will learn not to think in terms of items by themselves, out of context, so to speak, but rather in relationship to the many items of information obtained from the automated devices. He should learn to interpret and apply in combination with the automated systems the programmed methods laid down and suggested by the medical academician. Some medical technical experts may well become specialists in diagnosis, whereas others may become specialists in therapeutic techniques. Thus, as we stated before, we anticipate that the medical technical experts may become increasingly specialized in an ever narrowing frame of reference.

PHYSICAL STRUCTURE OF MEDICAL PRACTICE

As projected by Lesse and Wolf, the physical structure of medical practice is likely to become hierarchically structured to guarantee a maximum of efficiency and a minimum of duplication. The suggestion we wish to make is that medicine would function on three organizational levels: district general medical clinic (DGMC), regional specialty center (RSC), and zone specialty hospital (ZSH).

District General Medical Clinic

For medical purposes, the country could be divided into districts, their size determined by area and population. In a large megalopolis, there would be medical clinics that would function as part of huge organismic structures. In each district, the general medical clinic would supplant the present general practitioner as a source of initial consultation. It would be staffed primarily by medical technical experts.

The clinic would be fully automated and require a minimum of ancillary technicians and secretarial help. The patient's history could be taken by means of a standardized questionnaire, one that will be much more inclusive and sensitive than any now in use or available. Many kinds of biochemical studies, including the use of various tracer substances, recorded by scanners, will elucidate and correlate somatic and autonomic states and responses. Polygraphic recordings of the various body systems together with X-ray findings, soundings, and other measures of observation made by the medical technical expert could be fed into a computer programmed with an extremely broad compendium of medical knowledge.

Thus, the automated devices will replace in great measure the medical diagnostician and possibly, in some measure, the medical therapist. Medical scanners are likely to be far more accurate with regard to the examination of X-rays, electrocardiograms, electromyograms, electroencephalograms, and the like than the most highly trained physician. Highly sensitive scanners coupled with the results of various questionnaires also will probe intellect, affect, social adaptation, motivation, and unconscious psychodynamic mechanisms, the results of which will be fed into a computer, which will be programmed to contain far more information than could be elicited by any single man or group of men. Differential diagnoses too could be suggested by the computer, and therapeutic techniques could even be recommended or carried out.

One can visualize then that most illnesses will be treated at the level of the district general medical clinic. This would be in line with the present trend toward more generalized and nonspecific therapy, a trend that has been evident since the development of the sulfonamides and antibiotics, broad-spectrum metabolic therapy, endocrine therapy, and the like. It is conceivable that even certain types of psychotherapy based on educational, behavioristic, and reconditioning principles could be carried out at this broad general level. In the district general medical clinic we feel that the medical technical expert will have broad but not unlimited medical responsibilities, predetermined in great measure by the capacities of the automated system.

Not all patients would be handled in the district clinic, for patients with ailments too obscure or too refractory to therapy would not be handled at this level. They would be referred to a regional specialty center. If the patient is extremely ill, he might be sent directly to a specially equipped and manned zone specialty hospital, but only after the medical technical expert has consulted with superiors at the regional specialty center. Such a consultation would take the form of electronically transmitted reports that had been recorded, for instance, on video-audio tapes. With this information at hand and by means of closed-circuit television viewing of the patient, the representatives of the regional specialty center could decide whether or not the patient should be directly admitted to a hospital.

Severely traumatized patients could also be sent directly from the district medical clinic to the zone specialty hospital after closed-circuit television consultation with the representative of the regional specialty center had taken place. In emergencies, the district general medical clinic would merely perform life-saving techniques similar to present military aid stations or organized hospital emergency wards. In addition, the district general medical clinic would provide a service whereby certain patients could be brought to the clinic and returned home. Home visits, if they are necessary, may also be part of the duties of the medical technical expert in the district general medical clinic.

Regional Specialty Center

The regional specialty centers would receive patients from a number of district general medical clinics on the basis of area and population. They would be referrals from the district general medical clinic comprising those patients who could not be managed at that level. The regional specialty center would be equipped with facilities for more sophisticated history-taking, more extensive diagnostic procedures, and more complex therapeutic devices. The data obtained from the district general medical clinic, together with those gathered by the more sophisticated diagnostic devices, would be fed into more specifically programmed computers.

The regional specialty centers could be designed for optimal efficiency. They would be conveniently located to serve all the district general medical clinics in their particular regions. There would be a minimum of duplication of personnel and equipment. For example, there might be centers for surgery that would be very highly specialized. Subdivisions could exist for cardiac surgery, chest surgery, neurologic surgery, and the like. Similarly, there could be regional psychiatric, endocrinologic, and metabolic centers. It may well be that these terms will not be appropriate in the future, for, in general, illnesses will be viewed from a different point of view, as will be described later.

The regional specialty center would be supervised by a medical academician whose training and conceptualization of illness would prepare him to view sickness as a disturbance in the interrelationship between physiodynamic-psychodynamic and sociodynamic phenomena. The responsibilities in training of the medical academician will be described in detail elsewhere.[7]

In this plan, the regional specialty center would have a limited number of hospital beds where individuals may be treated as inpatients on a short-term basis. It may also act as a day hospital to which some patients could report during the daytime hours and then return home at night and others could go to their homes or jobs during the day, return to the hospital for evening therapy, and stay overnight. With the changing nature of illnesses and more efficient broad-spectrum therapeutic techniques, the majority of those patients who cannot be managed at the level of the district general medical center could be managed at the level of the regional specialty center.

Zone Specialty Hospital

Each zone specialty hospital would serve several regional specialty centers of the same discipline. It would be organized to manage patients who require long-term treatment or treatments that necessitate special intricate equipment or facilities. The hospitals would also serve as training and research institutes. As stated above, emergency patients would in some instances be sent directly to the zone specialty hospitals from the district general medical clinics after closed-circuit consultation with the medical academician stationed at the regional specialty center. These patients would be emergency cases requiring intensive care. The zone specialty hospital would also receive patients directly from the regional specialty centers for long-term therapy or for more definitive diagnosis than was possible on a short-term basis in the regional specialty center. The zone specialty hospitals would be highly specialized to avoid duplication, headed by a medical academician who would supervise the programming of the automated systems and act as the coordinator of teams of highly specialized medical technical experts.

In the surgical centers, medical technical experts would be highly skilled in certain surgical techniques, such as organ replacement or other standardized procedures. However, it would be the medical academicians who would have the broad concept of the patient as a physiopsychosociologic entity.

Zone specialty hospitals could also serve as regional clinical research centers. The regional specialty centers could have closed-circuit television communication for research purposes, for consultation, and for staff conferences and student teaching with zone specialty hospitals and they, in turn, with other zone specialty hospitals.

It would appear that the duties of the future physician may have little resemblance to those of the doctor as we know him today. Because the theory and practice of medicine of today are not likely to be applicable to the economic, political, philosophic, and technologic changes of the coming generations, it would appear obvious that the schedule and content of training the medical man of the future will be so designed as to prepare him for his future opportunities and duties. The medical student of today will be at his peak as a practitioner, research worker, or teacher at, or even before, the dawn of the next century. As such, he must be prepared to anticipate the social structure, the technological advances, and the very nature of disease that will be found a generation or two hence. For this reason, the medical educational planning cannot safely be delayed or confined to preparing physicians for the problems that exist today.

SUMMARY

In this chapter I have attempted to characterize the world of tomorrow as it is likely to be by focusing on three basic elements: socioeconomic and sociopolitical changes, overpopulation with tendency to limitation of available space, and automation. It was emphasized that these three elements must be viewed as an indivisible, interreacting group of forces and that it would lead to serious error if these elements were to be considered in isolation. In the conceptual framework used in this projection, an attempt has been made to design a medicopsychiatric system that would appear to be a logical outgrowth of the probable future technosocial structure. Similarly, some suggestions have been proposed as to the future role of the psychotherapist and the nature of some psychotherapeutic techniques, once again basing these on the cultural patterns that appear to be applicable to the not too distant future.

In the evaluation of any futurologic study or projection, one should have a conceptualization of how he believes the world is likely to be from a sociodemographic and technologic basis. If one does not have such a conceptual framework, a reasonable criticism of futurologic studies is most difficult and is likely to be fraught with personal prejudice.

REFERENCES

1. Flechtheim, O. "Is Futurology the Answer to the Challenge of the Future?" in R. Jungk and J. Galtung (eds.), *Mankind 2000*. London: Allen & Unwin, 1969. Pp. 266–269.
2. Hilton, A. M. "An Ethos for the Age of Cyberculture," *Proceedings of the Spring Joint Computer Conference of the American Federation for Information Processing Society*, Washington, D.C., April 1964, pp. 139–153.
3. Lesse, S. "Psychotherapy 1999: A Need to Prepare," *American Journal of Psychotherapy*, 18 (1964), 1–6.
4. Lesse, S. "The Relationships between Socioeconomic and Sociopolitical Practices and Psychotherapeutic Techniques," *American Journal of Psychotherapy*, 18 (1964), 574–583.
5. Lesse, S. "Psychiatry and Psychotherapy—Their Role in Futurology," *American Journal of Psychotherapy*, 21 (1967), 719–722.
6. Lesse, S. "The Influence of Socioeconomic and Sociotechnologic Systems on Emotional Illness," *American Journal of Psychotherapy*, 22 (1968), 569–576.
7. Lesse, S., and Wolf, W. Monograph in preparation.
8. Lesse, S., and Wolf, W. "An Exploration of the Basic Determinants and Trends of Medicine in Our Future Society," *American Journal of Psychotherapy*, 20 (1966), 206–227.

PART TWO

Clinical Contributions

[[9]]

ANOREXIA NERVOSA

Mara Selvini Palazzoli

THE TERM "ANOREXIA"

It should first of all be emphasized that "anorexia," the term most commonly used for this condition since it was first described, is an improper term. "Anorexia" etymologically means "lack of greed." It seems thus to include only the manifest symptomatology of these patients. We know very little about hunger and the awareness of hunger, about satiety and the awareness of satiety, about their biological and psychodynamic interconnections. Only recently has the experimental research of Stunkard and his associates[8] opened a fruitful avenue for the solution of these basic problems. Many who have written about anorexic patients without a detailed study of their behavior have accepted the patients' defensive explanations. The patients' attitude was believed to result from lack of interest in food. The habit of progressively insufficient food intake was believed to result from the digestive nervous disorders (feeling of fullness, constipation, and so forth) of which the patients complained. Anorexia was thus confused with depression or hypochondriasis.

Careful observation reveals that actually food is very important for the anorexic patients, frequently being the most important thing. In fact, these apparently detached and ascetic patients are excited by a casual conversation about food (as long as it is not their food that is mentioned). The same excitation is revealed by their hobby of cooking for others, their knowledge of recipes and delicatessen shops, their compulsive readings of the menus affixed to restaurant doors, and so forth. Anorexics have an extraordinary memory for food and meals served years before. It would be sufficient to study the oneirical world of these patients with their frequent, though often ambivalent, dreams about food to realize how greatly this so-called anorexia differs from the anorexia of patients affected by organic diseases. However, at a still deeper level, these patients give up food in order to reach the most important goal of all, as we shall see later. Consequently, food will become even more tempting.

DIFFERENTIAL DIAGNOSIS

An exact differential diagnosis between pseudoanorexia nervosa and true anorexia is necessary to avoid the uncertainty and confusions occurring in evaluating the case and, most important, to avoid therapeutic errors. Often, owing to the reticence and dissimulation of the patients, the diagnosis is very difficult. The following conditions must be considered forms of pseudoanorexia nervosa:

1. Depressive conditions, in which lack of interest in food is associated with lack of interest in any other vital need.
2. Schizophrenic conditions, in which refusal of food or bizarreness of eating habits is associated with delusional ideas concerning the symbolic meaning of food (for example, poison).
3. Neurotic reactions, most commonly of a hysterical type, which generally occur after a traumatic situation that proved humiliating or disappointing. In these conditions, food reduction is almost entirely brought about by the secondary gain of the anorexia, and the symptom is constantly aimed at controlling the environment—to attract attention, to blackmail, to obtain the desired responses, to escape from school, work, and existential involvement generally. The majority of the cases who automatically and precociously resort to vomiting belong to this group. After a brief period of reduced food intake, these patients cannot endure this renunciation. They are mostly inadequate personalities.
4. Chronic anorexias, who show an early onset in childhood on the basis of the typical conflicts of the oral and anal periods, improve temporarily at puberty, and later give rise to chronic conditions of an asthenic hypochondriacal type.
5. Simmonds' disease, which has inexplicably been confused for so long in the literature with nervous anorexia.

It is now clear that all forms of pituitary insufficiency, both primary and secondary (Sheehan's disease), almost never produce emaciation. Leaving medical and endocrine aspects out in the present context, the mental condition alone is sufficient for the differential diagnosis. Kind,[10] of Zurich, has conclusively shown that the psychic picture of apathy and abulia of these rare conditions is in marked contrast to that seen in anorexia nervosa.

In all the above-mentioned conditions, one characteristic of true anorexia nervosa, namely neuromuscular hyperactivity, is usually absent. I entirely agree with Hilde Bruch[4, 5] in considering as primary, in the pseudoanorexic condition, a concern with food or eating "which is used in various symbolic ways." In true anorexia, on the contrary, "the main issue was recognized as a struggle for control, for a sense of identity and effectiveness." The giving up of food serves the "singular goal of achieving autonomy and effectiveness through this bizarre control over the body and its functions."

This common goal for all real anorexic patients labels anorexia nervosa as a definite clinical entity, even though the Rorschach protocols, using the classical scoring, reveal features belonging to different diagnostic Rorschach categories.

As I shall mention later, I differ from Bruch only in proposing, within the area of true anorexia nervosa, a differentiation between two varieties: (1) a stable type, characterized by a constant limitation of food intake, and (2) a type that presents dramatic alternations between fasting and overeating. The latter group also includes, according to my experience, patients who show overt terror of overeating attacks that, however, nobody has ever been able to witness.

INTERPRETATION OF ANOREXIA NERVOSA

When we speak about anorexia nervosa, we actually refer to anorexic behavior. Anorexia implies real absence of appetite, whereas anorexic behavior implies that patients behave as if they had no appetite. In my opinion, the diagnosis of anorexia nervosa must be based on the careful observation of the specific behavior of the patients. This behavior reveals the conscious and stubborn determination to emaciate oneself, despite an intense interest in food, which reveals itself in many indirect ways. For example, they eat the peel of the apple after having carefully peeled it; they clean with the blade of the knife the paper that had contained the thirty grams of cheese it had apparently taken such an effort to eat, and so on. One's physical decay is looked on with great indifference, which the more cunning patients cover up by admitting their illness, without any real emotional involvement or any effective attempt to change the situation. This deterioration is actually accelerated by the typical neuromuscular hyperactivity, which, like amenorrhea, is present in the early stages.

In most of my cases, the onset of the disease took place at puberty in young girls, who until then had been considered physically and mentally healthy by their families.

Some writers, under the influence of Melanie Klein's ideas, have suggested that the anorexic patient by not eating can deny her impulse to destroy orally what she loves; in brief, she can repress cannibalistic impulses. I am rather skeptical about interpreting anorexia nervosa as a defense against the oral-sadistic impulse. I consider this interpretation arbitrary, because it does not take into account clinical and phenomenological observations, the only reliable foundations on which to base a psychodynamic explanation.

Patients who are in Klein's schizoparanoid position with oral-sadistic impulses organize their defenses against a reactivation of this position by developing either delusional ideas of being poisoned or an actual block in food intake. This block is entirely involuntary and is accompanied by strong irritation, preoccupation of starving, and intense feelings of bodily damage and physical decay. A patient of mine used to carry a bottle of milk. He would take advantage of any loosening of this block to sip from the bottle. The clinical picture of the true nervous anorexic is entirely different. She does not passively submit to a total and occasional block in food intake. With cold and consistent determination, she does not refuse but reduces food intake to absurd levels. The most important point is that, once she has introduced food, especially if in large quantities, by her standards, she does not feel that her body is threatened or destroyed. She actually feels at once that it is enormously increased, intrusive, and impending.

The basic phenomena of anorexia nervosa are, therefore, (1) persistence of hunger (which is either shown indirectly or is admitted only after long familiarity with the therapist), and (2) a willful and hard struggle against this hunger, (3) a consistent determination to emaciate oneself because of the feeling that the nourished body is expanding, threatening, and overpowering. An actual lack of hunger may be present in the terminal phases or when a too severe starvation and excessive use of vomiting or laxatives disturb the electrolyte balance and produce ketonemic intoxication.

The body is felt as a threatening entity that must not be brutally destroyed, but must merely be held in check. This central phenomenon of anorexia nervosa distinguishes it from any other similar syndrome. In my opinion, the Kleinian oral-sadistic position cannot explain why the anorexic, after having eaten, should feel that her body, far from being damaged or threatened, is unbearably enlarged, grown, and overwhelming.

Let us then ask ourselves whether the nervous anorexic is afraid of food or of her body. I strongly feel that she is afraid of her body, and therefore of food, which, once it has been swallowed, immediately becomes part of the growing body. She experiences food intake as an enhancement of her body at the expense of herself.

For the anorexic patient, to be a body means to be a thing. If the body grows, the thing also grows at the expense of the person. Her fight against the body-thing is her fight against being a thing. A desperate fight, because, paradoxically, though refusing to be a thing, she fights her battle not at the level of spiritual values, but rather at a material level, that of the body. We must now inquire how the anorexic patient could acquire this frightening experience of her body. I believe that she was able to do so by having completely equated the body to the incorporated object —namely, the mother, with its bad, disparaging aspects—in order to fight it and separate it from the self. I should like to emphasize that for the nervous anorexic the body does not contain the bad object, *but is* the bad object. From the phenomenologic point of view, the body is experienced as possessing all the features of the primary object as it was perceived in the situation of oral helplessness: it is powerful, indestructible, self-sufficient, growing, and threatening. If no active aggression is shown in the overt symptomatology and dreams, it is because unconsciously the object is experienced as being too strong to be destroyed. The despairing feeling of helplessness prevails. My patient Liliana had the following dream: "I am in front of my mother. I should like to do something, but I have two bleeding stumps." The ego of the anorexic is a pathetic ego who has felt and still feels helpless in every sense, biological and psychological, before the impervious object. The inner object has not merely frustrated generic drives and needs; it has frustrated the needs of the ego, above all the right to feel that inner sensations are one's own and legitimate, because they are consensually validated by the authority figures. As Rita says, "I have always been robbed of my own way of experiencing. This is the worst loss one can suffer. It leads to emptiness, lack of any affective link with life, of real vital intensity, of that which makes you feel yourself and not a thing, a heavy shapeless thing."

PSYCHOGENESIS OF ANOREXIA NERVOSA

A typical mother of the nervous anorexic may be aggressive, hyperprotective, and impervious, incapable of considering her daughter a person in her own right. It is often the parental couple, with its complementary pathology, or the whole family group that sabotages the basic needs of our patients' egos, especially those concerning the feeling of one's unique power and worth.

According to my observations, the most common basic interpersonal experiences of anorexic patients are the following: (1) During infancy, the ritual side of feeding is emphasized in the relationship with the mother who does not seem to derive pleasure from it. Control prevails over signs of joy and physical tenderness. "Parental stimulation disregards and overwhelms the initiatives coming from within the child."[5] (2) During childhood and the latency period, an impervious presence constantly interferes, criticizes, suggests, takes over the vital experiences and prevents them from being felt as one's own. These pathogenic interpersonal experiences give rise to a paralyzing feeling of ineffectiveness that pervades every thought and activity of these patients. In the childhood of these patients, even those who suffered no material deprivation, there was a conspicuous lack: their spontaneous and unique expressions were constantly questioned or disqualified. During the latency period, a life style of compliant surrender developed. The awareness of self, including body-self as being separate from others and from their expectations, was severely impaired.

The patient enters adolescence bound to her mother and obviously lacking any deep supportive peer relationship. In the turmoil of adolescent age, she undergoes traumatic experiences that are unbearable to her. She has to withdraw her libidinal cathexes from the parent figures and find new objects. She faces the difficulty of establishing new interpersonal relationships and of being accepted. Her body undergoes rapid changes: by growing and developing feminine characteristics, it seems a different body, yet it remains her own. There is, finally, the search for a definitive identity, which implies a disidentification from the mother. All these problems produce in the fragile premorbid personality of these patients a depression of the ego, which becomes afraid in facing and overcoming its tasks. The stage preceding the onset of the anorexic symptom should always be investigated. I have consistently found in it such signs as transient unreality feelings; boredom; the feeling of being different from others, from one's schoolmates, who appear either much older or much more childish; isolation; and, above all, an obscure feeling of helplessness, uselessness, and ineffectiveness. In this prodromic phase, uneasiness and depressed mood are often associated with an actual decrease in appetite that may draw the patient's attention to the problem of food. At this moment the depression of the ego faced by insurmountable tasks reactivates the shocking sense of helplessness experienced during the infantile period. An acute reactivation of the feeling of oral helplessness thus takes place.

The following dream of a patient of mine is like a parable that explains the typical development of an anorexic patient. "While it was very dark I found myself in a horrible dark house near the cemetery. I was hiding behind a cold radiator because I was afraid of many gypsies who were outside. However, Mother could follow every move of mine because she was behind, looking at me through a little window. Then Mother gave me a yellow dog, and suddenly I found myself on the road holding the dog by the leash. Only when I saw another huge dog coming toward me, I look at mine and I realized how horrible he was . . . his head was becoming increasingly larger and his body was extremely small . . . then he made me sick. I let the leash drop, and the dog stopped because without it he was not even able to walk any more." The little girl is shivering in the dark, owing to the lack of warm empathic contact with the mother (cold radiator). She is full of obscure fears (the gypsies represent the persecutive fantasies of the schizoparanoid phase according to Klein). At a certain moment, she realizes that the good and bad mother is always present (depressive phase according to Klein) but distant and controlling (looking through a little window). She realizes that she can gain her protection by becoming obedient and passive like a dog held by a leash (long, uneventful phase until puberty). When, in adolescence, she compares herself to the others ("I saw another huge dog . . ."), she senses the deformity of her own personality, resulting from her rational conformist split off from her own vital experiences (her dog has a big head and a very small body). She becomes panicky and unable to stand on her own feet (the dog cannot walk without a leash).

At this point I wish to stress, in agreement with Bibring,[2] that emphasis be laid not on oral frustration and the ensuing oral fixation, but on the infantile and childhood experience of the helplessness of the ego. The conception presented here "does not invalidate the accepted theories of the role which orality and aggression play in the various types of depression." It implies, however, that the oral and aggressive strivings are not so universal in depression as is generally assumed and that, consequently, the theories built on them do not offer sufficient explanation, but require a certain modification. At this point we can try to answer the puzzling question: Why does anorexia nervosa occur almost exclusively in the female sex and around puberty?* In my opinion, this tendency is owing to a process of concretization of a psychic process. Puberty is often a sudden and traumatic experience for a girl. Narcissistic libido cathexis has to be withdrawn from the infantile body and directed toward the new body, the adult, curved body that also has to be considered as belonging (belongingness of the experience of one's own body). This body, however, because of the permanent incorporation of the object, does not succeed in emerging as one's own and as distinct from the maternal object. On the contrary, owing to the development of the breasts and other feminine curves, the body is experienced concretely as the maternal object itself, from which the central ego wishes to distinguish itself at all costs. During this transitory phase of depression at puberty, a desperate defense is set up in our patients. The ego organizes the defense by means of a split within itself, in order to avoid the two major psychic catastrophes: deep depression and schizophrenic regression.

* The three cases of undereating I studied in males were cases of pseudoanorexia. One was a monk who had developed paranoid delusions: by fasting, he thought he could redeem the corrupt members of his order. Another was dominated by hypochondriacal ideas of a schizophrenic type, centered on the digestive system. The third was the closest to true anorexia, also because of the presence of neuromuscular hyperactivity. This patient, however, showed two atypical signs. In the first place, he explicitly declared a longing for food as for a "paradise lost," whereas true anorexics never admit such a longing. In the second place, he exhibited his fasting performances, unlike female anorexic patients, who constantly claim they have eaten a great deal.

The patient considers and experiences her body as a whole incorporated object that disparages her and forces a passive role onto her. Because of the comparatively advanced stage of psychic development at which she builds up a defense, the patient is able to distinguish between identification (which is an ego function) and oral incorporation (which is an instinctual process). In psychoanalytic literature, the two processes are considered correlated or even identical. But in the anorexic defense, the two processes are sharply distinguished. The incorporation of the bad object, which becomes one's own body, not only persists, but is actually reinforced for defensive purposes, in order to better control the object. The libidinal parts of the ego remain attached to the object and to the need of the object and, in splitting, are detached from the central ego. However, because the rejecting object is simultaneously bad and fascinating, an ambivalent attitude prevails. The central ego, associated with the superego components, then identifies itself with an ideal, desexualized, and acarnal image.

Whereas in the premorbid phase the object was unconsciously felt to be too strong to be destroyed, now that the bad object is equated to the body, active aggression can be consciously directed toward the body by grudging it food. The ego defense thus built up is characterized by the rejection of the body and of the food as a growing body. The ambivalent attitude toward the bad and fascinating object could also account for the fantasies of oral impregnation. Many who studied a few cases of anorexia nervosa found that their patients had the fear of becoming pregnant orally. They came to the conclusion that this particular fear is the core of anorexia nervosa. I seldom found impregnation fantasies. However, in the cases in which this fantasy was present, I am convinced that the fear of pregnancy is not to be interpreted as a sexual fear, but rather as a sexual symbol of a more primitive experience, that of being invaded by the object.

The pathological keeping-in-check of the body is synthesized by an attitude that I suggest be called body mistrust, whereas Hilde Bruch speaks of a perceptual and conceptual disturbance and of a body-image disturbance of delusional proportions.

At this point I think I may clarify how my view differs from that of Hilde Bruch. Bruch's clinical finding of a perceptual and conceptual disturbance only applies in my opinion to some of the cases of anorexia nervosa. I also suggest to amplify her concept of a body-image disturbance, as we shall see later.

PRELIMINARY RESULTS OF NEW RORSCHACH SCORING

In the course of research I have been carrying out for nearly twenty years on approximately forty cases of anorexia nervosa in young girls, fifteen of which have been treated for several years with intensive psychotherapy and subsequent follow-ups, I systematically administered the Rorschach test, in addition to other psychodiagnostic procedures. The data from the systematic analysis of twenty-four protocols were reported in my book *L'Anoressia Mentale*.[12]

Although the clinical picture of anorexia nervosa may be defined as monotonous, this is not true of the Rorschach finding. The protocols showed considerable variation in the number of responses (from nine to sixty-five), in their quality, and in the determinants of movement and color, which in some cases contrasted with the anxious or depressed appearance of the patients. I wish to emphasize here that a Rorschach pattern typical of anorexia nervosa was not found and that, after customary scoring, the grouping of the data according to classical diagnostic categories, such as hysteria, phobia, obsessiveness, and atypical cases, did not prove after follow-up to be prognostically reliable. The cases with fatal outcome were scattered throughout the four groups. Moreover, from a clinical point of view, the material under study was inevitably heterogeneous, for it consisted partly of cases of recent onset and partly of chronic cases, made stubbornly resistant by previous disastrous experiences, such as traumatic hospitalizations or coercive therapies (forced feeding). I was disappointed by the results of the tests and decided to adopt for prognostic purposes the clinical principle of the time of onset and the presence of the above-mentioned iatrogenic complications.

About two years ago I found unhoped-for aid in the paper by Lyman Wynne and Margaret Thaler Singer, "Thought Disorders and Family Relations of Schizophrenics."[20] I can make a brief mention only of the basic concepts of these writers. Their methodological basis was the concept of prediction as a research method, discussed by Benjamin.[1] The research was carried out by administering a battery of tests, including the Rorschach test, to the families of schizophrenic and neurotic patients. On the basis of the protocols of the parents alone, the predicting psychologists, who were unaware of the diagnoses of the patient-offspring, were asked to make the following predictions concerning the patients: (1) traditional global diagnosis (frankly schizophrenic, borderline schizophrenic, nonschizophrenic neurotic); (2) forms of thinking and communication; (3) severity of symptomatic ego disorganization.

As far as Rorschach scoring is concerned, the method used in analyzing the protocols was different from the traditional one and was later described by the authors in a special publication.[18] On the strength of lessons learned from errors, the authors reached the conclusion that, in order for the research to be fruitful and lead to accurate predictions, it had to be carried out exclusively in the style of thinking and communicating and that content had to be deliberately and strictly disregarded. Content of thinking and communicating must be relegated to a secondary role, for, as the authors point out, content may vary in time, whereas the ways of thinking and communicating have a permanent character. The families of schizophrenic patients (with marked statistical differences as compared to the families of neurotics) showed transactional thought disorders similar to those of the patient-offspring, varying in degree from the most severe forms of thought disorder (amorphous forms of thinking) to the least severe (fragmented forms of thinking). In other words, the form and structure of the transactions of the schizophrenic patient's family as a whole are comparable to those of individual schizophrenic thinking.

Therefore, the disorder in schizophrenic thinking and experience depends on how experience is differentiated, organized, and communicated, and this aspect is mostly learned in family relations. It should be noted that experience, thought, and communication are thus considered equivalent. A fragmented communication, for instance, is the expression of fragmented experience and thinking.

These concepts have enabled the authors to outline a classification of thinking disorders based on progressive cognitive disorganization. This classification includes four groups of decreasing severity:

Group 1. Amorphous form of thinking
Group 2. Mixed form of thinking (amorphous and fragmented)
Group 3. Fragmented form of thinking
Group 4. Stably constricted form of thinking

This classification is based on the developmental differentiation-integration principle, which was stated by Heinz Werner as follows: "Wherever development occurs it proceeds from a state of relative globality and lack of differentiation to a state of increasing differentiation, articulation, and hierarchic integration."[19] Obviously, orderly and hierarchic integration cannot take place if differentiation has been absent or faulty. The integration of experience is therefore based on its successful differentiation. Differentiation of experience includes, among other things, the capacity to differentiate self from nonself and the capacity to recognize and distinguish different kinds of feeling states, impulses, and wishes.

In the course of my research on anorexic patients who either had actual fits of overeating or expressed fear of fits of overeating that nobody had ever witnessed, I found clear clinical evidence of uncertainty, fragmentation, and confusion in bodily experience and conceptualization. When I asked them to describe the way and the intensity of their perception of their bodily stimuli, such as appetite and the feeling of satiety (but also sleepiness, fatigue, cold, even the need for micturition and defecation), they are strongly perplexed. If we make special reference, as we wish to make in the present context, to the perception of appetite and the feeling of satiety (especially the latter), their uncertainty is complete. They do not have an inner spontaneous awareness of these needs, as the rest of us have. They never "know" if and when they should eat, if they have eaten enough, and when they should stop. Every time they are overtaken by the fear, or terror, of not having controlled themselves. The history often reveals that the feeling of uncertainty first arose when departure for college or a vacation caused separation from the family environment, where an automatic and other-directed feeding ritual held sway.

In an earlier paper,[12] I ascribed these defects to an inadequate differentiation of body-self from nonself. From a genetic point of view, it appears that, from a very early age, the parents of these patients consistently forced on their children their own personal and arbitrary interpretations of their children's bodily needs. The parental interpretations had but few connections with the patients' actual subjective experience. This produced confusion and mistrust in the patients toward their own primary source of experience—their own body. The feeling of identity, including bodily identity, seems to consist in an explicit and implicit self-image that, in spite of the constant flux of internal and external stimuli, gives experience its continuity and consistency. Identity processes may be considered to be those ego functions through which the self is perceived to be differentiated from the nonself.

I applied the scoring manual of Lyman Wynne and Margaret Thaler Singer[18] to my own cases in order to check the clinical evidence and psychogenetic interpretations, namely, to check whether the patients who had clinically appeared to be most severe—the overeating anorexics, those with disastrous weight losses, and those with a fatal outcome—showed signs of perceptual and conceptual uncertainty and fragmentation under the external stimulus of the Rorschach cards, when their Rorschach data were reexamined according to this new method. According to my working hypothesis, such signs could be considered to be the expression of perceptual and conceptual uncertainty and confusion arising also under internal stimuli, that is, bodily stimuli. I realized that to reexamine the old Rorschach protocols was an unorthodox procedure, for the authors require for the application of their method a tape-recording that does not omit any behavior and any verbalization showing a transactional disorder. Yet, even by reexamining the protocols as they were originally recorded, I found differences significant enough to justify the division of my patients into two distinct categories: anorexics of the stable type and anorexics who oscillated dramatically between starvation and overeating.

Anorexic patients of the stable type, who had never had spells of severe bulimia or fear of bulimia or such rapid and dramatic weight losses as directly to endanger their lives, revealed a high degree focusing of attention and a stable and well-organized capacity for perception, experience, and communication. Not infrequently, they could be classified in the so-called restricted paranoid type of experience. Patients of this type presumably have an exact perception and recognition of bodily stimuli, but, in accordance with their type of defense, which consists in the persecutory mistrust of their own body, they interpret them in a persecutory manner. Once the body has been equated with the bad object, namely, with the threating entity, the logical consequence seems to be an attitude of mistrust toward the body, its stimuli and its needs. Like the bad object, the body is also fascinating and therefore cannot be abandoned and decathected (actually, in that case, a somatic depersonalization would take place). The body must merely be kept in check; it must not be allowed to dilate; it must undergo heavy work and strain. The master must be turned into a slave. However, what a frightening slave it is!

Paola, a severe anorexic of this type, would reach the point of purposely buying some savory food. She would smell it repeatedly, taste a morsel, and finally throw it in the ash can, exclaiming, as if she were speaking to another person: "You would like it, wouldn't you? Well, look at what I'm doing!"

I then reexamined the Rorschach protocols of patients who oscillated dramatically between spells of starvation and of overeating or who expressed fear of fits of overeating, which nobody had ever witnessed, but who at any rate showed rapid and life-endangering weight losses with dehydration (among them was a patient who died of an acute intoxication due to an actual food binge and one who became a drug addict and eventually died). These patients showed in the Rorschach transaction frequent signs of fragmentation of experience and thinking, perceptual uncertainty, and later denial of interpretations. In some cases, vague and indefinite percepts in the shape of anatomical stereotypes were present. These are the cases that, in my opinion, reveal a deeper perceptual and conceptual disorder, as indicated by Hilde Bruch.

These patients showed in their symptoms the same motivation as the stable anorexic, "the singular goal of achieving autonomy and effectiveness through this bizarre control over the body and its functions," yet their behavior was not equally consistent. Why is this? We can now try to find an explanation according to two points of view, a psychodynamic one and a developmental one.

From a psychodynamic point of view, the cases in which the patient undergoes crises of overeating as well as undereating may alternate between the battle against the object and the surrender to the object. To undereat is to rebel against the object and to overeat is to submit to the passive need of incorporating the object. The passive tie to the object is, of course, stronger than in anorexic patients of the stable type. But the battle to defend the autonomy of the ego is doomed to failure not only because of the stronger passive incorporative component. There has also been a defect in development, in learning, and in the differentiation and integration of experience. Defenses are thus precariously organized on the basis of the earlier distortions in perceptual and conceptual development, such as perceptual uncertainty, fragmentation of thinking and experience, marked deficiency in identifying emotional states (confusion of the feeling of hunger and that of anxiety, emotional emptiness, and loss of some existential meaning). In such cases I would speak not only of a body-image disturbance, as H. Bruch does, but also of a body-identity and body-cognition disturbance. By body identity and body cognition, I mean the result of a learning process during which the child has learned, in the transactional relationship with the caretaker, how to accurately perceive and conceptualize his bodily needs and how to satisfy them adequately, independently of the person who feeds him, out of a direct, consistent, and undisturbed contact with his own basic source of experience—his own body. In the case of these patients, I think one may speak of a psychotic development of body identity.

By way of conclusion, whereas traditional scoring and nosographic classification of twenty-five protocols did not yield any reliable indication of severity, the new method made it possible to divide them into two groups, including respectively fifteen and ten cases. The first group consisted of Rorschach protocols that did not show any appreciable thinking disorders; the second group consisted of protocols that showed clear and repeated signs of thinking disorder according to the scoring manual. To my surprise, all the patients with a fatal outcome fell into the second group, as the still-living patients who had the most unsatisfactory outcome. Those who reached complete recovery after a suitable long psychotherapy and achieved fundamental existential aims, such as love, sex, and procreation, all belong to the first group.

In spite of the shortcomings in the recording of the protocols, I considered these data a very stimulating encouragement to resume the research. Starting last year, I methodically began recording, with the correct technique, all cases of anorexia nervosa that come to me for consultation, with the aim of following their progress in psychotherapy and follow-ups. In order to yield sufficiently accurate findings, the research will have to continue for several years, thus making it possible to make a long follow-up and to collect reliable clinical data. It is quite often necessary to wait for months, sometimes years, for the patient to trust the therapist and provide sincere information, reflecting the facts. I can already state that the cases whose Rorschach protocols are free from thinking disorders more readily establish valid and consistent psychotherapeutic relationships, provided there has not been the previous trauma of a wrong treatment. The cases whose protocols show signs of thought disorder generally tend to refuse therapy or to enter therapy with such anguish and mistrust as to confirm the worst prognostic predictions.

CONCLUSIONS

At this point I wish to suggest my interpretative conclusion. Anorexia nervosa is a special defensive structure midway between the schizoparanoid position and depression. The incorporated bad object is neither broken up nor breakable, but remains a whole, just as the body with which it is identified is a whole. In accordance with the intermediate position between schizophrenia and depression, the experience of the body is also ambiguous: it is situated between the non-me and the bad me; it is at the same time alienated and one's own—persecutor and persecuted. The patient makes a projection, but defends herself against the schizophrenic's catastrophe by projecting the unacceptable within the structures of her own personality, into her own body instead of into others. The body thus becomes the persecutor, but a persecutor whom it is easy to spy on and control. This projection onto the body is a safeguard against interpersonal delusional ideas and thus somehow saves the capacity to socialize and to relate to the world. Anorexia nervosa is also a safeguard against the depressive catastrophe and actual suicide, which is very rarely carried out. The bad body, which must not be brutally destroyed but merely held in check, allows the ideal existence of a good self, idealized, enhanced, acceptable, and worthy of respect. When the anorexic system is organized, the patients actually emerge from the depressive phase.

The threefold meaning of the anorexic symptom may be synthesized as follows:

```
to keep  ─────────────┐
to keep out  ─────────▶ the good and the bad object
to keep in check  ────┘
```

To keep: the body as the good object is recognized by the patient as her own and is invested with libidinal cathexis—*no somatopsychic depersonalization*. To keep out: the body as the bad object is kept out of the self, which remains worthy of esteem—*no depression*. To keep in check: the body as the bad object is not allowed to grow larger than the patient. The patient can control it and the object world remains good—*no schizophrenia*.

This balance can also account for the exceptional stability of the anorexic syndrome in the many mild forms that escape the clinician but have an identical structure. In these mild forms, the ego defense is centered on keeping the weight at a minimum that is neither dramatic nor dangerous, but is rigidly determined and fixed. I am accustomed to calling this weight—also with my patients—"the magic weight." To go beyond it lights up the red signal of danger. Many so-called recoveries, as a result of various treatments, belong to this type of adjustment. Often this adjustment at the magic weight coincides with the resumption of the menstrual cycle: it provides a minimum level of biological and psychological security for the resumption of a typical feminine function.

I have called anorexia nervosa an intrapersonal paronia (intrapsychic paranoia). The research for power, experienced as impossible in interpersonal relationships, is carried out in the intrapersonal structure in controlling the body. The projection involves the body rather than the external environment. Can one therefore speak of an oral syndrome in anorexia nervosa? In a dynamic sense, no. One can merely speak of an oralized aspect of a problem of power and worth of the ego. In experiencing its primary relationship, the ego has found only these means of psychic survival: (1) preserving the object, (2) preserving the relationship with the object, (3) preserving the self. The price is a mutilated, often tragic, existence.

THE SOCIAL ENVIRONMENT

There are no statistics concerning the incidence of anorexia nervosa in Italy, but it is my impression that the illness is increasing in the country. In Italy, two radically different types of cultures exist, that of the north and that of the south. The culture in the north is to become more and more similar to that of other Western industrialized countries. It is characterized by the ambiguity of the role of the woman. The traditionally passive role of women in the rural patriarchal type of culture is gradually being transformed into a new many-sided and complicated role, a mixture of feminine and masculine characteristics, of submission and leadership, of passivity and activity, which does not find in the mother a valid model of identification. The new role is apparently matriarchal, but is actually assumed in an environment still permeated with patriarchal traditions, such as the conviction of man's superiority and the requirement of marked sexual inhibition in the woman.

If a higher incidence of anorexia nervosa were to be found in the northern culture, where the society expects much more from its women, and if a higher incidence were also to be found in middle and lower bourgeois classes as compared to the worker and farmer classes, then anorexia nervosa could be considered a largely socially determined illness.

It would be most interesting if large-scale comparative social anthropological research were to be carried out among the predominantly preindustrial migrants of the southern Italian culture and the emerging northern Italian culture. Such a study might be an important contribution to the clarification of the social factors connected with the epidemiology of anorexia nervosa.

PSYCHOTHERAPEUTIC SUGGESTIONS

I must say, first of all, that I disagree with the technique of early interpretation practiced by various analysts and explicity suggested by H. Thomä.[17] This German author suggests that the patients be immediately confronted with the analysis of their resistance to therapy and with the exposure of the tricks by which they hide food and throw it away, stimulate vomiting, or administer laxatives and enemas to themselves.

I am of the opinion that, especially in these cases, psychotherapy should not consist of an interpretative frenzy, but should rather aim at understanding the patients and especially at leading them to experience new, and therefore therapeutic, interpersonal situations. Why, then, repeat in therapy the impervious attitude they have always experienced in their environment, with their parents or their physicians?

The therapist should not concentrate on the symptom and overlook what lies behind it. These patients are basically incapable of real aggressiveness, unless it is directed against their own bodies. The therapist should therefore be careful not to reinforce in these superficially aggressive patients their basic defect, namely, their sense of helplessness and ineffectiveness. Faced with our astute interpretations, they will experience once again the well-known sensation of desperate helplessness, and they will defend themselves in earnest by an irrevocable refusal to establish relationships.

Having always treated these patients in an office setting, I know only too well how a single power struggle is enough to prevent these patients from returning for the next session. The analysis of their manipulation in terms of aggressiveness is then nothing but the therapist's way of venting his own aggressiveness, the frustrating feeling of therapeutic helplessness to which he is condemned for a long time. I have endured bravely (though also cautiously), and often successfully, the loss in weight of patients during psychotherapy. If I needed help in the form of medical therapies or hospitalization, I gave my colleagues, in the presence of the patient, the role of administrator and my full confidence, and I openly admitted the impending danger for the patient's life. However, if patients are referred for a suitable psychotherapy at an early stage, particularly before too many long years of illness or previous mistaken therapies have produced a hopelessly chronic condition, this point is generally not reached. From the very first session, I tell them with complete acceptance that I understand their reluctance to come to me. They never come of their own accord, they are always sent, not infrequently with threats, as an unpleasant alternative to hospitalization or to the dreaded tube-feeding. They are unaware of their severe personality deformation and are used to being fought at the level of the symptom. They mistrust therapy and consider it "a lot of chatter, which thinly disguises the only real purpose: to make them swell up like a balloon." It is, therefore, imperative from the very beginning for the therapist to be simple, unassuming, and sincere, so as slowly to induce the patients to cooperate. Like all adolescents, they are very sensitive to reticent, roundabout ways of speaking and allusions. They always fear hidden meanings. Though they themselves often use hypocrisy defensively, they detest it in others. It should be explained at once, clearly, in the terms most suitable to the individual case, that their problem is not that of food, though everybody seems to imply that "once they have got fat, everything will be all right." The problem of food is certainly serious, for it may endanger their lives. But what really matters is inside themselves, in their minds, in their pasts. What matters is their own histories, the series of remote and recent events, their difficult relationships with their environments, their ways of being-in-the-world, the ways in which they look at it, their solitude and fear, of which they are perhaps not even aware.

Even minor requests on the part of the therapist are not complied with for a long time. The patients rarely accept the couch. In my opinion, it is better not to use it. They do not follow the fundamental rule and seldom, if at all, associate. Even if they have dreams, they often do not report them. Faced with long spells of silence bespeaking mistrust, with the patient's large eyes pointed at him, the therapist often feels embarrassed and impatient. In such cases, the spells of silence should be interrupted. At times, one may remark sympathetically on their difficulty in expressing themselves and try to suggest what negative experiences in their relationships with others may have led them to this. Care should be taken, however, not to insist too much and not to offer help or affection. The patient may detect hypocrisy or, worse still, seductiveness.

Experience has often shown me that the interpretation of a dream, attempted without associations or with very few associations, has had a favorable shock effect. In such cases, far from insisting on a detailed analysis of repressed drives, I point out the hidden suffering of the patient, especially her feeling of helplessness. This should be done sympathetically and tactfully, taking care not to damage the already low self-esteem of these patients.

Proceeding in this direction, one may then invite the patients to make detailed reports of the present and of their everyday situations. Under what circumstances have they been unable to maintain their judgment, affirm their basic autonomy, and assert their human sovereignty, apart from the implicit, but unstated, sovereignty over their bodies?

The more severe cases that undergo alternate crises of overeating and undereating are so confused and alienated from their own bodies as a primary source of experience that rehabilitation is also necessary to lead them to pay attention to, describe, recognize, and ultimately have trust in their own internal and external perceptions. It is equally important to take into account, and to explain to the patients, that, as a result of their past and present interpersonal relations, something in them struggles on an emotional level against the new learning experience and the attainment of true autonomy of the body.

By means of this twofold psychotherapeutic approach, several cases, even very severe ones, have been able to arrive at complete clinical recovery.

I end by quoting one of my patients, Liliana, when she took leave of me before going back to her home town after her recovery. "I am grateful to you for not having exposed the lies and tricks of which I made such frequent use at the beginning. I must confess that for a time I thought you were dumb. Later, I began to feel the need to tell you the truth. One day, do you remember? I angrily threw onto your table the enema apparatus that I secretly used to employ. . . . To my surprise, you were neither triumphant nor indignant. You merely said: 'We must try and find out together why you still need it.' At that time it wasn't clear to me. Now I have understood that you saw through my lies and tricks from the beginning. But you also knew, as I know now, that at that time I had no other means to survive."

REFERENCES

1. Benjamin, J. "Prediction and Psychopathological Theory," in L. Jessner, and E. Pavenstedt (eds.), *Dynamic Psychopathology in Childhood*. New York: Grune & Stratton, 1959.
2. Bibring, E. "The Mechanism of Depression," in P. Greenacre (ed.), *Affective Disorders*. New York: International Universities Press, 1953.
3. Bliss, E., and Branch, C. *Anorexia Nervosa*. New York: Hoeber, 1960.
4. Bruch, H. "Transformation of Oral Impulses in Eating Disorders," *Psychiatric Quarterly*, 35 (1961), 458–481.
5. Bruch, H. "Perceptual and Conceptual Disturbances in Anorexia Nervosa," *Psychosomatic Medicine*, 24 (1962), 187.
6. Bruch, H. "The Psychiatric Differential Diagnosis of Anorexia Nervosa," in J. E. Meyer, and H. Feldman (eds.), *Anorexia Nervosa*. Stuttgart: Thième, 1965.
7. Fairbairn, W. R. *An Object Relations Theory of the Personality*. New York: Basic Books, 1962.
8. Jourdan, H. A., Wieland, W. F., Zelbley, S. P., Stellar, E., and Stunkard, A. J. "Direct Measurement of Food Intake in Man: A Method for the Objective Study of Eating Behaviour," *Psychosomatic Medicine*, 28 (1966), 836–842.
9. Kaufman, M. R., and Heiman, M. (eds.). *Evolution of Psychosomatic Concepts: Anorexia Nervosa; A Paradigm*. New York: International Universities Press, 1964.
10. Kind, H. "Psicopatologia dell'insufficienza del lobo anteriore," *Recenti Progressi in Medicina*, 24 (1958), 443–452.
11. Meyer, J. E. "Das Syndrom der Anorexia Nervosa. Katamnestische Untersuchungen," *Archiv für Psychiatrie und Zeitschrift, für die Gesamte Neurologie*, 202 (1961), 31–59.
12. Selvini Palazzoli, M. *L'Anoressia Mentale*. Milano: Feltrinelli, 1963.
13. Selvini Palazzoli, M. "Contribution à la psychopathologie du vécu corporel," *Evolution Psychiatrique*, 1 (1967), 149–173.
14. Selvini Palazzoli, M. "La strutturazione della coscienza corporea," *Infanzia Anormale*, 73 (1967), 9–30.
15. Stunkard, A. J. "Obesity and the Denial of Hunger," *Psychosomatic Medicine*, 21 (1959), 281–289.
16. Stunkard, A. J. "Hunger and Satiety," *American Journal of Psychiatry*, 118 (1961), 212–217.

17. Thomä, H. *Anorexia Nervosa*. New York: International Universities Press, 1967.
18. Thaler Singer, M., and Wynne, L. C. "Principles for Scoring Communication Defects and Deviances in Parents of Schizophrenics, Rorschach and T.A.T. Scoring Manuals," *Psychiatry*, **29** (1966), 260–288.
19. Werner, H. "The Concept of Development from a Comparative and Organismic Point of View," in Dale B. Harris (ed.), *The Concept of Development*. Minneapolis: University of Minnesota Press, 1957.
20. Wynne, L. C., and Thaler Singer, M. "Thought Disorders and Family Relations of Schizophrenics," *Archives of General Psychiatry*, **9** (1963), 191–206; **12** (1965), 187–212.

NEW VIEWS ON THE PSYCHODYNAMICS OF THE DEPRESSIVE CHARACTER

Jules Richard Bemporad

Clinical experience with depressed patients has led me to question the classical psychoanalytic theory of depression. Although the Freudian interpretation of melancholia was a significant advancement in its time and did much to open the way to the psychoanalytic study of object relationships, the theory nevertheless rests on metapsychological assumptions that today appear outmoded and in need of revision.

The classical psychoanalytic interpretation of depression is based on the theory of a pathological introject within the ego. It is maintained that the predisposition to melancholia resides in the formation of a pathologic ego introject following the loss of a love object in early infancy.[10] This early loss would free libidinal cathexes, which, rather than being redirected outward toward a new object, are directed inward to the ego, which takes on some of the characteristics of the lost object and becomes a reparative substitute. This introject becomes the intrapsychic effigy of this early, as well as later, cathected object, so that in adult life the depressive would react with the original infantile rage to subsequent losses, spending this rage on the internalized object rather than on environmental figures.

Freud thus accounted for the melancholic's self-recriminations, which he considered as evidence of anger directed at the ego introject. The presence of this self-accusatory behavior was also specified as one of the characteristics that differentiated depression from normal grief. The other major difference was that, whereas grief was a response to an external loss, depression represented an internal loss. Because subsequent losses reactivate the loss of the original love object, which had been incorporated into the ego, there results an impoverishment of the ego and a concomitant reduction of self-esteem.

Other contributions to the classical psychoanalytic theory of depression have retained the concept of the ego introject as an essential explanatory hypothesis. Abraham,[1] for example, gave a detailed account of the relationship between the clinical aspects of melancholia and the unconscious wish to incorporate a new love object. Three years later, Rado[23] interpreted the symptoms of melancholia as expressing the depressive's attempt to regain love from the powerful introject through painful expiation and self-abasement. Depression was seen as the result of complex unconscious events that gave the clinical manifestations their "meaning." The major features of melancholia resulted from retroflected anger directed at the ego introject. Other characteristics were interpreted as part of the over-all libidinal regression to the oral stage with its emphasis on incorporation.

On the other hand, some psychoanalysts outside of, as well as a few within, the orthodox circle have taken issue with various aspects of this formulation.[2, 6, 8, 21, 30] Some have suggested that depression be viewed as a primary affect, without any underlying meaning, that automatically arises in specific situations. Sandler and Joffee[24] exemplify this view by concluding that "if depression is viewed as an affect, if we allot to it the same conceptual status as the affect of anxiety, then much of the literature on depression in childhood (and this could be extended to adults) can be integrated in a meaningful way" (p. 90). Bibring has similarly tried to deemphasize the role of unconscious symbolism by stressing the importance of the ego in depression: "depression can be defined as the emotional expression of a state of helplessness or powerlessness of the ego" (p. 24). Bibring maintains that depression will be automatically experienced whenever the ego finds itself unable to live up to aspirations that are still strongly maintained.

Another area of disagreement has centered on the role of object loss in depression. Arieti,[2] Kielholz,[18] and, more recently, Hudgens[15] have all questioned the importance of an environmental loss in depressive states. Sullivan[28] went so far as to suggest that any so-called precipitating event was merely used to fixate and organize the depressive's symptoms on some concrete experience and did not merit any causative significance. The disagreement over the importance of object loss seems to center on what is understood to be actually lost. Freud defined an "internal" loss in melancholia as resulting in an impoverishment of the ego, which differed from the grief response, and so did not see depression as exclusively the result of a true environmental loss as much as the consequence of a specific predisposition to depression resulting from the formation of the ego introject. Nevertheless, the isolated experience of loss, whether internal or external, suggests the simple state of deprivation that belongs to a lower cognitive level than depression, which implies an awareness of finality and future suffering. The theme of the anticipation of one's own future, which Arieti[4] believes has been unfortunately neglected in psychiatric theory, seems to play a crucial role in depressive symptomatology. Phenomenological studies, as reported by Jaspers[17] and Minkowski,[22] certainly demonstrate the depressive's obsession with the horror of an empty and meaningless future, but have not incorporated this finding into a theoretical exposition of depressive states. It would appear that the emphasis on the instinctual or primitive aspects of the individual has been at the expense of an appreciation of the importance of cognitive and conceptual factors in psychopathology.

A final source of disagreement with the classical formulation results from the changing nature of depressive symptomatology over the last few decades. In the older literature, depressives were described as displaying an overwhelming sense of guilt and self-blame. Today, such patients are infrequently seen in the United States; depressed patients still present feelings of hopelessness and helplessness, but lack the excessive feelings of guilt and self-debasement. The absence of self-recriminations, as well as the lack of an overt sense of guilt and desire for punishment, led Weiss[29] to postulate a nonmelancholic form of depression. Harrow,[13] in a questionnaire study of fifty-two hospitalized depressed females, found a surprising paucity of guilt or self-blame. His sample differed so markedly from the older clinical descriptions that he questioned if the same diagnosis were applicable. Arieti,[3] as well, has not found self-accusatory behavior to be a consistent symptom of depression. He separates two forms of depression, the self-blaming and claiming types. The former resembles the traditional description of the melancholic, but the latter type exhibits a sense of blamelessness and unjust deprivation that the therapist is expected to rectify. The theoretical significance of this more recently seen claiming type is that it challenges the concept of retroflected anger directed at the ego introject, because the self-accusations, which were used as evidence of this anger, are absent. It would appear that the entire concept of introjection in depression is in need of clarification, especially in view of the development in psychoanalytic theory since the appearance of "Mourning and Melancholia."[10]

These questions warrant a reconsideration of the mechanisms of depression. In the following pages a view of depression that is less reliant on metapsychological theorizing will be described. Four major features of depression as well as the family background of depressives will be presented in an effort later to define the more basic pathology underlying depressive states. The role of anger in depression will be considered separately.

FOUR PSYCHODYNAMIC ASPECTS OF DEPRESSION

Dependency on a Dominant Other

Perhaps the one characteristic of the depressive that has been unanimously emphasized in the psychiatric literature is pathologic dependency. It was most probably this tenacious, demanding quality of melancholics that suggested to Abraham, in his pioneering work on depression, the existence of a libidinal regression to the oral stage. Although many authors have subsequently disregarded Abraham's formulations of unconscious dynamics, there has been a uniform acceptance of his excellent descriptions of the depressive's mode of object relations and character structure. The later contributions of Rado,[23] Fromm-Reichmann,[11,12] Jacobson,[16] and Bonime[7,8] have echoed the theme of dependency as central in depression, although considering this characteristic from vastly different theoretical positions. Arieti[3] has especially stressed the role of dependency in the etiology of depression, noting that, in his experience, decompensation of the depressive often occurs following the failure to maintain an ongoing relationship with a significant environmental figure. In contrast to the schizophrenic, in whom the psychotic transformation is in reaction to a failure of "cosmic magnitude involving the relation with the whole interpersonal world" (p. 401), severe depression seems to result from the loss of a relationship with one highly esteemed person in the immediate environment. Arieti called this idealized figure the "dominant other," whom, regardless of substitution in adult life, Arieti believes to be symbolic of the depriving mother.

The theme of dependency on a dominant other is indeed frequently seen in depressives. A forty-five-year-old bachelor, for example, who presented with a severe depressive reaction, described a life of exclusive emotional dependence on his mother. This patient spoke of his mother as an other-worldly, superior being in terms that were reminiscent of the "fatal woman" figure in the romantic literature of the nineteenth century. His father had left the household while the patient was still in his infancy, and the mother was remembered as the sole source of authority. In the course of therapy, it became evident that this idealized woman had tyrannically demanded obedience while ridiculing any attempt at independent assertion. The patient grew up believing himself to be a burden to his mother and undeserving of her love or attention. Her love or acceptance, in fact, was never freely given, but had to be earned by submission and self-effacement. He came to believe that he was really not good enough to merit her love, but that perhaps through great effort and perseverance she might eventually accept him. Her praise or support, sparse as it was, became essential for his seeing himself as worthwhile, whereas other achievements or successes brought him no pleasure or satisfaction. This pathetic individual continued to live with his mother in a near-servile capacity, although financially supporting her, until she died two years prior to his seeking therapy. After her death, the patient lapsed into a state of despair, leaving his home only to shop for groceries and later to visit numerous physicians with various somatic complaints. When his savings were gone, he sold articles of furniture, finally moving into a shabby, furnished room.

This man's history clearly demonstrates the role of the dominant other that in other cases may be hidden or disguised. The dominant other gives meaning to the depressive's activities; without this figure, life becomes pointless and devoid of pleasure. The dominant other is not solely utilized to obtain pleasure, but also to escape feelings of guilt and uncertainty for supposed wrongdoing. This patient's mother had served to reassure him that his conduct was acceptable and to provide a structure to his life so that he had merely to follow her commands. He had learned to fear the expression of his desires and to feel guilty over the possibility that he had somehow asserted himself.

It may be noted that, contrary to the classical formulation of depression, this man did not create an ego introject of the mother following a loss in infancy. He seemed to have accepted his mother's evaluation of him and to live the role that she created for him in that he required her continual presence in order to function adequately. However, this internalization of parental values does not mean the incorporation of a lost love object as initially intended by Freud. Certainly, all children adopt certain values and attitudes of their parents in the course of normal development without becoming depressives in adult life. The difficulty with the different meanings of internalization may be the result of a lack of reconciliation between the Freudian theory of depression and the later conceptualization of the superego. In the former, the infant incorporates the parent, whereas in the latter, the child identifies with the parent as a solution to the oedipal conflict. The classical theory, by wishing to trace the genesis of depression to the oral stage with the stage-specific defensive process of incorporation, had to differentiate this type of internalization from the postoedipal identification with the same-sex parent. It may be, however, that internalization of parental values occurs as a gradual process throughout childhood and that the concept of an introject is an unnecessary reification. More recent psychoanalytic contributions that stress infantile superego precursors seem to be postulating just this preoedipal acceptance of parental attitudes without having to hypothesize the formation of a pathological introject.

A further clarification of the process of internalization may also be needed. The difference between imitative learning, whereby the child models himself after the parent, and reactive learning, whereby the child is coerced to become an idealized model desired by the parent, should be specified in reference to such terms as self-image and superego. In the case of imitative learning, the self is automatically modeled after an esteemed environmental figure, often without any underlying conflict. Reactive learning, as intended here, is the process whereby the child is made to become a desired ideal, which does not necessarily resemble the parent, in order to win love or escape punishment. The attainment of this parental ideal leads to a sense of satisfaction, not because of any inherent gratifying quality, but because it ensures parental favor.

The depressive appears to be the product of excessive reactive learning and seems to have developed a reactive identity in that he functions best in a role that reflects the dictates of a dominant other rather than any independent standards. These individuals seem to require the presence of an external agency in order to derive satisfaction, being unable to gain pleasure from independent achievement. The patient described above, for example, was quite willing to go to any extreme to squeeze out a kind word from his mother, but reacted with fear and shame to the possibility of any behavior that might directly bring him pleasure.

Fear of Autonomous Gratification

The patient described above exhibited a marked inability and even dread of obtaining self-esteem or pleasure directly through his own efforts rather than through the medium of a dominant other. I have found this type of pathologic functioning, which may be called the "fear of autonomous gratification," to be a consistent feature of depressives. This characteristic may not always be immediately apparent, especially in view of the impressive achievements of some depressives. However, on further investigation, it is found that social or professional accomplishments bring the depressive little pleasure in themselves and are sought in an attempt to win love and acceptance from an external agency.

Nancy, a highly successful executive who began psychotherapy after years of visiting internists with vague pains and insomnia, exemplifies this fear of autonomous gratification. Although she held a position of considerable importance and made an attractive salary, she could not bring herself to furnish her apartment comfortably or live in a manner commensurate with her income. She considered anything spent on herself to be a shameful extravagance, but would buy inordinately expensive gifts for her parents. Nancy was equally self-sacrificing with her free time and would cancel social engagements if her boss asked her to work late or if her father asked to see her. In actuality, Nancy was unable really to enjoy a social evening unless she could somehow relate it to her work, just as she had to justify her buying clothes by saying that she had to dress well for work. She found it difficult to date and had a dread of any sexual confrontation. When she did go out, she tried to structure the evening so that she would be part of a group and thus escape being alone with a man. Even then she had to drink a good deal in order to fight feelings of guilt and degradation. Eventually, Nancy confessed that even her work, which seemed to be her major concern in life, brought her no pleasure in itself, but only served as a means of pleasing her boss. Whenever she gained recognition from him or was praised by her father, Nancy became ecstatic with a great sense of well-being and felt "vibrant" and "alive."

Although subject to mild depressive episodes for most of her life, Nancy became severely depressed when her boss decided to retire. She felt betrayed by his leaving her after her many years of self-sacrifice. This sense of desertion was intensified by her parents' coincidental plan to take an extended vacation overseas. Nancy felt that her only means of gratification and meaning were abandoning her, and the prospect of life without them was unbearable. Never having been able to gain a sense of self-esteem from her own efforts, but only through the presence of a dominant other, her life now seemed empty and pointless.

Nancy's early history can only be briefly outlined. Her mother was described as a shy, helpless woman who lived in fear of her husband who tyrannically ruled the household. Nancy was not allowed to form extrafamilial attachments, but was coerced to work hard and study arduously in order to bring "honor" to the family. She was sent to strict parochial schools, and her work was closely supervised by her father who made her feel guilty and ashamed if she did not perform according to his aspirations. She was repeatedly told how her parents were sacrificing themselves for her and how she frivolously squandered their hard-earned savings by not studying enough or by desiring to enjoy herself with school friends. Nancy grew up determined to win her father's admiration and to redeem herself against his accusations. Any activities that were not directed toward this goal were reacted to with apprehension and anxiety although superficially disparaged as childish or immoral. In keeping with this "pleasure anxiety," Spiegel[26] has commented that the depressive fears the experience of happiness and pleasure as much as the experience of anger. The only thing that matters is to be passively gratified by the dominant other, to be reassured of one's own worth, and to be freed of the burden of guilt.

Bargain Relationship

Implicit in the depressive's dependency and inhibition is what may be called the "bargain relationship," which typifies the depressive's mode of interpersonal relations. The bargain is simply that the depressive will deny himself autonomous satisfaction in return for nurturance from the dominant other. This relationship is initiated by the parent, but is later reestablished by the depressive on unwitting transference objects. This *quid pro quo* relationship ensures that gratification and acceptance will be forthcoming if willingness for self-sacrifice is properly demonstrated.

The significance of the bargain relationship and the sense of betrayal that it may engender is exemplified by a depressed young man who entered therapy with a feeling that he had been cheated by life. This patient felt that he had complied with all that had been expected of him, and yet he found his existence painfully empty and meaningless. As a child, he had been singled out as his father's favorite and had felt proud and superior because of his preferential treatment. However, he found that in order to maintain his status he had continuously to submit to his father's demands and expectations. He concentrated on being a model son for his father, believing that he would be grandly rewarded in adult life for his good behavior. Instead, as he approached maturity, he found himself unable really to enjoy anything or become absorbed in any career or interests. He had graduated from college in order to please his father, but had never really felt himself a part of university life. After graduation, he continued to work in his father's store in a fairly menial capacity and gradually came to the realization that he would remain there for the rest of his life. He had no close friends, interests, or hobbies. He was afraid of sexuality and suffered anxiety attacks whenever he tried to date. His one sexual encounter with a prostitute left him agonized with guilt and shame. Although his present situation was unbearable, he could not conceive of leaving his father and making a life for himself. He alternated between blaming his father for "cheating" him and despising himself for being a failure.

This young man expected his father and the therapist somehow magically to solve all of his problems. He had no sense of doing things for himself and saw any autonomous action as a betrayal of his father. The father had to share in the activity or approve of it for the activity to be free of anxiety and guilt; to attempt anything without the blessings of the dominant other was to betray a trust and to risk the loss of love and esteem. This patient, like many depressives, led an essentially ascetic life; the only things that mattered were those that ensured parental approval.

In this case, the positive or gratifying aspects of the bargain relationship have been illustrated rather than the more painful type of bond where coercion by guilt is prominent. In the latter case, the dominant other is needed to reassure against feelings of inherent evil and badness. In addition to an air of helpless resignation and a sense of worthlessness, these patients believe themselves to be inordinately vile and malicious, convinced that only the dominant other can free them from this self-image. One such patient, who required hospitalization, described herself in the most derogatory terms imaginable, whereas in reality she seemed to have led an exemplary life. Her mother was a selfish woman who resented any responsibility and detested the mothering role. When her husband left her, she blamed the patient and repeatedly told her that, if she had never been born, the father would have remained. The mother continued to blame her for her later misfortunes and in addition projected all sorts of sexual desires onto the patient, eventually making her believe that her incestuous desires had driven her father from the house. This woman accepted the blame for her mother's unhappiness and dedicated her life to seeking forgiveness. She could not tolerate her mother being cross or angry, but did everything she could to soothe or please her. For more than twenty years, this woman forced her husband and children to visit the mother weekly in another city; the patient would fuss over her and try to win her praise. The patient's mood for the following week depended on the success of these Sunday outings.

This woman became severely depressed when she developed intimate feelings for her employer. She could not tolerate her desires, which to her proved that her mother had been right in her estimation of her, that she was really wanton and base. All her efforts to redeem herself were now without meaning. She would never change; she had always been and would always be evil and worthless. She succumbed to an image of herself that she despised and disgusted her.

Inability to Alter Environment

It is of interest that, both in this and the former case, the depressive episode did not follow an environmental loss, but gradually developed from the painful realization of being hopelessly deprived of some necessary source of meaning and self-esteem. It would appear that depression is brought about by a sense of helplessness to alter oneself or one's environment, together with the awareness of a future devoid of meaning and gratification. This leads to a sense of hopelessness and despair, the cardinal features of depression.

As will be more fully elaborated below, the depressive becomes inordinately reliant on external agents for maintenance of self-esteem and gratification. Because of the concomitant inhibition of autonomous gratification and assertion, the threatened or actual loss of these needed agents results in an unbearable sense of futility and hopeless resignation.

This sense of hopelessness may also be at the core of the depressive reaction seen in schizophrenic patients. It is significant that these episodes of depression do not occur when the patient is actually psychotic, but rather during the period of recovery from the acute phase. The patient believes that he will again be subject to the terror of an acute psychosis and feels helpless in his efforts to prevent future decompensations. He sees himself as hopelessly ill and subject to a life of repeated torment, which will not allow for the attainment of normal goals and pleasures. I have seen a number of serious suicide attempts in just such patients who, having suffered through repeated episodes of psychosis, gave up the hope of a satisfying life and preferred death to the prospect of recurrent madness.

FAMILY BACKGROUND OF DEPRESSIVES

The families of depressives resemble those that Lidz[20] called the skewed type in his studies of the genesis of schizophrenia. In these families, parental authority is skewed toward one parent, either because of the other parent's absence or because of personality interaction, so that the children do not receive a blending of paternal and maternal values nor are they able to seek protection and support from one parent as a refuge from the other. In addition, the families of depressives demonstrate a great deal of cohesiveness and false pretenses of superiority that greatly restrict the influence of extrafamilial factors. These families overvalued achievement and worldly success that were to be obtained by hard work. Adult depressives often remember feeling that the dignity and honor of their family rested on their efforts and accomplishments and that this parental goal superseded any personal desire.

The mothers of future depressives, either from an overwhelming sense of helplessness or narcissistic egotism, were unable to impart a basic feeling of worth to these patients. Fromm-Reichmann,[12] in a study of twelve manic-depressives, found that:

> The mothers of these patients appear to have found the child more acceptable and lovable as infants than as children, when the manifold problems of training and acculturation became important. Our impression is that it was the utter dependence of the infant that was pleasurable to the mother and that the growing independence and rebelliousness of the early stage of childhood were threatening to her (p. 245).

On the other hand, Dince[9] in a study of adolescent failure of individuation, which he likened to severe depressive reactions, found that the mothers of his patients were often depressed or unavailable during the child's infancy. However, when the child developed into a toddler, these mothers selfishly clung to the child and attempted a reversal of the mothering role.

According to either type of mother-child interaction, there results a lack of comfortable autonomy and individuation in the child. Sandler and Joffee[24] report that in the childhood of depressives "it not infrequently happens that the child's parents are in unconscious opposition to progressive individuation and the influence of the parents may be perpetuated in their successor, the superego" (p. 94). The crucial factor seems to be that the mothers of depressives exploitatively try to derive strength and gratification from the child rather than to impart a sense of well-being and freedom. Many depressives remember that, as children, they felt obligated to make their mothers happy and content. They rarely experienced a spontaneous sense of joy from the parent, but always had to work at feeling appreciated or loved. These patients seem to have grown up believing that their simple existence was a burden on the mother for which they had to compensate by continuously trying to satisfy the parent who, in return, might respond in an assuring or loving fashion. Their own sense of worth became dependent on obtaining acceptance from the mother. In retrospect, many mothers of future depressives seem to have been depressed themselves and unable to take pleasure in their children.

Similarly, the fathers of these patients often used them to fulfill their own aspirations rather than allowing them to develop autonomous interests and satisfactions. The conditional love and acceptance could only be won by complying with parental demands for achievement and success. Extrafamilial involvements were forbidden as signs of disloyalty or ridiculed as mingling with "trash" and degrading the family name. Although indulgent and benevolent when their demands were met, these fathers could react violently when challenged or disobeyed. Spiegel[27] has found that a significant factor in the predisposition to depression in women is the father's rejection of his daughter's emerging sexuality at adolescence. Nancy's sexual maturation was seen, in fact, as a threat by her father, who feared she would become less dependent on him. However, the principal effect of the parent, whether mother or father, is to demand an unrealistic ideal that corresponds to personal needs and to punish the failure to realize this ideal by guilt and shame. Either parent, by tyrannizing the family, may become the dominant other; therefore, sexual factors appear to be secondary.

The depressive grows up in a highly restricted environment with little opportunity to validate the family's values and standards. He is given little sense of self-worth from either of his parents, who view the child as an agent of their own needs rather than a separate, self-willed entity. The future depressive is made to feel guilty and malevolent for behavior that does not correspond to the idealized model with which he is constantly confronted by the parent. Eventually, he begins to distrust his own impulses and to fear his own desires, so that he relinquishes control over his own gratification.

THE INTRAPSYCHIC STRUCTURE IN DEPRESSION

An interesting paradox exhibited by the depressive is the contrast between his infantile need of a dominant other and his many mature capabilities and superior achievements. The depressive is often an able, seemingly dedicated person who efficiently succeeds in whatever he attempts. He presents the façade of a reliable, responsible adult who can be counted on to fulfill his obligations. In short, he has learned to present himself as the idealized model so desired by the parent. However, the depressive, despite this veneer of independence, requires the presence of the dominant other—in the form of an actual person or transformed into an organization, social cause, or religious order—to function adequately.

This inability to achieve autonomous gratification and the persistent reliance on reflected gratification through the medium of the dominant other seem different from the intrapsychic situation in which a healthy ego is restricted by an excessively strict superego and must resort to symbolic or substitute maneuvers. For example, in some perversions, a specific object is used as a means to achieve gratification. In depressives, however, the other is not a means of gratification but the source of gratification. The dominant other is not used by the self to expedite gratification for itself, but figuratively replaces the self as the gratifying agency. The depressive seems to require an external object to function as the part of the self that bestows gratification and meaning. In this sense, depression might be categorized as an ego defect neurosis, as described by Hendricks.[14] In these disorders, according to Hendricks, "the symptoms are not primarily the result of a healthy ego's defense against an unresolved infantile conflict; they result from a fundamental inadequacy of some essential function of the ego itself" (p. 50). In depressives, the deficient functions would be in the area of autonomous gratification.

This need for another to assume ego functions may account for Freud's postulating an internal loss in melancholia. In effect, the depressive has lost a function that would normally reside within the ego when he loses the dominant other. However, this does not mean that the lost object or its predecessors had been introjected into the ego. Rather, it is just the failure of identification and imitative learning that causes the depressive to require an external agency to fulfill ego functions. As Arieti[5] has written in regard to the psychopath, the depressive has also been unable to transform the interpersonal into the intrapsychic. Thus, rather than the depressive incorporating the object into the ego, the reverse dynamic would appear more appropriate: the depressive must continuously externalize ego functions onto love objects and depend on them to perform these ego functions.

In any event, the depressive does not appear to have progressed beyond the mode of reflective gratification and has never learned independently to achieve satisfaction for himself. The exploitative use of these patients in childhood prevented their normally developing appropriate ego functions in the area of gratification.

In this sense, the depressive retains oral characteristics as described in the psychoanalytic literature. The application of the concept of orality, however, should be restricted to a metaphorical usage regarding one aspect of the depressive's life experience rather than being employed as a genetic explanation that implies specific etiological and metapsychological hypotheses.

The mode of reflective gratification evidences itself in the therapeutic relationship in the form of covert demands that override any desire for change. Although superficially cooperative, the depressive refuses to acknowledge the true goal of treatment. Instead, he parentifies and idealizes the therapist and devotes himself to obtaining nurturance and support. These patients merely re-create a dependent situation that they strive to perpetuate rather than form a true therapeutic alliance. As mentioned above, the need for reflective gratification creates the covert bargain relationship in order to ensure a reliable source of self-esteem. When the anticipated rewards are not forthcoming, the depressive may become inexplicably angry or lapse into petulant or self-recriminating behavior in the attempt to coerce the therapist into granting the desired support. This wish to be nurtured, and the various subterfuges that this demand may take, accounts for the irritating manipulativeness that has been described in the literature on therapy with depressives. The extraordinary aversion to influence[8] that these patients exhibit demonstrates that they do not want to solve their problems and leave therapy, but that they desire to hold onto the therapist who has become a new dominant other. The actual content of therapeutic sessions appears superfluous as long as the patient maintains, in his own mind, a satisfactory rapport with the idealized therapist. These maneuvers should not be viewed simply as a perverse use of therapy but as a pathologic mode of gaining self-esteem.

When one patient was convinced that he had to give up the mode of reflective gratification and was attempting to create avenues of independent gratification, he dreamed that he was walking between two women on a beach past a strong, very masculine man. In the dream, the patient felt that the man was ignoring him and looking at the two women. He felt intensely ashamed of his desire for the man to admire him, yet still was sorry that he was no longer pleasing to the man. This dream symbolized the patient's awareness of his pathologic tie to his father as well as the simultaneous desire to reestablish that tie. It also demonstrated this particular patient's competition with his mother and sister for the father's favor. Both the struggle to give up the mode of reflective gratification, in that the patient has the man ignore him, and the feeling of forlornness that would accompany this step are portrayed in the dream.

This patient had to fight against long-established and strongly entrenched methods of obtaining satisfaction in his attempt at autonomy. He also struggled with feelings of guilt as he began to explore independent interests and activities. As his determination increased, he reported fantasies that his father had died and that he should mourn his father's imagined death. He realized that he could not reestablish another relationship like the one he had had with his father without creating a pathological way of life, and he seemed to mourn the giving up of reflective gratification.

This theme of magically destroying the dominant other by acts of assertion is not uncommon in depressives and gives evidence of their extreme inhibition. As a child, the depressive believed that he had continuously to pay back a debt to the parent by pleasing him and proving his worth. He comes to see himself as valued only if he can elicit a positive response from the parent and so shuns any behavior that might cause disapproval. He sees every act as capable of catastrophic results and has carefully to consider the consequences of his behavior. It is thus not surprising that most depressives, although efficient, are rarely creative or remarkably original.

Some depressives who have become habituated to acting solely in accordance with the desires of the dominant other may find themselves overcome with apathy following the actual loss of the idealized other. Not only is their major source of meaning hopelessly gone, but, in some cases, their only chance at redemption or justification is lost. Occasionally, the dominant other is resurrected as a guiding spirit whose memory must be revered and whose directives must still be obeyed. The memory of the other replaces the presence of the other and allows the continuity of the bargain relationship, if only in fantasy. A more common sequence is seen in those individuals who, following the loss of the dominant other, devote themselves to a cause or join a rigidly demanding organization in order to restructure their lives according to external demands.

The need of an external standard of behavior is also reflected in the depressive's ignorance or naïveté about basic life functions.

Fromm-Reichmann[11] mentions that "the future manic-depressive, as a rule, grows up with an amazing lack of information about the important items of living, among them sex information" (p. 223). The cloistered childhood of the depressive and the severe restriction of extrafamilial influences, as well as the extreme parental intrusion into the everyday life of the child, result in a narrow view of life that the depressive later believes others cannot understand and that increases the tie to the dominant parent. The lack of sexual information, alluded to by Fromm-Reichmann, can be expanded to an over-all disinterest in sexuality, which is shunned as childish or vulgar. The concept of repression of libidinal drives does not do justice to the extreme fear of physical gratification in depressives. The denial of independent satisfaction was so repetitively rationalized as family loyalty or the expected expression of love and consideration that it becomes integrated into most aspects of everyday living.

The tragic aspect of this crippling of development is that it was never acknowledged by the family or child, but was strongly reinforced by moralistic rationalizations. The deception was fostered by the parent, who allowed the child to believe in his own ability and independence while actually sabotaging the child's attempts at autonomy. The future depressive strives to become the idealized image the parents hold up as a model, and he refuses to acknowledge his immature desires so that he is repelled by his own dependency. In some instances, it may be just the growing awareness of this aspect of the self that precipitates a depressive reaction, in that the individual feels ashamed of his dependent needs yet cannot give them up. He realizes that he is not the idealized model and that his behavior is a façade, covering up a repugnant yet persistent way of life. He envisions his future as hopelessly determined by a destructive and painful mode of being that is beyond his control. Against his better judgment, he finds himself compelled to perform and to please, and attempts at autonomy are paralyzed by feelings of anxiety and guilt. These feelings of powerlessness, of being caught in an unbearable situation with no hope of change, may bring about a clinical depression.

In summary, the predisposition to depression has been figuratively presented as resulting from an encapsulated ego defect that manifests itself in the inability to achieve autonomous gratification and to rely, in contrast to the rest of the personality, on passive or oral means of obtaining self-esteem. However, as indicated above, depression is a normal psychobiological response to the realization of irrevocable loss or the recognition of inescapable prolonged deprivation. The depressive appears more prone to episodes of melancholia because he is constantly in a vulnerable state of losing his sources of self-esteem and is less able to reestablish satisfying avenues of achieving a sense of worth. The need for approval and love from a dominant other, requiring constant replenishing, creates a cliff-hanging existence in which the expectancy of pleasure or meaning is wholly unreliable. This narcissistic investment of the self in external objects implies the possibility of the loss of these objects and the concomitant loss of future satisfaction. Therefore, the depressive must contrive and manipulate to maintain an ongoing relationship with a dominant other, of which the overt aspects may vary from complete subservience to brutal control. The interruption of this relationship through death, retirement, or career failure or advancement deprives the depressive of his only means of esteem and nurturance. Because of the intense bargain relationship, which sometimes approaches *folie à deux* proportions, the depressive believes that he can never find another gratifying object. He can see no point in doing anything now that the reason for performance—reward from the other—is no longer possible. There is no one to give him proof of his worth or to absolve him from his inner sense of evil and baseness.

Having accepted the dominant other's evaluation of himself, the depressive clothes the dominant other with magical, grandiose powers; the dominant other is always right, even in abandoning or rejecting him. This fear of having caused the loss of the other stems from the early fear of offending the powerful parent by independent behavior. Often, the depressive believes that he deserves to be abandoned or punished for not living up to the demands of the other. There is never a real sense of satisfaction in oneself or an inherent feeling of confidence. Every act must be carefully planned so as not to offend the powerful other.

Fromm-Reichmann[12] doubted that the suffering of the depressive resulted from any genuine feeling of regret or that this suffering actually produced any real desire for change. It may be that the depressive uses his suffering to manipulate others into supplying the desired sympathy and nurturance, but the pain is felt nevertheless. It is this tendency to self-blame and the concomitant inhibition of anger that is discussed in the next section.

THE ROLE OF ANGER IN DEPRESSIVE STATES

Because of the frustrating mode of existence that the depressive is subject to, it would not be surprising to find such an individual constantly bristling with anger and resentment. The failure to secure modes of satisfaction and the extreme self-sacrifice that these individuals impose on themselves would tend to provoke outbursts of fury and hostility. Although sudden episodes of aggression are sometimes encountered in severe depressives, only rarely do they display any overt signs of anger. Rather, the depressive is usually described as reacting to anger-provoking situations with feelings of self-blame. As mentioned above, this finding led Freud to postulate that the apparent self-accusations were really expressions of anger directed at the frustrating object, which, however, had been pathologically introjected into the ego. Depression was, thus, a problem of anger, whose misapplication accounted for the symptoms.

The depressive's lack of overt anger has more recently been interpreted in terms of his tenuous object relations. The expression of anger might antagonize the dominant other and jeopardize the sources of gratification. Arieti,[2] for example, describes anger in depressives ultimately leading to more depression in that it creates the fear that the dominant other might abandon the individual, leading to an increased sense of loss and hopelessness. Anger is seen as a highly dangerous affect that must be concealed and suppressed. Klein's[19] classic formulation of the depressive position emphasized the infant's fear of losing his inner good objects through his aggressive wishes. She interpreted the infant as attributing the pain and frustration of loss to his own angry behavior with a subsequent suppression of overt hostility. If Klein's basic formulations are extended to the interpersonal sphere, the depressive's plight of being angry while in a state of need for nurturance from the other and the resultant fear of the manifestation of that anger become more understandable. To express anger directly means to lose the all-important other who supplies the incorporated good objects, that is, gratification and self-esteem. Eventually, the depressive believes that any expression of anger will catastrophically result in the loss of gratification.

The depressive's lack of overt hostility might also be owing to his distortion of relationships. Some depressives so idealize the dominant other and so implicitly trust the other's judgment that they see no reason for resentment or anger. If they fail to obtain the other's acceptance, it is because they have not tried hard enough to be worthy, not because the other is stingy or unjust. They feel they have only themselves to blame and, thus, have no cause to become angry. A middle-aged depressed woman, describing the failure of her considerable attempts to win praise and love from her father, exclaimed, "What is wrong with me that he doesn't love me?" This woman could not conceive of her father as ungiving or unloving; it was her fault that she could not please him. Although married and the mother of three children, she still believed that her chief role in life was to please her father and devote herself to him. As in her childhood, her father was the only one who could make her happy and give meaning to her life. To alter her view of her father would have required an alteration of her entire mode of being.

Another possibility for the depressive's inability to express anger is that the capacity to feel angry and to use anger as a direct mode of achieving an objective implies a sense of autonomy and independence that is just the ability the depressive lacks. These individuals are tuned to the reactions of others rather than the expression of self, regardless of consequences. To become angry means to satisfy one's impulse without considering the effect on others and requires exactly the sense of self that the depressive has not developed. Thus, he resorts to more reliable manifestations of displeasure, such as pouting or suffering, which produce the appropriate impact on others—guilt and forgiveness. Some depressives, so aptly described by Bonime,[8] are stubbornly uncooperative in therapy, spitefully refusing to take their share of responsibility and taking pride in their resistance to change. Manipulation and control of others seem to be the cardinal features of their activity. This type of depressive, similar to Arieti's claiming type, may be understood as rebelling against the disappointments of past bargain relationships. These individuals feel themselves cheated by past dominant others who had not fulfilled their promise, real or imagined, in return for self-sacrifice. These patients then resolve never to show any signs of true mutuality or cooperation as a way of punishing the dominant other, whose role the therapist has transferentially assumed. They will demand all sorts of favoritism and support while refusing to take any initiative in therapy and ultimately desire to frustrate the therapist by not becoming what they believe he would wish them to be.

However, such patients never show anger overtly, but punish the therapist by continually reminding him of their lack of improvement in therapy—that is, the therapist's inability to change them. In this manner, they make the therapist feel powerless and frustrated, but never give him cause to terminate the relationship. Thus, they defeat the dominant other without losing him. Yet, these patients continue to center their existence around the therapist and in reality defeat themselves in order allegedly to control the other. Their activity continues to be judged in terms of the effect it will have on the therapist and the reaction it will elicit. Living in a world of reflective gratification, the depressive cannot conceive of himself as acting simply for himself. His every thought and act implicates the other and includes the other's reaction.

A talented college student who began experiencing episodes of anxiety and depression as she approached graduation described this type of other-dependent relatedness. She became immediately attracted to any man who showed her any attention and would rush into a close relationship without evaluating the other person. Her main concern was that the other be pleased with her, and she devoted herself to fitting into her boyfriend's preferences. Despite her efforts to hold onto the relationship and placate the other, she was often exploited and treated with little consideration. When this occurred, she persistently blamed herself for having been rejected. She believed that she had somehow offended the other or that she had not been sufficiently perceptive of the other's needs. The other was right, even in mistreating her. Each failure to maintain a relationship proved to her that she would be an old maid and condemned to a life of solitude. She believed that the only way she might escape abandonment was to surrender autonomy and spontaneity. Any display of assertiveness, especially anger or disagreement, would surely drive the other away. This young woman did occasionally get angry, but always after the fact; in the presence of esteemed others, she was overcome with the desire to please and to endear herself. Even her considerable gifts were at the mercy of others; a project that had taken her months to prepare became worthless if mildly criticized by a teacher. The teacher's judgment was never in question; if she had only worked harder, she might have pleased him.

The linking of the ability to express anger with a certain prerequisite sense of autonomy raises some questions as to the meaning of manic states. Aside from purely biochemical hypotheses, manic episodes have been interpreted as the massive release of hostility that had been repressed during the depressive phase. However, the manic patient is not simply angry; he is also terribly active, venturesome, assertive. The forced elation and the sudden self-importance in a previously dependent, other-directed individual betray more than a discharge of anger. The manic's behavior suggests an exaggerated attempt at autonomy as a solution to the painful mode of reflective gratification. The manic seems to be trying frantically to prove to himself that he is independent of the dominant other and able to gratify his own needs.

Freud[10] wrote that "the manic plainly shows us that he has become free from the object by whom his suffering was caused, for he runs after new object-cathexes like a starving man after bread" (p. 166). It is this freedom from the object, or as interpreted above, from the dominant other that the manic proclaims to such an exaggerated degree. Milder reactions, which in this light may be seen as analogous to manic states, are observed in all depressives. These consist of sudden and often inappropriate bursts of self-indulgence. Shopping sprees, eating and drinking sprees, or a variety of antisocial behavior in a depressive individual may represent feeble attempts to free himself from the dominant other and to prove his autonomy and independence. Yet, in both these minor spurts of pretended autonomy and the more pathological manic attack, the depressive fails truly to liberate himself from his need of the dominant other. Even in his most bizarre moments, the manic patient, in contrast to the schizophrenic, requires an audience alternately to impress and insult. Thus, the depressive, in his frantic yet deliberate attempt at independence, still needs someone else to be independent for or to confirm the validity of the attempt. Even in his extreme moments of self-proclaimed liberation, the depressive betrays his dependent needs.

The well-known hostility of the manic appears to be an effect of the inflated yet specious push for autonomy. Except for these rare circumstances, the depressive avoids anger at all costs. The conditioned inhibition of anger forms part of the dependent position of the depressive and ensures reflective gratification. Only after the depressive gains an internal and reliable sense of personal worth and frees himself from the need of the dominant other can he freely show anger. The evocation of anger in the course of therapy may thus be a good prognostic sign, not because a repressed affect is liberated, but because the ability to express anger spontaneously indicates a reduced fear of the dominant other and an increased capability to secure autonomous gratification. Actually, the depressive does not begin to express anger as a result of therapeutic intervention, but alters the mode and meaning of his anger. He ceases to dwell on feelings of hurt and resentment that exploit the use of anger for manipulating others and begins to employ anger in the service of impulse gratification, in the sense that Silverberg[25] intended by his term "effective aggression." This transformation of anger coincides with a growing self-assurance and a more realistic evaluation of the self and others. The depressive will feel free to show genuine anger and disagreement when he has established reliable and independent sources of self-esteem within himself.

CONCLUSION

Depression has been considered here as an affective reaction elicited by the individual's realization that an important source of self-esteem and meaning is lost. The sense of loss is intensified by the awareness that the deprivation is final; it cannot be repaired. What is lost is not simply a love object, but the source of meaning and satisfaction in one's life. Whereas for some the relationship with the environmental object is crucial, for others a specific cause, social position, or definite self-image may be important. What seems to be characteristic about the depressive is that he seems to depend almost exclusively on some external agency for his self-esteem. His entire mode of deriving meaning and pleasure from life is organized around someone else who then becomes essential to his ability to function. The situation is all the more serious when the other exists not only as the bestower of pleasure but as the reliever of guilt.

The more normal individual who contains within himself the ability to supply his own estimate of his self-worth and to take pleasure from his own activities has the assurance, even after a severe loss or failure, that he will again be able to achieve some modicum of contentment by his own efforts. These individuals may become transiently depressed if these resources are threatened by illness or incapacity. However, these depressive episodes are clinically different in that there is little shame and guilt or the overwhelming feeling of total helplessness and the reaction is commensurate with the loss. The depressive, on the other hand, has the backlog of the bargain relationship of which he feels ashamed and which causes him to see himself as cheated and unjustly deprived. In other instances, the orientation of guilt and self-blame makes him see his suffering as merited and just. He is further inhibited by fear of autonomous gratification and so totally reliant on obtaining self-esteem only through the medium of the dominant other that the world truly becomes empty and hopeless. In view of his lack of trust in his abilities and his anxiety about his assertiveness, the depressive feels incapable of undoing the loss and lapses into a state of apathy. The sense of helplessness is increased by intense feelings of guilt and betrayal that accompany attempts to find satisfaction without a dominant other. Occasionally, a new dominant other is preserved in near-psychotic fantasies; most often there is a paralysis of effort and a resignation to despair.

Clinical or pathological depression is thus seen as a primary disorder in the ability to derive meaning and gratification, which in turn produces distorted modes of relating and inaccuracies in the estimation of self. Treatment should center on correcting the pathologic manner of interpersonal relations and on convincing the patient of the availability of his own resources for preserving a satisfying way of life. It is this trust in one's ability to retain avenues of self-esteem and the capacity independently to evaluate self-worth that will protect the individual from falling into hopelessness and despair following the failures and losses that are part of everyone's destiny.

REFERENCES

1. Abraham, K. "A Short Study of the Development of the Libido, Viewed in the Light of Mental Disorders" (1924), in *On Character and Libido Development: Six Essays by Karl Abraham*. New York: Norton, 1966. Pp. 67–150.
2. Arieti, S. "Manic-Depressive Psychosis," in S. Arieti (ed.), *American Handbook of Psychiatry*, Vol. 1. New York: Basic Books, 1959.
3. Arieti, S. "The Psychotherapeutic Approach to Depression," *American Journal of Psychotherapy*, 16 (1962), 397–406.
4. Arieti, S. "Conceptual and Cognitive Psychiatry," *American Journal of Psychiatry*, 122 (1965), 361–366.
5. Arieti, S. *The Intrapsychic and the Interpersonal in Severe Psychopathology*. In press.
6. Bibring, E. "The Mechanism of Depression," in P. Greenacre (ed.), *Affective Disorders*. New York: International Universities Press, 1953.
7. Bonime, W. "Dynamics and Psychotherapy of Depression," in J. H. Masserman (ed.), *Current Psychiatric Therapies*, Vol. 2. New York: Grune & Stratton, 1962.
8. Bonime, W. "The Psychodynamics of Neurotic Depression," in S. Arieti (ed.),

American Handbook of Psychiatry. New York: Basic Books, 1966. Vol. 3, pp. 239–255.
9. Dince, P. "Maternal Depression and Failures of Individuation during Adolescence," in J. H. Masserman (ed.), *Science and Psychoanalysis,* Vol. 9. New York: Grune & Stratton, 1966.
10. Freud, S. "Mourning and Melancholia" (1917), in J. Strachey (ed.), *Standard Edition,* Vol. 14. London: Hogarth. (Also in *Collected Papers of Sigmund Freud.* New York: Basic Books, 1959. Vol. 4, pp. 152–170.)
11. Fromm-Reichmann, F. "Intensive Psychotherapy of Manic-Depressives" (1949), in *Psychoanalysis and Psychotherapy: Selected Papers of Freida Fromm-Reichmann.* Chicago: University of Chicago Press, 1959. Pp. 221–226.
12. Fromm-Reichmann, F. et al. "An Intensive Study of Twelve Cases of Manic-Depressive Psychosis" (1954), in *Psychoanalysis and Psychotherapy: Selected Papers of Freida Fromm-Reichmann.* Chicago: University of Chicago Press, 1959. Pp. 227–274.
13. Harrow, M. et al. "Symptomatology and Subjective Experiences in Current Depressive States," *Archives of General Psychiatry,* **14** (1966), 203–212.
14. Hendricks, I. "Early Development of the Ego: Identification in Infancy," *Psychoanalytic Quarterly,* **20** (1951), 44–55.
15. Hudgens, R. W., Morrison, J. R., and Barchka, R. G. "Life Events and Onset of Primary Affective Disorders," *Archives of General Psychiatry,* **16** (1967), 134–195.
16. Jacobson, E. "Metapsychology of Cyclothymic Depression," in P. Greenacre (ed.), *Affective Disorders.* New York: International Universities Press, 1953.
17. Jaspers, K. *General Psychopathology.* Chicago: University of Chicago Press, 1964.
18. Kielholz, P. *Diagnose und Therapie der Depressionen für den Praktiker.* Munich: Lehmanns, 1965.
19. Klein, M. "A Contribution to the Psychogenesis of Manic-Depressive States" (1934), in *Contributions to Psychoanalysis, 1921–1945.* London: Hogarth, 1948.
20. Lidz, T. et al. "The Intrafamilial Environment of Schizophrenic Patients: II. Marital Schism and Marital Skew," *American Journal of Psychiatry,* **114** (1957), 241–248.
21. Mendelson, M. *Psychoanalytic Concepts of Depression.* Springfield: Charles C Thomas, 1960.
22. Minkowski, E. "Findings in a Case of Schizophrenic Depression," in R. May, E. Angel, and H. Ellenberger (eds.), *Existence.* New York: Basic Books, 1958.
23. Rado, S. "The Problem of Melancholia" (1927), in *Collected Papers,* Vol. 1. New York: Grune & Stratton, 1956.
24. Sandler, J., and Joffee, W. G. "Notes on Childhood Depression," *International Journal of Psychoanalysis,* **46** (1965), 88–96.
25. Silverberg, W. *Childhood Experience and Personal Destiny.* New York: Springer, 1952.
26. Spiegel, R. "Specific Problems of Communication in Psychiatric Conditions," in S. Arieti (ed.), *American Handbook of Psychiatry,* Vol. 1. New York: Basic Books, 1959.
27. Spiegel, R. "The Role of Father-Daughter Relationships in Depressive Women," in J. H. Masserman (ed.), *Science and Psychoanalysis,* Vol. 10. New York: Grune & Stratton, 1966.
28. Sullivan, H. S. *Conceptions of Modern Psychiatry.* New York: Norton, 1953.
29. Weiss, E. "Clinical Aspects of Depression," *Psychoanalytic Quarterly,* **13** (1944), 445–461.
30. Whitehorn, J. "Psychodynamic Approach to the Study of Psychosis," in F. Alexander and H. Ross (eds.), *Dynamic Psychiatry.* Chicago: University of Chicago Press, 1952.

PSYCHOTHERAPY OF THE EMOTIONALLY ISOLATED WOMAN

Francis A. MacNab

There is a wide appreciation of the punitive and disturbing consequences of some forms of physical isolation. We do not yet fully appreciate the nature of emotional isolation and how physical symptomatology of the most complex order may be related to this inner experience of isolation. One woman who had suffered from frequent and extremely painful migraine for fifteen years found relief as she became aware of her deeply expressed reactions to her impoverished interpersonal relationships. Another single woman of thirty-five years manifested a neurosis that prevented her from holding a regular occupation. She had unsuccessfully sought marriage and despaired of having her own children. She developed fibroids in the uterus that necessitated a hysterectomy. She later married, and the apparently intractable neurosis disappeared.

This chapter discusses one case, the features of which are very common in the consulting rooms of those in clinical practice. Frequently, the attempts to treat the patient place her in such an objectified position that she is precluded from the basic experience of her personal confirmation. Often the unconscious attitude of the therapist to womanhood, women in general, or the woman in particular may affect his approach and involvement and the ultimate outcome of the psychotherapy.

I

The emotionally isolated woman and the various manifestations of her neurosis have been explored and interpreted in terms of her psychosexual conflict,[8] her unconscious fear of being a woman,[13] and her culture's continual denial of her emancipation and status.[9] The contemporary and apparently increasing incidence of this syndrome warrants a wider perspective.[11] In this chapter the problem of the emotionally isolated woman will be discussed in the context of the current lag in mental health education, the poverty of emotional nurturance, and the ambivalence regarding intimacy needs. It is necessary, also, to see the syndrome in the context of the phenomena associated with urbanization, increasing affluence, and the changing organization of society.

II

For two and a half years Mae was in intensive psychotherapy. When she first sought help, she was thirty-four years of age, married with three children aged nine, seven, and five years. Though she and her husband continued to be held in the marriage and felt a responsibility to it, they both felt that there was a basic incompatibility.

Sexual intercourse was repugnant to her and was always associated with shame. She said, "I always feel that a woman is not meant to enjoy it." She felt especially guilty when intercourse was accompanied by her orgasm. There had been premarital relations with men other than her husband, but though she felt disappointed that she did not enter marriage as a virgin, the guilt she experienced in this regard was minimal. The husband had his expectations—he wanted his wife to be like the alleged virgin he married. Irrespective of the atmosphere prevailing in the home, he wanted sexual relationships every night if possible, and he would become disgruntled and vindictive when refused. Mae found the sexual act a distasteful obligation "to keep him happy." The marriage situation became virtually a matter of *folie à deux*.

Her miserable state was reflected in her frequent episodes of depression in which she would imagine her husband was inflicting her with physical pain. Her husband was critical and difficult to please, and she was so affected by this that she felt she had lost all her confidence. Marital difficulty had become total interpersonal failure. Prior to marriage, she felt she had plenty of confidence, and her role as a librarian indicated an ability to organize and cope competently with a job of multiple demands. She recognized that the job, in a sense, was external to her intimacy conflicts. Since marriage, she said, "my husband always thought up better ways of doing things and cut me down to less than size."

At her most despondent, she developed a variety of skin ailments, which did not respond to the highly specialized treatment she sought. "The one good thing about my skin condition is that it frightens my husband off at night," she said.

Her husband was thirty-seven years of age and was an ambitious, hard-working middle executive of a large organization. It appeared that he was irretrievably involved in the affluent, materialistic, competitive commitments, with strong investments in vertical social mobility, and people—including a wife—became a means to an end. In a sense, his activity in business became a complex means of narcissistic gratification. His underlying attitude and values conveyed by his approach to life and to people pushed Mae into further isolation and despondency.

They lived eleven miles from his office; this meant many hours per week spent on traveling. There was also weekend work at regular periods and nightly paper work. Apart from the occasional symptoms of tension and fatigue, he assessed that he was able and competent, but regretted that his wife through lack of self-application had become such a tired, complaining burden.

Mae recognized that she had become a burden. She resented that her husband did not indicate that he needed her company. She tried to persuade him to spend more time with her on weekends, but she was afraid of the intimacy demands this would involve. She hesitatingly admitted relief when he was involved in work commitments. She felt distressed and guilty about her attitude and felt guilty about feeling guilty. It was as if all her emotional energy and psychic conflict had built up within, and she felt inadequate in her quest for some satisfying outlet and relief.

Mae's mother and father were both dead. They had died in advanced years soon after Mae had married. She was the second of a family of four. Her two brothers were enjoying successful careers, one as a teacher and the other as an architect. The youngest member of the family, a sister, prior to her marriage had been a social worker. They had been brought up in a country town where for many years their father had been a popular vicar.

She described an early strong attachment to her father, but "Father always seemed to be so disinterested in me and so distant from me, and I was never comfortable with him." Her remarkably accessible infantile memories revealed her profound disillusionment in her father. "It was as if beyond my father I had the image of a father that he did not fulfill." She readily recognized that her marriage could have been an attempt, on the one hand, to capture an ideal that she had entertained, but, on the other hand, to recapitulate the rejecting situation of her father. "Having sexual relations with my husband is like incest to me," she said.

She could recall the strong sanctions her mother had applied against the overt display of femininity and the recognition of sexual drives. Although a strong personality, Mae's mother had a limiting concept of the role of women and the potential of femininity. Mae, in her despondency, wept because she no longer had a mother, but nevertheless recognized her aggression toward her. Her mother, she figured, was reacting out of her own circumstances in which the husband performed a public role, while she had to be an auxiliary. It was a tightly controlled situation in which her mother knew her obligations and duties and complied with them. Mae felt this to be a helpless and fearful situation, and her overt aggression toward her mother became tempered with some compassion. "I think it had a lot to do with my resentment of my role as a wife and mother."

Mae's sense of loss, her growing helplessness, and damaged self-esteem merit further comment. It would be naïve to reduce this experience exclusively to its oedipal components. She had gradually lost all endorsement for her investment in love relationships so that her children, too, provided little satisfaction. With increasing loss of the love objects, there was an increase in narcissism and isolation.

The varying levels of anonymity, pretense, and depersonalization in suburbia, the social distance, and the daily isolation contributed to her sense of abandonment. Simultaneously, she was involved with the inarticulate conflicts pertaining to the moral and ethical questions of a pluralistic and changing society. In the past, she had made some disorganized attempts to clarify some of these questions, but she felt she lacked the resources to cope with the confusion. Likewise, she had tried to relieve her feelings of isolation. She had tried at intervals to sustain previous friendships, but family requirements and the suburban mobility precluded this. Her attempts to make both social and functional contact with kindergarten, school, and church groups had met with only perfunctory success. Her interaction with people on her street was friendly, but casual and without depth. All these factors added extra and external frustration to her intellectual and intimacy needs.

Mae wanted to become a creative person once again. She wanted to be able to make decisions, feel free in herself, and lead a life with more confidence and direction. Prior to this being a realistic possibility, it was necessary for her to relieve the tension and anger that had accumulated; it was necessary for her to clarify and reorganize her feelings and attitudes to people. These were not easy or short processes, for they had to be effected in the context of her diffuse and undefined sociological situation.

The reestablishment of Mae's personal identity and her sexual identity depended very greatly on the awareness of her intimacy needs within the therapeutic situation. This did not always, or exclusively, depend on what the therapist did, but rather on what he was and what he gave.

The therapeutic atmosphere.... includes and centers around the very person of the therapist; his living person and caring participation seemingly provide, above all else, for the fulfilment of the patient's intimacy needs. It is likely that this represents a basic dimension in the therapeutic process, a dimension upon which its very outcome may depend (p. 192).[7]

III

Psychotherapy can be regarded as a multiple process, parts of which can be simultaneously experienced by a specific person in specifically designated contingencies. We can determine areas of the patient's experience in which psychotherapy would be relevant and beneficial and then develop the form and method of psychotherapy appropriate to the patient's impoverished or distorted experience. This is to be distinguished from that eclecticism where technique and method seem to move with impression rather than planning. It may also be distinguished from the view that regards psychotherapy as a unitary, albeit varied, process to which the patient is applied.

In Mae's case, experiential areas of impoverishment and distortion were designated. Mae's emotional isolation, internalized aggression, and sense of abandonment had exceeded the point where she could allude to various external stresses as being the origin of her discomfort. Her discomfort had become internalized to such an extent that she was unable to cope with household chores and social situations. Her behavior and thinking were confused; she was miserable and without adequate emotional understanding, support, or nurturance.

It was decided by the therapist that the primary concern in Mae's psychotherapy would center around her intimacy needs, her confirmation as a person and as a woman, and the redirection of her behavior in a relatively refractory environment. She was asked to enter a psychotherapy experience in which the therapist would be relatively active in the relationship. She was asked also to attend group therapy in a group of eleven females, all of whom were experiencing varied and extreme manifestations of emotional isolation.

The beginnings of both individual and group psychotherapy were marked by timidity, weeping, a paucity of inner experiences, expressions of fear that the therapist would abandon her, followed by expressions of embarrassment. She appeared to have an overwhelming sense of inferiority, and her guarded violence seemed to alternate between a form of anal-sadistic demands to possess her husband and a masochistic denial of her womanhood and person generally. Though intellectually accepting her genitals, she often wished she was not a woman. These processes when interpreted to the patient brought a considerable broadening of her self-awareness and a realization of her distorted ego strengths.

The therapist gently but with encouraging firmness stated that he would not abandon her and that the direction of therapy would be toward a more trusting level of mutual dialogue. This meant that in the early stages it was necessary to endorse the patient as she was—a fearful woman fragmented in her organization and assumptions about herself and her world. It was necessary, too, to allude to the peculiar therapeutic partnership that would help her to move from a posture of isolated fragility to active participation in ongoing mutual dialogue. This entailed a growing and strong relationship with the therapist and with others in group therapy.

IV

The descriptive discussion that follows is built around a conceptualization that the author employed in his work with schizophrenic patients.[12] It represents one way of describing how Mae in particular was able to gain relief from her neurosis and gradually refind the initiative and courage to live affirmatively.

Being Present

In psychotherapy, the patient looks to the therapist. Implicit in this look is the belief that the therapist is aware of some of the possibilities of human health as well as human sickness. He can take into himself the tensions of the moral and ethical questions and the sociological environment and meet them in an integrated, satisfactory way. She looks to the therapist for an honest open encounter with another person who, having no investments (so far as this relationship is concerned) in subterfuge and camouflage, will meet her as a genuine person. Regrettably, many therapists use the therapeutic relationship as another situation—and often *the* situation—in which they can gain a great deal from their pretense and subterfuge.

Hans Trüb wrote that "only genuine partnership can save the sick person who has withdrawn from dynamic encounter with the world into isolation" (p. 145).[14] Mae had once enjoyed life, participated in it with a view of the world that seemed to evoke action, meaningfulness, and direction. When she came for help, she had withdrawn from vigorous interaction, was eluding meeting with others, and often distorted the world around her into what she feared it was. She described this dream: "I was wrestling my way through very tall dry grass. As I parted the grass, it would close over before I could get through it. It was a terrifying struggle, like walking through glue. In the distance, I could see large ants moving along the horizon, and crows sat watching my efforts from the dry trees."

A number of interpretations could be given to the dream. She saw it as an experience "in a terrifying wasteland." "It was as if I knew I had left home and could not find my way either back or forward—I was all exposed to the elements, without any real possibility of coping or finding a way."

It was important to help her, in spite of her alienation, ambivalence, and death wish, to move once again into the experience of being present to others and others being present to her. In the group, the encounters with one another and the interaction of one another's assumptive world brought cycles of inadequacy and fear, but also recurring flashes of her capacity to encounter the world with less ambiguity and incongruity in her experiences and communications. This was greatly assisted and confirmed by the group's warm, strong relationship with the therapist and the consequent empathy, coherence, support, and implicit hope that this relationship gave.

On one occasion, Mae wrote to me after the group session: "I think the group meant quite a lot though I remained so silent. I had a similar experience to Diana—perhaps more violent, but did not feel like talking to the group about it. But I feel I am beginning to understand a few more things each time I go through the trough." On another occasion, at a later date, she wrote: "Thank you for listening, but now I feel very frightened of the members of the group. I had no intention of saying anything about myself and feel ashamed that I have taken up time. I feel very inadequate and would like to hide from the group. I crave approval, but I have lost this by taking up precious time that others wanted." On a later occasion: "For the very first time I feel strongly, and I feel that what I say with deep and sincere honesty is me at last. This which you and the group have helped foster in *me* is a wonderful experience."

Psychotherapy was not only providing a situation in which she could gain some contact with her feelings, but allowed for some reorganization and reestablishment of herself. Instead of seeing herself and the world as bad, she began to experience an increasing warmth toward them.

There was the growing experience of self-realization that emerged from the human encounter. Implied in this experience was the encounter with the existential reality of her basic and inseparable relation with her world. This polarity (person-world) had all the potential for satisfaction and self-realization, but when the polarity became distorted, she experienced estrangement, isolation, and anxiety as the world drew away from her or threatened to abandon or overwhelm her. Alternatively, if the polarity became distorted in the other direction, she began to assume power, self-aggrandizement, and self-preoccupation.

Psychotherapy attempted to bring an awareness of the existential reality—the person's relation to her world, her estrangement, isolation, loneliness, and anxiety, her quest for power and self-preservation. If Mae could be helped to see how this polarity affected her sense of well-being, then in many instances positive action could be taken to ensure some balance was sustained.

Group psychotherapy greatly accelerated this process, for here the polarity and its potential were both experienced and observed within a controlled and supportive situation. The therapist can help the group learn and impart those ingredients essential for the therapeutic process—accurate empathy, genuine respect, and nonpossessive warmth, all closely related to the concept and the experience of the therapeutic encounter.[1] In addition, significant education for mental health and emotional growth can be effected in this group situation. It may seem superficial to make such reference to the part didactic work can play, but it needs to be emphasized repeatedly how important this is and how it can help confirm the person in her progress toward a sound and healthy life. Discussion of the elements of existential reality —the experience of estrangement, anxiety, loneliness, and so on— should not be neglected and, if done with empathy, will be greatly valued by the patient. The understanding of the positive and negative aspects of human relatedness can prevent the destruction of many relationships and actually promote a greater readiness for a shared experience within the conflicts of the relationship. "Only men who are capable of truly saying *Thou* to one another can truly say *We* with one another" (p. 32).[10]

There are psychotherapists who find tolerance and psychotherapy possible for vindictive neurotic women only so long as there are substantial monetary compensations. Even among the most highly trained and long experienced, wide latitudes of preconception and prejudice can be detected as far as women are concerned. There is the myth that tends to posit as one mark of effective training the purity of thought; but our humanity intervenes. This should not entirely mar our intention of trying to be present to our patient in such a way that the patient experiences us as fully present to them rather than partially present or simultaneously present to others. When one person is genuinely present to the other, pretense and appearance are minimal; each attempts to make himself present in the fullness of his personal being. As the one experiences the other as "present," and more especially present to *her*, she can begin to experience her own self-becoming or self-realization. The possibilities of decisions, direction, and creativity become real once again.

We saw in Mae how she had withdrawn from being present to others, how others had pushed her out of being present into someone or something that was distant, or something that once was present but had become past. Her condition made it virtually impossible for her to present herself as present. Psychotherapy required the warm and unreserved involvement of the therapist: the initiative must always fall on him, and by his presentness he encouraged the patient to move back toward the world she felt had abandoned her, the world she had grown to fear.

In the group, the members quickly came to appreciate the way they could be present to one another and to the group as a whole. They tested this, at first, for they openly admitted how in all other groups they had found it necessary to pretend and live behind a mask. It was notable how much therapeutic value or personal benefit ensued from this experience of being present to others. Some, as they wept over their horrible past and contemplated the hopelessness of their present situation, discovered that the most exhilarating present situation was the presentness of the group. They thus felt able to enter that basic movement of the life of dialogue—what Martin Buber called "the turning toward the other" (p. 22).[3]

Self-Disclosure

The turning toward one another implied openness and directness in self-disclosure. Instead of concealment and fretting about the impression being made on others, instead of preoccupation with one's inadequacy and estrangement, there was a gradual awareness that she could disclose who she was and, though still flinching with internalized wounds, could experience the acceptance of the group, its symbolic representation of continuity and belief in the approaching future.

Psychotherapy helped Mae dare to be a real person. From time to time, the therapist would assure her that she was a woman so that she could relinquish the controls and defenses by which she was tenuously protecting herself. For this to occur, much depended on the therapist, his warmth and active engagement. Mae—as each other member of her group—had to see in him the epitome of trust and commitment; as each group member realized this experience, it was reflected in the group itself. This was not achieved readily. The neurotic isolate fears commitment and closeness, especially after a long history of uncertainty; she attempts to deny the principle of continuity. Mae would protest repeatedly that her whole identity was being threatened, her identity as a person, a woman, a wife, and mother. Hanna Colm wrote:

> A neurosis is stifling in so far as it makes the patient unable to affirm himself as a worthwhile person in relation to other persons because he is not able to accept, and is threatened by, the negative in himself, in others, and in life itself. He withdraws to a limited area of living to avoid facing the negative and its risk. His sickness prevents him from coping with the anxieties which the healthy person can deal with affirmatively. It is his own secret self-condemnation that has made him neurotic, lonely and isolated—his own condemnation of the negative feelings which various situations or people call up in him, his failure to live up to ideal concepts or perfectionistic standards. Freeing his courage for self-affirmation means helping him to accept these things for which he has condemned himself; this courage also helps him to accept as meaningful the negative in his fellow man and in all life, and out of this comes respect, tolerance, and often love for the other person (p. 183).[5]

Mae's psychotherapy became, at depth, a process toward a mode of being of affirmation. In addition to affirming herself, it was necessary for her to affirm existence. Her life would inevitably involve the positive and negative, love and violence, hope and misery, wanting to be and negating all that would help her to be. The critical task was to recognize and affirm these ambiguities and in spite of their most destructive possibilities determine to be. Martin Buber wrote: "Sent forth from the natural domain of species into the hazard of the solitary category, surrounded by the air of a chaos which came into being with him, secretly and bashfully he watches for a YES which allows him to be and which can come to him only from one human person to another" (p. 104).[4]

Confirmation

Mae's self-affirmation and confirmation were to involve three aspects in unity: (1) the aspect of self-attribution, the striving for her self-identity; (2) the aspect of endorsement, which comes only from another person; and (3) the aspect of mutuality, which arises out of the first two. On the basis of this confirmation, she would be better able to affirm the ambiguities of her situation and deal creatively with them. Confirmation involved fear and anxiety, conflict and uncertainty, each in its destructive aspects reflecting how a satisfactory solution could not be found in isolation or individualism. Mae's confirmation was found in the therapeutic relationship, both with the therapist and with the group. Confirmed here, she was better able to cope with the negative and destructive aspects of her other relationships.

Ultimately, she came to see that confirmation could not take place in any other milieu than that in which two persons commit themselves to community so that there is the constant challenge to develop both oneself and the other. In this mutuality, both can move forward to the experience of sharing and enjoyment.

Part of our universal estrangement is that we are always exposed to the menace of the loss of mutuality. Mutuality can become artificial or altogether absent. Genuine mutuality, fundamental to confirmation, has been described as follows: "Each brings a sense of his own meaningful, positively valued identity, and, out of experience or participation, together mutual recognition of identity develops, including a growing recognition of each other's potentialities and capacities" (p. 207).[15] Genuine mutuality constantly fades into various shades of pseudomutuality, which means that although a person may not enter a relationship, he tries to maintain the impression that the relationship exists. There is, therefore, a failure to affirm one's estrangement, and with it there is the pretense that relatedness is sustained. This is one of the recurring menaces for the isolated woman. Her social situation among other women, and in the eyes of men, does not permit a ready acceptance of her isolation. Her own image of herself and her defenses also resists this acceptance and its accompanying misery and dread. In some instances, when the realization of isolation comes, it can be accompanied by such other affect that she extracts herself from relationships, and a situation of nonmutuality prevails. People become objects. Concern for another's life or encounter with life fades away.

The group in group therapy presented a constant challenge to the nonmutuality of isolation and distance. It was common for pseudomutuality to prevail there, with concealment of actual thoughts and desires, but this too seemed to challenge itself, so that, as Emil Brunner put it, "the self no longer merely regards life from the point of view of the 'I,' but also from the point of view of the 'Thou' " (p. 320).[2]

As Mae made her sometimes timid, sometimes torrid, journey toward her confirmation, she began to cope with her life situation and began to present a different image to her husband. At one group session she said: "I began talking with my husband. I was overwhelmed to find I could really find myself wanting to love him." On another occasion she said, "I must have really stepped out of myself. I actually put my husband in the witness box; I told him who I was and how I wanted things to run from now on. After all these years, I—his little gray mouse—actually spoke up. But it was different. I was as nervous as if I was making my first public speech. I felt angry, but the old feeling of bitterness had gone. I don't feel trapped any more. In a way I was trapped in myself and using all kinds of vetoes against my husband. I feel more active and realistic in my feelings, even though the situation has not changed much."

Mae's experience of confirmation came through an understanding of her intimacy needs, an awareness of the possibilities of her interpersonal relations, and the acceptance and affirmation of both the positive and negative aspects of her existence. The experience of confirmation was an experience of herself in dynamic relation with others, and this evoked the possibilities of action, creativity, and transcendence within her situation.

Her skin complaint was less evident, and she was able to predict its course according to the comfort and discomfort of her interpersonal relations. The symptoms of her neurosis were relieved. Her isolation continued, but she had adopted different attitudes, values, and methods of management. In the latter stages of her psychotherapy, I suggested she read Antoine de Saint-Exupery's *The Little Prince*. Eighteen months after her therapy had been terminated, she rang me to tell me she was coping well. She added: "What makes the desert beautiful is that somewhere it hides a well . . ." (p. 89).[6]

REFERENCES

1. Berenson, B. G., and Carkhuff, R. R. *Sources of Gain in Counselling and Psychotherapy*. New York: Holt, Rinehart & Winston, 1967.
2. Brunner, E. *The Divine Imperative*. London: Lutter-work, 1937.

3. Buber, M. *Between Man and Man*, trans. R. G. Smith, London: Routledge & Kegan Paul, 1947.
4. Buber, M. "The William Alanson White Memorial Lectures, Fourth Series. (1) Distance and Relation," *Psychiatry*, **20** (1957), 97–104.
5. Colm, H. *The Existentialist Approach to Psychotherapy with Adults and Children*. New York: Grune & Stratton, 1966.
6. De Saint-Exupery, A. *The Little Prince*, trans. K. Woods, London: Penguin, 1966.
7. Ferreira, A. J. "The Intimacy Need in Psychotherapy," *American Journal of Psychoanalysis*, **24**, no. 2 (1964), 190–194.
8. Freud, S. (1946), *Collected Papers*. Vol. IV, Third Edition. London: Hogarth.
9. Friedan, B. *The Feminine Mystique*. New York: Norton, 1963.
10. Friedman, M. S. "Dialogue and the 'Essential We,'" *American Journal of Psychoanalysis*, **20**, no. 1 (1960), 26–34.
11. Horney, K. *Feminine Psychology*, ed. H. Kelman, New York: Norton, 1967.
12. Macnab, F. A. *Estrangement and Relationship*. London: Tavistock, 1965.
13. Rheingold, J. C. *The Fear of Being a Woman*. New York: Grune & Stratton, 1964.
14. Trüb, H. Quoted in H. Colm, *The Existentialist Approach to Psychotherapy with Adults and Children*. New York: Grune & Stratton, 1966.
15. Wynne, L. C., Rycoff, I. M., Day, J., and Hirsch, S. I. "Pseudo-mutuality in the Family Relations of Schizophrenics," *Psychiatry* **21** (1958), 205–220.

THE MARGINALLY ASOCIAL PERSONALITY: THE BEATNIK-HIPPIE ALIENATION

Robert E. Gould

Although the marginally asocial personality appears in many guises, it always presents a basic core factor: the feeling of alienation. The marginally asocial individual feels estranged—from society, from himself, or from both. The problem of alienation has long been recognized; the term itself has become a catchword of the past generation. The self-alienated may complain of boredom, chronic malaise, unhappiness, the meaninglessness of life, or the injustices heaped on him. The society-alienated has rejected —or been rejected by—some important part of the world in which he lives. The reasons for this rejection may have been subjective ("healthy" or "unhealthy") or objective and beyond his control—racial, social, or economic. In either case, the society-alienated person finds himself in a minority position and an "outsider." The way his alienated feeling is expressed will depend on idiosyncratic individual experiences, intrafamilial dynamics, and his particular social milieu. These factors will also determine whether he will seek psychiatric help or adopt one of several marginally asocial types of behavior through which he can express his real self and/or the anxiety accompanying his estrangement from others.

All minority group members who are discriminated against or disadvantaged—economically, socially, or culturally—in an affluent culture belong, by definition, to the marginally asocial group.

Discrimination also alienates those whose behavior deviates markedly from "accepted" mores, and those who stand apart from the majority by reason of age—both youth and the elderly.

The largest marginally asocial group is youth. The adolescent naturally goes through a period of feeling marginal, isolated, strange in relation to society, his family, and even himself. This feeling is intensified when his needs clash with the institutional styles and practices of the prevailing culture. Today's adolescent faces an increasingly complex, automated, and depersonalized world, which makes his search for identity and purpose even more difficult and often intensifies or prolongs his alienation.

One dramatic expression of marginally asocial behavior among the alienated young has led to the phenomenon of "beatniks" and, more recently, "hippies." The hippie has been often described, but not really well understood. This discussion presents a definition and history of the hippie—what he is and why he is there —and traces the social and cultural forces and intrafamilial psychodynamics behind his development. An analysis of various aspects of hippie belief and behavior follows, along with suggestions for management of this special type of alienation.

THE HIPPIE SCENE: A DEFINITION AND HISTORY OF THE MOVEMENT

The hippie movement, viewed from a narrow literal perspective, officially began in January 1966, when Ken Kesey,* a vagabond novelist, began a cross-country (United States) trek in a flamboyantly decorated bus, accompanied by a gaily costumed band of footloose men and women who had decided to form a new society and set their own standards for living. From a larger, broader view, one can trace hippie roots back to ancient philosophers and Christian martyrs and to such disparate moderns as writers Henry David Thoreau, Albert Camus, Aldous Huxley; poet Allen Ginsberg; novelist Jack Kerouac; philosopher Alan Watts; and the musical Beatles. The hippie, in one form or another, has, in fact, always been with us. He has been the rebel of his times, changing as the times have changed, and demonstrating, as his culture does, a varying mixture of health and pathology.

* One history of Kesey's trip, which also offers one of the best descriptive pictures of the hippie scene, is in Tom Wolfe's *The Electric Kool-Aid Acid Test*.[28]

These rebels belong primarily to the same segment of alienated youth in every generation. They lack a sense of identification with prevailing institutions, yet they need to make their presence not only felt but somehow meaningful—by changing their own lives and structuring their own private world or by restructuring the world surrounding them. As the angry young men of each era, they are the highly vocal and visible nonconformists who challenge or reject the mores of their elders or the "Establishment" itself.*

The so-called Lost Generation following World War I dedicated itself to the reckless pursuit of mindless pleasure; the hippie of the 1920's was called a "bohemian." The Depression generation of the 1930's embraced left-wing ideology in a passionate effort to improve society; the hippie of this group was called a "radical," "pinko," or "communist." After World War II, cold war disillusionment gradually replaced hope for lasting peace in a brave new world. The lost rebel of this generation gave up on the world and decided to live for himself. He began to seek the basic rhythms of life in sensuality and transient, rootless solitude; the hippie of this era was called a "beatnik."

The beat personality, immediate predecessor of the current hippie, was instantly recognizable by his chosen external badges—beard, dirty jeans, general unkemptness. The still-evolving hippie of the late 1960's has added longer hair and more colorful adornments. The beatnik's private pursuits, such as promiscuity, alcohol, drugs, and jazz music, were similar to those of today's hippie, except that the hippie consumes less alcohol than the beats did and more drugs (new and old). His music has also changed from jazz to "rock," although it may be evolving back to jazz in the 1970's.

Two early literary spokesmen for the beat era, Jack Kerouac[17] and John Clellon Holmes,[12] described the beatnik's philosophy and way of life as a serious and dedicated search for self-awareness. One poetic portrait of the beat life was dramatically expressed by Allen Ginsberg's *Howl*.[6] True "beatness," these writers declared, must be sought in a highly disciplined manner; it

---

* Also called the "System," this refers in general to the people and institutions having political and economic power. It implies a traditional, conservative, or middle-of-the-road status quo philosophy and behavior. In the United States, it also represents the upper and middle classes and those most influential in establishing policy and control of the major elements in the society, such as schools, law, government, and the general mores and customs, which are most acceptable and, as the anti-Establishment views it, conventional, obsolete, or harmful.

is *organized* disorganization, and it requires wholehearted and serious devotion to the ideal of beatification. The word "beat," in fact, is nothing more than an abbreviation of "beatific" or "beatified." As the original beat writers and poets saw it, their chosen way of life—disheveled though it may have been—was fuller and more significant than anyone else's. They campaigned for the right not to work, not to settle down, not to raise a family, not to become status-seekers. To be truly beat, according to Holmes, meant achieving a "nakedness of mind, and ultimately of soul; a feeling of being reduced to the bedrock of consciousness."[12] This definition of the beat *by* the beat differs markedly from that offered by most nonbeats, typified by a recent article on the beatnik by Masserman,[18] who defines the term "beatnik" as implying "an accusatory assumption on their part of having been 'beaten' into martyrdom." This is not at all its meaning or derivation. Nor was the term "beatnik" adopted by them (the beats themselves) with "defiant avidity."[18] Rather, it is a word created by the media, in this case, by a newspaper columnist—Herb Caen of the *San Francisco Chronicle*. It was popularized by a national magazine[24] and then picked up by almost all the nonbeat world.

As originally conceived, the beat life was one of noninvolvement, political and personal detachment from anything lasting, meaningful, or responsible. Most beats stated that they had no wish to shatter organized society, only to elude and prevent society from contaminating their free style of life. (Their unconscious desires were, of course, more complicated.)

At the beginning of the 1960's, the beat world began splitting apart; in response to the onrushing civil rights movement in the United States and the controversial war in Vietnam, activism claimed many of the alienated young. In fact, only the beat appearance remained the same; they were still unkempt, unwashed, and unshaven, if no longer uninvolved. A small minority remained true to the earlier beat attitude of voluntary withdrawal from societal pressures and regulations. Some of this group emigrated to Europe where they continued to pursue "kicks," living as nomads and working only enough to keep alive. (It is not surprising that malnutrition was common among the beats, who apparently preferred hunger to the routine of daily labor.) Another emerging splinter group was the "surfers," mostly West Coast youths for whom the "kick" of riding an ocean wave on a surfboard had become a way of life. These beachcombers later took to roaming other coasts as well as the Pacific—in search of the perfect wave, the hallucinatory revelation (via drugs), the great sexual experience.*

These two groups, direct descendants of the original beats of the late 1940's and 1950's, scorned the new activist, "involved" group of the 1960's and refused even to accord it "beat" status. Nevertheless, the traditional beat rapidly lost ground in the cities and on college campuses and was succeeded by a new rebel, similar in appearance but very different in philosophy. Instead of withdrawing from society, the new beat suddenly found himself allied with a sizable segment of the nonbeat population in the battle for Negro civil rights and the protest movement against the war in Vietnam.

Today's hippie, a descendant of yesterday's beatnik, derived his name from the slang expression of the 1940's "hep," which meant in on, or up on, the latest trends or ideas. (Today's equivalent would be "with it.") The term "hep" originated among professional jazz musicians (mostly Negro), who later converted "hep" into "hip" to preserve the term as their own. A "hep" or "hip" individual became a "hipster" during the 1950's, when jazz music became "bebop." The word fell into disuse from 1958 to about 1966, when it was resurrected for the hippies. As with the term "beat," there is much misunderstanding of its origins. For instance, Stubblebine notes that the term hippie "does not derive from the underworld term 'hipster.'"[23] Hipster is not an underworld term, but a jazz term, and hippie *is* derived from it. Stubblebine further states (from a definition offered in the *American Dictionary of Modern Slang*) that "the hippie is denying the need for emotional interaction." This is, in fact, almost the direct opposite of the hippie creed. Again as with the term "beatnik," most hippies do not use the term "hippie" in describing themselves or do so reluctantly. For lack of a better descriptive term, I, too, will use the term throughout this chapter, but reluctantly.

Sharing the beat's philosophy of living now and not for the future, sharing the same scorn for current sexual mores and the resulting hypocrisies, following the drug use, wanderlust, and fascination with Oriental mysticism—Zen and Yoga—the hippies tried to find themselves through an even wider assortment of techniques. Sex, music, and drugs, although still basic methods for withdrawing from life or for trying to get more deeply into life, were supplanted by a violent, intense assault on all the

* A chronicle of the surfing life is well portrayed in the movie *The Endless Summer* and in two magazine articles by Tom Wolfe.[26, 27]

senses—overwhelming displays of dazzling light, color, music, dance, movement, art. This mixed media explosion is, in the hippies' phrase, designed to "blow the mind"—to release it from the controls of middle-class convention, to expose and free the real self. An espousal of fun, joy, love, nonviolence, beauty, freedom, self-expression, creativity, spiritual over material values, and mutual respect along with his mind-blowing sensuality made the hippie at least more attractive, if not more acceptable, than the old-line beatnik with his dour disposition.

Hippiedom and its communes, in which groups of males and females lived together, sharing food, possessions, and at times sexual partners, flourished in the Haight-Ashbury section of San Francisco and the Lower East Side of New York City during 1967 and early 1968. Other large American cities also had hippie centers, and the phenomenon spread to the capitals of Europe and even such faraway places as Katmandu, Nepal. But even as public attention focused on these hippie centers (via television and the press), they lost much of their original flavor and spirit. Harassed by tourists, police, the underworld, such "rightist" rebel youths as the motorcycle gangs, and such hostile disadvantaged minorities as Negroes and Puerto Ricans (mainly in New York City), hippies could no longer survive on love and nonviolence in the big cities. Available sex had turned into rape, "free" drugs were being fought over by criminal elements seeking them for profit, and murders and muggings finally forced an exodus. Hippies found refuge in the desert and hills surrounding San Francisco, near Indian reservations in the Southwest, rural areas in upstate New York, and in Canada and other parts of the world.

In 1968, the presidential campaigns of Eugene McCarthy and Robert Kennedy inspired some hippies to become actively involved in social and political life and to form their own political party, the Youth International Party (YIP). Its members were called "Yippies." The Yippies, led by ex-hippies Abbie Hoffman and Jerry Rubin, borrow generously from the hippie traditions of serious social criticism and the "put on" (kidding the Establishment by caricaturing, satirizing, and exaggerating its faults). Yippies campaigned to end both war and pay toilets and to legalize psychedelic drugs, free food, and a heart transplant for President Johnson. (Hoffman,[11] in a book published in late 1968, describes the Yippie program and its origins in detail.) But the main objectives of combining hippie and New Left philosophies and the development of an alternative society were paramount.

The Yippies made their first appearance by staging a demonstration in New York's Grand Central Terminal in March 1968 as a militant antiwar statement. During the Democratic National Convention, Yippies and other groups staged noisy protests against what they felt was a "closed" convention, with the candidate picked beforehand. When the protesters were savagely beaten by Chicago police,[23] world attention focused on the episode, and perhaps for the first time hippies won widespread public sympathy.

Both the hippie and Yippie movements are still flourishing because the social conditions that bred them have not fundamentally changed.

SOCIAL AND CULTURAL FORCES

The psychodynamics of the marginally asocial hippie personality involve not only psychological and genetic determinants, but also a number of social and cultural forces beyond the intrapsychic and interpersonal. America and its institutions have created certain conditions that inescapably increase youth's "normal" quota of alienated feelings. For example, the more intensely an individual opposes the Vietnam war on moral grounds, the more marginally asocial he must be, because the consequence of such acts as draft-card burning and draft resistance or evasion is to make an outlaw of anyone who commits them.

The civil rights struggle, and glaring hypocrisies and injustice in many areas of U.S. life set the stage either for active rebellion by the young or for withdrawal from a world they hate yet feel powerless to change. Sit-ins, demonstrations, riots, and hippieism are all expressions of youth's alienation. And these activities in turn aggravate the estrangement between the young and the parent culture.

Still another sign of youthful ferment is evident in the colleges. As these institutions have grown, so has the distance between the students and the adult campus Establishment—faculty and, more especially, administration. Again, the student has felt increasingly powerless (much as the Negro has in U.S. society), with no voice at all in policy-making decisions that directly affect his critical years of formal education. Academic alienation has been crucial in setting off a wave of campus rioting, beginning at the University of California in Berkeley in 1963 and gradually spreading across the country. Finally, at Columbia in 1968, students not only rebelled against a university system that made them feel dehumanized, but also joined protest forces with the outside (Negro) community to thwart a university building plan that failed to consider the neighborhood's needs.

Though some of the young fight to reverse this alienation by direct activism against the system, others choose withdrawal from it—and their primary means of withdrawal is through drugs. The reasons for this choice need to be carefully examined.

Again, to begin with, we must consider the culture. America has long been a highly drug-oriented nation. Alcohol, nicotine, amphetamines, barbiturates, and tranquilizers had been part of the scene for many years before marijuana, LSD, and the other psychedelics appeared. This increasing dependence on drugs (that is, on any relatively pure chemical agent that exerts a reasonably predictable effect on the user's physical or psychological dependence) was forecast most clearly, accurately, and dramatically by Aldous Huxley in his *Brave New World*[13] back in the 1930's.

Besides progress, the culture also emphasizes and glorifies speed. Americans want fast airplanes, faster cars, fast-fast-fast relief of pain and tension. Is it any wonder that one of the fastest-acting drugs used by the young to relieve *their* pain, methedrine, is called, simply, "speed"?

Many of today's young feel that alcohol and tobacco are more harmful than marijuana (although the long-term effects of marijuana are just now beginning to undergo serious study). Poet Allen Ginsberg, among other hippie leaders, has been active in campaigning to legalize the use of marijuana. Its use and defense fit many psychological needs of many of today's young, not only hippies. (This point will be further developed in the specific discussion on drugs.)

Still another important American tradition, closely related to the increasing emphasis on drug usage, is its great moral emphasis on the Protestant Ethic, a principal now undergoing rapid change. Past emphasis on the virtues of work and chastity and forsaking immediate pleasures until they are somehow "earned" has given way to anxiety about extinction via nuclear holocaust, to a lack of belief in a future that one can plan for, to unacceptable wars and their ambiguities, to a technocracy that reduces man's need to labor long and hard for his livelihood, to the lack of confidence in the values and way of life of their elders.

The welfare state, the shorter work week, rapid social and technological change, increasing affluence, emphasis on spending rather than saving and on consuming rather than contributing—all have undermined the foundations of our old work ethic. We seem to take from life rather than build for the future. We are careless about conserving our resources and protecting our air and water from pollution. We build obsolescence into our cars and houses, so that nothing we have is meant to last—it is just for now. It is only logical that our young should be called the Now Generation and that they too should want their satisfactions now. Each of these general sociological conditions has contributed importantly to the growth of the hippie movement. The same factors, interacting with specific combinations of family and psychic experience, then form the individual hippie personality.

INTRAFAMILIAL PSYCHODYNAMICS

Clearly, a wide variety of intrafamilial psychodynamics can contribute to a youngster's development of a hippie adaptation to life. Nevertheless, some general observations can be made from the families I have seen in practice, as well as from interviews with hippie nonpatients on New York's Lower East Side. The following is an extract from an illustrative and typical family history.

Jerry, a twenty-year-old boy, was referred because he had dropped out of college, was smoking pot, did not want to work, and wanted to spend all his time in New York City's East Village hippie center.

The father, who had been quite poor in his youth, had had to go to law school at night and work during the day. He became a labor lawyer, dedicated to fighting for the underdog, helping struggling unions to get started against powerful and oppressive employers. Having begun his career at the height of the Depression, he now, at fifty-two, still claimed to be acutely aware of economic and social injustices. Jerry's mother, fifty years old, also had been poor and had dropped out of college to help support her younger brothers. Later, she had become a writer and shared the same political and social philosophy as her husband.

The father's law practice prospered; he began to represent insurance companies and now-powerful labor unions, in marked contrast to his old efforts for the working man. The couple had a son, Jerry, and a daughter, moved to a fashionable New York suburb, and enjoyed all the materialistic advantages of upper-middle-class life. The children grew up hearing a great deal of their parents' liberal social views and philosophy, but the family's life style did not match the ideals they expressed.

Jerry entered therapy, not because he wanted to be cured or to change his values, but because he felt unhappy, at times uncontrollably angry, and emotionally empty. He had no close relationships, and several girls with whom he had had sexual relations had told him they did not feel he was warm or could love.

What emerged in therapy was a peculiar ambivalence in Jerry's feelings toward his parents. He had identified with their ideals and stated beliefs. Much of this was internalized and ego syntonic. Now he felt cheated and angry about the hypocrisy he sensed in them. Their liberalism, he felt, was only cocktail party philosophizing and contributing money to civil rights groups, such as SNCC (Student Nonviolent Coordinating Committee) and CORE (Congress of Racial Equality). As he saw it, his parents did little to change conditions for the disadvantaged. Furthermore, he believed that they felt unfulfilled in their own lives, and although committed to the "good" things (material comforts), he was convinced they felt guilty about "selling out" their principles. They quarreled frequently, but in several family treatment sessions it was clear that even their quarrels never touched on what was really troubling them. I found that, on confrontation, they used rationalization, intellectualization, and denial to keep from facing the fact that they were not living according to the values they were preaching.

What faced their son, Jerry, if he continued on the conventional path of college and professional school, was a life like theirs —which seemed to him sterile, empty, and banal—yet undeniably society would say that they had "made it." Jerry had no rebuttal for their arguments about the importance of college to prepare for a good job and all the things that would make life comfortable.

Dropping out of college and gravitating to the East Village hippie world was Jerry's escape from a setting in which he felt stifled and trapped. At the same time, he was also acting out the socialistic ideals his parents had preached but failed to practice.

Living in a commune, sharing meager goods, and espousing brotherly love, Jerry, in effect, was gratifying several needs. Although his parents expressed strong disapproval of his behavior,

Jerry covertly hoped to win their respect by living according to standards they had so warmly praised. At the same time, he sought to hurt them for betraying him by selling out to materialism and personal gain. By defecting to hippieism, he could express his anger, renouncing what his parents had achieved and hurting them by going against their wishes. The hippie commune came closest to a way of life that could answer most of his current needs.

Further along in therapy, when college activists were winning victories for students' rights, and greater opportunities for disadvantaged youths, a dormant but visible desire to be a part of this movement led Jerry into the Yippie area of the hippie scene and finally back into college as a political activist. Therapy had helped bring to the surface his buried identification with early parental ideals. He had succeeded in working through his anger against his parents and could now emerge from his hippie refuge. He reentered college, where he really felt most comfortable. The social changes on campus helped him to identify more positively with college life, and, at our last meeting, he was doing well—within the system—but still retaining his hippie ideals.*

Another hippie patient did not fare so well. Susie P. was a runaway whose father had found her in the East Village but could not persuade her to return home. After several family interviews, Susie agreed to enter psychotherapy. Although barely sixteen, she had experimented with almost every drug available (marijuana, amphetamine, methedrine, and so forth) except heroin. Her older brother, eighteen, was living somewhere in the East Village, virtually out of communication with his parents. The family lived in a New Jersey suburb forty minutes from Manhattan. Both the mother and the father were in therapy with the same psychiatrist. The parents were extremely status conscious, living far beyond their means, and, although socially they presented a fairly good front, both were privately quite miserable.

The family was well to do, but deeply in debt because of their chronic overspending. They were very active in local civic and social activities, belonged to several clubs, and went out frequently. The father also worked long hours at his job (establishing his own advertising agency). His work often kept him in

---

* It should not be inferred that returning to college per se is necessarily the best solution for every dropout. It happened to be so for Jerry.

Manhattan at night, entertaining clients. By chance, Susie had recently learned that her father engaged in extramarital affairs. She also discovered that her mother knew all about her husband's habitual infidelity, but found it more convenient to remain quiet and uncomplaining.

The parents were generally civil to each other, but the marriage was obviously empty and unsatisfying for both. Their interest in the children focused on what looked right rather than what was right. Although they made sporadic attempts to "do" more with and for the children, they were essentially unemotional and concerned largely with material aspects of life. They had little interest in political or social issues.

Susie found herself more and more isolated. She took to playing rock group records all night in her room until, when introduced to the East Village scene by a girlfriend, who also turned her on to drugs, Susie found freedom, friends, and a new life. She soon began going to the Village every night and truanting from school (in which she had no interest and was doing badly). Finally, she decided not to return home. Her father came for her immediately and called his own psychiatrist, who referred the girl to me.

Susie was extremely immature and virtually insatiable in her need for mothering. Drugs with which she was now freely supplied filled great oral dependency needs and produced feelings of euphoria and relief from depression, anxiety, and tension. She expressed both hatred and indifference toward her parents, often wishing them dead or declaring she didn't care if she never saw them again. I could find no positive identification in the several sessions we had together. Among her hippie friends in the Village she was the "baby." They fed and cared for her. She did not have to do anything, although she did occasionally panhandle "for fun." Even in this activity, she seemed to be asking people to care for her, love her, pity her.

Susie could not tolerate psychotherapy, which was not nearly so appealing as drugs and her particular hippie supports. At last report Susie was living in a pad with about ten other young people, quite unreachable by anyone outside the East Village. She almost never leaves that area, which functions as a permissive, accepting, nurturing mother, gratifying primitive and yearning needs that she has not outgrown and until now never had satisfied.

A composite picture emerges from the family histories of fifty-five other hippie patients and nonpatients. Of the thirty patients whom I have seen clinically, five represent only one or two interviews, usually at the request of the parents, to which the youngsters agreed as part of a bargain; the others ranged from six months to two and a half years in treatment. Interviews with the twenty-five nonpatient hippies were from forty-five minutes to one and a half hours; through several of these contacts I have maintained lines of communication with the hippie community on an informal basis.

At least some characteristics of the typical hippie can be drawn.* He is likely to be a college dropout, from a white, middle-class, comfortable or prosperous family, who has never lacked the so-called advantages of mid-twentieth-century life in the United States. Although his parents may be separated or divorced, they are more likely to have remained together, often in a loveless marriage —a tired, resigned habit, in which each partner follows a busy, separate path except for the evenings they spend together. The parents of some hippies (a minority, but by no means negligible) seem to have good marriages, in which there is a reasonable amount of love and harmony. But among the good marriages that produced a hippie, the positive facets of the parents' relationship had not extended to good parenthood. In almost all cases, the hippie adolescent feels deeply critical of the way his parents lived. "They are nowhere" is a typical description. The youth feels, and sometimes the feeling is bone-deep in intensity, that with all their material comfort, they are spiritually empty, hypocritical, bored, and boring.†

Because these parents seem more or less content with their lot, they generally erect defenses of denial and rationalization so that, even if a youngster tries to express his doubts and anxieties about the aspects of their life that he views so critically, he cannot get through to them. A communication gap, cliché as that term has become, does occur. If the youth attempts to be open about his feelings, his parents tend to be preachy, angry, or simply devoid of understanding.

---

* There is of course no typical hippie, except as created by such media as the press or as a stereotype by those who are concerned only with the superficial aspects. The description here is meant only to be a broad general guideline, not a definitive portrait of all, or even most, hippies.

† For a comparison of different familial patterns contributing to two other alienated types, committed and uncommitted college students (nonhippies), see Keniston's perceptive study in depth of two small groups at Harvard University.[15, 16]

Family life was often characterized as unpleasant (the mildest reaction) or intolerable (a common reaction). This complaint seldom involved physical abuse; the term was generally used in a psychological sense. All these hippies had been unhappy at home and felt a lack in their family life. One mother was described as extremely dominating and smothering; another was said to have been excessively permissive, an attitude that her son felt was merely a thin disguise for her true feelings about him—indifference and rejection. Many parents were described as liberal and permissive. Under proper conditions, this can encourage freedom and independence, but in most of the parents in the group I studied, it appeared that the permissiveness involved a subtle form of rejection or, in some cases, a veiled invitation to act out in a way their parents secretly wished they themselves could. Some parents were described as living a loveless, but civilized, life together. In one household, the parents seemed to get along quite well together, but were too busy to give the attention their daughter needed. There were many types of family constellations, but the common factor was a lack of warmth and family closeness, or else there was an apparent closeness that actually cloaked rejection or disappointment. Some hippies felt that their fathers had not spent enough time at home when they were young, either because of long hours at work or excessive socializing. Descriptions of some fathers were vague and shadowy, and the father seemed distant and emotionally detached from the family. Parental values were either openly materialistic or, if idealistic and humanitarian principles were professed, they were not practiced. In either case, the youngster developed the feeling that his parents had sold out and that the good life they had sold out for was sterile and unfulfilling. The hippie's response was to run away from his parents' home and from the parent culture as well. In his view, society had also failed to understand him and to answer his needs; society was guilty of false values and hypocrisy (as evidenced in the Vietnam War, the civil rights struggle, de facto segregation). Society, too, had, in effect, rejected him by espousing values different from his own. The combined influences of these societal and parental forces, which complemented each other, seemed necessary to form the full-fledged hippie.

The following section examines various aspects of the hippie life style and how each relates psychodynamically to his needs.

PSYCHODYNAMIC ASPECTS OF THE HIPPIE LIFE STYLE

Extended Family, Tribal, or Communal Living

Joining a hippie commune provided each of its members with a substitute family and a chance for family closeness and sharing that they felt had been lacking in their own homes. For some, the hippie commune represented an escape from an inhibiting environment to one that was more open, yet still within a family setting.

Although, on one level, almost all these youngsters were looking for close relationships, many, feeling rejected and hurt or betrayed by a parent, could not tolerate genuine closeness for fear of being hurt again. The commune offered protection for such a youth, because with a group of surrogate parents, his need for mothering could be answered by many, yet the risk of his becoming dependent on any one individual was diminished. The nonjudgmental acceptance of the hippie commune was especially inviting to the more severely rejected youngsters. Because of the protective atmosphere in which one could count on being fed and taken care of, even if he contributed little or nothing to the group, some quite dependent and immature youngsters have found their way to a hippie commune. Indeed, without a commune to run to, such adolescents could not leave home and survive on their own. The tolerance and protection and acceptance of the group extend occasionally to a quite sick schizophrenic who finds in this milieu perhaps the most comfort and support he has ever experienced.

So, in the extended family setting, a youngster may appear to be having one or more close relationships though actually keeping himself at a safe distance from real intimacy; similarly, he may appear to be very independent (leaving home and living on his own), though actually placing himself in a highly dependent state, in the total caring and accepting atmosphere of the commune.

The Love and Nonviolent Ethic

The core philosophy of the hippie movement is that there should be more love and less hate and violence in the world. Banal as this sentiment may sound, it has energized the movement and has had the distinction of an attempt to practice what most of the world merely preaches.

The hippie's tremendous emphasis on love and nonviolence results from his conviction that these constitute the only means of saving the world (and himself). Love, say the hippies, will neutralize hate and violence and will also revive human relationships that have, as noted earlier, grown so increasingly inhuman.

In most cases, these young people are seeking the love they have missed at home. A discernible pattern indicates that those who have least experienced love have sought it the most fervently in their hippie wanderings and proved least able to feel it in their relationships.

In cases when the search for love attempted to fill a void in the hippie's personal life, it also often appeared to be a reaction formation designed to keep under control the hostile, angry impulses he originally felt toward the parents who failed him. If a hippie is on the verge of "blowing his cool" (getting angry and ready to do violence), some member of the group may invoke the sacred word "love," which actually serves to restore his temper and inhibit an overtly hostile act. For the most part, these youngsters have been consistently nonviolent. (Most of the violence involving them has been committed against them by authorities, such as police, in breaking up their "be-ins," or demonstrations, or by individuals of other minority groups, such as Hell's Angels,* who for different reasons used the hippies as scapegoats.) One is tempted to speculate on at least two reasons for the hippies' impressive record of nonviolence. First, the constant reaffirmation of love and nonaggression keeps hostile impulses repressed and out of awareness. Second, the group solidarity in upholding this principle projects a kind of group image or ideal that represents the aspirations and values of all members. As an ideal, it may stand at variance with the sicker, more aggressive qualities in any one individual, but the youngsters identify with it and draw strength from it, so that, together, they are enabled to live up to their love credo. This interpretation is drawn from a group therapy experiment which Sadock and I conducted with adolescents at Bellevue Psychiatric Hospital.[22]

"Make Love Not War," a slogan widely adopted on the hippie front, was nothing more than a slogan. Sexual activity among

---

* A rightist, belligerent group for whom the motorcycle is a symbol of its daring, violent, exhibitionistic style. Members often carry guns and knives and although anti-Establishment, they are "hawks" on the Vietnam War.

hippies was no more exaggerated than among the general population. Promiscuity, a term that hippies would reject as pejorative, generally occurred among those using sex as a way to achieve closeness. Some of the most vocal protesters against hypocrisies in sexual mores and campaigners for sexual freedom were those with sexual problems for which they were trying to compensate. Others were fully potent and enjoyed their sexual activity. (My patient group did not include the latter type.) Sexual activity varied as much in the hippie scene as in the general culture. Reports of wild, prolonged orgies seem to be mostly a fantasy of the press and other mass media, which reveals more about the needs of the myth-makers than it does about the hippie. Sex is not nearly so central or constant in hippie life as is commonly supposed. For many patients and some nonpatients, sex was not even primarily an orgastic sensual experience, but rather an act of offered comfort and a means of obtaining a cared-for, belonging feeling. Some hippies desired greater numbers of sexual partners in order to rebel against the hypocritical social traditions of chastity and monogamy—to dispel the air of sacrosanctity and to make sexual activity acceptable for its own sake, unfettered by false and repressive restrictions.

Psychedelic (Mind-Expanding) Drugs

Drugs and the psychedelic experience have occupied a front-and-center position in the hippie's life. In these activities, no single explanation holds valid for all hippies. Some, whose lives have been meaningless, sterile, banal, who have found parental values unacceptable, and whose identifications with parents are ambivalent, seek drugs and any mind-changing stimulus to help them find their "true selves." Depending on the particular youngster and his special life experiences, the hippie might be searching for a sense of self he had never developed, trying to blot out anxieties, fears, and the feeling of alienation. Running away and changing one's style of dress and appearance as, for example, through longer hair and beard, can symbolize the death of the old personality and the starting of a new life. The drug and psychedelic experience may also symbolize this dying and rebirth; in fact, this is precisely how the experience has been described by some of my hippie informants. This finding has been noted also by Brickman.[1]

Drugs are not necessarily the center of most hippies' philosophy, though some observers of the hippie scene have believed otherwise. The fact is that many hippies have given up drugs or sharply reduced their use, explaining that drugs became less necessary when they found other meaningful ways to escape from their unfulfilled past lives and to find purpose and relevance in the present. Many have found artistic and sensual fulfillment through creating or enjoying mixed-media experiences—complex aesthetic combinations of light, sound, color, form, and movement that reproduce the psychedelic experience found through drugs. This has created a base for new and quite exciting frontiers in creative expression. Various forms of Eastern religions and practices based on transcendental meditation have allowed some to feel that they have transcended the mundane trivialities of our society to reach new levels of self-awareness and in-touchness. Still others have found that commitment to social and political activist groups brings a sense of aliveness and meaning to their existence. In these individuals, drug use is relegated to a minor role, indicating that it served merely as a way station or temporary means to attain their goals, until other, more effective and perhaps less dangerous ways could be found.

There is, in most of these activities, a common search for answers and revelations about life and the purpose of one's own existence.

Alienated from society, not sure he wants to be a part of it, the hippie is seeking a different way. He does not like what he has seen and wants to see beyond or above (and so to transcend) the culture to which he is so strongly bound by the old links of identification with parents and institutions. Despite his conscious rejection of this culture in adolescence and afterward, he must use dramatic and radical means to free himself. Drugs fill this need exceedingly well. The literature is well supplied with detailed descriptions of individual reactions and feelings under the influence of drugs,[3, 5] which need not be examined here.

The drug experience offers a form of social fulfillment that many of these youngsters could not otherwise achieve. For many of the lonely, unrelated hippies yearning for, yet fearing, closeness to others, any act of sharing holds great attraction. Marijuana smoking in a group setting (often with a single joint passed from person to person) is felt as a shared experience. It may also produce the feeling of harmony with the universe—and fellow man. This feeling, when experienced, appeals to almost everyone, especially to the alienated youth who, being further removed than others from this state of being, yearns more intensely for it.

Almost all hippies have tried marijuana and are users to some degree. A wide variety of other drugs have been sampled, the most popular being LSD and methedrine. At one end of the spectrum is the hippie who takes only marijuana; at the other end is the hippie who tries and uses every drug he can obtain so long as it affects his mood in some positive way, despite concomitant negative effects. Significantly, I know of no hippies who use heroin and only a few who have ever tried it. They have, in general, contempt for the heroin user and put the drug down because —as a surprising number express it—"I can get 'hooked' on heroin." They are aware that the drugs they do use do not have the strong addictive qualities that heroin does.

The use of drugs by hippies (as well as many youths who do not fall in this general category) has many meanings, some of which apply to almost all youth; others, to only a few individuals. Among the common meanings is that the use of drugs (especially marijuana) has become a symbol of rebellion against the older generation, a rejection of parents' values and of the Establishment. That the drug is illegal, whereas tobacco and alcohol remain legal and protected by those who use them, illustrates dramatically, in the eyes of youth, the hypocrisy of their elders. Rebellion and demonstrations by the young for legalizing pot then fall in line with their demonstrations and cries against the Vietnam War and for civil rights.

But the use of marijuana, as well as other drugs, such as LSD, represents more than revolt against parents and the Establishment. People, even idealistic youngsters, seldom transcend their culture or its values even when they consciously deny and reject them. Because, as mentioned earlier, youngsters today have been reared in a drug-centered society, there is identification with their parents and with the parent society that has made the consumption of drugs a daily and important ritual. If alcohol is the adult's "thing," the youngster chooses something else for his—marijuana. So the youngster is able to imitate his parents while rebelling against them. Smoking pot thus constitutes an act encompassing many dynamic qualities. The illegality of marijuana obscures the understanding of its use, because the mere fact of illegality has significance for every user. The dynamic meaning may be the desire to break a law that the youth considers terribly unfair or a desire to be caught and punished, in which case other complex motivations are involved. Many users smoke pot in circumstances that increase their chances of being apprehended; others take precautions that make their activity virtually safe from detection by authorities. What the youth does in terms of the legal risks must, of course, be considered as part of the full meaning of his use of pot. With this in mind, I will mention several categories of marijuana users.

The first group, and I have found it to be a very large one, is composed of youngsters whose main reasons for using marijuana are curiosity, adventurousness, and, to some extent, the desire to conform to their peer group. This category of marijuana users is the healthiest. These are the ones who can take it or leave it, who do not go on to hard narcotics, and who, in many ways, use it as the social drinkers use alcohol. The cocktail-before-dinner drinker or the one who has a few every Saturday night has his equivalent in the youngster who, instead of going to a party where liquor is served, goes to a party where marijuana is passed around.

A second group, or possibly a subgroup of the first, includes those youngsters who, in using marijuana, are expressing rebellion and growing-up pains. Here the behavior is reminiscent of what many present-day adults did when they were adolescents—sneaking cigarettes and drinks to act like their parents.

Another group, which does manifest psychopathology, is one whose members are withdrawn, passive, shy, and inhibited; they suffer feelings of inadequacy and insecurity (all characteristics long ago described and labelled "drug addict personality").[28] With this group, psychological dependency on marijuana is more likely to develop, as is the potential for going on to other drugs of a more dangerous nature.

One of the many categories of marijuana users would include the hippie who is looking for an inner truth, salvation through love, and a way to avoid such evils as hypocrisy, the "rat race," competitiveness, and false values. This is anything but a uniform group, because one sees among its members the most regressed of schizophrenics, who consume enormous quantities of pot and other drugs to conjure up another world, however unreal, because it seems better than the one they are living in. At the other end of the hippie spectrum, one sees some who have the ego strength and security to try another way of life within the dominant culture—despite that culture's hostile attitude toward its deviants.

"Do Your Thing"

Along with the love ethic, the life style of the hippie is expressed in his exhortation, "Do your thing, man," which in essence means doing whatever is right for you, so long as it fulfills your potential and needs and does not actively interfere with another person doing *his* thing. The young have seen how much adult activity, in both the business and social scenes, is performed for many reasons other than self-fulfillment. They see the paradox in having more free time, yet less freedom; they see this as a root cause for the "hang-ups" that prevent their parents and other adults from getting any real pleasure out of life.

This conclusion, in turn, leads to the anti-intellectual stance of so many hippies, who believe that overmechanization and decreased personalization of life have obscured and covered up man's ability to be in touch with his own real feelings. Again, the hippie using drugs, music, meditation, or whatever, is basically trying to find himself and a meaning to his life. In this sense, many hippies are not running away from life, but searching for an alternative to a hollow (or "plastic") existence.

Style of Dress

Even the hippie's style of dress—his gaudy, colorful, sometimes bizarre clothes and grooming—constitutes another means of breaking loose from the confines of conventional society. "The system" forces everyone to look and act alike—button-down shirts on Madison Avenue, pin stripes on Wall Street. (Some big companies, including IBM and several major brokerage firms, even forbid employees to grow beards.)

The hippie dresses individualistically, although most members of hippie groups tend to adopt similar clothing styles. Love beads are now an almost universal hippie badge, as are Indian headbands, old army uniforms, and articles of Indian or other primitive cultures. A significant minority also indulges in body painting. Almost all hippies wear their hair long, although a fair number have now adopted the bushy "Afro" hair style, still another expression of hippie alliance with the alienated minorities.

Again, the hippie style of dress has different meanings for specific individuals. I have found the following motives most common:

1. To symbolize revolt or rebellion against conventional authority (parents, schools, the business community).
2. To express individuality and independence.
3. To express identification with "primitive" and "natural" man (Indian and gypsy attire). This symbolizes rejection of modern society, with its automated, mass-produced artificiality, and a return to simplicity, innocence, oneness with nature—and by extension, with oneself. The adoption of Indian clothing also may express identification with a minority, oppressed, underdog group. Some "fun games" hippies play make the American Indian the "good guy" and the cowboy the "bad guy." Some of the drug-using hippies also identify with the Indian's liturgical use of peyote, a drug whose effects are not dissimilar from those of LSD.
4. To return to the free, irresponsible, happy times of childhood. Such regression is facilitated by wearing costumes, especially Indian and cowboy, which are so closely identified with childhood in America.

Hippie attitudes and rituals are often contradictory, as are those of all adolescents. Dressing in costume may express rebellion against middle-class conformity, but the costume itself is a hippie uniform, and wearing it indicates conformity to standards set by their peers. Their very rejection of—and rejection by—the majority intensifies their need to belong to one another and to show that they *do* belong.

In my studies with another alienated group—juvenile delinquents from disadvantaged and broken homes—I have found that, where ties to parents were weak or negative, peer group attachments meant more to these youngsters than did relationships with their parents. Like the hippie community, the delinquent gang offered more support and sustenance to its members than any member received at home, and its members responded by feeling greater loyalty to the gang than to their families.[9]

Music—Acid, Folk, Raga, Soul, Art, and Revolution Rock

The musical expression of a group reveals a great deal about its nature and also yields important clues to the personality structure of individuals within it. Today's still-evolving revolution can be traced almost directly from its origins in Negro spirituals and jazz to the acid, folk, raga, soul, and art rock of the current hippies. Each stage has expressed the theme of alienation and personal need and has stirred the deepest emotions both in the musicians and in those who respond to their music.

Jazz evolved into "rhythm and blues" during the 1940's and early 1950's, but it remained one of the few areas of life in which the black man could express himself, despite the surrounding climate of oppressiveness and discrimination. These early forms of "soul" music flourished first in the ghettos and then beyond, as black political movements became more open and radical. Although called "race music," such music expressed feelings shared by all the alienated and the oppressed, including another, quite different, minority group—the young white rebels called "beatniks," and later "hippies." Rhythm and blues music, evolving into rock 'n roll, emphasized vitality, sexuality, and individual freedom.

During the 1950's, U.S. singer Elvis Presley spearheaded the rock music explosion, with dramatic emphasis on sexuality and free body movement. It was a freedom cry to the alienated young, expressing both a reaction to repression and hypocrisy and an invitation to break loose. Breaking the barriers of formal music, the new sounds suggested sexual freedom in rhythms, then in explicit lyrics, finally in expressions of social as well as sexual protest. This burst of musical freedom was both an echo and a call to battle for the alienated minority.

In England, the Beatles, who, in many ways—music, style of hair and dress, various experimentations with drugs and Oriental philosophy—could be classified among the first true hippies, embraced rock music as a means of self-expression and, like Presley and later rock performers (essentially hippies), reached responsive chords in many of the youth of the United States and other countries. Of course, not all who respond to this new music are hippies. But I believe that the youth—and it is largely the music of the young—who "dig" this music most intensely are responding to its deep appeal for freedom in sexuality and self-expression and the search for self-identity.

Acid rock is the most formless form of rock music—a fantasy jumble of sounds presumably re-creating the surrealistic aural and visual experiences of psychedelic drug trips. The heavier drug users are most responsive to and understanding of this music.

Folk and art rock, another variation, is notable for lyrics of social protest. As exemplified by poets and singers, such as Bob

Dylan and Joan Baez, it involves social and political commentaries skillfully woven into a rock ballad form. Other hippie groups, such as the Rolling Stones and the Fugs, have become enormously popular along with the Beatles, as they all added sharp notes of irony to their lyrical protests.

In blending Middle Eastern and Indian sounds and rhythms, raga rock expressed feelings of and explorations into the mystic, the timeless, the search for peace and tranquillity—especially in opposition to violence, competitiveness, materialism, and intellectuality.

Revolution rock is really a kind of folk rock, emphasizing the need for or the inevitability of revolution. The assassinations of Martin Luther King and Robert Kennedy, two leaders with large followings among the alienated young; the prolonged agony of the Vietnam War; increasing violence in the battle for civil rights; the contagion of frustration and bitterness—all have led to music calling for more dramatic and radical action.

Whatever its artistic or aesthetic merits, rock music has psychological significance as an expression of personal needs and conflict, some of it on a nonverbal and unconscious level. Words alone could never convey so much, especially for the less articulate members of the hippie group. A hippie movie is entitled *You Are What You Eat*. In essence, the message of rock music is "You are what you feel."

Theater

Hippie philosophy and style have also pervaded current theater, contributing significantly to the social revolution. The Radical Theater Repertory has over twenty groups (and is still growing rapidly) throughout the country. The most notable example is the Living Theater, led by Julian Beck and Judith Malina, an ensemble group comprised mainly of young men and women who qualify as hippies, having set up their own communal life, living and traveling as well as performing together and sharing everything equally, including whatever money their performances earn.

The Living Theater has developed an intensely realistic style that breaks down the traditional boundary between audience and actors. The desire to make the theatrical experience a shared one, to make actor-audience communication closer and more reciprocal, fitted their offstage philosophy, which demands that life and art become a unified whole. It is a theater of confrontation; in portraying reality, which can be tedious and painful, they spare the audience nothing. If the play is about suffering, as is *The Plague*, the players try to make the audience feel the pain, experience it, share it. Performers roam freely among the audience to argue and provoke reaction, to urge everyone to take off his clothes, as they do (*Paradise Now*), symbolizing the stripping away of inhibitions so that spectators become participants—in spiritual union with the actors. It is noteworthy that in the recent marathon group therapy sessions—lasting two days—on the West Coast, patients and therapist conduct their sessions in the nude. In *Hair*, a successful rock musical, for the first time on the Broadway stage, a frontal view of nude figures is presented—not for the sake of shock or sensation, but rather to show that it *can* and *should* be done to abolish false modesty. Symbolically, again, it stands for a stripping away of all false masks and hypocrisies. It also shows the actor exposed (in both senses)—vulnerable, helpless, unarmed, and nonviolent—in his most natural state of being.

Mixed Media

In the mixed-media displays, dance, movement, music, color, film, and light are programmed in combinations—for total assault on all the senses. These productions are designed to produce new feeling sensations by breaking through and breaking down the normal boundaries—"blowing the mind."

The reports from those who have undergone these experiences are that they can be like taking LSD—a trip without drugs—a way of engaging a part of the self that has been locked up and unreachable by other means. These mixed-media trips are described as being beautiful, profoundly moving, and offering new insights and truths (presumably by tapping areas of the unconscious that have never been reached or else have been repressed). Many hippies who have had difficulty feeling deeply and who have complained of boredom, malaise, and "not being alive" were touched by this shotgun assault, when a less intense stimulus would not get through to them. Others, better integrated to begin with, were able to achieve fresh, exciting sensations by an artistic combination of various art forms into a creative single unity. This mixed- or multimedia effect is consistent with the hippies' style of breaking down barriers (not just between people, but between art forms as well) and synthesizing all creative forces into a unifying whole.*

"Tell It Like It Is"—The Communications Media

To fill the widening credibility and communications gaps, caused by distortions and omissions in the nation's conventional press, dissident young people have established an underground network of newspapers and periodicals in almost every big city and on many college campuses. In discussing topics it feels are being suppressed or misrepresented, the Movement (for this group is an amalgam of hippies and radical activists) presents its views in a completely uninhibited new journalistic style, marked by free use of four-letter words that have never been printed in the straight media and liberally spiced with cartoons and seriocomic strips depicting nudity and diverse sexual acts (signifying that sex can be fun and also funny). Again, as in other art expressions of the Movement, it is an attempt to profane the sacred cow and strip away hypocrisy.

At its best, this radical journalism has been creative, provocative, and diverting in its approach to social issues of the day, its serious confrontations with institutions and public policies, and its deep comic thrusts and brilliant satiric diatribes. It has, on occasion, unearthed news of importance to everyone and has scooped straight journalism (as in the article exposing the activities of the CIA on college campuses throughout the United States).[21] Paul Krassner, founder of *The Realist*, a forerunner of uninhibited underground journals, is one of the media's leaders. Other influential and highly regarded journals are *Rat* (New York City), *Avatar* (Boston), and the *Express Times* (San Francisco). The journals also serve to keep members of the movement in touch with one another. It is their own thing in communication.

---

* In a series of interviews, members of the Group Image in New York City, a group of some forty young people, including college graduates and dropouts, expressed to me the gratifications they achieved as artists by working together, pooling their individual talents into something more than any one individual could produce alone. Although they live in about eight different "pads," they spend a large part of the day together in a big loft, working on various artistic projects combining a number of different disciplines and talents.

TREATMENT

Because the consensus of the middle-class population, both lay and psychiatric, is that the hippie is mentally disturbed, the question of whether treatment is indicated, and, if so, what kind, is an important one. A complicating factor is the presence of social as well as psychological determinants in the psychological makeup of the marginally asocial personality, as exemplified by the beatnik-hippie type.

At one extreme is the blatantly psychotic hippie, who finds in the supporting, tolerant hippie community a benevolent, nonthreatening atmosphere, in which he offends no one and no one takes critical or punitive action against him. Indeed, the community often has been so protective that, in effect, it provides such a youngster with the kind of support he might receive from one of the more benevolent state hospitals. At the other extreme of hippiedom are relatively healthy youngsters, quite intact, who have felt keenly the wrong or unsatisfying aspects of their lives and who have needed to experiment with this more adventurous life style to see what it might do for them. A few show strong confidence, self-esteem, and self-awareness, which help them tolerate the extra stress of a minority or unpopular position.

The majority of youngsters I have encountered belonged somewhere between these two extremes, showing a wide spectrum of emotional difficulties and strengths and cutting across all diagnostic lines. The hippie is clearly not an asocial stereotype characterized by a single set of superficial signs and symptoms and treatable or untreatable according to a single set formula.

If one bears in mind the fact that, in general, the hippie style of a troubled youth is employed as an adaptive maneuver to make up for and counter the gaps and distortions of his previous living experiences, the pathology revealed often centers on the hippie's inability to communicate with others on a level that permits any real emotional gratification. As a result of his emotional loss of family, he feels loneliness and a profound depression. The hippie attempts to mask these sensations behind bizarre, exhibitionistic, and wild antics. His life style attempts to compensate for the loneliness and depression, a finding also noted by Heilbrunn.[10]

The motivations for the individual hippie's pattern of behavior must be studied and clearly determined before any evaluation of their true meaning can be made. This will then dictate whether therapy should be recommended and, if so, along what lines. In a recent panel meeting involving six hippies and an audience of psychiatrists, I emphasized this key point: to be deviant is not necessarily to be sick.[7] The society-alienated person may or may not be mentally ill; the self-alienated person assuredly is. In the latter case, treatment would proceed along traditional lines, but not necessarily using traditional methods. Uncovering areas of conflict, working through and understanding the material associated with anxiety, identifying and clarifying the factors in past and present experiences and behavior that have contributed to the warps (as well as the strengths) of his personality, and breaking through defense patterns are all necessary to allow the greatest latitude for growth and resynthesis of the personality.

The therapist must then be prepared to explore alternative ways of living to which the hippie might comfortably adapt, or which the therapist must learn to accept as valid. The therapist should be in touch with the ways in which various social structures relate to the particular individual's life style if he is to be helpful in exploring with the patient those paths that may be constructive to follow and those that would lead to further conflict and difficulties in living. What is needed is not a cure for the hippie's way of life, but a means of helping to eradicate difficulties in his search for a sense of identity and self-esteem. If this goal is achieved, the youth may continue to live in the hippie world—and successfully—or he may return to more conventional society, still retaining various elements of his hip values. Again, he may eschew the hippie style altogether, viewing it as an adolescent phase to be passed through on the way to a more mature identity. I have had hippie patients in therapy where success, or cure, was noted in those who subsequently followed one or another of these paths. The point is that the therapist should take care not to let his own value judgments and biases cause him to view deviance per se as a symptom of general or specific mental illness. Too often he unwittingly acts as an agent of the Establishment (although he may consciously protest this), and this blind spot may interfere with his effectiveness in being truly helpful to the patient. A psychiatrist who feels that beatniks have "an attitude particularly irritating to those of us who regard many of them as poseurs . . . who have been pretty well spoiled by foolishly overpermissive parents and an excessively indulgent milieu . . . execrable esthetics (raucous cacophony, miscalled music; clonic convulsions, miscalled dance; or monstrous montages, miscalled art . . .)"[18] is certainly entitled to his opinion, but he ought not to work with this type of patient.

In therapy, it is virtually impossible to treat a hippie by means of orthodox psychoanalysis. The patient will not stand for it. He wants to "rap"* and to have a dialogue. He will ask questions, such as whether or not the therapist ever turned on with marijuana or LSD. One can and should explore the covert meanings of the question and what is being looked for and needed in the answer. But after all that is done, there are those who still need to know the answer before they can discuss freely their drug use and other subjects. Alternate methods to more active therapy could be employed to get the patient to open up, but they would be very time-consuming (and therefore wasteful), fraught with possibilities of failure, and would certainly incur the possibility of the patient not waiting around for circuitous methods to work.

It is my belief and experience that therapy can be accomplished by engaging in a dialogue, by referring to personal example, and by many other techniques that must be considered modifications of standard therapy. The style of the therapist must be made suitable to and congruent with the style of the patient, rather than the reverse. Too often the therapist with a limited and inflexible method ends up saying "the patient was not a good therapeutic case," whereas the more correct assessment would be that the techniques of the therapist were not appropriate for this patient. I found an analogous situation in working with blue-collar, or working-class patients.[7]

Each therapist may find his own way, verbal and/or nonverbal, to establish rapport with a group who, whatever other pathology it may have, has a style of "paranoia" (a phrase hippies often use, but with a different connotation from the psychiatric definition). The slogan that originated on the Berkeley campus—"Don't trust anyone over thirty"—would include psychiatrists. One can gain these youths' trust by being understanding of what they are and why they are. Even so small a matter as understanding their jargon, a special language with which they set themselves apart from unsympathetic outsiders, would be helpful. To make them speak in an unnatural (to them) way would create a barrier to communication and trust. This is not to imply that the therapist should employ their language himself, except for the few to whom it may come naturally (the same can be said for drug experimentation), because this kind of artifice or implicit condescension

---

* To be able to talk freely, but with a two-way active interaction.

would turn off the hippie who wants honesty in the person who may want honesty of him.

I have not found that referring to personal example or using other essentially nonneutral material interferes with or distorts transference. The inappropriate carryover of distortions in perceptions of current figures and situations resulting from earlier, traumatic relationships with significant people in the patient's life need not be altered by the therapist's activity, so long as the therapist is aware of the purpose of his own actions, and so long as they are not a manifestation of neurotic tendencies or countertransference on his part.

In helping to increase a patient's self-awareness (working through defenses and symptoms and expanding ego boundaries), no one method of therapy would suit all circumstances. This is why any psychoanalytic technique with the hippie and, especially, the adolescent hippie, should be modified as the occasion dictates. If the therapist chooses to engage in more active participation (a greater risk for greater gain), he must be extremely careful to avoid burdening the patient with additional problems, and he must guard against making irrelevant or anecdotal comments without a goal or purpose in mind.

DISCUSSION AND SUMMARY

Many authorities, in evaluating the plight or flight of the hippie, argue that he has dropped out of society, that he is passive and lacks a positive, constructive program. This position, I believe, is inaccurate, because it misses the more dynamic, motivating force (whether sick or healthy) behind the hippie style. To leave college, family, and the comforts of conventional middle-class society, move to a slum or distant, rural commune, and defy so many traditions and mores, may be evidence of anxiety, associated with his psychopathology, of such a high level that he must flee from this oppressive (to him) environment. On the other hand, these same acts may reflect the courage and strength to go against the mainstream whose values and mores are not relevant to the youth's needs. In either case, it is decidedly active, not passive, behavior. A hippie youth may, in fact, be more active than one who glides docilely into the way of life his parents want for him, whether or not that way is stultifying. The conventional youngster who conforms may do so automatically, without thinking, or may be afraid to veer from the accepted path.

Nor does the hippie drop out of society. Indeed, seldom has so small a group (numerically) been so much in the public eye or roused society to such great extremes of outrage and compassion. In trying to counteract established society, hippies have, in fact, produced a vital counterculture.* Their acts of defiance are committed within the social order and are meant to change it. They rely heavily on ridicule and denunciation (throwing money from the gallery of the New York Stock Exchange, exorcising the Pentagon, nominating a pig for President, and so forth). They confront the system by refusing to follow its orders and following instead the group philosophy of love, nonviolence, sincerity, freedom (of speech and sex), creative self-expression, nonconformity, simplicity, fun. Their creed seems, at least to this observer, to contain some elements of a positive alternative to the admittedly imperfect world they reject. But, even if they do not put forth a totally cohesive and constructive program, their protest is not rendered wrong or meaningless, as many critics have argued. It overlooks the significant fact that recognizing the evils of a system and refusing to play its game or obey its rules is a quite positive and healthy action. Had more Germans refused to participate in the Nazi government program or to remain innocent bystanders, the incredible annihilation of six million Jews might not have occurred. To ask the right questions or to make accurate criticisms forms the basis for further change, even if the questioners and critics may not themselves follow through.

The hippie's relationships with other marginally asocial groups are ambiguous, and his identifications and empathies are largely unreciprocated. An important and illustrative example is his uneasy alliance with the black community. Hippies, although sympathetic to the black man's cause, did not, at the outset, become actively involved in his political protests, primarily because the blacks were then fighting for equal rights and justice within the Establishment. Later, when the more militant Negroes began their black power, separatist movement—outside the Establishment—hippies joined their battle for civil rights and better economic opportunities. The Negroes, however, did not welcome them, and very few black youths have found their way into the

---

* "Counterculture" implies activity, challenge, and more confrontation than does the usual term, "subculture," and so better expresses the nature of the movement.

hippie groups. The many causes for this can only be mentioned briefly here.

The hippie, who generally comes from a comfortable home and has been fairly well educated, deliberately adopts a disadvantaged way of life that Negroes live, but *not* by choice. The fact that the hippie can physically pull out of his poverty and unemployment whenever he chooses causes the Negro to react with bitterness and resentment at what seems to him like game-playing and mockery. Also, because most Negroes (and lower-class whites) have regarded the middle-class value system and way of life as goals to be desired and achieved, if possible, the hippie's voluntary rejection of such material and social advantages threatens the Negro's belief that they are really worthwhile. The result is that the blacks feel hostile and scornful of hippies and unwilling to join their movement. Although both are fighting against the same power groups, and often for the same causes (as in the anti-Vietnam War protests), their motivations remain fundamentally dissimilar.

The hippies' message in music, their composing and performing heroes—the Beatles, Dylan, Baez, and others—have now won acceptance in the adult music world as an authentic, creative, and cultural contribution. Hippie innovations have also been welcomed by the movies, theater, art, and the fashion world. Long hair and flamboyant clothing styles are being worn by some of the stanchest pillars of the Establishment.

Significantly, even though many hippies may be individually sick in varying degrees, the movement as a whole is socially healthy. A treatment program must inevitably direct itself to the individual hippie who is troubled, but treatment must also be addressed to the sociological conditions that breed hippies, so that the problem can be prevented as well as cured. To begin with, a drug-centered society such as ours cannot hope to stop youth from experimenting with new drugs of their own. Similarly, violence, war, hypocrisy, discrimination, crass materialism, and a decline in spiritual values cannot prepare youth to enter an adult society with respect for its standards and a desire to conform to them.

The hippie and the radical left seek to revolutionize society. If this is to be forestalled, society must reorganize its own system so as to be more relevant to the needs of today's youth, and it must do so with considerably greater "deliberate speed" than has been shown, for example, in implementing the 1954 Supreme Court decision on civil rights.

The world as ordered is not to the liking of the alienated—all the alienated, not just the hippies. Other groups disaffected and disillusioned with society (and/or themselves) express their deviancy from the system in ways other than the hippie style. It is beyond the scope of this chapter to describe them all or to delineate the dynamics that distinguish each, but among others counted as marginally asocial, alienated youth groups are the campus rebels and political activists, many of whom are part of the New Radical Left[9, 14, 20]; the Black Panthers, a militant separatist movement led by Eldridge Cleaver,[2] Stokely Carmichael, and H. Rap Brown; Hell's Angels, representing the rightist, gun- and knife-wielding motorcycle set[24]; Peace Corps and Vista volunteers, who are idealistic and somewhat romantic youths looking for valid, human commitments on a people-to-people level and who hope to find their own personal identity as well. All the marginally asocial contribute mixtures of pathology and health in their various assaults on the traditional system of Western culture.

As a consequence of this dissatisfaction, the world is undergoing a social revolution. In restructuring a society, to change customs and mores and overturn tradition, a period of disorder necessarily occurs. If one merely focuses on the disorder in progress (for example, the hippie movement), one may say it is nihilistic and unconstructive, but history has shown us that change from one kind of order to another inevitably involves a chaotic transition period.

So long as unjust and "sick" conditions exist in society (the personal society of family as well as the impersonal outer society), hippies will develop to challenge these conditions. Even if, in the next generation, he is called by yet another name, the hippie (beatnik, radical, bohemian) will remain the alienated rebel of his time.

REFERENCES

1. Brickman, H. R. "The Psychedelic 'Hip Scene': Return of the Death Instinct," *American Journal of Psychiatry*, December 1968. Vol. 125, pp. 766–772.
2. Cleaver, E. *Soul on Ice.* New York: McGraw-Hill, 1968.
3. Cohen, S. "Pot, Acid and Speed," *Medical Science*, February 1968.
4. *Cox Commission Report: Crisis at Columbia.* New York: Vintage, 1968.
5. DeBold, R. C., and Leaf, R. C. (eds.). *LSD, Man and Society: A Synposium.* Middletown, Conn.: 1967.
6. Ginsberg, A. *Howl.* San Francisco: City Lights, 1956.
7. Gould, R. E. "Dr. Strangeclass: Or How I Stopped Worrying about the Theory

and Began Treating the Blue Collar Worker," *American Journal of Orthopsychiatry*, **36,** no. 2 (January 1967), 78–86.
8. Gould, R. E. "The Hippie Scene," *Medical Times*, **96,** no. 5 (May 1968), 449–510.
9. Gould, R. E. *Society's Child: The Making of a Delinquent*. New York: Praeger, 1968. (Adapted from "The Delinquent Adolescent," presented at Hillside Hospital, February 25–26, 1967.)
10. Heilbrunn, G. "How 'Cool' Is the Beatnik?" *The Psychoanalytic Forum*, **2,** no. 1 (Spring 1967).
11. Hoffman, A. *Revolution for the Hell of It*. New York: Dial, 1968.
12. Holmes, J. C. *Go*. New York: Scribner's, 1952.
13. Huxley, A. *Brave New World*. New York: Harper & Row, 1932.
14. Jacobs, P., and Lander, S. *The New Radicals*. New York: Random House, 1966.
15. Keniston, K. *Young Radicals*. New York: Harvest, 1968.
16. Keniston, K. *The Uncommitted*. New York: Dell, 1960.
17. Kerouac, J. *On the Road*. New York: New American Library, 1957.
18. Masserman, J. H. "The Beatnik: Up-, Down-, and Off-," *Archives of General Psychiatry*, **16,** no. 3 (March 1967).
19. "Movie Review of *Pull My Daisy*," *Time Magazine*, December 14, 1959.
20. Newfield, J. *A Prophetic Minority*. New York: New American Library, 1966.
21. "The NSA and the CIA," *Ramparts Magazine*, March 1967.
22. Sadock, B., and Gould, R. E. "A Preliminary Report on Short-Term Group Psychotherapy on an Acute Adolescent Male Service," *International Journal of Group Psychotherapy*, **14,** no. 4 (October 1964), 465–473.
23. Stubblebine, J. M. "Health Hazards of the Hippies," paper presented at the Annual Meeting of the American Psychiatric Association, Boston, Mass., May 1968.
24. Thompson, H. S. *Hell's Angels: A Strange and Terrible Saga*. New York: Random House, 1967.
25. Walker Report, *Violence in Chicago*. New York: Bantam, 1968.
26. Wolfe, T. "The Pump House Gang Meets the Black Panthers—Or Silver Threads among the Gold in Surf City," *The New York Herald Tribune*, February 13, 1966.
27. Wolfe, T. "The Pump House Gang Faces Life," Part II, *The New York Herald Tribune*, February 20, 1966.
28. Wolfe, T. *The Electric Kool-Aid Acid Test*. New York: Farrar, Strauss & Giroux, 1968.
29. Zimmering, P. et al. "Drug Addiction in Relation to Problems of Adolescence," *American Journal of Psychiatry*, **109,** no. 4 (October 1952).

EREUTHOPHOBIA AND ALLIED CONDITIONS: A CONTRIBUTION TOWARD THE PSYCHOPATHOLOGICAL AND CROSSCULTURAL STUDY OF A BORDERLINE STATE

Yomishi Kasahara
and Kenji Sakamoto

I

Since the first half of the eighteenth century, studies have been conducted on ereuthophobia, in which the sufferer fears blushing in the presence of others and, consequently, tries to avoid being in a situation where this can happen. Since the turn of the century, in particular, a number of significant researches have been made public. Among others, the outstanding findings of Janet and Fenichel are meaningful even today.

Because ereuthophobia and allied conditions constitute the neurosis most frequently observed in Japan, ereuthophobia has been the focus of interest in this country since the inception of the study of neuroses half a century ago.

Although this line of study has been pursued in Japan for half a century, the more severe cases have hithertofore been neglected; this chapter focuses on them. This essay aims, first, to consider psychopathologically and phenomenologically borderline features* shown by these types of disorder and, second, to submit data to facilitate a comparative study of these conditions in different cultural contexts.

II

It is generally agreed that Casper[5] gave the name "erythrophobia" to this variety of neurosis in 1848. It was Pitres and Régis,[31] however, who attempted its clinical classification in 1896. They divided erythrophobia into three types—*ereutose simple, ereutose emotive*, and *ereutose obsessionale*—and claimed that only the last should be called "ereuthophobia" ("fear of blushing") rather than "erythrophobia" ("fear of red").

Janet made the pioneering contribution toward clarifying the characteristic features of this syndrome. He placed ereuthophobia along with its allied conditions, including Morselli's dysmorphophobia and the like, under the comprehensive category of "phobias of social situations," thus setting them apart from other types of phobias. Not only did he differentiate this from the phobias of objects, in which dangerous objects or animals are feared, but he also demarcated it from such phobias of physical situations as agoraphobia and claustrophobia, in which space, as perceived in purely physical terms, is feared. In this chapter, references to ereuthophobia and allied conditions signify Janet's phobias of social situations. Of late, some prefer to call this, as Ey does,[8] "phobias of human contact."

In Japan, Morita, at just about the same time as Janet, paid close attention to this pathological phenomenon. (Morita's name is well known in our country, as a result of a school of psychotherapy having been named after him.) The types of neurosis, which he chose as susceptible to his psychotherapeutic approach, were what are generally called neurasthenia, anxiety neurosis, and a limited variety of obsessional neuroses, following the current diagnostic criteria of Western countries. Because he consid-

---

* The definition of the borderline state varies according to author. In Japan, the following criteria are generally accepted: (1) It is a clinical entity, which borders on neurosis and on schizophrenia. (2) It is not just quantitatively halfway between them. In part, the symptoms are something qualitatively different. (3) As a rule, these patients remain substantially the same throughout their life. Our definition is more or less similar to M. Schmideberg's.[33]

ered that such neuroses derive from a common constitution, he placed them into the general category of *shinkeishitsu* (*shinkei* means nervousness, *shitsu* means temperament). He indicated in his therapeutic efforts that, to facilitate the removal of such symptoms, one should accept, not fight, them. This method appealed to the Japanese sufferers of these symptoms and developed into a school of psychotherapy unique to Japan—Morita therapy.[22]

So much for the historical account. It remains to be pointed out, however, that the symptoms central to *shinkeishitsu* are ereuthophobia and allied conditions. Morita[25] recorded a great number of the symptomatic variations of this, such as fear induced by one's own facial expressions, fear of eye-to-eye confrontation, fear of being ugly, fear of stammering, fear of emitting bodily odor, fear of a crowd, fear of one's superiors, and so on.[24] It is established psychiatric practice in Japan to bundle these up and give them a comprehensive nomenclature, *taijin-kyofu*. When translated into European languages, it is customary to use such words as "anthropophobia" or "homilophobia." This practice may be misleading in that it might imply that the subject is fearful of others in the same way he is afraid of a horse. In fact, the subject is fearful that he might make a bad impression on others.[20] Therefore, it would be more appropriate to use, after Janet,[17] the phrase, "fear of social situations."

What interests us here is that practically all the Japanese psychoanalysts at the early stage of psychiatric study endeavored to clarify the dynamics of these symptoms. Yamamura grappled energetically with this problem. It was through his efforts that the views on ereuthophobia held by such psychoanalysts as Freud, Ferenzi, Steckel, Fenichel, Alexander, and Numberg were introduced to Japanese psychiatric circles.

To the best of our knowledge, few references have been made to the more severe manifestations of these symptoms, which we would like to discuss in this presentation. The following have been all we succeeded in garnering. Murakami, who has been one of the leading psychopathologists in Japan since 1940, stated that "it is at times difficult to differentiate between obsessional ideas regarding interpersonal behavioral patterns of which ereuthophobia is one manifestation and 'idea of reference' or 'persecutory delusions' or otherwise," and, accordingly, "in order to make clear the process through which obsessional experiences transform themselves into delusion of influence, it is best to take up such obsessional experiences in interpersonal relationships as fear of blushing."[27] And he described several cases, in which phobias are transformed into delusion of influences and hallucinations. A similar description was made also by Yamamura from the vantage point of psychoanalysis.[42] In the West, Fenichel stated that "severe cases may be inhibited to such an extent that they withdraw from any social contact. They anticipate possible criticisms to a degree that makes them hardly distinguishable from persons with paranoid trends."[9]

This chapter also aims at a description of transient states toward delusion in severe cases. The most eloquent symptoms are fear of one's sight being transfixed with those of others and fear of emitting bodily odor. Both these may develop as transitions from ereuthophobia or may be present simultaneously with ereuthophobia. In any event, they are closely related to ereuthophobia. As a rule, they are, however, a shade more serious than ereuthophobia in their incapacitating inhibitions and show definite borderline features. Therefore, studying these severe cases, it is possible to clarify several psychopathological features that are obscure in cases of simple ereuthophobia. To resort to the established terminology, these are to be categorized under dysmorphophobia, or fear of being ugly and at the same time repulsive. Discussed individually, the former is akin to what is called "stage fright" (Ferenzi)[10] or "scopophobia" (Fenichel),[9] the latter directly corresponds with "phobische Geruchsillusion" (Gebsattel),[14] "paranoische Eigengeruchspsychose" (Tellenbach),[37] and "das phobische Beziehungssyndrom" (Walter).[40]

III

A typical case of eye-to-eye confrontation complains: "In the presence of others, I get more tense and ill at ease than is warranted by objective circumstances. I am self-conscious at being looked at. At the same time, I am at my wit's end as to where to direct my sight. I cannot decide whether I should look away from another's eyes or not. If not, I cannot tell to what extent I should stare into the other's eyes. Thus wavering, my looks lose their naturalness, and I end up by staring into the other's eyes with unwarrantedly piercing looks. It would be more accurate to say that my eyes become automatically glued to the other's eyes."

When this happens, rather than feeling that he himself is being looked at, what pains the subject is that his own eyes stare at others in an unnatural manner. This is because he thinks his unnatural, piercing look hurts others by depriving them of their mental liberty. This is not merely speculation; it is a fact for the patient. He intuits this fact by the way others behave toward him. Others may look away from him, get fidgety, make grimaces, or leave his presence. In short, others lose self-possession and avoid his presence. It is psychologically extremely painful for him to embarrass people in this way, so he ends up by trying not to see people as much as possible.

The foregoing is a rough outline of the complaints commonly lodged by the severe cases of this disease. Subjects usually develop these symptoms between puberty and early adulthood. It is rather rare for these symptoms to persist with unabated intensity after the subject passes the age of thirty. Their onset, in those who are older than forty, is extremely rare. In this sense, it can indeed be called a disorder peculiar to adolescence. The more severe the symptoms, the more restricted the subjects' spheres of activities are. Despite the persistence of their complaints and the intensity of their delusions, subjects appear to be perfectly normal. In fact, they tend to be more sociable than the average youth. Few cases border on schizophrenia.

Whereas in mild cases fear to be looked at by others is predominant, in severe cases, as was indicated in the case cited, they clearly suffer more from the fear of unintentionally staring at people with strange looks than from the fear of being looked at by others. It goes without saying that, even in the latter case, the fear of being looked at coexists with the former fear. Thus, the combination of staring at and being stared at forms one of the pathological foci of this syndrone. As this has already been discussed by many psychoanalysts since Freud[12] as the problem of exhibitionism in relation to scopophilia, we shall refrain from delving into it.

Somehow or other, little mention has been made of this phobia in Western psychiatric literature. The only references we found are one of the case reports on two cases of obsessive neurosis made by Westophal in 1877[41] and the somewhat corresponding morbid state described by such psychoanalysts as Ferenzi[10] and others[11] as stage fright or scopophobia. It is, however, possible to interpret the concept of dysmorphophobia, or the fear of being ugly and repulsive, in broad terms to consider this as a special variety of dysmorphophobia in which the subject is overly concerned with his own eyes.

In any event, the subject experiences fear in the presence of others. Therefore, it should do us well to pay attention to his further complaints in order to determine what kind of characteristics these others possess. The subject does not experience any fear in the presence of his own relatives, of those with whom he is on intimate terms, or of doctors and counselors. Conversely, neither does he experience fear when he finds himself among total strangers, as on a crowded street. Fear is induced on his part in the presence of those who are neither particularly close nor totally strange, in other words, those of intermediate familiarity. This is especially so when he finds himself in a large group. To be more specific, he is most susceptible to fear in a group composed of people of about his same age and background. If they happen to be members of the opposite sex, he is stuck in a particularly agonizing bind.

It is not at all pleasant for him to make a speech on a stage in the presence of a large audience or be in the presence of his superiors. Compared with a small group situation mentioned above, however, these situations are a lot easier to bear. This is because, compared with enduring the complex interpersonal relationship of being seen and being unable to help seeing, it is a great deal more bearable only to be seen, say, on a stage.

The foregoing, hopefully, serves to show that it is most difficult for the subject to be forced to pass time chattering, without concentrating on any specific topics, in a small group comprised of people of intermediate familiarity who are neither close nor alien, as differentiated from a crowd. We will try to observe in detail what is happening when he grows phobic in this kind of small group.

To cite an extreme example, they all feel relatively at home when talking tête-à-tête with any person. If a third party enters the dialogue situation, his presence cannot fail to upset them, no matter who he is. The ereuthophobic automatically directs his sight to this third person. This sort of sideglancing action is indeed repulsive and greatly hurts the other's feelings. If the third person should start talking to the person with whom he himself had so far been talking, he feels ostracized and develops an acute sense of inferiority.

The foregoing can be interpreted in the following manner: the ereuthophobic is able to form a dialogue situation in which a tête-à-tête interpersonal situation is the rule. He cannot, however, form a triangular interpersonal constellation (a community of three, or a group of three, or a triumvirate situation that can justifiably be called the prototype of all the varied social situations). In such a social situation, he automatically shifts his eyes away from the person facing him to the third party. And the person at the side, rather than the one in front, engages his central concern. Actually, be it in a train situation or in a classroom situation, those who concern him most are those seated by his side. Some subjects go so far as to say that in such a situation, metaphorically, they look from the sides of their eyesockets and their sight pierces the persons sitting right next to them. Also, they frequently complain that their sight field is too expansive or that they can see farther to the side than they want to and suffer from their sideglacing obsession. Their measures to cope with this vary. For example, a certain student tries to prevent people from entering his sight by seating himself at the very end of the foremost row in a classroom; some others, by wearing sunglasses. Still others try to stare straight ahead in order not to glance sideways and end up by actually developing a piercing look. For all practical purposes, let us call this characteristic "fear of sideglancing," borrowing the subjects' nomenclature. More will be said later as to the cultural implications of this fear of sideglancing.

There is another point in the foregoing statements to which we would like to draw the reader's attention. Namely, a subject feels relatively at home when talking tête-à-tête with whomsoever happens to be with him, but he gets upset in a triangular situation no matter who the third person happens to be. That is to say, the identity of the particular "who" does not pose a problem. Arieti, in discussing the differences between a phobia and a delusion, said that "whereas in delusions the threatening objects are other human beings (the persecutors), in phobia there is a dehumanization of the source of fear."[2] Here again we can observe, in some degree, dehumanization of phobogenic objects.

Here let us cite another set of complaints that makes us feel that it is proper to associate this particular phobia with dysmorphophobia. To quote, "in such a [social] situation my own eyes are not under my control, and move automatically as if they were objects foreign to me. My eyes become on such an occasion so unbelievably ugly and become so piercing as to hurt people."

Dysmorphophobia is nothing but a variation of hypochondria in the sense that its subject is overly concerned with his bodily self. What sets dysmorphophobia apart from other manifestations of hypochondria is the fact that the feeling of one's body being a foreign object does not remain merely one's own private concern, but it comes to seem simultaneously repulsive to others. As a matter of fact, the subjects complain in a wide variety of manners on this score. Their complaints range from such simple ones as embarrassing others to such extreme ones as that one's strange look is infectious or that something radiates from one's body to paralyze others. In any case, what is of central concern in this context is the fear of hurting others. Therefore, we may be justified in labeling this as an "altruistic phobia" after Kaan[18] and Dietrich.[6] This is to be set apart from egoistic phobia in which external intrusion by phobogenic objects is exclusively feared.

Notwithstanding, the most serious problem posed by these severe cases is, as was pointed out by Murakami and Fenichel, that the distinct demarcation line with paranoid conditions often disappears. Actually, certain subjects display clear-cut, acute onsets of paranoid states under some stressful conditions. In the great majority of cases, however, these onsets are transitory, with the subjects recovering from the onsets within two or three weeks at the longest. Thus, they are akin to micropsychosis, or short-lived psychotic attack, as suggested by Hoch.[16] The following is one example of this micropsychosis.

The subject is a seventeen-year-old male high school student. He voluntarily sought hospitalization owing to his fear of eye-to-eye confrontation. One year after his hospitalization, he seemed to be making smooth progress toward recovery. It just so happened, however, that an eruption developed under his pubic hair. He secretly tried to cure this eruption himself, but in vain; he then grew anxious, fearing that he might have contracted syphilis. He finally confided his apprehension to one of the nurses and received proper medical treatment. Immediately after this episode, however, he began to hear gossip and laughter directed at him by the nurses in the nurses' station. Foremost among them was a pretty nurse toward whom he had secretly entertained a fond feeling. In due course, he came to believe that the whole staff and all the inmates of the hospital considered him as being syphilitic and that all were bent on driving him out of the hospital. At long last, he had an open confrontation with the nurse in question.

His was a full-fledged persecutory paranoid state in which delusions were rampant, without, however, developing into a delusion of influence. After a mere reassignment of ward, his excitement subsided after one week. After four weeks' time he was receptive to having his misjudgments corrected. It required another half year before he was persuaded to return to his former ward. Not only in this extraordinarily morbid state, but also in his usual phobic state, he was firmly convinced that his own sight hurt others so much so that others avoided his presence, and he was insistent that he could intuit this from manifold gestures others showed.

These delusions are by no means readily susceptible to corrections even when the subject has improved enough to be able to better adapt himself to the external environment. As Cameron[4] says, "he lives with endless tension over mutual misunderstanding and misinterpretation, and is plagued constantly by ideas of self-reference," and the subject undoubtedly shows paranoid characteristics.

The idea of self-reference that may appear in this disorder will disappear if the subject is separated from the situation in question, excepting, however, such extreme cases as the aforementioned high school student, without ever tending to form a pseudo-community.[4] Insofar as this holds true, it is also clear that this differs from the typical paranoid delusion. As has been discussed above, the phobia seems to claim a place for itself in the spectrum of psychiatric disease. In further establishing this unique position, we would do well to use the fear of bodily odor—in which delusional content is more obvious—as the material of our investigation.

IV

The subject, a nineteen-year-old university student majoring in natural sciences, is convinced that the odor his body emits offends others. Thus convinced, he tries to avoid people as much as possible: in a classroom, he invariably seats himself in the back row and leaves the classroom the moment the lecture is over. However, he cannot actually smell the odor he emits. At times, he feels that the odor is peculiar and extremely difficult to describe. Most often he cannot even understand the nature of this odor. Therefore, the conviction that his body emits the odor is derived, not from his own perceptions, but from observing the way others behave. That is to say, he intuits that he is emitting the obnoxious odor by observing people around him touching their noses with their hands, or coughing, or laughing. Sometimes he can ascribe the sources of this odor to such specific parts of his own body as the anus or genitals, but not always. In any case, what is self-evident is that something comes from inside his body that causes a feeling of displeasure in others and makes them avoid his presence.

The case reports of this nature far exceed in number those on fear of eye-to-eye confrontation. Yet, the peculiarity of the present syndrome probably accounts for multiple nomenclatures accorded by various authorities. To cite a few examples, there is such a variety of names as "phobische Geruchsillusion" (Gebsattel),[14] "exocentrique" variation of "olfactive hallucinations" (Durand),[7] "mitwelt-abhängige Eigengeruchs 'Halluzination' mit Beziehungswahn" (Walter), and "paranoische Eigengeruchspsychose" (Tellenbach).[39] In Japan, since the early days of psychiatric study, attention has been paid to this syndrome as one manifestation of phobia of social situations. During the past decade, however, attention came to be focused more on the fact that they have the characteristics peculiar to borderline cases, and many researchers submitted their respective opinions, one after another, on this syndrome.[23, 29, 34, 38]

The subject to this fear of emitting bad odor exhibits clinical characteristics that are almost similar, in many important ways, to those of the above-mentioned fear of eye-to-eye confrontation, for example, the fact that the subject does not give an abnormal impression despite his deep delusional convictions.

As to the characteristics of this phobia of emitting bodily odor:[19]

1. They can be roughly divided into two categories, one that has its initial onsets during puberty, the other during menopause.
2. Those who undergo initial onsets in puberty can be divided into three categories: those who develop this phobia as an initial symptom of schizophrenia, those who remain in a prolonged monosymptomatic state, and those who develop this phobia merely as a passing phase in puberty.
3. Even those who follow a smooth course toward recovery may sometimes shift to schizophrenia after the lapse of one or two decades. Even when they fall short of this extreme, it often happens that they experience more than one acute attack of a schizophrenialike psychosis during the same period of time. In this regard, this phobia subtly differs from fear of eye-to-eye confrontation, in which the subject may undergo, at worst, short-lived episodes, even in the eventuality of his becoming psychotic. In other words, in terms of functional difficulties, fear of one's bodily odor is some degree more

serious. This observation is clearly endorsed by the findings obtained from the Rorschach tests and the like.
4. The majority of those initial onsets taking place during the menopause fall into the category of depressive psychosis, in the broad sense.
5. With the exception of a certain category of cases who undergo their initial onsets during puberty and who recover without undergoing any large-scale treatments, they are, on the whole, difficult to cure.

The task that confronts us in this context, however, is to consider the characteristics peculiar to borderline state in this disorder. Delusions of reference on the part of these subjects are firmly established. Although they cannot clearly perceive it, they remain convinced that a strange odor emits from their own bodies to make others feel unpleasant and shun their presence. This morbid conviction is extremely insusceptible to correction. Even when those psychiatrists in whom he puts his confidence voice such suggestions, he remains quite immune.

However, this phobia can be differentiated from ideas of reference observed in schizophrenia and paranoia in at least the following three respects. First, there is no tendency toward the systematization of paranoid trends, in other words, formation of pseudocommunity.[4] Second, as Arieti has pointed out,[2] the threatening objects as far as the subject is concerned are not any specific human beings, as is the case with typical persecutory delusions: what exists between the patient and his phobogenic source is nothing other than the I-it relationship (Buber).[3] Third, it can be pointed out that this phobia cannot be fully accounted for by the mechanism of fully established delusional projection. To elaborate the last point, in the case of fear of one's bodily odor, as is the case with fear of eye-to-eye confrontation, the reason why people ostracize a subject lies in himself. Unlike persecutory delusions, others do not persecute him without any reasons.

Having said that the reasons for being persecuted lie in oneself, it must be noted at the same time that this phobia differs in the following regard from depressive psychosis with its delusional self-accusation or delusional expectation of punishment. That is to say, in case of depressional delusions, one's own morals and behavior are to blame, whereas for those who suffer from the fear of their own bodily odors or their own eyesight, their own bodies or, more specifically, the particular parts of their bodies are to blame exclusively. Insofar as their bodies pose problems, it cannot be denied that they are hypochondriacs: nevertheless, as has already been pointed out, the very concept of dysmorphophobia involves the mental posture that one is being repulsive in relation to others. This is to be contrasted with simple hypochondriac symptoms that do not involve, in general, any object relationships. On the other hand, the abnormalities of one's bodily odor and eyesight are sensed intuitively from the way others behave far more frequently than by being perceived by oneself. Therefore, it is untenable to propose that this phobia has nothing to do with the mechanism of delusional projection. Seen in terms of defense mechanisms, this halfway character is apparent in the phobia. As we see it, they do not identify excessively with the projected objects until they feel themselves affected and ruled by them, in reference to Klein's concept of projective identification.[21] Therefore, we separated this kind of delusional mechanism from the usual full-fledged paranoid delusion and tentatively called it an incomplete type of delusional projection from the above-mentioned point of view. Particular attachment of these patients to their bodily selves might be one reason for their incompleteness of projection and steadiness of these symptoms.

So far we have attempted to indicate that fear of one's bodily odor represents an intermediate state without corresponding directly with paranoia, phobia, depression, or hypochondoria. By being intermediate, however, this phobia is by no means transient. Rather, it is stable in its own way. This is clear from the fact that these phobias persevere for a decade or two with minor fluctuations. Roughly speaking, all these severe cases might very well be called borderline patients. As a matter of fact, Hoch,[16] who proposed the concept of pseudoneurotic schizophrenia, hints at the presence of these cases in the following passage taken from his volume on symptomatology. "In these patients we often see imperceptibly a day-dream emerging into a hallucination or a vague hypochondriacal idea becoming a somatic delusion, ideas on relationship with other people, in the frame of social anxiety, developing into ideas of reference."

Finally, let us point out another fact to show that these severe cases share so much in common that they are a distinct entity. In brief, their pathological conviction of destructive influences emanating from their bodies indicates an underlying change of bodily ego feeling that is confined to their neurosis. "Actually, however, it is not accurate to say that the odor goes forth from my body. Superficially this may smell akin to the bodily odor. In actuality, however, this is a discrete odor that is to be set apart from my bodily odor, which I can detect. Rather, more precisely speaking, 'nerve' or 'my atmosphere' may be more appropriate than the word 'odor.' What remains certain in any event is that some such thing goes out from inside to outside. Actually, however, I cannot very well tell which particular parts of my body are its sources. At times, it seems to come out from around my loin; at other times from all over the body. Compared with this, those who are able to pinpoint the parts of the body, such as their eyes or their faces, that harass them, are lucky."

The foregoing is a statement made by a patient after having recovered to a considerable degree. Although the expression "bodily odor" is employed for the sake of convenience, the subject is clearly aware that this is something vague that cannot be ascribed to any specific part of his body. He is at the same time singularly well aware of the direction of the odor emitted, that is, from inside his body to the outside. This particular subject states that fear of eye-to-eye confrontation is the lesser evil. In actuality, however, those who fear eye-to-eye confrontation are in exactly the same boat; they have the same kind of experiences and call this indescribable something "nerve" instead of "sight" and state that it issues forth not only from their eyes but also from their backs.

Some cases we have treated successively showed fear of eye-to-eye confrontation, fear of their bodily odor, fear of their conversations or sleep-talking being eavesdropped on, and fear of magical dissemination of their ideas. All these symptoms share one common feature—their inside to outside direction. This is in contrast to delusion of influence, which is directed from outside to inside and is observed in its most full-fledged form in what Tausk[36] calls the "influencing machine." In our close scrutiny of clinical processes of each individual case, the overboard conversion of symptoms with the from inside to outside direction to those with the from outside to inside direction are far fewer than anticipated. However much symptoms may change, the from inside to outside orientation itself is maintained with a considerable degree of independence throughout these varied symptoms in the great majority of the cases. Therefore, Fujinawa and others[13] tentatively conclude that this from inside to outside orientation of symptoms is one of the earmarks of the borderline state.

V

In this last section, we would like to make a few remarks from the vantage point of crosscultural psychiatry. As has already been discussed, this type of borderline case is frequently encountered among neurotic Japanese youth. In the first place, I must say with regret that no reliable data are at our disposal that would enable us to determine quantitatively to what extent ereuthophobia and allied conditions are present, including mild cases, among contemporary young neurotics. It might serve our purpose, however, for us to make use of the statistics on mental health prepared by the student health center of our university. Incidentally, the number of college students in Japan today is 1.4 million, which corresponds to 19.5 per cent of their age group. This particular university is attended by students who are comparatively brilliant.

According to the previously mentioned statistics, of the 430 students who received psychiatric care at this center within the time span of one year, one-half were neurotic. Of this one-half, 18.6 per cent can be classified into the category with which we now are concerned. This percentage ranks third after depressive reaction accounting for 24 per cent and psychophysical reaction accounting for 20 per cent. The rest comprises schizoid personality, obsessive neurosis, transient maladaptation, hypochondria, and the like, each accounting for about 5 per cent, with the matrix group being 10,000 in number.

The responses to the annual inquiry directed to all the students entering this university also may be of some reference value. This questionnaire consists of sixty itemized questions concerning psychic or somatic abnormalities. Among these items, those entries checked most frequently by the students range from purely physical difficulties, such as headache or eyestrain, to purely personality or psychological difficulties, such as overanxiety about the future. There are no significant differences observed at several other universities or between males and females. What is noteworthy is that the items popular by large percentages include such items as "liable to blush" and "worried about others' looks." Needless to say, this indicates that a certain type of tension is liable to emerge in interpersonal situations, regardless of their severity or morbidity. Table 1 compares those items considered relevant to ereuthophobia with those purely physical items, such

TABLE 1

Statistical Data Gathered from 2,481 Students Entering the University in the 1967 School Year.

QUESTION ITEMS	NUMBERS OF STUDENTS RESPONDING AFFIRMATIVELY	PERCENTAGES
Liable to blush	995	40.1
Worried about others' looks	798	32.2
Stammers or gets a tremulous voice	239	9.6
Emits a strange bodily odor	51	2.1
Difficult to fall asleep	458	18.5
Suffers from a headache	597	24.1

as headache. One can tell at a glance the high degree of popularity enjoyed by those questions related to ereuthophobia as well as fear of eye-to-eye confrontation.

One should not immediately infer from these data, however, that roughly one-third of the college students today are suffering from interpersonally oriented phobia of one kind or another. This questionnaire instructs the students to check those items applicable to their experiences if the student had the experience in question even once during the preceding year. Still, we may not be missing the mark widely when we infer that there is a marked tendency for university students to maintain ereuthophobic mentality subclinically.

This naturally makes us wonder whether there are any differences in the respective ratios concerning the occurrences of these neurotic types between the past and the present in Japan. Regrettably, we have no data reliable enough for this purpose at our disposal. The only statement we may be justified in making, in light of the above data, is that even today ereuthophobia and similar symptoms remain one of the most representative neuroses among the Japanese youth.

There are no clear-cut differences between males and females. According to Janet,[17] Douboux reported in 1847 that more females than males were subject to these disturbances. In present-day Japan, we observe decidedly more cases of males suffering from this in the clinics. Perhaps, for females blushing is more socially acceptable than for males, so that the former may not suffer from this so much as to motivate them to visit doctors.

One also wonders what the incidence of this syndrome in different cultures is as compared with that in Japan. There are reasons to believe that in foreign countries this neurosis may not occur so frequently as it does in Japan. It is true that scattered references to the fear of one's bodily odor are observed in Western literature. As to the fear of eye-to-eye confrontation, however, to the best of my knowledge, practically no literature exists. The symptom as such no doubt exists, but it may fail to attract doctors' attention. Even when we deal with ereuthophobia and its allied conditions as a whole, as far as literature is concerned, these do not seem to be limelighted in the West. Dietrich,[6] the exception to this rule, took up dysmorphophobia of late. He notes that in Europe during the past two decades there has been only one dissertation dealing with this phobia as its main theme. He goes on to say that ereuthophobia is very rare in Germany. Even in the Orient, countries other than Japan do not pay much attention to this. As a matter of fact, its incidence seems to be quite low. According to our investigation, leading psychiatrists in Formosa agree that in their country there are practically no phobia of social situations, such as ereuthophobia. Some Thai psychiatrists had had experiences similar to them.

It is extremely difficult to establish fully that a particular neurotic type is in the foreground in a given culture at a given period. Our data being limited, we do not mean to assert that phobias of social situations are in the absolute majority in Japan. In order to establish clearly this hypothesis, more precise comparative study of neuroses is absolutely necessary. It may be most effective for this purpose to compare neurotic types prevailing among college students belonging to various cultures. College students can be considered as forming a social stratum that is comparatively alike in many important respects crossculturally. In any case, it seems to be more useful for our present purpose to compare the data furnished by campus psychiatry rather than to compare statistics gathered from inpatients and outpatients. Although precisely numerical, statistical comparisons are not feasible as yet, on the above-mentioned grounds, if a particular variation of phobia of social situations is more liable to occur in a given culture, what is left for us is to consider this phenomenon in relation to its background culture.

When dysmorphophobia is mentioned in Western psychiatric literature, the common objects of concern enumerated are the nose, skin, hair, teeth, chin, shape of skull, breast, and body weight. Few and far between are mentions of bodily odor. As far as we have researched, the eye has not been taken up. In contrast to this, for Japanese psychiatrists the fears of eye-to-eye confrontation and bodily odor are kinds of neuroses encountered almost every day and little mention is made of the skull, breast, nose, skin, and so forth.

For reference we would like to present the breakdown of the thirty-nine cases with this syndrome now being treated among the students of the university; those who suffer from their bodily odor number 11; exclusively from blushing 6; from their sight 5; voicing 2; hair 1; excessive coughing 1; negligible scar in their face 2. Without bothering ourselves with the absolute number of the cases subject to phobia of social situations, in view of the foregoing, we believe that it can be stated with a considerable degree of probability that the sight and odor types abound.

It then seems to be in order to consider, in sociocultural terms, reasons, if any, why Japanese people have a marked propensity to the themes of sight and bodily odor when they display phobia of social situations.

Let us consider, first, the reason why sight is chosen. In our everyday interpersonal relationship, the act of staring at the person one is talking to is something quite extraordinary, and not an everyday occurrence. This act more often than not is considered to be rude. To be stared at induces in the minds of the Japanese a certain sense of displeasure that the onlooker, with the exception of extraordinarily intimate relations, is suspicious. To look intently at the person one is talking to does not, as far as the Japanese are concerned, signify respect. On the contrary, looking downward tends to be appreciated even today, especially on the part of the female, as being suggestive of a certain elegance.

There is a Japanese cultural characteristic by which people are hypersensitive about looking at and being looked at. As the great majority of us even today discipline our infants, as a rule, by saying that "neighbors are watching whatever you do." The neighbors, after all, signify the world at large, this intimidation reflecting an average criterion of value judgment. Thus they end up by growing into a personality that incessantly watches whatever those outside their family circles say or do, either consciously or unconsciously. At the same time, they maintain an anxiety of being looked at by others. For example, in Japan, we have a traditional game called "Nirammekko" (game of eye-to-eye confrontation), in which two persons try to outstare and embarrass each other. What this hypersensitiveness about interpersonal relationships tells us explicitly is that multiple variations of the words "I" and "you" are employed, depending on the nature of the interpersonal relationship between oneself and one's partner prevailing in a given situation. In concert with this interpersonal attitude, the Japanese mode of communication is markedly nonverbal, emotional, and nonrational. The Japanese tend to esteem roundabout expressions, avoiding the point. What those who fear others fear is to face others' rude, pointblank remarks in a given interpersonal situation. At the same time, they themselves fear lest they say something pointblank that does not conform with the established code of etiquette.

In any event, it is not impossible, should one try, to detect some cultural influences in the morbid state of the phobia of sideglancing of those who fear eye-to-eye confrontation. The sideward direction they in particular concern themselves about has its own intrinsic meaning, just as above, below, front, or hind have their own respective significances. To the Japanese, the side is a direction where, in contrast to above or below, equals stand hand in hand, or, as it were, a space of friendship. In addition, however, to these positive implications, it also implies something negative in that it could be a space where envy and competition lie. The authors hope, in making this point, that the reader may recall their previous statement that the very people whom the subject of phobia of social situations finds most difficult to deal with are those of background similar to his. Morita has also pointed out that, behind the fact that the subject of phobia of social situations fears particularly the emergence of a sense of shame, there lies a deep-rooted desire to surpass others. To elaborate further, to look sideways is one of the most detestable behavioral patterns for the Japanese, as is shown in such an idiom as "without looking aside," which relates itself to diligence. (Diligence is so important for the Japanese that it almost replaces practically all the ethicoreligious principles.)

In the second place, we cannot help pondering why bodily odor means so much to the Japanese when they develop a phobia of social situation. It can at least be advanced that the Japanese appreciate odorlessness more highly than fragrance. The idea of being clean ordinarily reminds the Japanese of a state where there is no odor rather than one where there is pleasant odor, perhaps owing to our indigenous religion, Shintosim, rather than to Buddhism. Of all the variety of odors, to emit the bodily odor degrades one's social standing. In contrast to the West, where people tend physiologically to emit a stronger bodily odor and where, to go a step further, it is an established code of social etiquette to enhance one's bodily odor by sprinkling perfume over one's body, Japanese take baths as frequently as possible to keep the body clean and never dream of emphasizing the bodily odor apart from burning incense to give fragrance to rooms or clothing. In the light of this, Japan may very well be a cultural setting where the theme of bodily odor looms large in phobia of social situations.

We have described severe cases of ereuthophobia and allied conditions seen frequently among the Japanese youth of today, and discussed them in relation to the Japanese cultural background only. We wish to conclude on the hopeful note that more precise comparative studies between multiple cultures will be conducted on this borderline state.

REFERENCES

1. Adachi, H. "Sur le maladie qui se croit d'être puant." *Juntendo Medical Journal*, 7 (1961), 901.
2. Arieti, S. "A Reexamination of the Phobic Symptom and of Symbolism in Psychopathology," *American Journal of Psychiatry*, 118 (1961), 106.
3. Buber, M. *I and Thou*. New York: Charles Scribner's Sons, 1958.
4. Cameron, N. "Paranoid Conditions and Paranoia," in S. Arieti (ed.), *American Handbook of Psychiatry*. New York: Basic Books, 1959. Vol. 1, pp. 508–539.
5. Casper, J. V. "Biographie d'une idée fixée, *Archives de Neurologie*, 8 (1902), 270.
6. Dietrich, H. "Über Dysmorphophobie (Missgestaltfrucht)," *Archiv für Psychiatrie*, 203 (1962), 501.
7. Durand, V. J. "Hallucinations olfactives et gustatives," *Annales de Médico-psychologique*, 2 (1955), 777.
8. Ey, H. et al. *Manuel de psychiatrie*. Paris: Masson, 1960.
9. Fenichel, O. *The Psychoanalytic Theory of Neurosis*. New York: Norton, 1945.
10. Ferenzi, S. "Stage-Fright and Narcissistic Self-observation," in *Further Contributions to the Theory and Technique of Psychoanalysis*. London: Hogarth, 1926.
11. Flügel, J. C. "Stage Fright and Anal Erotism," *British Journal of Medical Psychology*, 17 (1938).
12. Freud, S. "Three Essays on the Theory of Sexuality" (1905), in J. Strachey (ed.), *Standard Edition*. London: Hogarth. Vol. 7, pp. 123–243. (Also published as *Three Essays on the Theory of Sexuality*. New York: Basic Books, 1962.)
13. Fujinawa, A. et al. "On the Experience of Exuding Something from Inside to Outside," *Proceedings of the Fourth Annual Meeting of Japanese Association of Medical Psychotherapy* (1967).
14. Gebsattel, V. *Prolegomena einer Medizinischen Anthropologie*. Berlin: Springer, 1954.
15. Hesnard, A. *Les Phobies et la névrose phobique*. Paris: Payot, 1961.
16. Hoch, P., and Polatin, P. "Pseudoneurotic Forms of Schizophrenia," *Psychiatric Quarterly*, 23 (1949), 248.
17. Janet, P. *Les Obsessions et la psychasthénie*. 2 vols.; Paris: Alcan, 1903.
18. Kaan, H. *Der Neurasthenische Angstaffekt bei Zwangsvorstellungen und der Primordiale Grübelzwang*. Leipzig: Deuticke, 1892.
19. Kasahara, Y. et al. "On Experience of Exuding Bodily Odour" (in preparation).

20. Kato, M. "On the Problem of Anthrophobia (Taijin-Kyofu) in Japan," (in Japanese), *Japanese Journal of Clinical Psychiatry (Seishin-Igaku)*, **6** (1964), 107.
21. Klein, M. "Notes on Some Schizoid Mechanisms," *International Journal of Psychoanalysis*, **27** (1946), 99.
22. Kora, T. *Morita Therapy*. Tokyo: Jikei Medical School, 1964.
23. Miyamoto, T. "On Fear of Exuding Bad Bodily Odour" (in Japanese), *Shikai-Tenbo*, **25** (1966), 461.
24. Morita, S. *Treatment of Neurasthenia and of Obsession* (in Japanese). Tokyo: Hakuyosha, 1926.
25. Morita, S., and Kora, T. *Treatment of Ereuthophobia* (in Japanese). Tokyo: Hakuyosha, 1953.
26. Murakami, M. "Transition of Clinical Symptoms of Chronic Schizophrenia," *Psychiatria et Neurologia Japonica*, **46** (1942), 110.
27. Murakami, M. "The Relationship between Schizophrenia and Neurosis," *Psychiatria et Neurologia Japonica*, **5** (1951), 55.
28. Murakami, M. *Abnormal Psychology* (in Japanese). Rev. ed. Tokyo: Iwanami, 1963.
29. Nakazawa, A. "Von der Mentalität Kranker, die über Körpergeruch klagen," *Psychiatria et Neurologia Japonica*, **65** (1963), 69.
30. Ogino, K., and Mizutani, T. "An Interesting Case of Stare-Phobia," *Japanese Journal of Psychoanalysis*, **6** (1959), 21.
31. Pitres, A., and Régis, E. "Obsession de la Rougeur (Ereuthophobia)," *Archives de Neurologie*, **3** (1897), 1.
32. Pitres, A., and Régis, E. "Obsession de la Rougeur ou Ereuthophobia," *Archives de Neurologie*, **13** (1902), 177.
33. Schmideberg, M. "The Borderline Patient," in S. Arieti (ed.), *American Handbook of Psychiatry*. New York: Basic Books, 1959. Vol. 1, pp. 398–416.
34. Shikano, T. "Clinical Study on Chronic Olfactory Hallucination" (in Japanese), *Japanese Journal of Clinical Psychiatry (Seishin-Igaku)*, **2** (1960), 37.
35. Takahashi, T. "Sur la phobie du contact humain—Une étude microsociologique," *Psychiatria et Neurologia Japonica*, **68** (1966), 26.
36. Tausk, V. "On the Origin of the Influencing Machine in Schizophrenia," in *Psychoanalytic Reader*. New York: International Universities Press, 1948. Vol. 1, p. 52.
37. Tellenbach, H. "Der Oralsinn und das Atomosphärische," *Jahrbuch für Psychologie, Psychiatrie und Medizinische Anthropologie*, **12** (1964), 254.
38. Tsutsumi, S. "A Clinico-Statistical Study of Olfactory Hallucination in Endogenous Psychosis," *Psychiatria et Neurologia Japonica*, **67** (1965), 60.
39. Walter, K. "Über mitweltabhängige Eigengeruchs-Halluzination mit Beziehungswahn," *Nervenarzt*, **33** (1962), 325.
40. Walter, K. "Über das 'Phobische Beziehungssyndrom,'" *Nervenarzt*, **36** (1965), 7.
41. Westophal, C. "Über Zwangsvorstellung," *Berliner Klinische Wochenschrift*, **14** (1877), 699.
42. Yamamura, M. "Psychoanalytische Studien über Erythrophobie," *Arbeiten aus dem psychiatrischen Institute der Tohoku Universität*, **2** (1933), 69.
43. Yamamura, M. "Über Menschenscheu," *Arbeiten aus dem psychiatrischen Institute der Tohoku Universität*, **5** (1936), 45.

[[[14]]]

PSYCHOTHERAPY AND FAMILY INTERVIEWS

Alberta B. Szalita

> Though in one sense our family was certainly a simple machine, as it consisted of a few wheels, yet there was this much to be said for it, that these wheels were set in motion by so many different springs, and acted one upon the other from such a variety of strange principles and impulses—that though it was a simple machine, it had all the honor and advantages of a complex one—and a number of as odd movements within it, as ever were beheld in the inside of a Dutch silkmill.
> —LAURENCE STERNE[49]*

INTRODUCTION

Primarily, this is a chapter about the clinical use of family interviews as an addition to individual psychotherapy. Basic to the views stated in this work is the belief that family interviews add a unique dimension to individual therapy and the belief that individual therapy, without an attempt to see the patient in action, proves to be an incomplete and, therefore, a less effective exercise of the profession.

Family interviews are not new. At the beginning of this century, relatives brought a mentally sick patient to see a doctor, and in many places this practice still continues. If the patient was lucky enough to be present during the interview, he was treated as a thing; one talked in his presence as if he did not understand what it was all about—as if he did not count. The family history given by the family members was considered objective, whereas the patient's account, if he was asked to give one, was considered subjective and, therefore, unreliable. It might not be an exaggera-

---

* I am indebted to Murray Bowen[19] for bringing Sterne's most interesting work to my attention.

tion to say that the patient was looked on with fear and disdain. To talk to a psychotic patient as one human being to another, with a wish to understand him, was the exception rather than the rule. Perhaps this practice is not so outdated as it may seem. In time, with the spread of psychoanalytically oriented psychotherapy, the reverse took place—the family was excluded and the patient was the one on whom attention was focused. Finally, we have arrived at the point where the family and the patient are seen as a unit with appreciation of the mutual impact that the participants have on the course of illness as well as the impact that the illness has on the whole family.

The nature of severe mental illness remains unknown. What is genetically determined and what is culturally produced has yet to be discovered. Most workers in the field, however, recognize the importance of environmental conditions and learning processes on the development of mental disturbances, in general, and schizophrenia, in particular.

Most recent contributions to family therapy come from investigators who devoted their thought and research to families with members suffering from overt schizophrenic disorder. And all are committed to the idea that some specific family interactions are connected with the etiology of schizophrenia.[19, 36, 61] The general tendency is to view schizophrenia as a disease of the family unit. I am not in full accord with these views. Lidz[36] is of the opinion that "limitations of the 'mind' are often not deficiencies of the brain but of the linguistic and experiential symbols required for thinking, and that distortions of mentation can derive from the family environment" (pp. 9–10). Contrary to Dr. Lidz, clinical experience compels me to assume some physiologically determined obstacles in the communication system of the brain in the etiology of schizophrenia.[51, 52] But this assumption does not prevent me from agreeing with Lidz that the development, not the cause, of schizophrenia is due to untoward environmental influences. A potentially schizophrenic child may be prevented from developing a full-blown mental disorder by appropriate family environment and schooling, particularly when the defect is recognized early.

Human transactions are complex and can be much easier understood when dealt with in their precise, concrete emergence. For example, the content of schizophrenic production often becomes comprehensible when viewed within the family context; the oddities appear as a logical result of the family interactions.

The temptation to make an exact science out of the psychiatric field hardly leads to anything more than obscurity. The ambition of a scientific rigor, laudable as it may be, often removes the clinical experience from its veritable nature. The tendency to borrow terms from sociology, which in turn borrows from physics, inundates the literature on family therapy, which is currently booming. In the words of Nathan W. Ackerman, "The impact of the expanding discoveries of family study and treatment will exert a profound effect on all known forms of psychotherapy, psychoanalysis included."[7] Family therapy is the fashion of the day. Promising as it may be, there is an inherent danger in the indiscriminate use of this form of psychotherapy.

More often than not, I think of family therapy, and psychotherapy in general, as belonging to the performing arts rather than to the sciences. It is essential, therefore, for the practitioner of any form of family therapy to have vast knowledge of the humanities, personal experience in small-group dynamics, and thorough training in individual therapy.

Diagnoses of family disturbances seem to be feasible at this point only in terms of identification of discrete, limited interactions. Perhaps, in time, we shall be able better to formulate diagnostic criteria and classifications of types of family disorders. At present, the model for individual therapy predominates in the conceptual formulations currently in print—however disguised—because it corresponds more closely with therapists' perception of clinical settings. It is worth noting that implicit in the individual model is the fact that all communication is interpersonal.

We have to be reminded that classical psychoanalytical theory, as well as the interpersonal, assumes the social nature of the individual mind.[24] As one example, I shall quote Glover:[30] "After the first months of what we may call somewhat loosely 'narcissistic function,' there is no such thing as individual psychology. Not only is the child from early infancy a social animal, which means a recognized member of a small family group, but the pattern of his mind is in human group patterns. The group mind is by no means a fiction" (p. 182).

Family interviews consist of various combinations of dyadic sets, combined with observations of the response and effect of the other members of the family present during the interview. The bridge between the conceptual formulations of family processes and individual psychodynamics is yet to be made and integrated into a comprehensive clinical theory and practice.

HISTORICAL NOTE AND DEFINITION

Interest in family therapy began in the 1930's and has been increasing since, especially in the last few years with so much attention being given to community-centered psychiatry. Family interviews, as well as family therapy, are natural consequences of expansion of modern psychiatry over the past fifty years. It converged, I think, from four sources: (1) child therapy, (2) group therapy, (3) revolution in family life owing to industrial and sexual revolutions, and (4) the disappointments in individual psychotherapy of schizophrenia.

Nathan W. Ackerman is the father of family therapy. He also was the founder of the Family Mental Health Clinic of the Jewish Family Service in New York City. His writings encompass every aspect of family therapy. He is foremost a clinician, devoted to the well-being of the patients more than to concepts about them. It is not easy to conceptualize his approach to family therapy. He believes in change, and he believes in people. He emphasizes the strength of the family. In his own words,[7] "The strength of family therapy derives from its capacity for joining forces with the spontaneous healing powers of the family group" (p. 7). His unique style is hard to describe. He uses himself freely, spontaneously, and, like a good actor, displays a quality of presence that enables him to engage the family in a meaningful dialogue. His penchant for embarking on territory that people usually consider private, namely sexual content, stirs up considerable controversy. However, this is one way, and his inimitable way, of establishing contact, intimacy, or a kind of entrance into family life.

"Family psychotherapy," as defined by Ackerman,[7] is

a method of intervention which involves an on-going emotional engagement and interchange in face-to-face contact with the entire family ... it may be that some family members are temporarily excluded from some sessions, but the focus remains on the totality of the family. ... The process involves a continuous concern for the relations and interchange between family and individual members (p.2).

He does, unabashedly, participate in family transactions, changing roles from that of a father, grandfather, teacher, doctor. He is versatile in assuming different roles and switching from one role to the other, and he does not hesitate to enter into the family "as if a member of it."

"The family interview," says Dr. Ackerman, "permits the appraisal of specific units of pathogenic experience within the frame of total experience with special emphasis on the potentials of restoration of health"[6] and thus offers an invaluable source of information and guidance in individual therapy, plus being an extremely valuable diagnostic procedure. He formulates his goals for family therapy as follows:[7]

(1) define and reduce the focus of most destructive conflict and fear; (2) heighten the mutual complementation of need, thereby strengthening family against critical upsets; (3) promote harmony and balance in family functions, strengthen the individual against destructive forces within himself, surrounding him in the family and in the community; (4) influence family identity and values toward health and growth (p. 4).

My interest in family interviews in combination or as an adjunct of intensive psychotherapy in schizophrenia started accidentally about twenty years ago, when I was working in a hospital setting. Inadvertently, I interviewed the father of a schizophrenic patient in the patient's presence.[57] I found that my understanding of the patient's pathology increased enormously and that the interactions between father and son gave me a new view on the patient's life. My interest in the family unit as a subject of study, and particularly of systematic interviews as therapeutic interventions, came as a second step.

The knowledge of the family enables the therapist to avoid countertransference problems and enlightens him as well to particular aspects of transference. Patients have a tendency to instigate, in the therapist, prejudicial attitudes toward other family members in order to avoid responsibility for their actions, allay guilt, fix blame, or assure approval and affection. Some of their idiosyncrasies are not always discernible in a one-to-one setting.

Experience in family interviews has a definite impact on the nature of individual therapy, for family dynamics becomes a part of the therapist's orientation. It becomes evident in the kind of questions he might ask and the tendency to examine in greater detail the minute interactions between the individual patient and his immediate environment. Such orientation helps the therapist to avoid dealing with generalizations and makes the therapy more specific. It also has a direct influence on all the members of the family.

Finally, it is good when family members know the person who

indirectly influences their lives for a number of years. Individual therapy, as we well know, is a lengthy business and has, at times, a profound impact on the life of an individual and his family, not to speak of the financial burden it carries.

My own attitude toward family therapy, particularly the combined use of family interviews, can be summarized as follows: I do not insist on the presence of all members, other than for diagnostic purposes. I even find it more useful to see members of the family in a variety of combinations. My participation is that of an interested outsider. My aim is to get the family to think together about their life predicament and to increase their awareness of themselves as well as their impact on others. I endeavor to concentrate on the strength of the participating individuals in helping them to organize their forces to meet the challenge of their limitations.

Because of the underlying interdependence of the family and its hunger for "togetherness," a unitropism, as I would call it, pervades a family in spite of the apparent centrifugal forces and discord. This tendency is utilized for minute examination of infinitesimal aspects of behavior,[18] differentiation of intention and effect, reorganization of thought processes, and comparison of thoughts with the verbalizations.[4] All this leads to increasing the integrative abilities, attention span, and adaptability.[36] I call this approach "psychointegration."

FAMILY INTERVIEWS COMBINED WITH INDIVIDUAL PSYCHOTHERAPY IN SCHIZOPHRENIA

No attempt will be made at a systematic review of literature on family studies in schizophrenia; because there is no comprehensive theory of schizophrenia available, there can be no specific approach to psychotherapy. Each investigator makes a choice as to what he considers most important. The differences are as varied as the person who applies the particular approach.*

The temptation to study families of schizophrenics is understandable in that (1) it affords an opportunity to study all known

---

* The best summary of the current theories is to be found in "Family Interaction Processes and Schizophrenia: A Review of Current Theories," by Elliot G. Mishler and Nancy E. Waxler.[38] This article concentrates on Bateson, Lidz, Wynne, and their followers.

mental pathology in an exaggerated form, (2) schizophrenia remains the most pressing problem of the day, and (3) individual psychotherapy of severely afflicted schizophrenics does not easily, if ever, meet the patient's needs, no matter how interested or devoted the therapist may be to his patient.

There is usually, if not always, a need to enlist the cooperation of the environment or the family, be it a hospitalized or an ambulatory schizophrenic patient. Studies of families only reaffirm the clinical observations of various workers[12, 28, 37, 50, 57, 60, 61] that every case of a serious disorder that comes to the clinician's attention shows disturbances in parental relationships. Foremost stress is on inadequate mothering. The role of the father in rearing children has only recently grown in importance in light of current studies,[36] the third industrial revolution, and the present sexual revolution.

The familiar difficulty arises when one wants to apply the concepts evolved from these studies to the etiology and diagnosis of schizophrenia. Valid as the observations derived from these studies are, descriptive and felicitous as some of the terms invented might be, they are ubiquitous in all families that come to our attention, regardless of the diagnosis. For example, Bateson's "double bind," which has received wide acceptance, and Wynne's "pseudomutuality," or the "rubber fence," are not, I think, specific enough for the schizophrenic process. These phenomena, which they so neatly describe, are also present in patients with hysterical and obsessional character structures and their relations with their families.

I shall briefly discuss Lidz's views, which are essentially very congenial with mine. But, whereas his views are integrated into the body of psychoanalytic theory, mine are not, as I favor integrated eclecticism. His attitude seems to be a direct extension of the psychoanalytic triad, with which I do not argue. After all, the fact is that analytic therapy is based on family dynamics. The oedipal constellation, with all its implications, is nothing more than variations in a family situation. Lidz emphasizes the ill-defined age and sex boundaries that I speak of as a lack of capacity that affects structure, organization, and sense of time.

The following passage exemplifies some of his views pertinent to this discussion:[37]

The dynamic organization of all of [these families under study] was seriously disturbed by the marital schism or skew, the failure to maintain generation boundaries, and by failures of the parents to maintain their sex-linked roles. . . . The father is involved as well as the mother, and it is difficult to assign responsibility for such failures. The controlling and dominating wife must have a husband who can be dominated, and some such fathers might be considered to force their wives to assume instrumental leadership of the family (p. 332).

These remarks are applicable to all families that come to my attention in both private practice and at the Family Mental Health Clinic. These are very important observations, but not specific for the etiology of schizophrenia, though they are constant features of families examined. The deficiency in leadership that Lidz mentions I consider one of the most distinct characteristics of every family that requires outside help for the solution of its difficulties.

In 1952, I expressed a view,[52] which I perhaps asserted with too much conviction at the time, but one that remains a pivotal concept in my approach to therapy, mainly that:

While it is true that an exaggerated quality of defensive processes brings about a difference in the quality, one cannot escape the feeling that with a schizophrenic there is a primary difference in the quality itself . . . based on a discontinuity in the experiences . . . . a parcelled organizational structure with its proneness to dissociative processes. . . . One can compare the self of the schizophrenic to a sea in which there are a great many small, separate islands, with almost no means of communication between them. This disjointedness gives a feeling of unreliability on oneself and a lack of confidence in one's own conscious and unconscious tools (pp. 146–147).

Confirming my assumptions (if these findings are reliable), there was an article in the June 1968 *Psychiatric News* titled, "Chemical Variations Found in Schizophrenic's Blood," in which is stated:

Evidence collected independently by three laboratories indicates that the blood of schizophrenics contains excess amounts of a component of the alpha-2-globulin. Researchers theorize that the excess may result in perforation of brain cell walls with resulting accumulation of outside materials within the cells, as well as leakage from the cells of important substances. . . . Their accumulation in the cells . . . could explain the disruption of the normal communication processes.

Recent clinical observations lead me to believe that the basic schism in schizophrenia consists in a difficulty in decoding body language from within and without. There is the well-observed discrepancy between the patient's mimicry and verbalizations.

Body language may be more crude than verbal language, but it is immediate and more universal. The schizophrenic patient often assumes that what he reads in someone else's face is his own feeling or that he is the cause of it. Perhaps the most important aspect of his difficulty is in differentiating between himself and others. Having made this observation, I shared it with some of my ambulatory patients and found that it proved to be therapeutically useful. Making the family members aware of this and/or other difficulties also has a great therapeutic impact, because the awareness allows for the continuation of corrective experiences so essential for the schizophrenic patient.

For example, an ambulatory schizophrenic entered a store to get some photographic equipment. A woman was standing in front of him taking a long time to ask endless questions of the salesman. The patient became impatient. He moved closer and stood directly behind the woman. At this point, she turned toward him. He noticed that she had a tense and seemingly angry expression. A sudden anger surged within him as if her facial expression referred directly to him. He related that he was about to do something violent when he heard his doctor's voice telling him: "It has nothing to do with you." He moved to the side and discreetly continued to watch her, as if to check. Her facial expression continued to be tense; she apparently had difficulty in trusting herself with a new camera. The patient relaxed, so he said. Arieti reports similar experiences in different contexts than this and perhaps with different theoretical assumptions.[11] Fromm-Reichmann's therapeutic skill was largely enhanced by her uncanny capacity to decipher the patient's mood and preoccupation from his facial expression and posture. Her appropriate formulation of them was always met with great relief by the patient, as I have also observed.[53]

Among the various other psychotherapeutic interventions there are a few I consider pivotal for the treatment of schizophrenia and that are most accelerated when used in combination with family interviews. They are:

1. Differentiation among feeling, thought, and action. Everybody has some areas where this differentiation is not sufficient, but the schizophrenic has more difficulty in this field than does the rest of humanity. It is a difference between saying "I have a feeling" vs. "a feeling took hold of me." It is a truism to state that a patient feels helpless and unable to trust himself when he has no control over his feelings. The therapist begins by making the

patient aware of this difficulty and convincing him that this is a common human problem. Family members are often unaware of this difficulty in themselves and particularly in the identified patient. This capacity to differentiate among one's feelings, thoughts, and actions is essential for the acquisition of self-knowledge and the development of spontaneity with direction and purpose and is a quality worth cultivating—as important for the therapists as for the patients.

2. In order to know one's feelings, reflect on them, and decide on an appropriate action, one must be able to be an observer and operator at the same time. To a considerable extent, this capacity is needed for good adaptability. I assume that if we were able to devise a means to ascertain the ratio of the capacity of "thinking and talking at the same time," "thinking on one's feet," and "thinking and doing," we could measure degrees of adaptability. The family interview provides the schizophrenic patient with an opportunity to observe himself and others in action. It also gives him a chance to verify his impact on the family members. This exercise can be enhanced if the therapist is explicit about the task at hand. Candor, well intentioned and appropriately timed, never gets the therapist into trouble with schizophrenics and/or their families. Therapeutic interviews have to have a design and direction. The therapist has to exert his leadership to prevent too much confusion, uncertainty, and multidirection.

3. The most important and spectacular results come from differentiation between intention and effect. Every communication has an intention, form, content, and effect. To be aware of one's intention and to convey it in an acceptable form to the listener enables one to notice the effect and modify the form of communication to meet one's ends. Thus, the individual sharpens his capacity to use feedback from the responder. Proficiency in this direction helps to sharpen the discrimination of perception[42] and nuances of feelings. It also trains the patient in sustained attention.

It is characteristic of a schizophrenic to be unable to deal with more than one person or one item at a given time. This is probably owing not only to anxiety, but to a limited and scattered attention span. He has to practice the capacity of shifting attention from person to person. This opportunity is more readily available in a family interview. The quality of attention is decisive for learning from experience. The schizophrenic often meets similar situations as if they have just happened for the first time. Many patients have accounted for it as a lack of consciousness.[57] What is not noticed remains a sensation and not a perception and can hardly be integrated into experience.[43] Objectivity depends on the refinement of perception and this, in turn, on the quality of attention.

Many have called our age the "Age of Anxiety." I prefer to call it the "Age of Awareness." Whatever increases the margin of awareness and consciousness contributes to improvement of the faculties, which can be defined in terms of presence of mind, the development of which, after all, is the main task of therapy.

It is evident that all these interventions are designed to increase the integrative capacities of the ego.[27] To exhaust this subject, one would have to include all the principles of psychotherapy. Concepts used in individual psychotherapy are, by and large, applicable to family therapy.

DEFICIENCY IN LEADERSHIP

The major defect in family life requiring attention and correction is deficiency in leadership. Each family that seeks help shows a deficiency in leadership. " 'A family without government,' says Matthew Henry, 'is like a house without a roof, exposed to every wind that blows.'—He might better have said, like a house in flames, a scene of confusion, and commonly too hot to live in" (Henri F. Amiel, p. 205).[23]

Lack of leadership gives the family a haphazard, amorphous quality. Cohesiveness is often maintained by tradition and family life goes on until some crisis occurs. Then the lack of organization and the lack of direction show up and lead to a disintegration of the family; this is usually when it applies for help. The most frequent precipitating causes are a rebellious, delinquent, nonconforming child, a difficulty in school, deterioration of the relationship between the marital partners, and an outsider threatening to enter a family group. The delicate balance disintegrates because the family members lack the capacity to deal with such patterns of behavior.

Organization and structure are often confused, even by professional workers, with rigidity and authoritarianism. So it has become the fashion, nowadays, to run the family on self-demand principles that are only too often a mistaken notion of freedom.

Freedom implies discipline and responsibility. There are also some authors who assume that the ever-increasing organization of life is a menace to individuality.[46] Well-organized family life leaves only more space for individual development—if it results in more automatic habits, it leaves the mind free for individual variations. The issue is whether organization is used to afford greater freedom and leisure or whether it is used to manipulate, intimidate, and control. The family identity depends on a sense of direction and on the ability to use autoexecutive faculties—for example, selection of what is appropriate or inappropriate for a given situation, freedom of individual variations in choice, and the responsibility for one's decisions that goes with it. A good leader in a family allows each member to make his decisions when he is capable of doing so, and he knows when to step in and if and when there is a necessity to take over. He also imposes and maintains a hierarchy of responsibility.

Possessiveness is sometimes confused with leadership, but it actually deprives an individual of an opportunity for individuation. A couple, both analyzed, came for consultation on account of a problem with their thirteen-year-old daughter. Both teachers, they watched their daughter while she was doing her homework, criticizing her compositions, calling the school when there was an examination, and watching over her work constantly. They assumed this to be a way of fulfilling their parental responsibility. The girl, a bright youngster, started to fail at school, became irritable and depressed. The parents were seen with the daughter. After a few interviews, the parents understood that the girl's schoolwork should be her responsibility. And, it was suggested that if they wanted to be helpful, they should allow her to turn to them for help.

Another example was given to me by an adult man who failed in a postgraduate course because he was watched by the instructors. He recalled that, when he was young, his mother used to watch him doing his homework. He would sit with an open book, fingering the pages, and mumbling to himself, "Mama thinks I'm studying. I'm not studying. Mama thinks I'm studying. I'm not studying." In the meantime, she thought he was working.

Freud commented that only very few civilized persons are capable of existing without reliance on others or are even capable of coming to an independent opinion. "You cannot exaggerate the intensity of man's inner irresolution and craving for authority."[26] This craving for authority increases with illness, particularly in depression, and all the more in advancing age. What Freud described is tantamount to a lack of confidence in one's personal authority, a lack of reliance in one's capacity to lead oneself (a fault, so to speak, in the steering mechanism, or in what I have earlier referred to as the autoexecutive faculty).[56]

The problem is complicated by the fact that when the head of the family has difficulty in leadership, he takes refuge in opposition, negativistic or passive attitudes, and passing the buck. The impairment of the autoexecutive function amounts to the incapacity to direct one's affairs. The diminution of this faculty is accompanied by a diminution of trust in others. The individual, then, is not only incapable of using his own judgment, but also that of others. He cannot lead his life, but is also refractory to leadership.[56]

During the family interview, the therapist is often called on to assume leadership by providing conditions in which decisions can be made. He accomplishes this by questions and examples of clear thinking and weighing of alternatives that lead to a solution of a discernible conflict. His function does not stop at supplying the deficiency, but in eliciting dormant forces within the family enabling some of the family members to assume responsibility and to give direction to their lives in the absence of a natural leader. Such directed thinking stimulates all members, thus dividing the responsibilities, and, also, encourages them to support the one who dares to offer a suggestion or to make a decision. The reluctance to take a stand most often stems from fear of blame, fear of consequences, fear of being wrong. If there is no differentiation of roles and no hierarchy of responsibility, chaos, confusion, and disorganization reign within the family.

RELATIONSHIP BETWEEN INDIVIDUAL AND FAMILY INTERVIEWS

In an individual interview, the focus is on the experience of the patient in relation to his own needs and desires and his effect on others, including the effect of the patient on the therapist. In viewing the patient within his family setting, the focus is divided. In other words, there is a considerable shift in focus, resulting from the greater opportunity to observe the patient's effect on others and their effect on him.

The family interview permits the therapist to observe the patient in action. This allows the therapist to familiarize himself with various sets of the patient's behavior, depending on who participates in the interview, in a short span of time. A number of clues to the transference reactions can also be picked up from one or a few interviews. It can be argued that in individual treatment it is possible to find out the important relationships with relatives and nonrelatives who influence a patient's life. But, at best, the process is lengthy, and some of these patterns will be excluded in the one-to-one relationship, no matter how long the treatment takes.

In addition, the reliability of the information is questionable. When the patient talks about his relationships with members of his family, or other persons, the description, even when very reliable, is biased by his perception. His vision, motivations, the degree of self-deception, and the time lapse will distort his memory and color the narrative. He rarely, if ever, fully describes a situation—at best, it can be a more or less accurate approximation of the real state of affairs. The "real," to him, is the way it affects him. It is true that the therapist can check the information as the patient externalizes the inner conflicts and projects one part on to the therapist. For example, he may treat the therapist as he has been treated by the parent or as he treated the parent. This is what analysis of transference is, after all. But rare is the case when the therapist is able to discern all the intricacies of interactions that the patient needs to dramatize because of the unresolved conflicts of the past. It should be noted, also, that the therapist rarely can extricate himself sufficiently in his role of the participant observer.* The balance between observation and participation is indeed delicate. If the two participants are attuned to the type of thought processes that are representative of dreamlike subjective experiences, it is hard to switch to the kind of clarity needed for appreciation of mutual interaction. The shift of attention is decisive and requires considerable practice.

The therapist operates differently in a family interview than he does in individual sessions. He encounters a greater variety of impressions that engulf him. He is trapped by the interplay between the family members, as when he watches a drama on the stage. But, unlike a spectator at a play, he has to let the action

---

* "The expertness of the psychiatrist refers to his skill in participant observation of the unfortunate patterns of his own and the patient's living, in contrast to merely participating in such unfortunate patterns with the patient."[50]

affect him and also think about it and to put it to therapeutic use. He cannot postpone the critical evaluation and think later. A beginner may find himself acting out a part that the family unit may design for him. He may fall into a pattern that a given family uses on meeting a stranger. He may not immediately be able to differentiate himself from the family. He needs to learn to become relatively aware of the impact of the bewildering, at times, diversity of characteristics and relationships. There is always a period of confusion and a lack of a clear idea of how different situations relate to one another. He has to select among the various impressions accessible and relevant to an immediate conflict and amenable to change. With tolerance for uncertainty and anxiety and with tolerance for the unknown, the therapist will find a focus. Once a focus is found, the therapist's anxiety diminishes, and he then may be able to feel, hear, see, and impart what he sees to the participants. He may also diminish the anxiety among the family members once he gets them to participate and to think together.

When a therapist has a patient in individual therapy and he deems it necessary to have an interview with a spouse or with the rest of the family, his task is easier than interviewing an unknown family. Even if he has seen the patient only a few times, there is a certain familiarity already established that facilitates meeting the group. He is then less likely to be trapped into the interactions. The therapist does not need to use any information previously obtained from his patient; professional confidence is preserved. He uses only the material at hand, that is, what he sees and hears, and responds to what unfolds before him. The guidelines are actually the simplest interactions; the most obvious are frequently neglected. It is a known fact that simplicity is the most difficult thing to achieve. One cannot overemphasize the problem professionals in our field have in using generalizations that are invulnerable, boundless, and perhaps pretentiously omniscient. Very often it is nothing else than hiding behind words for fear of intimacy, fear of being wrong, fear of being helpless, fear of being inadequate—the very same fears prevalent in every family and every individual that comes to us for help. These fears, in principle ubiquitous, take a variety of forms and disguises in each family. Yet, these are the first types of interactions that a therapist has to pay attention to, pinning them down in specific form and making the participants aware of their harmful and contagious qualities, along with the effect they have on each member of the group. The family interview is designed to stimulate the interest of the participants in scrutinizing their behavior. The therapist aims to induce the participants to examine the intentions of their utterances, verbal and nonverbal.[25] It is important that the family members notice the form their communications take, that they follow the content and observe the effect, that they receive the feedback and correct the ineffective patterns in order to put their point across. Before one can relearn, one has to first become aware of the ineffective and destructive interactions. The therapist has to learn to talk to "a point" that is usually candid and brief, diminishing the distance between language and thought.[41]

The way family members listen to one another is never so blatantly illustrated as when it is observed in action. It is indeed amazing how little awareness people have of the effect they produce. I interviewed a couple in which the wife was known to interrupt everybody. The husband was not aware that he never listened to anybody, was impatient with and contemptuous of his wife. I noticed during the interview a number of instances when he did not allow his wife to complete a sentence and brought these to his attention. The patient was thoroughly surprised, as he never thought of himself as the one who did not listen. This confrontation made a difference to both of them: he stopped to reappraise his behavior; she felt understood and her facial expression relaxed. Husbands and wives very often look for an opportunity to fight with each other. Fencing is what they want and is more important than what they fence about. The content is irrelevant. Fighting is a substitute for intimacy—in anger they are together. When fear prevails, affection cannot be experienced.

These well-known aspects of family interactions have been amply illustrated in our contemporary drama, for example, *Who's Afraid of Virginia Woolf?*, where the humiliating invectives that each dishes out to the other is a way of avoiding helplessness and despair. It is rather a power struggle than a desire to hurt and annihilate the partners, as Edward Albee tries to tell us.

The value of a conjoint interview very often rests in the fact that the presence of the therapist as moderator enables the couple and the children finally to say something to one another they had wanted to say for a long time but did not dare do. This often clears up a misunderstanding, heals a long-standing hurt, and makes it clear to all how much support they need from one another. When they learn, as a result of such interviews, to drop some of the pretenses, be simply themselves, accept one another, then a dialogue between family members becomes possible and meaningful. Patients have to learn that there is no need to like everything about one another. This necessitates a differentiation between the totality of the person and some of his objectionable qualities. There is also a childish misconception many couples harbor that a loving spouse has to guess what is needed without making the desire explicit and to have it satisfied without asking for it. The asking diminishes the value when given. It is construed as being not out of full-hearted accord. One often hears a patient say, "If he (or she) really loved me, he (or she) would know what I need or want." This is the longing of the unconditional acceptance a baby has in the crib—when an infant cries, a mother guesses what his needs are and tries to satisfy them. Take as an example a couple I interviewed in which the husband reproached his wife for not giving him 100 per cent of her attention, even though they had four children. The wife said she was able to give him only 80 per cent. I am not sure how they managed the statistics.* In this particular instance, a jealous husband and only son never learned to share his wife with his four boys.

CONJOINT FAMILY INTERVIEWS IN CONSULTATION PRACTICE

In the last few years I have frequently conducted family interviews in consultation practice. Colleagues refer patients who are seen with their spouses with some apparent benefit in fostering improvement in the individual therapy as well as improvement in the relationship between the marital partners. I have conducted these consultations with one or more family members, separately or in varying sequence, and have, at times, included the treating therapist. Experience shows that this procedure could be recommended as routine. I think it unfortunate that such interviews take place only in a crisis.[47] For example: I was consulted by a couple whose marital discord had become unmanageable. The

---

* A Hassidic saying, which I like to quote to patients, goes: When two people quarrel and one is 55 per cent right, that's very nice and he should be content. If he is 60 per cent right, then he should feel very fortunate and thank God for that. What are you going to say about one who claims that he is 75 per cent right? Wise people say that it is very suspicious. Now, what about one who claims he is 100 per cent right? Such a man is a ruffian and a good-for-nothing cheat.

husband and wife had both been analyzed, apparently with considerable individual benefit. Thereafter they used their so-called free associations on each other. Although these were limited to accusations, invectives, and obscenities freely larded with four-letter words, they were surprised that this "complete candor" led only to attacks and counterattacks that demonstrated ever-sharpening skills at humiliating the other. Since they cared for each other, they were bewildered by their inability to change this pattern of behavior. The conjoint interviews gave them their first opportunity to learn that a difference of opinion need not signify rejection and that contempt is not conducive to congenial conversation. They also became aware that they reacted to sneers, gestures of impatience, and facial expressions but scarcely listened to each other's words. In these interviews, they heard each other out for the first time in twenty-five years of marital life.

Another example: A patient whom I saw in consultation complained that whenever he came home from work he invariably found his wife busy with the children and paying little or no attention to him. He would have liked her to have prepared some hors d'oeuvres and have had a cocktail with him. He could afford help and would have liked her to be free when he was home. He stated that his wife stubbornly refused to yield to his desires in spite of explicit requests, and for this reason he looked for satisfaction in extramarital relations. I wondered about the reason for his ineffectiveness. Why didn't his wife want to spend time with him? The complaints are usually the other way around. I then asked to see him with his wife. On seeing them together it became clear that she saw the situation quite differently. He would come home with a gloomy face and would bury himself behind a newspaper studying the stock market reports. He never asked her for the cocktails. He always reproached her and complained, expecting rejection and thus provoking it. This was an unresolved transference situation with his mother, notwithstanding his five years of analytic treatment.

This is a rather common occurrence in family life, and one should be able to take up such issues in individual therapy. The patient may become aware of how he bites the bait and, yet, continue to interact automatically with the spouse in the habitual way, irrespective of his awareness, because the tone of a request and the tone of a response evoke an automatic reaction without regard to content. Whenever a patient relates such a situation, the therapist may respond in the mood of the patient and side with him, whereas, in viewing the couple together, the therapist is relieved of such participation. He has his attention totally free to observe the two participants and see the complementarity of their interaction. And it is this interaction that is not accessible in individual therapy.

I have already stressed above the importance of being an observer and an operator at the same time, manifesting a quality of attention and a quality of presence.

Another example relating to the area of differentiation between intention and effect: A couple on the point of separation or divorce was seen. Every time the husband started to say something, the wife interrupted with either "It's not true" or "It's a lie" or she shook her head, negating whatever he was saying. This would stop the husband short, and then he would withdraw. The therapist brought it to their attention as a statement of fact, without implied reproach. The wife was surprised and was ready to look at why she reacted the way she did, what she wanted, and what she got from it.

Still another example: A couple went abroad for a vacation with their children. The husband said, "Next year, we will take a baby-sitter along with us so we can have dinner alone and spend some time together." The wife, before she heard the end of the sentence, got furious with him. "You can't stand the kids!" He was hurt and felt misunderstood. She didn't hear that he wanted to be alone with her. The mood of the evening was spoiled. In a conjoint interview with this couple, the therapist tried to initiate between them a kind of dialogue that made it possible to understand and accept that each was entitled to a different response to a given situation and that rejecting a viewpoint did not have to be equated with the rejection of the person who voiced it.

THE FAMILY INTERVIEW—INDICATIONS AND CONTRAINDICATIONS

There are no contraindications to having a family interview at the start of individual therapy or in the early stages. An initial interview with family members can be explained to the prospective client as an attempt to acquaint the therapist with those immediately concerned with his life. As was mentioned before, such an interview may help the therapist to understand the patient better and may even shorten the length of therapy and deepen the nature of the individual therapeutic relationship.

More often than not, such interviews take place as a result of a crisis or when therapy does not progress satisfactorily. If at such a time the patient or the therapist requests a family interview, then thoughtful consideration should be given to the wisdom and timing of such an interview. For example, I treated a patient for whom it was his second analytic experience and who complained about his wife's frigidity. The wife also had undergone analytic treatment. I suggested that I would like to see him once with his wife. His response, if not totally negative, was that of surprise or apprehension. He asked me why I wanted to see his wife, and I replied that I would like to see how they got along with each other. It seemed to me they were scared of each other, and I wanted better to understand the nature of the discomfort between them. The husband suffered from premature ejaculation, which disappeared during treatment, but his wife's sexual inhibitions and frigidity continued. He then told me she did not want to come to see me. I inquired how he presented my request to his wife. His answer was that she did not want to have sexual relations with him, and so he said to her, "By the way, my doctor wants to see you." It was evident that he took the opportunity to extend the invitation to come to see me in the form of a threat. Subsequently, they both came and found the interview quite revealing—namely, they became aware of how tentative he was in approaching her, how sexual relations were perceived as a contest as to whether he would be virile enough or she would be receptive. Each one engaged in intercourse as a test and to "get it over with." The wife then insisted she would like to come to see me a few more times. My patient was not particularly happy about such a possibility, and I suggested that we first work it out by ourselves and left it up to him to bring her when he felt like it. I later saw them together four times. These interviews facilitated the deeper analysis of the sibling rivalry between my patient and his younger sister.

This is a mild example of how a patient might misuse an invitation by the therapist to see his spouse or member of a family in midstream of the therapeutic process. Patients sometimes ask the therapist to see their spouses because they want to use the therapist in manipulating their conjugal partners. In such situations, the therapist would do well not to yield to such pressure unless he is confident he will not fall prey to manipulation. I would advise against conjoint interviews if the patient in treatment shows strong paranoid tendencies unless the therapist is well equipped to handle paranoid trends.

Contraindications to the use of this method may arise under certain conditions, and Ackerman lists a number of them: (1) when "the evidence indicates the existence of an irreversible and progressive trend toward disintegration and break-up of the family union"; (2) when there is "dominance within the group of a concentrated focus of malignant destructive motivation"; (3) when there is "incorrigible dishonesty of the individuals"; (4) when there is an "unyielding cultural or religious prejudice against this type of intervention in the private affairs of family life"; (5) when there is "danger of an outbreak of physical assault or where intervention on the defense operations of the family and its members may precipitate a critical psychosomatic breakdown"; and finally, (6) when "organic disease or disablement of a progressive nature" interferes with the use of psychotherapy.[4]

TRAINING IN FAMILY THERAPY

Family interviews and family therapy are not easy tasks and require a good deal of preparation and skill. The Family Mental Health Clinic (of Jewish Family Service) conducted an experimental training program in 1964–1965 as an introduction to family therapy. The program consisted of a thirty-five-week course, six hours weekly. There was (1) a course in family therapy theory and practice, using demonstrations of interviews by senior staff members that were viewed *in vivo* (through the one-way mirror) by the trainees, in addition to live supervision of families in the process of treatment that were shown to training candidates; (2) a course in family dynamics and individual psychotherapy; and (3) a course, The Family in Literature and Drama.

The program did not provide training in small-group dynamics, which I think is indispensable to round out training in family therapy. A proper training course in family therapy would have to take three years in addition to preliminary training in individual therapy, although it is possible that individual and family therapy could be learned simultaneously.

Recently, the clinic added extensive use of video tape recordings as a means to study family interactions, to supervise therapy, and also for therapeutic use. We had families watch their own tapes and found that seeing themselves made a considerable impact and drove home aspects of behavior that required changing. As an illustration: A sixteen-year-old adolescent, with an outbreak of an acute schizophrenic episode, was unaware of his mimicry, gesticulations, and paucity of language until he saw himself on a video tape playback. As he watched himself on the monitor, he kept mumbling, "I have to learn to control myself. I have to learn to control myself. I have such a limited vocabulary." Viewing this tape changed his perception of himself, and he was able to restrain his behavior and verbal outbursts in the subsequent weeks as witnessed at home, in school, and further video tape sessions. Apparently, the use of video tape increases the self-awareness more than verbal exchanges in psychotherapeutic sessions.

As mentioned in the introduction, I believe it is essential for a psychotherapist to have knowledge of the humanities, which requires continuous study of literature and drama. This has been advocated by many psychologists, among them William James, Rollo May, and particularly Cyril Burt (pp. 18–19).[35] Scientific psychology, emulating science, draws on physics, cybernetics, and ethology to advance knowledge of how man adapts to his environment. This knowledge, though fascinating and essential for integrated eclecticism, will fail of its purpose if it crowds out the humanities. For precision of thought and richness of insights into the vicissitudes of family life, we need to study the cumulative experience of the great thinkers of the world.

REFERENCES

1. Ackerman, N. W. *The Psychodynamics of Family Life.* New York: Basic Books, 1958.
2. Ackerman, N. W. "Theory of Family Dynamics," *Psychoanalysis and Psychoanalytic Review*, 46, no. 4 (Winter 1959), 33–49.
3. Ackerman, N. W. "Psychotherapy with the Family Group," *Science and Psychoanalysis*, 4 (1961), 150–157.
4. Ackerman, N. W. "Family Psychotherapy Today: Some Areas of Controversy," *Comprehensive Psychiatry*, 7, no. 5 (October 1966), 375–388.
5. Ackerman, N. W. "Family Therapy," in S. Arieti (ed.), *American Handbook of Psychiatry*. New York: Basic Books, 1966. Vol. 3, pp. 201–212.
6. Ackerman, N. W. *Treating the Troubled Family.* New York: Basic Books, 1966.
7. Ackerman, N. W. "Developments in Family Psychotherapy," in J. H. Masserman (ed.), *Current Psychiatric Therapies*. New York: Grune & Stratton, 1968. Vol. 8, pp. 126–136.

8. Ackerman, N. W., Beatman, F. L., and Sherman, S. N. (eds.). *Exploring the Base for Family Therapy*. New York: Family Service Association of America, 1961.
9. Ackerman, N. W., Beatman, F. L., and Sherman, S. N. (eds.). *Expanding Theory and Practice in Family Therapy*. New York: Family Service Association of America, 1967.
10. Allen, F. H. *Psychotherapy with Children*. New York: Norton, 1942.
11. Arieti, S. "The Schizophrenic Patient in Office Treatment," in *Psychotherapy of Schizophrenia*. New York: Karger, 1965. Pp. 7–23.
12. Arieti, S. "Creativity and Its Cultivation: Relation to Psychopathology and Mental Health," in S. Arieti (ed.), *American Handbook of Psychiatry*. New York: Basic Books, 1966. Vol. 3, pp. 722–741.
13. Ashby, W. R. *Design for a Brain—The Origin of Adaptive Behavior*. New York: Wiley, 1960.
14. Auerbach, A. (ed.). *Schizophrenia—An Integrated Approach*. New York: Ronald Press, 1959.
15. Bach, R. O. (ed.). *Communication: The Art of Understanding and Being Understood*. Toronto: Saunders, 1963.
16. Bell, J. E. "A Theoretical Position for Family Group Therapy," *Family Process*, 2 (March 1963), 1–14.
17. Benedek, T. "The Emotional Structure of the Family," in R. N. Anshen (ed.), *The Family: Its Function and Destiny*. Rev. ed. New York: Harper, 1959. Pp. 353–380.
18. Boas, G. *The Inquiring Mind—An Introduction to Epistemology*. LaSalle: Open Court, 1959.
19. Bowen, M. "Family Relationships in Schizophrenia," in Alfred Auerbach (ed.), *Schizophrenia—An Integrated Approach*. New York: Ronald Press, 1959. Pp. 147–178.
20. Cassirer, E. *Language and Myth*, trans. S. K. Langer. New York: Harper, 1946.
21. Cassirer, E. *An Essay on Man—An Introduction to a Philosophy of Human Culture*. New Haven: Yale University Press, 1944.
22. Edman, I. (ed.). *The Philosophy of Santayana*. New York: Scribner's, 1936.
23. Edwards, T. (compiler). *A New Dictionary of Thoughts; A Cyclopedia of Quotations*. New York: Standard Book Co., 1960.
24. Freud, S. "Letter 59—Extracts from the Fliess Papers," *Standard Edition*. London: Hogarth Press. Vol. 1, pp. 244–245. (Also in M. Bonaparte, A. Freud, and E. Kris (eds.), *The Origins of Psychoanalysis; Letters to Wilhelm Fliess*. New York: Basic Books, 1954. P. 193.
25. Freud, S. "The Forgetting of Names and Sets of Words" (1911), in J. Strachey (ed.), *Standard Edition*. London: Hogarth Press. Vol. 6, p. 24.
26. Freud, S. "The Future Prospects of Psychoanalytic Therapy" (1910) in *Collected Papers*. London: Hogarth Press, 1933. Vol. 2, p. 290. (Also in J. Strachey (ed.), *Standard Edition*. London: Hogarth Press. Vol. 11, p. 146.)
27. Freud, S. "On Narcissism: An Introduction" (1914), in J. Strachey (ed.), *Standard Edition*. London: Hogarth. Vol. 14. (Also in *Collected Papers of Sigmund Freud*. New York: Basic Books, 1959. Vol. 4, pp. 30–59.)
28. Fromm-Reichmann, F. Sections IV and V, in D. M. Bullard (ed.), *Psychoanalysis and Psychotherapy: Selected Papers*. Chicago: University of Chicago Press, 1959. Pp. 221–321.
29. Gibson, R. W. "The Family Background and Early Life Experience of the Manic-Depressive Patient," *Psychiatry*, 21, no. 1 (1958), 71–90.
30. Glover, E. *War, Sadism and Pacifism*. London: Allen & Unwin, 1946.
31. Hamilton, G. *Psychotherapy in Child Guidance*. New York: Columbia University Press, 1947.
32. Hebb, D. O. *The Organization of Behavior*. New York: Wiley, 1959.
33. Jung, C. G. *The Undiscovered Self*. Boston: Little, Brown, 1957.
34. Kaplan, B. "The Study of Language in Psychiatry: The Comparative Developmental Approach and Its Application to Symbolization and Language in Psychopathology," in S. Arieti (ed.), *American Handbook of Psychiatry*. New York: Basic Books, 1966. Vol. 3, pp. 659–688.
35. Koestler, A. *The Act of Creation*. New York: Macmillan, 1964. Introduction.

36. Lidz, T. *The Family and Human Adaptation.* New York: International Universities Press, 1963.
37. Lidz, T., Fleck, S., and Cornelison, A. R. *Schizophrenia and the Family.* New York: International Universities Press, 1965.
38. Mishler, E. G., and Waxler, N. E. "Family Interaction Processes and Schizophrenia: A Review of Current Theories," *Merrill-Palmer Quarterly,* **2,** no. 4 (October 1965), 269–317.
39. Mumford, L. *The Myth of the Machine.* New York: Harcourt, Brace & World, 1967.
40. Parsons, T. and Bales, R. *Family, Socialization and Interaction Process.* Glencoe, Ill.: The Free Press, 1955.
41. Piaget, J. *Six Psychological Studies.* New York: Random House, 1967.
42. Read, H. *The Forms of Things Unknown.* New York: Meridian Books, 1967.
43. Russell, B. *My Philosophical Development.* New York: Simon & Schuster, 1959.
44. Schecter, D. E. "The Integration of Group Therapy with Individual Psychoanalysis," *Psychiatry,* **22** (August 1959).
45. Schimel, J. L. "Parents of Problem Children," in G. L. Usdin (ed.), *Adolescence: Care and Counseling.* Philadelphia: Lippincott, 1967. Pp. 119–129.
46. Seidenberg, R. *Anatomy of the Future.* New York: University of North Carolina Press, 1961.
47. Simmel, G. *Conflict.* Glencoe, Ill.: The Free Press, 1955.
48. Simmel, G. *The Web of Group Affiliations.* Glencoe, Ill.: The Free Press, 1955.
49. Sterne, L. *The Life and Opinions of Tristram Shandy.* New York: Modern Library. Book V, Chap. VI, p. 372.
50. Sullivan, H. S. "The Theory of Anxiety and the Nature of Psychotherapy," *Psychiatry,* **12,** no. 1 (1949).
51. Szalita, A. B. "Remarks on Pathogenesis and Treatment of Schizophrenia," *Psychiatry,* **14,** no. 3 (August 1951).
52. Szalita, A. B. "Further Remarks on the Pathogenesis and Treatment of Schizophrenia," *Psychiatry,* **15,** no. 2 (May 1952).
53. Szalita, A. B. "The 'Intuitive Process' and Its Relation to Work with Schizophrenics," *Journal of the American Psychoanalytic Association,* **3,** no. 1 (January 1955).
54. Szalita, A. B. "Regression and Perception in Psychotic States," *Psychiatry,* **21** (February 1958).
55. Szalita, A. B. "Some Psychiatric Aspects of Rehabilitation of Physically Handicapped," *Nordisk Psykiatrisk Tidsskrift,* **18,** no. 5 (1964).
56. Szalita, A. B. "Psychodynamics of Disorders of the Involutional Age," in S. Arieti (ed.), *American Handbook of Psychiatry.* New York: Basic Books, 1966. Vol. 3, pp. 66–87.
57. Szalita, A. B. "The Combined Use of Family Interviews and Individual Therapy in Schizophrenia," *American Journal of Psychotherapy,* **22** (1968), 419–430.
58. Whitehorn, J. C. "Types of Leadership Involved in Psychotherapy," *American Journal of Psychotherapy,* **16,** no. 3 (1962).
59. Whitehorn, J. C. "Education for Uncertainty," *Perspectives in Biology and Medicine,* **8,** no. 1 (Autumn 1963), 118–123.
60. Will, O. A. "Process, Psychotherapy and Schizophrenia," in A. Burton (ed.), *Psychotherapy of the Psychoses.* New York: Basic Books, 1961. Pp. 10–42.
61. Wynne, L., Ryckoff, I., Day, J., and Hirsch, S. "Pseudo-Mutuality in the Family Relations of Schizophrenics," *Psychiatry,* **21** (1958), 205–220.

PSYCHOANALYTIC CONSIDERATIONS IN A CASE OF CARDIAC TRANSPLANTATION

Pietro Castelnuovo-Tedesco

At the time of this writing, there are as yet no published reports on the psychiatric aspects of cardiac transplantation, but one can be sure that this is only because heart transplants are still very new and because, understandably, the focus so far has been on the technical aspects of this outstanding surgical feat. Also, a number of the patients who have been operated on have died during the early, critical phases of the postoperative period before complications, other than those fundamentally physiologic, could occur. Yet, it can be anticipated that as more heart transplant operations are carried out and as these patients' survival after surgery gradually increases, more and more will be noted about the psychological import of these operations and about their attendant psychiatric complications.* Numerous reports already have emphasized the significance of psychological factors in the transplantation of other organs (in particular, the kidney)[5, 6, 7, 14, 21] and in other types of cardiac operations (mainly, open-heart surgery[1, 2, 3, 4, 8, 9, 11, 12, 15, 16, 17, 19] for chronic valvular disease). Note has been taken of the not infrequent occurrence, especially in the latter cases, of transient, postoperative psychotic reactions.

In the instance of renal transplantation, the usefulness of routine psychiatric screening of recipients and particularly of donors

---

* Shortly after this article had been completed, I became aware of a report by Lunde,[18] given at the 1969 annual meeting of the American Psychiatric Association, in which he reviewed the experience with heart transplantation at Stanford University. In their series of nine patients, three had suffered postoperative psychotic reactions. The nature of these psychotic disturbances was not described in detail.

has repeatedly been described.[5, 6, 7, 14] Severe depression and concern with damage to the body, especially the sexual organs, have been observed.[14] Recipients tend to have difficulties with their sense of obligation to the donors, and some donors showed unconscious resentment toward the recipient or toward those who had recommended the transplant.[5, 6, 7] After surgery Cramond's[5] patients manifested considerable regressive interest in food and in eating, whereas interest in sex generally declined. Cramond[5] also noted other features that emerged during the follow-up period:

1. Ideas of a "second chance." He says, "In general, the recipients see the operation as giving them symbolic rebirth and can describe the feeling that in some way they have some special task or role to carry out. There is some evidence that religious conviction intensifies, and one patient appears to have had a religious conversion following this experience."

2. Socioeconomic fears, based on a variety of real financial difficulties and on anxiety about the future.

3. "Graft-traumatic" anxiety, that is, concern lest the grafted kidney suffer injury and a tendency to avoid aggressive or sexual activities.

In the case of open-heart operations, the occurrence of psychiatric complications, often serious, has been described repeatedly.[1, 2, 3, 4, 8, 9, 11, 12, 13, 14, 15, 16, 17, 19] Emphasis has been placed, more than for kidney transplants, on the awesome threat to life that these procedures involve.[1, 9, 15] Kennedy,[15] for example, has given a dramatic representation of the heart patient's predicament, noting that "from the moment he enters the hospital, he must live constantly with the prospect of immediate death and with the assaultive knowledge that while he will lie powerless and unconscious, his heart will be held in a stranger's hand, at the mercy of a knife that will be put to it, and at the price that any error could result in something worse than amputation or impotence—total extinction."

Why in these cases the threat to life should loom larger than in those of renal transplantation is not altogether clear, except that there is much more folklore and mythology about the heart than about the kidney: for everyone the heart is *the* vital organ par excellence, and its malfunction entails the danger of sudden death. The heart is a more strongly cathected part of the body image than the kidney, not only because of its significance (real and imagined), but also because its action is directly and sometimes forcefully experienced; the kidney, by contrast, works silently. Thus, the heart is perceived (and cathected) much more like an external body part than like other internal organs. One who is sensitive and easily hurt is said, in fact, to wear it on his sleeve. Realistically, also, the life expectancy today is greater after renal than cardiac transplantation.

If we compare the psychiatric complications in the two situations, we notice that the former seem different in quality and less severe than the latter. Mainly depressions and other pyschoneurotic manifestations have been observed after renal transplants,[5, 6, 7, 14] whereas after open-heart operations, psychotic reactions have been prominent.[1, 2, 3, 4, 11, 12, 16, 17, 19] The nature of these psychotic reactions usually has not been described in detail, and it is often not at all clear whether they are mainly organic, or psychogenic, in origin, that is, whether in response to disturbances of body chemistry and physiology or to the symbolic significance of the experience (or, in what degree, to both). Attention has been directed primarily at the *psychotic* manifestations, which are always more dramatic and arresting, whereas the *psychoneurotic* reactions have, with few exceptions,[9, 15] been overlooked or at best given scanty consideration. Finally, much has been made of sensory deprivation[1, 2, 4, 8, 11, 12, 16, 17] and sleep deprivation[1, 2, 4, 8, 11, 12, 16, 17, 19] as etiologic factors in many of the severe postoperative reactions. However, there has been apparently limited realization that sensory deprivation refers to a particular set of circumstances that induce and facilitate psychological regression by artificially removing the environmental supports needed for the maintenance of secondary process thinking. Similarly, sleep deprivation has been considered mainly in terms of its physiologic manifestations, although it also describes conditions that promote a pathological and disorganizing regression by preventing the regression in the service of the ego that characterizes normal sleep. In short, an exhaustive, in-depth review of this whole area appears very much in order.

CASE REPORT

A fifty-eight-year-old white, married grocer had suffered for ten years from heart disease that had become progressively more incapacitating and had resulted in repeated hospitalizations. In fact, during the past year, he had led a bed-to-chair existence, unable to walk and troubled by severe breathlessness and angina on the slightest exertion.

For many months, the patient had been eager to have a heart transplant. From the beginning, he had followed the development of this new procedure and had kept abreast from the reports in the press of the outcome of the various patients who had been operated on. He had had little difficulty dismissing the fact that most of these patients had died soon after surgery. He felt that the operation would work for *him* and, in any case, that it was very much worth the risk. Without it, he knew he would soon be dead, and so he had pleaded with his general practitioner, who was also his friend and next-door neighbor, to help him obtain the operation. His physician at first had been skeptical of this request, because the procedure was still so new that it had never been performed in Southern California. However, at the patient's insistence, he placed him in contact with the transplant team. The patient's wife also strongly favored the operation. Both the patient and his wife were sure that it would be a success and at no point—before or after the transplantation—did either acknowledge having had contrary thoughts or serious doubts about its advisability. In fact, in the several months that elapsed between the initial evaluation and surgery, the patient, whose symptoms were steadily progressing, began to despair that he might die before a suitable donor could be found; his wife repeatedly approached members of the transplant team urging them to "find us a donor" and expressing fears that the team had forgotten about her husband.

Finally, one night in February 1969, a heart became available when a young married woman, who had had a fight with her husband, shot herself in the head and was brought, dead on arrival, to the Harbor General Hospital. Immediately, a call went out to the patient who was driven promptly to the hospital by his wife. He was so elated at the prospect of receiving a new heart that he hummed and whistled as he left his home in the early hours of the morning. The operation was started within an hour after his arrival, so that he had very little time to acquaint himself with his new surroundings and with several of the staff (especially the nurses) who were to care for him. He had, however, met the key members of the surgical team when they had evaluated him for cardiac transplantation in October 1968 during his admission to a nearby hospital.

Medical History

Although in childhood the patient had had an attack of rheumatic fever, he had been quite free of symptoms of heart disease until 1956, when, at forty-six, he suffered a myocardial infarction. A second, massive infarction occurred in 1967, and thereafter he remained gravely ill and restricted in his activities. Cardiac catheterization in 1968 revealed advanced chronic rheumatic heart disease with calcific involvement of the mitral and aortic valves and coronary occlusive disease. There had been no other significant illnesses or operations.

Family History

The patient's father died young of unknown cause, possibly tuberculosis. The patient's mother, brother, and sister died of arteriosclerotic heart disease. Three other sisters are living and well. There was no other history of familial disease, including psychosis.

Social History

The patient was born in California in 1910, the youngest of six children. His father died when the patient was five years old, leaving the patient's mother to support the family. She became a cook in the fields for migrant farm workers, but the work was seasonal and uncertain, and this meant that the family had no stable home and moved about a good deal. Occasionally they went hungry. According to his wife, the patient "never had a real home" until his marriage to her. The patient had been very close to his mother, had clung to her for protection, and had spent long hours watching her while she cooked. He was not particularly close to any of his siblings.

The patient completed only two years of high school, but later in the navy managed to obtain a high school diploma. On returning from the service, he went to work as a bartender and restaurant manager, and, a few years later, at forty, he married his present wife, who was the owner of the restaurant and who had just recently been widowed. She points out that although he had

had a prior, brief (and unsuccessful) wartime marriage, he seemed very much an "old bachelor" and that his experience with women had been quite limited. With his wife he soon established a dependent relationship, which became characteristic of their marriage even before it was confirmed and reinforced by his cardiac illness. He called her "mother," and she rather openly hovered over, and protected, him. Their sex life had been fairly regular in the very early part of their marriage, but soon had decreased sharply. He had never been sexually passionate, and this troubled his wife, who on several occasions sought the help of physicians for her husband. To the patient, however, his sex life was not a problem, and he would say that he was not very interested simply because he was very tired from overwork. He did, in fact, work very hard and in this way managed to build his grocery store into a small but thriving business which gave him a good income and of which he was keenly proud. Besides his work, he enjoyed reading, the comforts of his home, and the good food his wife prepared for him. He did not care much for conversation or social gatherings, and even with his wife he was emotionally undemonstrative. He was, in short, a quiet, soft-spoken, rather inhibited man with many obsessive-compulsive and schizoid features, dedicated to his work and to the simple routines of his life. He had never shown any sign of mental illness.

The Operation

The transplant operation lasted six hours and proceeded without significant complication. The excised heart revealed heavily calcified aortic and mitral valves and severe occlusive disease of the whole coronary system. One of the surgeons later recalled that as the transplanted heart had belonged to a woman, there was at first a tendency at the operating table to refer to it as "she." They might say, for example, "She is beating all right." Later, after the chest had been closed, "she" became "he" once more.

The Early Postoperative Period

The patient spent the first postoperative day in the recovery room and was then transferred to a special room where strict isolation technique (cap, mask, gown, gloves, and so forth) was observed and where complex electronic equipment continuously monitored the patient's heart action. Wires from electrodes attached to the chest connected the patient, as if by an umbilical cord, to the cardioscope. Here, on a screen, the patient's EKG was represented, and it was visible to him as well as to a nurse who was constantly in attendance. Immediately after awakening from the anesthetic, he was noted to be alert and intellectually quite intact (he remembered, for example, the name of one of the physicians whom he had met only a few minutes prior to surgery), indicating that cerebral circulation had been well maintained throughout the operation. He said he felt "fine" and, except for a little initial discomfort at the site of the incision, he was free of pain. It is important to emphasize that throughout the postoperative period (until the final, terminal phase) he had no major *physical* complaints (although he was somewhat bothered intermittently by hiccoughs) and that he gained daily in appetite, strength, and motility. On the second postoperative day, he was allowed out of bed for a few minutes. By the fourth day, he was watching television, and by the end of the first week, he was spending some time in a chair and was able to take a few steps about the room. This represented more ambulation than he had managed in more than a year. During this early postoperative period, there were, however, several episodes of arrhythmia which were promptly and effectively controlled, but which must have raised considerably the patient's anxiety. One such episode (on the thirteenth postoperative day) was treated with an electric shock to the chest, under general anesthesia.

During the first two or three nights, he was very much afraid to go to sleep and clearly felt that if he stayed awake he would stay alive, whereas if he fell asleep he might well die. This soon passed, and he became, in fact, mildly euphoric, expressing confidence and exultation over the outcome of the operation. He smiled contentedly, repeatedly saying that it all seemed almost too good to be true, but also that he had known all along that everything would turn out all right. He was much interested in knowing about the donor, and several times asked who she was, why she had died, what her situation had been, and so forth. Once he expressed his thoughts about the intensive care unit and recommended that the nurses give more physical care (for example, back rubs, which he enjoyed) and pay less attention to the cardioscope and other monitoring equipment. Such outspoken comments, however, were atypical and most rare; gradually, it became apparent to those caring for him—physicians and nurses —that he had become extremely dependent on the staff: he doted on them, was profusely grateful and full of extravagant praise for their efforts.* Sometimes, he would take the hand of the chief surgical resident, hold it, and tell him how much he appreciated everything that was being done for him. He regarded the surgeons as practically godlike and only as something slightly less than miracle men. He felt and expressed the thought that he was as reborn. He looked forward to going home soon and to enjoying his wife's cooking, but he gave little conscious thought to what his life now would be like. In particular, he could not approach at all the question of the final outcome of the operation or of how much life was still ahead of him. His wife shared his massive denial, and once, when the author pointedly brought this up, she remarked that, as experience with the operation still was so limited, perhaps he would live another ten, fifteen, or more years. At any rate, death was placed in the distant future. It is interesting that—even in his precarious circumstances—he did what everyone else does, namely, place death somewhere far off in the distance.

The Psychotic Episode

The author first met the patient on the twentieth postoperative day. Physically he was progressing very well, but it was noted that he seemed moderately depressed and lacked his previous euphoric confidence in his progress. Several factors suggested themselves to account for this change. First, the daily dose of prednisone, which probably had contributed to his euphoria, gradually was being reduced. Also his wife, who since the operation had been in constant attendance at his bedside, decided, in view of his markedly improved state, to return to their home (two or three hours away from the hospital) for several days. Simultaneously, the staff, concerned about his evident dependence, had begun to "wean" him by emphasizing how well he was doing

---

* The only complaints he allowed himself were about the food. This, incidentally, is a time-honored and institutionalized displacement by which hospitalized patients often convey the negative side of their feelings they cannot express directly to the staff.

and by telling him that soon he would be discharged. Visits by the staff became a little less frequent and detailed than they had been in the immediate postoperative period. His anxiety about himself and the eventual outcome of the operation remained untapped, and it was probably intensified by the news that soon he would be sent away from the hospital where the doctors, his powerful protectors, resided.

On the evening of the twentieth postoperative day, while watching a television newscast, he heard a pronouncement by a prominent physician that heart transplants should not be performed because they are ineffective, costly, and wasteful; many patients needing ordinary, accepted therapies could be treated with the funds required to carry out one transplant. The patient was very upset by this. He failed to eat and appeared quite restless as well as depressed and withdrawn. He spoke very little, but commented to the nurse that possibly he would not be around very much longer. He experienced some heart palpitations and said "I think she is calling me, she is coming after me," referring to the woman whose heart he had received. He had thoughts about being reborn, about having a new heart, and whether it was right for the woman (the donor) to have been left without a heart. How would she manage without one?

On the following day, he appeared still quite withdrawn and depressed. He looked puzzled and preoccupied and complained that his thoughts were confused and that he did not seem able to "get his bearings." He felt "a lot of mental pressure," and at one point, with tears in his eyes, said, "I can't seem to attach myself to anything." He requested that his wife be called, and, when she arrived, he seemed somewhat comforted. At first, there was some superficial brightening, but basically he remained withdrawn, tense, and self-preoccupied. Occasional, brief comments had a hollow, inappropriate ring, others indicated suicidal ruminations. He remained unchanged for the next several days and was difficult to involve in conversation. He was tense, hyperalert, suspicious, and now also had developed marked tremor, the somatic expression of his extreme anxiety. However, when asked how he felt, he would say "fine," which obviously was anything but the case.

On the twenty-sixth postoperative day, the patient became acutely psychotic, unmanageable, and combative, demonstrating surprising strength. He refused all oral medication and was repeatedly incontinent of both urine and feces. He appeared very frightened. Combativeness and hyperactivity alternated with periods when he was mute, rigid, catatonic, staring fixedly with apprehension and suspicion at the activities about him. He was sedated first with intramuscular Librium and later with oral Thorazine. I visited him frequently and was able to acquaint myself with some of the content of his psychotic state. He said that his thoughts were racing wildly and that he was very confused, yet he remained oriented in the usual sense of the word. He expressed the belief that the operation had not been carried out and, on the other hand, also the idea that, because the operation *had* been carried out, all the staff (doctors and nurses) had lost their positions at the hospital. He wondered how they would manage without salaries. In particular, he was convinced that the surgeons' research grants had been "cut off," so that all their work would come to an end. He also had thoughts of being pauperized and of not being able to afford the visits of the doctors.

Gradually he improved, and by the thirty-fourth postoperative day, he appeared quite recovered from his psychotic episode. His tremor also had completely disappeared. He was able to recall that the experience had been like a nightmare, and he remembered particularly having been very frightened and very confused by the jumble of his thoughts, which seemed so intense and so real. He had refused to take his medicines because something told him that he should not, but he did not know why, and this further intensified his anxiety. He also was able to explain the episode of sphincter incontinence. He "knew" (as if he had received an order), he said, that he was not supposed to move his bowels or pass urine, and therefore he held them in as long as possible until finally, unable to control himself any longer, he had soiled himself and the bed. Now all these memories were fading away and becoming dimmer day by day, so that at times he wondered whether they had really happened or whether they had been a dream or the product of his imagination. He was concerned about a possible recurrence of the episode and did not wish to think about it any more. He had no awareness that his psychosis was related to intense mixed feelings and anxiety about the operation. It is important also to clarify that during his psychosis effective cardiac action was maintained (even though there was recurrent arrhythmia) and that laboratory tests were unremarkable. The psychotic reaction had the features of an acute schizophrenic reaction rather than of an organic delirium.

The Late Postoperative Period

As already indicated, the patient recovered fully from his brief psychotic episode, and plans for discharge from the hospital were again entertained. He began by going out for car rides or for supper at local restaurants and spent the night with his wife at a motel nearby. He tolerated these activities very well, enjoyed himself, and felt emotionally much closer to his wife than he ever had. He was impressed as he never had been before by the joy and excitement of being alive, and, on one of these occasions, he actually *told* his wife that he loved her, a sentiment that previously, in his inhibited way, he had failed to express. He spoke with relish and anticipation of his plans for returning to work, part-time, in his store. However, he could give no thought to the future or to his prognosis. All that mattered was that he was going home.

Suddenly on the thirty-seventh postoperative day, as plans for discharge were being readied, he developed a shaking chill and a fever. A pleuritic friction rub was noted. Chest X rays revealed evidence of pulmonary embolization. There was increasing depression of the white cell count, soon followed by rising fever and other signs of generalized infection. Rejection of the heart also had set in: the circulation became compromised and anuria ensued. Despite total efforts, the deterioration could not be reversed. He gradually became comatose and died on the forty-second postoperative day.

I then learned that he had requested that his body be cremated and his ashes scattered at sea from an airplane. It is a testimonial to the complexity of the human personality that so plain and unromantic a man should have envisaged such romantic funeral plans. His wife arranged to have them carried out. Prior to the time when the heart transplant had become a possibility, he had spoken of wanting to "leave his body to science," wishing his death to serve some positive purpose for humanity. I also learned that in earlier years he had never wanted to visit his mother's grave. As he put it, it would do no good, as she was dead anyway, and it would only upset him.

DISCUSSION

A number of conclusions and conjectures may be drawn from this case material. They not only have relevance for understanding this particular patient, but highlight problems present in some fashion in other cases of cardiac transplantation.

One perceives that the operation entailed enormous psychological stress and unspeakable threat for the patient and that he dealt with this by massive denial of the danger and of his own mixed feelings and fears. His "confidence" that all would work out all right and his inability to consider, and speak of, the outcome and eventual prognosis certainly are in keeping with this. It is clear that this degree of denial had relevance for the development of the psychosis. Yet, one is simultaneously led to consider whether some measure of denial may not actually be helpful and even necessary in order that the patient be willing to consider and undertake the transplant operation. How else could he take part in a procedure where the risks are so great and the odds so unfavorable? It also brings up a question, which must be answered as well for other patients who undergo this procedure, namely, why did he not choose to let his life take its natural course? There is, no doubt, the "realistic" wish to survive, the expression of a persistent libidinal attachment to life. In this case, it would seem that there were also phobic concerns about dying and specifically about permitting events to take a natural course. The need to maintain control appears closely entwined with his compelling desire to live. (In his psychosis, he experienced an imperative command to control his sphincters and a subsequent inability to do so. Dying meant letting go, being swallowed up.) Everything about dying and particularly about a *natural* death was distasteful to him (his earlier preference for "giving his body to science," his later quest for the transplant, his insistence on cremation, and so forth). One surmises that the threat came not only from the fear of final dissolution (which everyone shares), but also from the unconscious idea that in this physical dissolution he would be reunited with his mother, something that he both longed for and feared (in the end, he requested that his ashes be scattered at *sea*). There was no peaceful acquiescence to the inevitable, but rather a need to prevent this reunion by all available means, which included seeking out a new and still experimental operation.

Ideas of dying and of being reborn apparently were closely connected in his mind. The latter would prevent the former, yet there was constant danger that the two states would merge or replace each other. In order that he live, the other had to die. In order to live, he needed the heart of the woman, but once he had the woman's heart inside him, his body image was no longer the same, and his capacity to remain separate from her became impaired (she could "call" him, as she did during his psychosis, reminding him that he—and her heart—belonged to her). Regressively oral incorporative trends were stimulated which suggested to the patient that he had robbed the woman (that is, mother) of what belonged to her, namely, her heart. The patient repeatedly had expressed guilt over this. He had incorporated part of her, but she could—projectively and in retaliation—engulf him. We recall that his psychosis began after hearing on television a medical opinion to the effect that he had taken more than his share, that his expensive operation had deprived others of their due. Regarding the prevalence and deep-seated nature of these concerns, one is reminded both of statements by current critics[10, 13, 20] of transplantation about its "cannibalistic" features and also of the popular folklore about vampirism and Frankenstein-like monsters who live on at the expense of other beings. The literature is already full of discussion and dispute about the ethical problems of transplantation; but *ethical* problems quickly become *psychological* problems for all concerned—the patient (and his family), the surgeon (and his associates), the donor's family, and (in the case of kidney transplants) the donor as well.

It is evident that the patient handled the massive threat to his bodily integrity not only by denial, but also by regression. The latter process, unstemmed, finally culminated in psychosis. In the beginning, the patient tried to manage these regressive pulls by establishing an outspokenly dependent, compliant, and "grateful" transference to his physicians, whom he regarded as all-powerful saviors. When this stance was inadequate to contain his fear, his ambivalence, and—in particular—his aggression, he became depressed. (One surmises that his aggression must have been activated by his position of extreme passivity—before, during, and after the operation—and as a result of deneutralization, consequent to regression.) When depression also proved insufficient, he regressed still further into psychosis. *Then* he was no longer grateful and compliant but became negativistic and combative, thought that the operation had not yet taken place, and "punished" the doctors by having them all fired and cut off without a penny. This was also, by projection, an expression of his guilt for having robbed the mother. In his delusion, the patient as well as the doctors had been pauperized.

On the other hand, one wonders whether the psychosis also did not serve adaptive functions, by permitting an emergency discharge of intense feeling, which might not have been adequately dissipated if he had consistently maintained a relatively mature ego state. Certainly, after he recovered from the psychotic episode, more genuine and substantial progressive trends came into view. His convalescence quickened, he seemed to have less anxiety about leaving the hospital, and he was able even to tell his wife that he loved her and to experience a degree of emotional intimacy that he had never before permitted himself.

Questions arise as to how these very important issues might be handled more effectively in a future case. Undoubtedly, it would be helpful if a psychiatric evaluation could be carried out *before* the patient is operated on rather than afterward. However, to speak of psychiatric evaluation does not do justice to the requirements of the situation. The function of the psychiatrist should be not only to evaluate the patient so as to screen out those who are psychologically unsuitable, but also to provide a therapeutic relationship that would help anchor the patient during this very major trial. The psychological threat is so great that even the normal patient needs to be protected from it in every way possible. (Incidentally, I believe that our patient, despite his share of the usual peculiarities of character, had been a reasonably normal man.) It would be helpful for the patient to meet and get to know the staff (nurses as well as doctors) who will take care of him sometime before the operation rather than enter the hospital just as surgery is about to get underway. This would help him to establish with the staff a less stereotyped and infantile transference, one less likely to promote regression. Although the prognosis of the operation had been discussed with the patient in great detail in the course of obtaining his informed consent, it is clear that repeated review of these issues is needed to deal at least to a degree with the denial that inevitably will be part of the picture. Despite the enormous difficulties all of us have even considering the possibility of our own nonexistence, it would seem important to help the patient handle the experience as much as possible at the level of secondary process rather than at that of irrational hopes and primitive fears. As more transplant operations are carried out, the prognosis will not only improve but also become better known, which will help give a greater measure of reality to the experience. It has been suggested that these operations may become less frightening when they become better known and more generally accepted. For example, serious psychiatric complications appear to have been more frequent with the early open-heart operations than later on.[4, 5] Of course, one cannot exclude that improved surgical technique and operative conditions also contributed to this.

One is reminded also of a procedure that for many years has been found useful in arranging the adoption of children, namely, keeping the donors anonymous. Similarly, much might be gained in cases of transplantation if the anonymity of the donor were carefully safeguarded whenever possible. This anonymity should extend not only to the personal circumstances of the donor, but also to his sex. The transplantation has a different significance, depending on whether donor and recipient are of the same or the opposite sex. One anticipates that this would reduce the complications engendered by guilt, resentment, and the need for gratitude. It might also tend to make the transplantation a less personal transaction (as with blood transfusions), thus, perhaps, decreasing the impact of regressive incorporative fantasies.

Finally, it may be useful to distinguish between *life-saving* and *life-extending* procedures. The former remove a diseased part and, if successful, permit the patient to achieve—completely or nearly completely—his normal, or allotted, life span. By contrast, the latter—regardless of their eventual outcome—carry the implication that the patient's life span has been extended beyond its normal limits. Here the patient's situation is not unlike that of the owner of an old car, who replaces its engine and then fancies that he has a *new* car. It involves, truly, the idea of a new lease on life. Life-saving operations, then, generally mean the loss of a part which is highly cathected, but, having become diseased (that is, "bad" or "waste"), has to be extruded and dispensed with. Psychologically, this means restricting the body image and gradually de-cathecting something previously valued and making non-ego out of what earlier was ego. That this is difficult to achieve is evidenced by the occurrence of postoperative depressions and in some cases (especially when the lost part was external and visible) by a stubborn retention of the part in fantasy, as occurs in phantoms. Instead, with life-extending operations, a part of the body—also highly cathected—is replaced with a similar part, usually from another human being. Something, in other words, is added. Psychologically, this means expanding the body image by incorporating into the ego what previously was nonego, a part object that at the most primitive level is ambivalently regarded as life-giving on the one hand and lethal on the other. This is the matrix in which one finds, besides depression, blissful euphoria or paranoid dread.

In sum, the most basic and interesting problems pertaining to survival, body image, and ego integrity appear to underlie the development of these new operations.

NOTE: The author is indebted to Dr. Richard J. Cleveland, Assistant Professor of Surgery, UCLA, and head of the Harbor General Hospital heart transplant team for his helpfulness and consideration, and to Miss Evangeline Dominguez, R.N., who spent much time with the patient, for her thoughtful observations.
The clinical work was supported in part by NIH grant No. HE–12490.

REFERENCES

1. Abram, H. S. "Adaptation to Open Heart Surgery: A Psychiatric Study of Response to the Threat of Death," *American Journal of Psychiatry*, **122** (1965), 659.
2. Blachy, P. H., and Starr, A. "Post-Cardiotomy Delirium," *American Journal of Psychiatry*, **121** (1964), 371.
3. Bliss, E. L., Rumel, W. R., and Hardin Branch, C. H. "Psychiatric Complications of Mitral Surgery," *AMA Archives of Neurology and Psychiatry*, **74** (1955), 249.
4. Burgess, G. N., Kirklin, J. W., and Steinhilber, R. M. "Some Psychiatric Aspects of Intracardiac Surgery," *Mayo Clinic Proceedings*, **42** (1967), 1.
5. Cramond, W. A. "Renal Homotransplantation—Some Observations on Recipients and Donors," *British Journal of Psychiatry*, **113** (1967), 1223.
6. Cramond, W. A., Court, J. H., Higgins, B. A., Knight, P. R., and Lawrence, J. R. "Psychological Screening of Potential Donors in a Renal Homotransplantation Programme," *British Journal of Psychiatry*, **113** (1967), 1213.
7. Cramond, W. A., Knight, P. R., and Lawrence, J. R. "The Psychiatric Contribution to a Renal Unit Undertaking Chronic Haemodialysis and Renal Homotransplantation," *British Journal of Psychiatry*, **113** (1967), 1201.
8. Egerton, N., and Kay, J. H. "Psychological Disturbances Associated with Open Heart Surgery," *British Journal of Psychiatry*, **110** (1964), 433.
9. Fox, H. M., Rizzo, N. D., and Gifford, S. "Psychological Observations of Patients Undergoing Mitral Surgery," *American Heart Journal*, **48** (1954), 645.
10. Harken, D. E. "One Surgeon Looks at Human Heart Transplantation," *Diseases of the Chest*, **54** (1968), 349.
11. Hazan, S. J. "Psychiatric Complications Following Cardiac Surgery: Part I. A Review Article," *Journal of Thoracic Cardiovascular Surgery*, **51** (1966), 307.
12. Hazan, S. J. "Psychiatric Complications Following Cardiac Surgery: Part II. A Working Hypothesis—The Chemical Approach." *Journal of Thoracic Cardiovascular Surgery*, **51** (1966), 320.
13. Jouravleff, N. "De la désacralisation ou allons-nous vers un canibalisme rénové?" *Presse Médicale*, **76** (1968), 333.
14. Kemph, J. P. "Psychotherapy with Patients Receiving Kidney Transplant," *American Journal of Psychiatry*, **124** (1967), 623.
15. Kennedy, J. A., and Bakst, J. "The Influence of Emotions on the Outcome of Cardiac

Surgery: A Predictive Study," *Bulletin of the NY Academy of Medicine,* **42** (1966), 811.
16. Kornfeld, D. S., Zimberg, S., and Malm, J. R. "Psychiatric Complications of Open-Heart Surgery," *New England Journal of Medicine,* **273** (1965), 287.
17. Kornfeld, D. S. "Psychiatric Complications of Cardiac Surgery," *International Psychiatric Clinic,* **4** (1967), 115.
18. Lunde, D. T. "Psychiatric Complications of Heart Transplants," paper presented at the 122d annual meeting of the American Psychiatric Association, Miami, Florida, May 7, 1969. Later published in *American Journal of Psychiatry,* **126** (1969), 369.
19. Nahum, L. H. "Madness in the Recovery Room from Open-Heart Surgery, or 'They Kept Waking Me Up,'" *Connecticut Medicine,* **29** (1965), 771.
20. Shambaugh, G. E., Jr. "Medical Ethics, Heart Transplantation and Otolaryngology," *Archives of Otolaryngology,* **87** (1968), 453.
21. Wilson, W. P., Stickel, D. L., Hayes, C. P., Jr., and Harris, N. L. "Psychiatric Considerations of Renal Transplantation," *Archives of Internal Medicine,* **122** (1968), 502.

LATE SYMPTOMATOLOGY AMONG FORMER CONCENTRATION CAMP INMATES

Paul Matussek

As the mass media brought the terrors of the German concentration camps to the attention of the world at the close of World War II, a scientific as well as a human interest arose for the fate of those persons who survived the camps. In an increasingly more active concern, the medical and, in particular, the neurological and psychiatric disciplines began a conscientious attempt to ascertain, describe, and explain the long-term physical and mental health problems wrought by this extraordinary stress experience, many of which problems persisted as many as five and ten years after the liberation. It is unfortunate that the otherwise comprehensive medical literature treating this problem used a variety of selection methods that seriously impaired the objectivity and generality of the findings and consequently the empirical foundation from which theoretical inferences could be drawn. A review of the literature revealed that in nearly every case the investigations were conducted either with the special populations of patients seeking medical treatment or applicants for indemnification. Earlier studies fell prey to three major sources of bias:

1. The investigator saw only patients, those survivors who sought medical attention, and did not examine the larger population of survivors who felt equally sick but did not seek treatment nor those survivors who were healthy.

2. The investigator saw only those patients who belonged to his particular medical specialty. Symptoms and complaints that fell

into other specialty areas received little and often no attention or recognition.

3. Investigators who examined applicants for the indemnification commissions could not determine to what extent the complaints they heard as well as those they attended to were influenced by the context and pressures of this special interviewing situation.

This investigation, the partial results of which are reported here, was designed to avoid the sources of selection bias discussed above and to provide answers to the following three issues: (1) How high is the percentage of persons among former concentration camp inmates who do not feel that their health has been impaired? What are their characteristics? (2) Are the symptoms mentioned in connection with reparations different from those mentioned in a scientifically oriented interview? (3) What disease patterns or dimensions can be ascertained from the complete somatic and psychic symptom picture with the use of factor analysis?

MATERIAL AND METHODLOGY*

Every thirtieth applicant for internment indemnification was selected from the files of the Regional Office for Indemnification. Because of this selection procedure, the resulting groups of religiously persecuted and emigrants (persons now living in Israel and New York) were too small. We therefore obtained several further names from other official sources as well as from former persecutees. The final sample of 155 persons was distributed in grounds for persecution and land of residence groups (see Table 1).

The subjects were interviewed in their homes during the years 1959–1963 by psychotherapeutically schooled and experienced psychologists and medical doctors (Cohen, Geröly, Halbach, Köhler, Mickans, Vardy). The average length of the interviews was five hours. Questioning concerning the contemporaneous physical and mental complaints comprised only a part of the

* Space limitations allowed for the presentation of only the most important methodological issues. A detailed methodological discussion can be found in our forthcoming publication in which the relationship between concentration camp incarceration and interpersonal contact, marriage, occupation, emigration, and Weltanschauung is also included.

TABLE 1

Grounds for Persecution	
Racially persecuted*	n = 113
Politically persecuted	n = 30
Religiously persecuted	n = 12
Land of Residency	
Germany	n = 120
Israel	n = 24
New York, U.S.A.	n = 11

* We have used the word "racially" because of its special application by the Nazis as a description of Jews, that is, for historical reasons alone.

interview. To satisfy our criteria and thus to have been included in the list of late disabilities, the complaint must have arisen five years after the liberation and have persisted for several years. The interviewer emphasized that the interview would not be made available to any official agencies and that it would not be possible for the interviewee to incorporate the interview into a medical report for private purposes.

In order to assure the reliability as well as the comprehensiveness of the complaints voiced in the interview, at least one, and, in most cases several, medical reports were used. In eleven cases no medical records were available, because these persons had not applied for compensation of illness and injuries.

NONAPPLICANTS FOR HEALTH COMPENSATION

In the case of eighteen former concentration camp inmates, it was possible to determine clearly that they had not applied for the compensation of illnesses and that they would in all probability not do so in the future. Because of the small size of this group and our inability to determine whether they were representative of the larger and unknown population of nonapplicants, we did not intend any general statements from our analysis of them. The results of this subgroup analysis should therefore be viewed within this restriction. Our justification for this analysis was that this special subgroup has received little attention in the previous literature.

Of the eighteen persons in this group, sixteen were racially persecuted emigrants and two were German priests living in Germany. In order to determine the degree to which these persons were disturbed by somatic and psychic disabilities, the voiced complaints are presented in Table 2.

TABLE 2

Absolute Number of Somatic and Psychic Complaints Mentioned by Nonindemnification Applicants in the Research Interview.

SOMATIC COMPLAINTS	ABSOLUTE NUMBER	
Dyspeptic	5	
Headaches	2	
Visual and auditory disturbances	2	
Spinal cord	3	
Rheumatic	1	
Gynecological	1	
Sterilization	1	$s = 15$
PSYCHIC COMPLAINTS		
Nightmares	6	
Nervousness, irritability	5	
Depressive moodiness	4	
Anxiety	3	
Memory disturbances	1	
Tiredness	1	$s = 20$

The complaint frequency contained showed that the nonapplicant subgroup was in no way free from complaints. Psychic complaints predominated over somatic ones. A comparison between the nonapplicants and the total sample found that the former averaged 0.9 somatic complaints and the latter 37 complaints, a substantial difference indicating that the nonapplicants were somatically healthier. In regard to psychic complaints, however, no differences between injury reparation applicants and nonapplicants could be found.

Of the eighteen nonapplicants, only four were free from both somatic and psychic complaints. The remaining fourteen nonapplicants produced a list of complaints sufficiently pronounced and serious to have secured an indemnification. The explanation of their reasons for not seeking an indemnification relied on an independent and psychologically bipolar motivational and behavioral pattern that was isolated in the general exploration of the attitudinal and emotional working-through process of the inmates' concentration camp experiences ("KZ Verarbeitung"). These poles have been named "living the role of the concentration camp inmate" and "denying the role of a concentration camp inmate."

Living the Role of the Concentration Camp Inmate

Characteristic of this person is his constant preoccupation with his past. Both the persecution and incarceration have become fundamental elements in his present self-concept and world outlook. In addition, he seeks such nontangible rewards as higher social standing in the community in the form of special consideration, concessions, and recognition. This group was composed of five persons. The priest belonging to this group is a good example of this pole.

In reply to the question concerning the usefulness and ability of financial indemnification to compensate for and to help the individual overcome the consequences of the concentration camps, one priest replied: "Money could never serve as an indemnification or compensation for me. I find even the application for this to be contradictory to the nature of the priesthood. I also consider the idea of being paid for one's sufferings to be basically false." Father S suffers from ulcers, depressive moodiness, nightmares, and nervousness. He considers all these symptoms to be consequences of his persecution and incarceration.

A fifty-six-year-old racially persecuted inmate gave the following reasons for his rejection of an application for health damages: "I will not take any blood money from the Germans, in any case, not until everyone has been compensated." During the persecution, he had been sterilized and suffered from dyspeptic complaints, depressive moodiness, nightmares, and nervousness.

The attitudes toward indemnification illustrated in the above two examples are characteristic for the working-through process variable "living the role of a concentration camp inmate." The financial compensation for health impairment is rejected in order to give greater weight, credence, and respectability to the claim for social acknowledgment. The portrayal of this role is so important to the person's self-respect that all forms of reliance or dependence on the former persecutors, that is, through medical examination, pension applications, and so forth, are avoided. The psychological stability of these persons is so limited that the application for a pension is experienced as an encroachment on their definition of themselves as former concentration camp inmates.

Denying the Role of the Concentration Camp Inmate

The remaining nonapplicants represented this pole. The comparative infrequency of this pole was explainable by the social needs of this group, which necessitated their acceptance by the larger community. Their replies to the question of the suitability of money as a compensation for their persecution and the ability of a financial compensation to aid in overcoming the consequences of the persecution illustrated this attitudinal pole.

A thirty-seven-year-old persecuted female inmate living in Israel reported no illnesses or disturbances with the exception of chronic migraine headaches. Although she denied having suffered any psychic effects from the persecution, she remarked that "one does not lose the memories." This statement and several others indicated that she has occasional nightmares. She made an overall tense impression. She appeared intent on removing all vestiges of her concentration camp past from her life. A second person, a thirty-five-year-old, also living in Israel, didn't believe that he could have obtained a pension nor did he make an effort to inquire into the matter. He expressed the opinion that the public pays too much attention to the sufferings of the concentration camp times. He said that this became evident during the Eichmann trial. Although he had dyspeptic complaints as well as depressive moodiness, he denied that his health had suffered in any way from the incarceration. He hardly thinks about these events any longer and avoids all newspaper articles dealing with this period.

On the basis of the above descriptions, it was assumed that these were not only persons who were unable to overcome their concentration camp past, but who also attempted to avoid any and all interest and notice of this subject from the outside world. Although they were both somatically and psychically impaired, they made no effort to receive compensation. Their energies were devoted to repressing their past. The tiring and strenuous procedure of filing for compensation would endanger the attempt, undertaken with great strain, to achieve a workable psychic stability.

In summary, the percentage of nonapplicants in our sample was small. Although the nonapplicant subgroup was healthier somatically, it was not psychically healthier. The rejection of an application for financial compensation was not a consequence of minimal illness, but rather a consequence of the particular motivational and attitude patterns that have been defined as "living the role of the concentration camp inmate" and "denying the role of a concentration camp inmate."

THE INFLUENCE OF THE COMPENSATION-ORIENTED EXAMINATION FOR THE INVESTIGATION OF CONCENTRATION CAMP RELATED COMPLAINTS

Von Baeyer, Häfner, and Kisker, in their review of the literature on the late effects of concentration camp incarceration,[16] reported a level of disagreement among the different investigators that is hard to explain. Although one would assume that the varied times of investigation, the varied patient populations, as well as the varied techniques used are partly responsible, this did not seem to be an adequate explanation for all the discrepancies. It was our opinion that the kind of interview situation itself and its purposes were also elements that determine the complaints that were voiced and registered. The interviewee orients himself to the situation and reports not only those symptoms that he feels he possesses but those that would interest a surgeon, a psychiatrist, or an internist. Similarly, the complaints voiced and emphasized in an interview for financial compensation are likely to be different from those declared in a scientifically oriented interview. This assumption, which Matussek[10] called "the coercion to symptom suitability," was tested in this investigation by comparing the complaint type and frequency patterns noted in the compensation as opposed to the scientifically oriented interviews. In both situations, the interviewer clearly stated his interest in all kinds of complaints. We have intentionally pursued this question with the complaints themselves rather than diagnoses, owning to the

TABLE 3

Absolute Frequencies of Somatic Complaints in Two Interview Situations for 106 Male and 38 Female Concentration Camp Victims.

COMPLAINT CATEGORIES	FREQUENCY IN MEDICAL INTERVIEW	FREQUENCY IN SCIENTIFIC INTERVIEW	SIGNIFICANCE LEVEL*
Vegetative	86 (59.7%)	48 (33.7%)	.01%
Dental	53 (36.8%)	19 (13.3%)	.01%
Rheumatic	48 (33.7%)	24 (16.8%)	.1 %
Heart–circulatory	95 (66.0%)	68 (47.2%)	.1 %
Head	64 (44.4%)	42 (29.3%)	.1 %
Liver–gall bladder	35 (24.3%)	16 (11.2%)	.1 %
Urological	24 (16.8%)	8 (5.6%)	.1 %
Back injuries	48 (33.7%)	30 (20.8%)	.5 %
Visual and auditory	35 (24.3%)	21 (14.1%)	.5 %
Lungs–bronchial	57 (39.6%)	41 (28.7%)	.5 %
Internal	27 (18.7%)	13 (9.1%)	.5 %
Stomach	61 (42.6%)	50 (34.8%)	—
Angina pectoris	29 (20.1%)	20 (13.9%)	—
Complaints from concentration camp injuries	22 (15.3%)	19 (13.3%)	—
Neurological	11 (7.6%)	8 (5.6%)	—
Chronic angina neck complaints	9 (6.3%)	0 (0 %)	—
Bleeding from frost wounds	5 (3.5%)	4 (2.8%)	—
Dermatological	1 (0.7%)	0 (0 %)	—
Gynecological	14 (37.8%)	10 (27.0%)	—

* The significance levels reported here were obtained with a 2 x 2 chi-square analysis.

frequency of conflicting diagnoses stemming from identical symptomatologies. The complaint list was a more objective foundation for the comparison and also served subsequently as a diagnostic framework.

Tables 3 and 4 present the somatic and psychic complaints registered by doctors serving the indemnification commission and interviewers working on this project ($n = 144$).* These tables showed that substantially fewer somatic complaints were mentioned in the scientific interview. In nine of the nineteen complaint categories, the difference was statistically significant. This result was primarily owing to the great emphasis placed on so-

* The medical reports that accompanied the case records from the indemnification commission were obtained in the compensation interview. Our material was collected in the scientific interview.

TABLE 4

Absolute Frequencies of Psychic Complaints in Two Interview Situations for 106 Male and 38 Female Concentration Camp Victims.

COMPLAINT CATEGORY	FREQUENCY IN MEDICAL INTERVIEW	FREQUENCY IN SCIENTIFIC INTERVIEW	SIGNIFICANCE LEVEL
Mistrust–shyness, contact disturbances	6 (4.2%)	62 (43.4%)	.01%
Feeling of isolation	2 (1.4%)	54 (37.8%)	.01%
Nightmares	28 (19.4%)	75 (52.5%)	.01%
Hate feelings	0 (0 %)	31 (21.6%)	.01%
Paranoid tendencies	1 (0.7%)	21 (14.7%)	.01%
Irritability and internal unrest	41 (28.5%)	72 (50.2%)	.01%
Depressive moodiness	43 (29.9%)	61 (42.6%)	.5 %
Sleep disturbances	45 (31.3%)	46 (32.2%)	—
Anxiety	29 (20.1%)	33 (22.9%)	—
Memory and concentration impairment	32 (22.2%)	39 (27.3%)	—
Tiredness and apathy	30 (20.8%)	36 (25.2%)	—
Vitality disturbances	11 (7.6%)	9 (6.3%)	—
Suicidal thoughts	6 (4.2%)	5 (3.5%)	—

matic complaints in the compensation interview. The indemnification commission was concerned with somatic and not with psychic injury. In the scientific interview, the somatic complaints were not described as often or as comprehensively.

The scientific interview, having been conducted by psychotherapeutically experienced personnel and having shown a greater interest for both the general welfare and psychological problems of the interviewee, obtained a substantially higher frequency of psychological complaints. The only psychic complaints mentioned with equal frequency in both interview situations were those directly connected with physical injuries, such as tiredness, apathy, concentration, and memory disturbances.

Striking by comparison was the fact that seven complaint categories were recorded statistically more frequently during the scientific interview. Particularly illustrative of the effects of different interview situations was the finding that whereas 21.6 per cent of the interviewees mentioned hate feelings in the scientific interview, such remarks were either not made or not registered in the compensation interview. Though one might want to discredit the significance of hate feelings in the shaping of clinically relevant symptoms, such a view would simultaneously neglect its possible correlation to other psychic symptoms, such as mistrust and shyness, as well as overlook the significance of situational cues in eliciting clinically relevant material. It would seem that if this view were taken, an essential factor in the attainment of a complete understanding of the symptom picture[16] would be overlooked.

This becomes clearer when the scientific and psychiatric interview situations are compared.* It was assumed that of all the medical exploration settings mentioned so far, the psychiatric interview approximated our scientific interview most closely. Nevertheless, it was found that the four following symptoms were voiced substantially more often in the scientific interview: mistrust, shyness, disturbances in interpersonal contact ($\chi^2 = 2.88$, 10 per cent); feelings of isolation ($\chi^2 = 8.73$, 1 per cent); paranoid references ($\chi^2 = 3.44$, 10 per cent); and hatred ($\chi^2 = 6.64$, 1 per cent). This comparison provided an additional confirmation for the assumption that the interview setting can and does have a pronounced effect on behavior of the interviewee. The former concentration camp inmate did not feel comfortable enough before the doctors representing the indemnification commission to uninhibitedly report the changes in his personality since his concentration camp incarceration. How many applicants found the examining doctors, particularly the German doctors, to be so objective and understanding that they could express their mistrust and hatred, which included the doctors, and in a situation in which they wanted something from the doctor, namely, that he write a report that would advance their compensation claims for health damages?

In summary, the kind and frequency of disturbances voiced in a medical interview situation depends on the purpose of the investigation, the questions asked, and the orientation of the doctors. In order to gain a fuller perspective of the late effects of concentration camp incarceration, this influence must be considered. The insufficient control and consideration of interview setting effects in the earlier literature is a further reason for the inconsistency of the research findings in this area.

---

* Forty-four persons had also been examined by psychiatrists working for the indemnification commission. The symptoms registered in the psychiatric interviews were compared with those from our scientific interview.

FACTOR ANALYTIC INVESTIGATION OF ALL PSYCHIC AND SOMATIC COMPLAINTS IN TWO DIFFERENT INTERVIEW SITUATIONS

The earlier literature has shown that there are nearly no medical problems or diagnoses that have not been found among former concentration camp inmates and classified as late effects. In the neurological-psychiatric field, in which the largest literature on this subject is to be found, the question arose as to the suitability of the usual diagnostic categories for the classification of symptoms. This literature contains two contrary points of view. On the one side are the proponents of the standpoint that all symptoms arising in the postliberation period can be understood within the traditional psychiatric-neurological diagnostic system.[1, 8, 9, 10, 14] The opposing standpoint has emphasized the uniqueness of the postliberation symptomatology among former concentration camp inmates and the necessity of developing a special nomenclature to describe it. The authors taking this position have coined such term as "concentration camp syndrome,"[5, 7] "the asthenia syndrome among deportees,"[15] "asthénie postconcentrationaire et troubles psychiques,"[13] and "concentration camp neurosis."[3] These authors do not contest the fact that other illnesses besides the concentration camp specific illnesses are also present. However, they imply that the more familiar illnesses among former concentration camp inmates are of less significance than the typical concentration camp illnesses and are consequently of peripheral rather than central importance.

The earlier literature has not been able to settle this dispute. The situational aspects of the investigations, the times at which they were undertaken, and the special interests of the researcher were much too variable to have offered comparable material. The evaluation of the symptomatology by specialists in different disciplines also caused the somatic and psychic complaints to be considered separately. Consequently, it was not possible to decide as to the relative importance of the somatic and psychic complaints. In addition, the preferred methodology among these investigators was clinical judgment, an unreliable and heavily biased procedure, which not only lacked objectivity but was incapable of getting beneath the external symptomatology to examine the illness dimensions that lay at the heart of the matter. The major question in this regard was whether there are one or several illness dimensions and whether they are psychic, organic, or psychosomatic.

To answer this question, we used a factor analysis of all the psychic and somatic complaints recorded in the scientific and compensation interviews. The demographic variables "age" and "sex" were included as control variables. In this way, it was possible to isolate age and sex-specific illness dimensions. The inclusion of other demographic variables was judged as unproductive as previous factor analyses of clinical data showed that the resulting factors were too heavily laden with nonclinical variables. In other words, in order not to obscure the relevance of clinical symptoms, only the demographic variables "age" and "sex" were included in the factor analyses. All remaining demographic and psychological variables as well as the objective stress data were analyzed with correlational and chi-square methods. The results of these computations cannot be discussed in this context because of space limitations, but are presented in our forthcoming monograph.

The factor analysis, in addition to age and sex, took account of fourteen somatic and twelve psychic complaint categories that met the statistical criterion of having been registered in at least 20 per cent of all interviewees. The $n = 144$, with 106 men and 38 women.

The factor extractions from the correlation matrix used the principal axis procedure.[6] The Varimax principal rotation provided a four-factor structure as most plausible. (See Table 5.)

TABLE 5

		RELATIVE PERCENTAGES OF VARIANCE
Factor 1	Psychosomatic syndrome (state of exhaustion)	.32
Factor 2	Gynecological illness	.26
Factor 3	Internal illness	.22
Factor 4	Psychic syndrome (mistrust)	.21

Factor 1: Psychosomatic Syndrome

The symptoms comprising this factor and their respective loadings were:

Head complaints	.61
Memory and concentration disturbances	.58
Tiredness, apathy	.56
Depressive moodiness	.53
Nightmares	.49
Sleep disturbances (insomnia)	.49
Irritability, internal disquiet	.39
Vegetative disturbances	.38
Vital disturbances	.38

Among the four factors derived from the factor analysis, factor 1 possessed the greatest similarity to the symptom complex described in the literature under a variety of names, such as the typical syndrome among former concentration camp inmates. The previous literature has also demonstrated the fruitlessness of disputing the name of the syndrome. A uniform nomenclature is not to be expected nor even a relative agreement concerning the symptomatology itself. Different investigators will undoubtedly continue to offer different opinions reflecting their personal, educational, and disciplinary experience and outlook.

For these reasons and also because factor 1 is not comparable to any of the clinical syndromes mentioned in the literature, we have refrained from labeling factor 1 with any of the designations previously used. Had we relied on earlier designations, we would have cast suspicion on our own methodology by suggesting the similarity or even the correspondence between our factor analytically derived syndromes and those put forth on the weight of clinical judgment alone. Had this been done, we would have sacrificed an opportunity to infer etiological relationships through the unjustified attention to superficial symptoms, which receive the aura of etiological relevance by being replaced by obstruse clinical terminus.[1] For these reasons, we preferred the label "psychosomatic syndrome" for factor 1. The factor is composed of both psychic and somatic complaints. However, it does not contain any special psychosomatic illnesses, such as ulcers.[2] The designation "psychosomatic syndrome" also took account of the composition of the other factors that were either purely somatic factor 2 (gynecological illness), factor 3 (internal illness), or a purely psychic illness, factor 4 (psychic syndrome).

The label "psychosomatic syndrome" was not only justifiable by the combination of psychic and somatic complaints it contains. It also had to offer evidence that a psychogenic component was operative in the emergence of this condition. In this regard, psychogenic is not to be interpreted as "imaginary" or "manipulatable," but rather as a primarily unconscious, personality specific form of the working-through process for particular kinds of problems. In other words, the working-through process of the sufferings incurred in the concentration camp is dependent not only on the actual conditions of the incarceration that precipitated the psychogenic problems, but also on the individual's past history of problem-solving as well as the contemporary situations with their specific psychological challenges in the family, on the job, and in social relations. Each former concentration camp inmate developed an individualistic form of response to the concentration camps. This reaction pattern cannot be properly explained by either the traditional model of trauma adaption or Selye's stress theory.[1]

This assumption was strengthened by the finding that nightmares were contained among the symptoms in factor 1, but not anxiety during the waking hours. Theoretically, one might have expected the reverse. However, because nightmares prevailed over daytime anxiety, it was possible to conclude that particular problems may be worked through in the unconscious rather than in the conscious state. It is therefore not surprising that the so-called concentration camp nightmares are not always connected with experiences stemming from the German concentration camps but also with communist concentration camps. A communist, who experienced the socialist countries and Russia as a paradise of freedom and also experienced the terrors of the German concentration camp on his own body, finds himself a captive in a Russian concentration camp in his dreams. We assumed on the basis of this experience that the terror situation in dreams is not only connected with the real experience of the past but also with a great number of unconscious determinants of the contemporary situation. In psychodynamic terms, the events of the persecution and tortures, insofar as they appear in the relatively frequent symptoms of concentration camp dreams, are not simple repetitions of these experiences. They use components of the concentration camp period as well as contemporary experience.

Once these implications have been fully realized, the symptomatology of factor 1 would then be viewed in a not typical fashion. Hermann and Thygesen,[7] Eitinger,[5] and others attribute the symptom picture, which one would most probably describe as a depressively colored state of exhaustion, exclusively to the cerebral injuries resulting from the concentration camp incarceration. This assumption was not confirmed by the majority of investigators, even those who undertook their research at the same time as Eitinger.[5] Von Baeyer et al.[1] have offered further evidence contradicting the assumption that a neurological injury lies at the root of this symptom complex, for example, the fact that in comparing their group of former concentration camp inmates with young draftees between nineteen and twenty-one years of age, there was no difference between these populations in the incidence of the state of exhaustion symptom.

We inferred, therefore, that the symptoms in factor 1 were connected with both the incarceration and the contemporary life situation. It was consequently not surprising that in our sample of former concentration camp inmates some interviewees suffered more seriously from these symptoms than did others. We found that Jews of prewar Polish nationality (1 per cent) and those inmates less than thirty years of age in 1945 (1 per cent) as well as the racially persecuted (5 per cent) were more frequently suffering from the symptoms in factor 1 than the remaining subjects in our sample.*

The frequency with which the psychosomatic syndrome appeared in our sample as well as the number of psychosomatic symptoms found in each subject are shown in Figure 1.

The distribution shows that this symptom complex, which of the four factors has the greatest similarity to those symptoms that

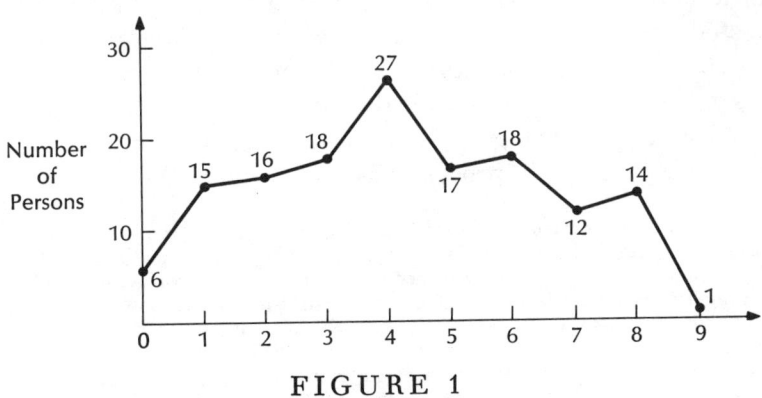

FIGURE 1

Frequency distribution for the nine complaint categories contained in factor 1, among 144 former concentration camp inmates.

* These differences are discussed at length in our forthcoming publication and were mentioned in this context only for illustrative purposes.

have been described as typical concentration camp injuries, does not arise nearly as often as is usually assumed. Only one person possessed all nine complaint categories. A further six persons possessed none of these symptoms. The most frequent complaint combinations, 7, 8, and 9, were found among twenty-seven, or 18.8 per cent, of the sample, and the combinations of 1, 2, and 3 symptoms were found among forty-nine subjects, or 34 per cent of the sample.

The number of symptoms, which in factor 1 means the number of complaints expressed by the subject in the interview, is neither to be confused with symptoms objectively assessed by a doctor nor a measure of severity of illness. A person with only headaches can be more seriously ill than someone with a variety of complaints. However, the frequency of complaints in Figure 1, which approaches a normal curve, shows that the often-described factor concentration camp syndrome in a more fastidiously selected sample is an exception rather than a rule.

Factor 2: Gynecological Illness

This factor was represented primarily by the variable "gynecological complaints" and indicated that a sex-specific illness was present among former concentration camp inmates.* The appearance of gynecological complaints as an independent symptom pattern deserves special attention. It was distinctly plausible to have expected the appearance of other sex-specific factors. Men might have reacted with heart disease or women with migraine headaches rather than with genital disturbances. The fact that women reacted with gynecological complaints strongly indicated that in the working-through process among women the appearance of

* The factor "gynecological complaints" was in fact composed of three highly intercorrelated variables: "female sex" (.79), "gynecological complaints" (.76), and "no dental complaints" (.44). The relevance of the first and last variables requires an explanation. The presence of the variable "female sex" in this factor was a redundant and self-evident relationship. Aside from saying the obvious, namely, that gynecological complaints are specifically female concerns, the loading of .79 indicates that being female does not necessitate the presence of gynecological problems. The third variable, "no dental complaints," which at first glance must strike the reader as an unusual correlate, was in fact a further confirmation of the sex-specific nature of factor 2 although in no way related to or seen as a supplement to the gynecological symptom complex. The relationship of no dental complaints among women and frequent dental complaints among men most probably stems from the generally harder camp conditions experienced by male inmates as well as the greater frequency of abuse and head injuries suffered by the male inmate. As such, the variable "no dental complaints" is at best a negative indicator of sex specificity.

gynecological disturbances predominated over all other symptom forms. This finding justified the inference that the predominant form in which women reacted to the extreme stress of the concentration camp was through disturbances of their sexual functions. The earlier literature documented the short-term, sex-specific reaction of women under the emotional and physical pressures of the camp situation citing the high incidence of the amenorrhea. However, this early and often-repeated finding failed to indicate that what seemed to be a short-term sexual malfunction in the immediate postwar years developed in many cases into a permanently irreparable disability. The significance of this illness is also readable from its frequency. The fact that the gynecologist Döring[3] found that seventy-four of seventy-nine former female inmates examined by him during the years 1958–1961 suffered from gynecological disturbances was in part a product of his medical specialty. That seventeen, or 47 per cent, of thirty-eight women examined in a nonbiased sample also complained of gynecological disturbances underscored the fact that women react primarily with disturbances of their sexual functions rather than with other kinds of health problems.

Factor 3: Internal Illness

This factor was composed of the following complaint areas:

Heart-circulatory disturbances	.62
Liver-gall bladder disturbances	.56
Lungs-bronchial disturbances	.50
Older persons (1960, more than forty-five years of age)	.47

Factor 3 also consists exclusively of somatic complaints. The possible role of psychic components in the development of this symptom complex was not apparent. The subjects complained of physical illnesses that the examining doctor in the compensation interview was able to corroborate. The two characteristics of this syndrome deserving special attention were that it dealt with internal illnesses and that it possessed an age-specific component.

In relation to the specific illnesses themselves, it was found that there was a connection between heart-circulatory and lung-bronchial disturbances and age, as well as between heart-circulatory and liver-gall bladder complaints, but not a high correlation between liver-gall bladder and lung-bronchial complaints and age. It was also worth noting that no other internal somatic illnesses, for example, ulcers and high blood pressure, appeared as illness syndromes in our analysis of all somatic and psychic complaints.

The age specificity of factor 3 lay in the finding that this symptom constellation appeared more frequently with advancing age. One could find a parallel here with the sex specific factor 2.

The distribution of the complaints within the entire sample is shown in Figure 2. The extremes of no symptoms and all four

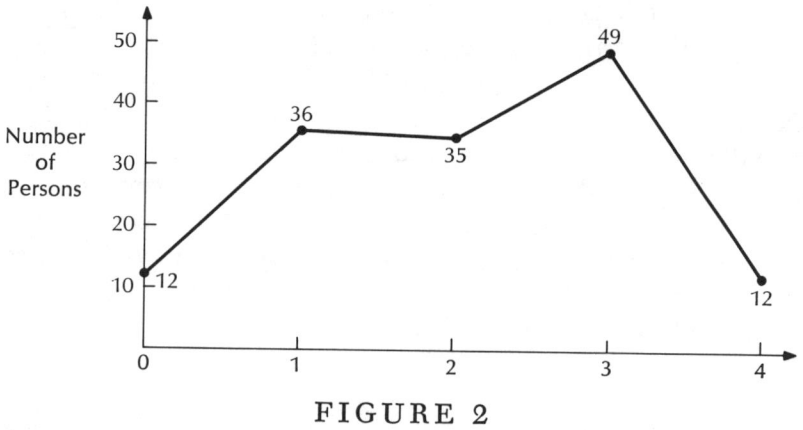

FIGURE 2

Frequency distribution of four complaint categories of factor 3 among 144 former concentration camp inmates.

symptoms appeared with equal frequency, with twelve subjects mentioning none of these complaints and twelve all four. The most frequent symptom combination, three, was represented by forty-nine persons or 34.0 per cent of the sample. In terms of the relative significance of this symptom complex, it is clear that internal illnesses do not occupy a less important position among the illnesses found among former concentration camp inmates than the so-called typical concentration camp syndrome.

Factor 4: The Psychic Syndrome (Mistrust)

The complaints appearing in this factor were

Mistrust	.65
Feeling of isolation	.48
Paranoid ideas	.48

In contrast to the three previous illness factors, factor 4 was composed exclusively of psychic symptoms. This could be called a "social illness" as it contains variables that deal with the relationship between the individual and his fellow men. Mistrust correlated with the feeling of isolation and with paranoid ideas. However, the relation between feeling of isolation and paranoid ideas was not significant. These two variables, which were independent, grouped around the symptom "mistrust."

In the evaluation of the significance of mistrust for the contemporary situation of former concentration camp inmates, it would be easy to overlook a highly relevant clinical aspect of this syndrome. Matussek[11, 12] and Von Baeyer et al.[1] have discussed the significance of the mistrust as a permanent symptom of the concentration camp oppression. From our factor analysis, it can be assumed that the symptom "mistrust" appears in two different forms. One person is mistrustful, particularly in contact with Germans, because, for example, he has the ever-present suspicion that there is likely to be a Nazi murderer among a group of pedestrians and consequently avoids such anonymous encounters through social isolation. This condition is often accompanied by paranoid ideas. Another person is also mistrustful, distances himself from social contacts, but does not react with paranoid tendencies in his self-chosen isolation. These possibilities represent a plausible, statistically secure relationship and as such are in no

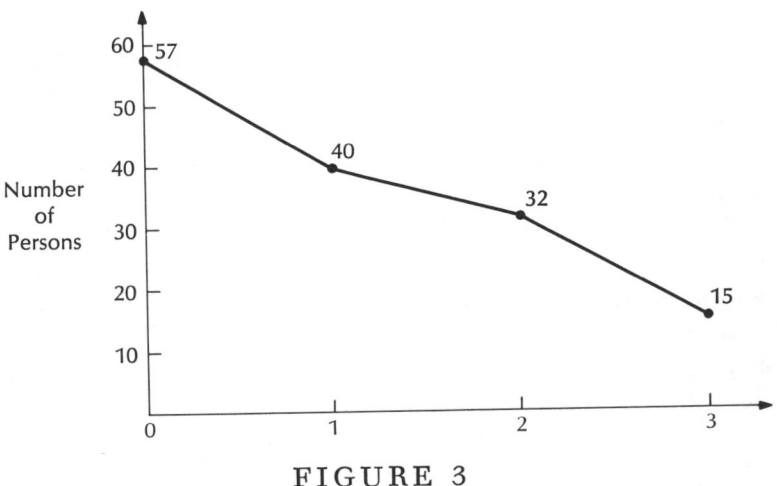

FIGURE 3

Frequency distribution for three complaint categories of factor 4 among 144 former concentration camp inmates.

way necessarily valid for any particular person. Mistrust and paranoid tendencies can also be related in other ways.

The essential aspect of this factor was that it emerged as an independent illness syndrome from the complete picture of physical and psychological complaints. The strongly emphasized experience-reactive disturbances of the incarceration by Venzlaff[15] and Von Baeyer et al.[1] has received confirmation in our investigation. Mistrust played the central role in this syndrome. The distribution of the symptoms in the sample is shown in Figure 3. No symptoms were found among fifty-seven subjects (39.6 per cent), one symptom among forty subjects (27.7 per cent), and two or more symptoms among forty-seven subjects (32.6 per cent).

SUMMARY

1. The percentage of persons who were able to come through the terrors of the German concentration camps without damage to their health was very small in our material. Even those persons who made no compensation claims were not completely healthy. They decided to do without indemnification because of a special set of motivations concerning their identity as former concentration camp inmates.

2. The disunity in the findings of the earlier literature on the late effects of concentration camp incarceration was owing to the peculiarities of the investigating situation and its influence on the types of complaints communicated in particular contexts. The comparison in this study between the complaints voiced in a compensation and scientific interview showed substantial and statistically significant differences in many symptom categories.

3. The factor analysis of all somatic and psychic complaints voiced and recorded in two different types of exploration interviews provided four illness dimensions—one psychosomatic, one gynecological, one internal, and one psychic. The assumption, stressed in the earlier literature, that one definite syndrome is typical among former concentration camp inmates could not be supported by our findings. Two factors, the gynecological and the internal, were respectively sex and age specific.

The illness dimensions discussed in this chapter supplement the existing literature in that for the first time it has been possible to discuss the structural relationships among complaints. However, it should not be forgotten that the results of this study must also be viewed within the context of this particular sample and our methodology. The heterogeneity of the methodologies involved as well as the different times of investigation restrict the generality of these findings.

The relationship among the four illness dimensions to the stress experiences of the persecution period as well as to the demographic and psychological variables of the pre-persecution period has not been discussed here. These issues have been presented in detail in our forthcoming book. It was possible to show statistically that the intensity and extent of the stress conditions during the persecution and particularly within the concentration camps were primarily responsible for the development of the illnesses discussed. In addition, but of secondary etiological significance, were the psychological and sociological characteristics of the inmates dating from the period prior to the persecution and incarceration. These variables were more closely responsible for the particular form and relative success of the largely psychological working-through process of the stress experiences.

In the interpretation of the possible connections between stress experiences and health injury, we have consciously avoided all theoretical models proposed to date. None of them, neither the concept of the traumatic neurosis nor the various stress theories, was capable of tying our findings together in a systematic and convincing way.

REFERENCES

1. Baeyer, W. von, Häfner, H., and Kisker, K. P. *Psychiatrie der Verfolgten*. Berlin: Springer, 1964.
2. Bastiaans, J. *Psychosomatische gevolgen van onderdrukking en verzet*. Amsterdam: Noord-Hollandsche Uitgevers Maatschappij, 1957.
3. Bensheim, H. "Die KZ-Neurose rassisch Verfolgter. Ein Beitrag zur Psychopathologie der Neurosen," *Nervenarzt*, 31 (1960), 462–469.
4. Döring, G. K. "Spezifische Spätschäden der weiblichen Psyche durch die politische Verfolgung," in H. Paul and H. J. Herberg (eds.), *Psychische Spätschäden nach politischer Verfolgung*. New York: Karger, 1967. Vol. 2.
5. Eitinger, L. "Pathology of the Concentration Camp Syndrome," *Archives of General Psychiatry*, 5 (1961), 371–379.
6. Harmann, H. H. *Modern Factor Analysis*. Chicago: University of Chicago Press, 1960.
7. Hermann, K., and Thygesen, P. "KZ-syndromet," *Ugeskr. für Laeg.*, 116 (1954), 825–836.
8. Kluge, E. "Über die Folge schwerer Haftzeiten," *Nervenarzt*, 29 (1958), 462–465.

9. Kolle, K. "Die Opfer der nationalsozialistischen Verfolgung in psychiatrischer Sicht," *Nervenarzt*, **29** (1958), 148–158.
10. Levinger, L. "Psychiatrische Untersuchungen in Israel an 800 Fällen mit Gesundheitsschaden-Forderungen wegen Nazi-Verfolgung," *Nervenarzt*, **33** (1962), 75–80.
11. Matussek, P. "Die Konzentrationslagerhaft als Belastungssituation," *Nervenarzt*, **32** (1961), 538–542.
12. Matussek, P. "Die Rückgliederung von Verfolgten—die Bewältigung ihres Schicksals," *Therapiewoche*, **13** (1963), 1109–1113.
13. Segelle, P., and Ellenbogen, R. in C. Richet and A. Mans (eds.), *Pathologie de la Deportation*. Cannes: l'Imprimerie Aegitna, 1958.
14. Strauss, H. "Besonderheiten der nicht-psychotischen Störungen bei Opfern der national-sozialistischen Verfolgung und ihre Bedeutung bei der Begutachtung," *Nervenarzt*, **28** (1957), 344–350.
15. Targowla, R. "Syndrom der Asthenie der Deportierten," in M. Michel (ed.), *Gesundheitsschäden durch Verfolgung und Gefangenschaft und ihre Spätfolgen*. Frankfurt-am-Main: Röderberg, 1955.
16. Venzlaff, U. *Die psychoreaktiven Störungen nach entschädigungspflichtigen Ereignissen*. Berlin: Springer, 1958.

PART THREE

Psychiatric Studies of Childhood and Youth

A PSYCHOTHERAPEUTIC CONSULTATION IN CHILD PSYCHIATRY: A COMPARATIVE STUDY OF THE DYNAMIC PROCESSES

D. W. Winnicott

My aim is to give an exact account of a psychotherapeutic consultation with a child to illustrate the work that can be done in one interview. In order that this work may be done, the circumstances of the case need to be favorable, but not more favorable than they are in the vast majority of cases that come to a psychiatrist for help. When clinics develop waiting lists, it is the difficult cases that push themselves forward, with the result that the work becomes oriented to the difficult cases and there is then no room for the common, amenable disorder. Were it not for the children of our colleagues, who gain priority not through clinical urgency but through our relationships to one another, we might almost forget the existence of the amenable case.

The psychiatrist who wishes to train to do psychotherapy must learn his technique thoroughly. The details of such a training can be studied in the prospectus of any of the psychoanalytic training centers. The basis of such training, apart from the study of theory, is the analysis of children under supervision. Usually, the work is undertaken on the basis of five interviews a week, which is the nearest possibility to a daily session. Such treatments certainly go very deep, and when they are successful they produce lasting and favorable changes. These changes are in the direction of emotional development according to the inherited potential of the individual, and according to the environmental provision that has been a feature and that may be expected to be a feature in the child's immediate future. The aim in psychoanalysis is to release the patient from hold-ups and blocks in emotional development. The treatment does not produce health; but when it works well, it does facilitate healthy development.

One thing is certain. If the student analyst has a student's mind, then he or she learns a great deal from each such case. After the training in psychoanalysis, the analyst works in a clinic or in private and then finds that adaptation must be made according to the ability of those who care for the child to comply with what is needed optimally. It often happens that a one-session-a-week treatment is the best that can be arranged, and good work can be done by this arrangement in certain cases. There are other forms of therapy, such as play therapy and group therapy, and the analyst who has been trained in analysis needs to be able to bring what he knows from the intensive daily treatment of one child to whatever kind of treatment is appropriate in the circumstances of any one case.

EXPLOITATION OF THE FIRST INTERVIEW

In my own work, in which I have had to adapt my technique learned in the psychoanalytic school to the treatment of cases of all kinds, I have had one big surprise, and it is this that I wish to report and to illustrate: in the first interview with a child, that which might be called a diagnostic interview, a deep-going therapy can be extremely effective. Whatever the theory of such a treatment, the fact remains that a great deal of opportunity for giving treatment is wasted by the therapist's fear of going deep quickly. In other words, the caution it is proper to exert at the beginning of a psychoanalytic treatment may seriously hamper the therapist who has an opportunity of seeing a child only once or perhaps in a run of a few sessions spread over months. Though I remain convinced that the right training for this work is the psychoanalytic training, I find it important to draw the attention of those who are so trained to the work that they can do in one session, if they will study the necessary modifications in technique.

A certain amount of hostility to this work may arise from various sources; for instance, the psychologist in a team may feel left out because it is important not to queer the pitch of the therapist by an insistence on an initial intelligence test or a personality assessment. Also, the social worker may feel that the social work on the case is by-passed. I have often adopted the procedure in my clinic of inviting one or two social workers to be present during the psychotherapeutic interview, the result of this being not only that the social worker feels included in the case, but also that there is no need to report to the social worker what has happened. This leaves time for discussion on the basis of the experience that has been shared. Owing to the fact that it is not possible to predict exactly which case will respond to this kind of psychotherapy, the way needs to be kept open for any one case to turn into an ordinary case in which the entire clinic team participates, each member of the team contributing to a general build-up of an understanding of the total problem.

In predicting, it is best to take it as axiomatic that the child who is to be helped in this way is able to go home from the therapeutic consultation to a satisfactory environment. No high standard of satisfactoriness need be assumed; it is simply that, in the type of case that can benefit from the kind of work that I am describing, the family situation needs to be such that a good-enough environment can be provided if the child becomes able to make use of it. In other words, in a fairly good home setting, a child is distressed because of personal conflicts, and these conflicts make it impossible for the family to perform its function properly or fully.

It should be noted that it is not a question of looking for cases in which the child's illness is slight. The symptomatology may be noisy and blatant, and indeed one gets to learn that the silent hidden illness is particularly difficult to treat quickly because the silence implies that the child knows that the family cannot tolerate personal conflict and the difficulties that belong to emotional development. In this way, a child who is quite normal except for bed-wetting may be much more difficult to help than a child who is destructive, is stealing, or is ill-treating his brother as in the case that I wish to describe.

In order to illustrate my thesis, I must describe a case. It will be clearly seen that there is an advantage for teaching purposes in having this kind of case to present to students. In describing a case under psychoanalysis, so much has to be omitted in any description that the student may become suspicious lest what is not being told should be more important than what is being reported. In this kind of case, it is possible to describe to the student all that one knows of the case, with the result that discussion starts on a fair basis.

The inherent disadvantage that follows from giving a case in illustration is that there is only room in this chapter for this one case. It is necessary for me to make it clear that each case stands alone. The student of this kind of work may study other cases that I have published, and such a study will show that the technique does not implant a pattern on the case and that no two cases are alike. Unfortunately, these publications are scattered in the literature, but an attempt is being made to publish a group in one book. (See the References at the end of the chapter.)

What follows is the description of one therapeutic consultation. The result in this case was satisfactory in terms of the clinical picture. I do not claim that the child was cured of an illness; nevertheless, a child who is released from blockages in emotional development goes home from the consultation to a changed world. The various members of the household find themselves with a child who is released and who can use them more freely, and they behave differently toward the child. In a way, it is they who do the cure or what there is of a cure in the course of the subsequent weeks and months, although without the therapeutic consultation, they would not have been able to do this, but would have remained available but unused.

CASE OF M

Family History

M is an eight-year-old boy. His siblings include six-year-old twins—a boy and a girl—and a four-year-old girl.

The mother of this boy wrote me a letter in which she stated the problem as seen from her point of view. The main trouble as she saw it was that M, who was the eldest child, had never really accepted the arrival of a twin brother and sister, who were born when he was two years old. She wrote: "Their birth threw him into utter turmoil that manifested itself in many obvious and wretched ways. He is heavily dependent on me and involved with me." There were certain other pathological features, such as a predilection for sadomasochistic situations and the beginnings of a pleasure in the idea of whipping. Also, he showed a potential for perverted tendencies such as a compulsion to look at and to feel girls' pants. Though he tended to be bullying and aggressive at home, he was on the whole placatory and nervous at school, and not very popular. In his school work, he was doing well, showing a special interest in history and English. The mother added that she had had some treatment herself and that, although this had enabled her to deal better than previously with the other children, her improvement had not made a difference to the tendencies in M that she was reporting.

The Session

The parents brought M to the therapeutic consultation. After a few minutes in which we all talked together, they retired to the waiting room and patiently waited the one and one-quarter hours that elapsed before M finished his contact with me. They had to go home without having a talk with me, but I had warned them of this. Several weeks later, I saw the parents together and was able then to give them my full attention; it would have been detrimental to have done this immediately after my interview with M.

The Interview

I found M to be very lively, and one could almost say that he was eager for something. He was restless, and, during the drawing games, he was often standing rather than sitting, and the game was always liable to degenerate into an activity that contained winning and losing. My aim was to enable him (if possible) to play at squiggles, but first I had to concede a period of noughts and crosses, a game that (I soon found out) he did not really understand. A distorted form of this game appeared later. (See Figure 1.)

It seemed to me at the time to be unlikely that we could make use of the session in terms of playing of the kind that would naturally lead to contact between him and me of a deepening kind. I went forward, however, and in the end I was rewarded.

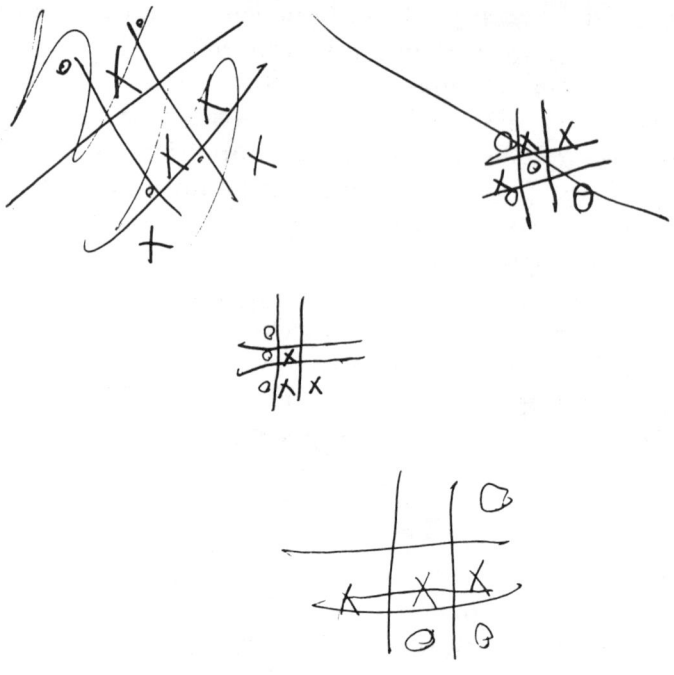

FIGURE 1

Squiggles

I explained the game to him, letting him know that first I make a squiggle that he can turn into something if he wants to do so, and then he makes a squiggle for me to turn into something. Then I made my first squiggle. (See Figure 2.)

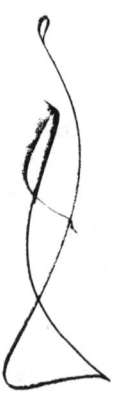

FIGURE 2

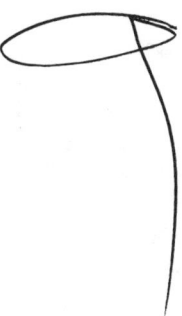

FIGURE 3

He said: "It's like an eight," and he had no impulse to turn it into anything. On this occasion, perhaps because of his restlessness, I deemed it advisable immediately to make a comment that might or might not lead to a development in our tenuous relationship. I said: " That's you"—because he had just told me that he was eight years old. He immediately entered into the game and made a squiggle. (See Figure 3.) This was a vigorous squiggle done like mine, as if undirected and not deliberate. He looked at it, and quickly said: "That's me too; it's a nine, and I will be nine in a week's time." We were now in communication with each other in terms of the game, but there was still much restlessness. I became hopeful.

Figure 4 shows my next squiggle. He had no desire to alter this or to make it into anything. He just said: "It's a cloud or a piece of lace." This made me think of the whole area of fantasy and of what I have called transitional phenomena, things that belong to the transition from being awake to being asleep, and I explored around this area, fishing for information from him about transitional objects or techniques that he might remember. This led to nothing in his particular case (although it might have done in another case), except that he told me of a teddy bear that he had had when he was three. So we continued with the game.

I noted that he did his next squiggle (Figure 5) in two separate parts, so I turned one part into a head and the rest into a figure that eventually resulted in a drawing of a girl with a handbag. He made a comment in two layers. In the superficial layer, he said: "You draw well!" and then with more conviction

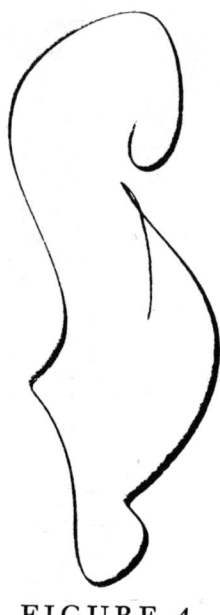

FIGURE 4

he said: "Really it was a lantern." He meant that, if I had let him turn the squiggle into something, he would have made it into a lantern. This implied that therefore, I was not magically in touch with his thoughts. Incidentally, he made the handle of the hand-

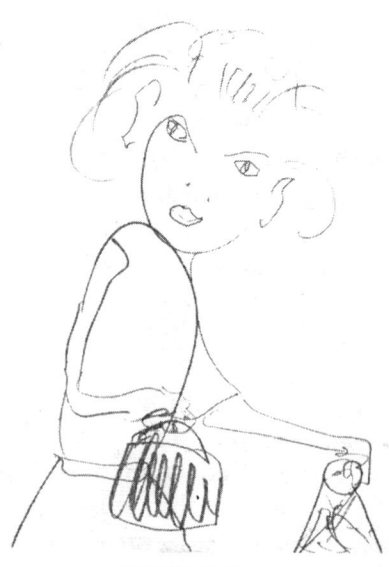

FIGURE 5

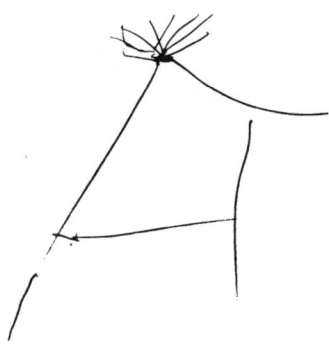

FIGURE 6

bag more securely joined to the bag. He was restless here and walking around, bending down to draw on the low table without sitting.

He sat down to do his next squiggle (Figure 6). It was simply four lines, and he immediately said, "I know what it is," and he turned it into a volcano. I said, "Well, that's you again," and he seemed to accept this idea with good grace.

He said my next squiggle (Figure 7) was a bush or a snail, and the only thing he would do about it was to decide which way up it ought to be. (Note the laziness that indicates that he feels that the result should come by magic, not by work and skill. This squiggle game allows for the operation of this principle, until the child begins to feel like active participation.)

His next squiggle is shown in Figure 8. I made this into a plant in a pot, but he said that was quite wrong. He said: "It is a whirlwind." I said: "Well, that's you again." I added: "They all seem to be about you, except perhaps the girl, but I drew that one." We talked a bit about his being a boy or a girl and his preferences. He came down heavily on the side of being a boy. When asked for reasons he became rational and said: "Well, girls are all right but I happen to be a boy."

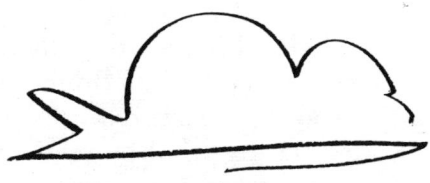

FIGURE 7

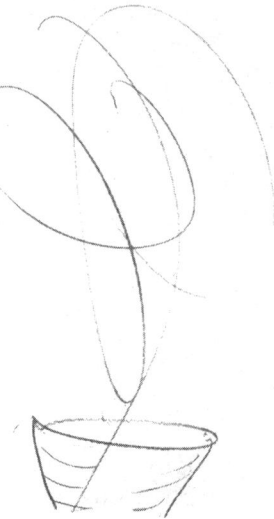

FIGURE 8

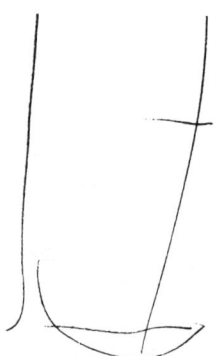

FIGURE 9

His next squiggle is shown in Figure 9. He was now quite happy to be playing the game that I had instituted. He said: "That's a book; that's me again because I love books, and I read all the time."

He said my next squiggle (Figure 10) was a funny plant. I said: "Well, if that's you there is something funny about you. What could it be?" And he answered: "My sister's always laughing at me." Contemplating what he might make this squiggle into he said: "Do you recommend anything?" I said: "No, I had nothing in my mind when I did it." I felt that there was an indication here of his having some fear of spontaneity and free fantasy and of his wanting the support that I might offer by giving ideas of my own.

He said, in reference to his next squiggle (Figure 11): "It's got

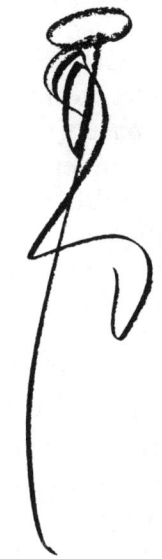

FIGURE 10

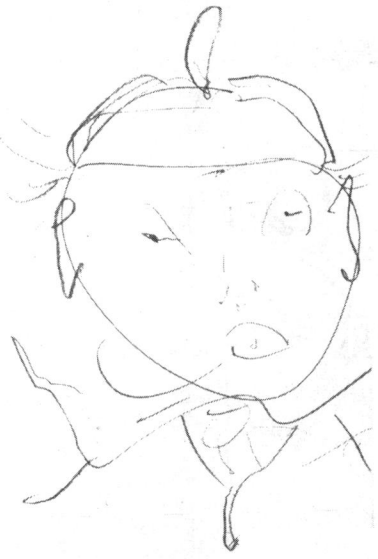

FIGURE 11

a collar." This gave me the clue, and I filled in the face, and again we decided that it was a picture of him.

The Period of Reassessment

We were now in a period that occurs in nearly all these therapeutic consultations, in which nothing much seems to be happening. At one time in the past, I might have thought that we had come to the end of our contact, but I have learned that this is a phase during which the child is reassessing the situation. On the basis of what has happened, the child is (unconsciously) weighing up the reliability of the professional relationship and is taking a little time to decide whether to accept the risks that belong to deeper involvement. It is a kind of changing gear, and, if the consultation proceeds, one finds regularly that the work goes on at a deeper level. There may be more than one of these reassessment areas in a consultation of this kind.

During this period, we played a type of game that is his own distortion of ticktacktoe. (See Figure 12.) He called it "crosswords." I could see here that he was nearer to dream than to

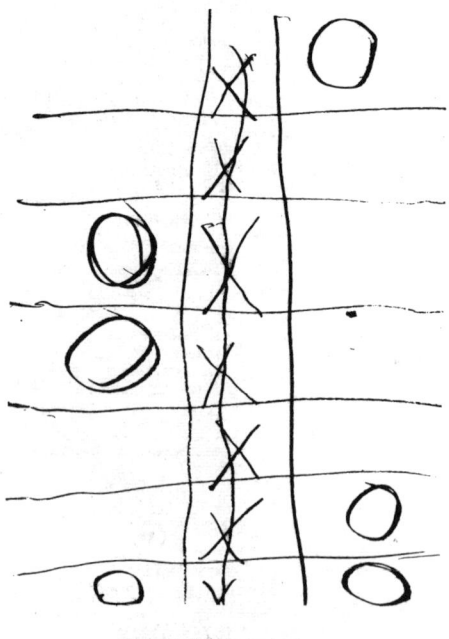

FIGURE 12

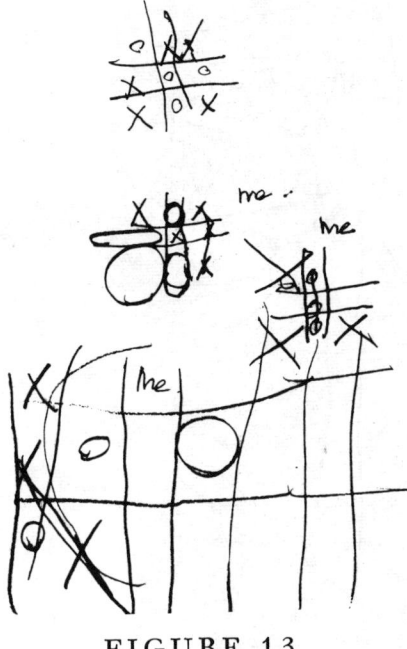

FIGURE 13

reality and therefore entitled to be in control, and I let him win. He shouted: "I've won!" and was very pleased. Figure 13 shows his continuation of this distorted game.

I now began to fish around for dreams, knowing full well that we were on a knife edge. His restlessness would very easily take him away from manageable discussion, yet he was near enough to fantasy and to dream for me to be able to invite him to look into himself. As it turned out, he responded positively to my query about dreams, and from that moment the consultation proceeded without my having any more anxiety about its turning into a fiasco. I knew that I could leave the dynamic of the interview to the process in the child, which would drive him to communicate with me in terms of his main problem.

Work at a Deeper Level

In response to my query about dreams he said: "I have one dream every night, but I don't know what these dreams are. I could tell you a funny dream"—and he liked my suggestion that he should take a large sheet of paper to illustrate it. He started

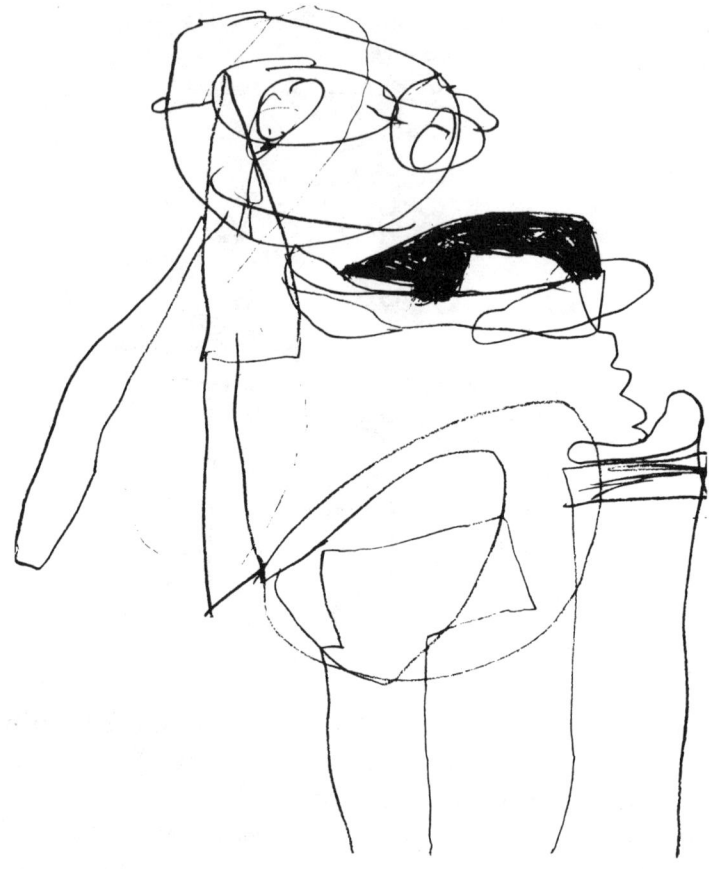

FIGURE 14

to draw on one side (Figure 14) and then turned the paper over and continued as if doing the second attempt on the back (Figure 15). (I have learned that these tiny details have to be taken seriously and that this meant that he was talking about his own back. From the mother, afterward, I learned that M compulsively asks about the birth of babies and that he has a fixed idea that they come from behind and not from the front as he has been repeatedly told.)

The thing about this dream is that he dreamed it when he was "very little, probably three." He said: "At the time when I dreamed it, it was very frightening, but in the course of the years it has become funny." I made an attempt to join up this early age of the dream with the arrival of the twins, although I knew that he was two when the twins had arrived.

The dream as given by him at this stage was obscure. First, there is a chandelier and there is a "red lady" hanging down from it. As the dream goes on, there are toboggans down the sand that slopes to the beach and to the sea—"and they all landed in the sea." There appeared to be lots of red ladies in the dream. The red, he said, was the color of blood. He kept saying how silly it all was, and from this I could infer that he knew that although the dream had turned into a funny dream, originally it was not funny and was of great significance. He went on: "These characters in the dream do acrobatics and things with skipping ropes; that is not in the dream though; that is what came into the dream later when it became funny. When I dreamed the dream at the beginning, I was very little, and there was nothing nice about it. It was only frightening. Everything was red."

At this point I got the feeling that he was remembering having the dream and being very frightened, and he was only a little

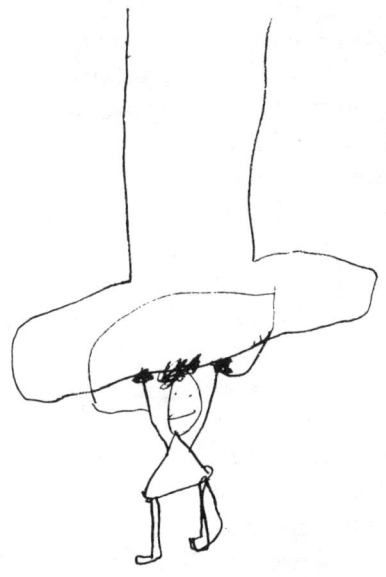

FIGURE 15

boy. He now turned the page over and continued drawing (Figure 14). (This was the side of the page that he used originally, before he turned it over to draw on the back.) Here he drew an eight (obscure in the picture because of the subsequent elaboration). I said: "Oh, that's you again." And he filled in the details of the face, giving himself glasses. I made a comment about this, and he said: "Well, I may have to wear glasses one day because, you see, I read such a lot. I really do love books. I read in the night all the time; history and the men and women in history." He went on to talk about Lord Nuffield "who gave away £30 million; so what he must have made I don't know. He was an experienced engineer."

For the moment I abandoned the dream, feeling that he had gone as far as he could for the time being toward being frightened again. So I asked him what he was going to be, taking up the idea of Lord Nuffield as an engineer. "Well, maybe a scientist. But at school science is not very interesting." He then told me about the literary occupations of his father and mother, obviously being proud of them. While he was talking, he was doing something very dark on the drawing (Figure 14). I asked him about it, and he said: "See me picking up the telephone." But it seemed to me that the original idea was to have something very dark on this page. I assumed that this was an obscurantist move, a symbolic representation of repression, an almost deliberate blackout to deny something frightening, for instance, the blood-red ladies. The telephone, however, has a positive meaning as a symbol of communication.

(It will be observed that I am not making interpretations. I allow the rich material to develop in its own way, and work in confidence that he will use his trust in me and in the professional setting to reach to the reliving of being frightened of the dream as it was dreamed when he was three years old.)

We were in a second tense period, but I could guess that there was another stage to be reached. I occupied the time by saying to him: "Whom do you love best?" I followed this up quickly with the comment: "I know." I think I did this because I could see that he was not going to answer my question in terms of mother and father of whom he had just been speaking. He was at a loss, and I wanted to make use of the fact that he had not yet decided how to deal with my question. If I had waited, he would have given an answer based on rationalization. He seemed puzzled at my saying that I knew, and he asked me to tell him.

So I said: "Yourself." Naturally I was influenced by the many ways in which he himself had come into the material of the drawings. He reacted to my answer with a display of indignation. "No, I don't love myself at all; I don't love anbody." He went on with the theme, however, and told me that he probably does love his grandparents, and no one else. He gave me a picture of home life in which the girl twin plays with the little brother and the boy twin is of no use. "He never plays with me. I have no one to play with." He then told me about one boy friend. The basis of this friendship seemed to be that the boy bullied him. We were now heavily on the masochistic side of the sadomasochistic organization. Apparently, these boys do achieve quite a lot of playing together, but the playing is liable to degenerate into some kind of antisocial activity. He illustrated this: "Once I got into trouble climbing into school through the window and opening the teacher's desk, but there was nothing in it." I followed this up with the question: "Do you ever pinch (steal)?" "No, but I play at pinching things, and I always give the things back."

He now returned spontaneously to dreams with the statement: "I have a dream every day of my life but the dream never comes into my vision." This seemed to be his way of describing a consciousness of dreaming without consciousness of the content of the dream, or alternatively the way that he can remember a dream, but when he wakes fully he forgets it. He went on: "I have only seen two dreams in full vision in my life; one had to do with horses and carts, and it was nice and was connected with the book *Black Beauty*; the other one I only half saw, and it was very nice indeed, about Norse gods who all came true; it was great." And he went on to tell me that he had read about Norse legends. He had obviously collected a great deal of information from the books that he read in bed.

Things were still a little tense, and I said: "Are you a happy person?" to which he replied: "Not at school; I get bullied." And he went on to describe the way in which the boys are beastly to him. On the other hand, on the particular day that he was talking to me the boys had voted for him to be one of the editors of the class magazine. I said: "Do they actually hurt you?" "Oh, no," he said boastfully, "they can't hurt *me*; I know judo, but they say nasty things, and they don't believe things that I have said that are true. They go about saying I am a liar." And then he confessed: "I used to boast a lot."

We talked about school a little while, but I was waiting for an opportunity to get back to the drawing of the dream. At last he got back to it on his own. He said: "It was a shock when the twins were born. You see, I was not very old; I was about two. It brought about a change in my life." He then made the comment: "I don't really remember, but Mother thinks I am still affected by this"—showing that he was not really back in the situation of having his life upset by the twins. But he went on: "I don't like the world, and I don't like living, and it is horrible at school." And then he gave me a rather excited account of the way that a belief in God is needed at his school, and he cannot manage this himself.

I said: "Do you believe in anything? Do you believe in yourself?" He shouted: "What do you mean? I don't really understand." At this point he was trying very hard to come to grips with the idea that I was putting forward about a belief in himself as something that was related to the belief in God. I tried to help him out by saying: "Well, do you feel that you are important to someone?" To which he answered: "No." Then he tried to get out of the position that he was in by boasting: "Oh, I can have fun; I know the right television program to turn on." And then he became very serious about God again and discussed the philosophical problem that if God is the Father then who is God's father and who is the father of God's father? He ended up by saying: "You could go on for millions of years like that till you were dead." So I said: "Is your own father important to you?" "Well naturally he likes having a son, but I like nagging my father." And then he went back to the question of belief in God. (I found out later that the parents, who agree on most matters, have a permanent disagreement in terms of religion and a belief in God. Here, perhaps, comes the word "crosswords" that he used to describe the game he had invented.) He told me that he had read all about religion "in the encyclopedia where they do try to be scientific."

At this stage he entered a phase in which it could be said that he was identified with God. For a while he was saying things like: "I found out for myself all about everything, how all the planets work, how everything was formed, and so on and so on," which led me to make the remark: "So in a way you are God and God is you." He reacted to this sharply. "No, I don't want to be God! I hardly know anything! I don't know a trillionth of one of what the world knows!" After this extreme retreat from an identification with God he gave me a description of Leonardo da Vinci, the cleverest man, as he said, because he invented things that were beyond his time. He gave me a very good description of Leonardo's position. Then he returned to something more personal and said: "My brother never plays with me; I am lonely."

It was now necessary for me to make a final attempt to get to the analysis of the dream, and I knew that I must get M to reach over to the sadistic side of the sadomasochistic organization because, as we were at that moment, the main defense was that he was liable to get bullied and badly treated and neglected. In answer to something I said, he told me that he used to be always teasing his brother so that the fact that his brother never played with him could be put down to the brother's defense against being bullied by M. Then he went on to say that he used to thwack his brother when he was little. M was now right back at three years old, with a little brother of one year, and (this time not quoting his mother) he said: "You see, I wanted to be the only one."

He was now ready to look at the dream again, operating from the sadistic side. He seemed to know what everything meant, but he was not able to convey it all to me. "The chandelier—well, not really a chandelier, a sort of lamp hanging down. It's bosoms. A breast like a man's." He was seeing what he had called the chandelier as the torso of a man or woman looked at from the point of view of a baby on the lap. He was now able and willing to talk about the red ladies. He said they were torn-off breasts. This was quite spontaneous. I think that he was using the idea of his brother at the breast to express his own very primitive sadistic fantasies toward the actual breast of the mother, ideas that dominated him when he was three years old.

He was now showing very great anxiety, and he was able to convey some but not all of the fantasy content. The tobogganing and the sliding down to the sea had to do with birth. So the dream was now a mixture of a birth dream and a sadistic attack on the breasts. His mind was working at a terrific rate: "Oh, yes, there was another thing in that dream; it was like a film; there was an interval. Actually I loathe custard but, you see, I did love custard when I was a baby" (that is, before the birth of the twins and the changed attitude to his mother). "This waiter came along; there was a piano there. Funny, isn't it! These people were dining. They called out: 'Waiter!' and the lady said something, only in the dream there were no words, and the waiter brought the custard." (He was in the preverbal era of his life.) He interrupted himself here to say: "Me! Ugh! Custard!" And he went on: "And they suddenly came to the chandelier; there were bosoms in a sort of a way on the tummy; a bosom or a breast." He was pointing to the drawing and saying that he had the idea of the swollen belly of pregnancy as a central breast and that this was the object of his attack in the dream leading to the blood or the raw surfaces. (He was superimposing his attack on the pregnant belly onto his sadistic attack on the breasts.) He added: "There were six or eight ladies really, all red."

He was right there in an infantile relationship with his mother's body, and he went on about bosoms (breasts), and then about man who, as he said, "gathers it all together in the penis, the thing that holds the seed." (So now he had the sequence quite clear in his mind: breasts; pregnant belly; male with no bosoms but a penis. Everything was blood red because of the sadistic attack.) He went on: "Yes, they were bosoms, I remember now," and I had the feeling that he had now reached the frightening three-year-old version of the dream, a dream that in the course of the years had gradually become funny. He was sufficiently in touch with sadistic fantasy and impulse for me to cease to worry about his masochism. He had reexperienced his angry attacks and had got behind these to his oral sadism that belongs to the primitive love in the object relationship to the breasts; moreover, he had reached to the preambivalent object-relating to the breasts in the recapturing of the love of custard, which had turned into a phobia of custard.

We had now spent one and one-quarter hours together, and we were both glad to finish.

Sequel

A month later both parents came to talk to me about M. I went over the details of the consultation with them, and they found their view of their son very much enriched as a result of this information. I felt reasonably certain that they were mature enough not to let me down by reporting even indirectly what I had told them. It has to be remembered that parents have no knowledge of what is going on when we do psychotherapy of a child, and they are liable to feel that the whole thing is a mystery. When they hear a factual account of what transpires, they can make use of the information that it gives about aspects of their child that do not become evident in ordinary home life. Incidentally, these parents were able to add one or two significant details that enriched my understanding of the case.

The parents were very much impressed by one thing: although it had always been evident to them that the birth of the twins had been a disaster from M's point of view, the first time that M ever actually said this himself was after he came back from the consultation. Also, both parents had noticed a lightening of tension, especially between M and his brother. The very evening of the consultation they found M and his brother playing and fighting together in a boyish way on the sofa, and this was quite a new feature. The parents were well satisfied with the result and were willing to wait for further developments.

A month later I found the parents extremely pleased with what had happened. The father said that somehow or other M had "found a key" in his consultation with me. The mother said that she kept on expecting something horrible to happen because she is so used to an unbroken series of disasters, but somehow or other the whole atmosphere had changed, everything centering around a great improvement in the relationship between M and his brother.

Soon after he came home from the consultation, M said to his mother in astonishment: "Dr. Winnicott said I only love myself!" The mother described the change in M: "It is as if he was turned inside out." She explained that whereas formerly he was always boasting about what he could do, he was now talking about things that he was actually planning to do, and the whole thing had become realistic. For the first time they were able to tease him without being afraid of his flaring up in a rage. He had been working well at school as before, but there was now less of a sense of pressure, and he seemed to be more relaxed about such secondary matters as marks and place in his form. The parents realized that only two months had passed and that there was still opportunity for a return to the former condition, but they could not help noticing that the change in M had produced favorable changes in the whole of M's environment, so that in a way he was now for the first time using his family and what the family could offer. Especially, he seemed released for making use of his mother.

Comment

A therapeutic consultation is described that illustrates the sort of work that is appropriate in child psychiatry. This is different from psychoanalysis and from prolonged and regular psychotherapy. In child psychiatry, the slogan must be "How little need be done in the clinic?" and obviously this slogan belongs to a type of case in which the family and the school are ready waiting to be used if the child is enabled to get past some block in his or her development so as to be able to use them. In this particular case there were unfavorable signs at the beginning of the consultation, restlessness indicating that the child had a great fear of deep feelings. Gradually, by the technique employed, the boy was able to gain confidence in the relationship and so to be able to play. Thus, he not only could remember a significant and frightening dream, but he could reach back to a reliving of the time when he was having it, at the age when he was highly disturbed by the birth of the twins, that is, when he was two or three years old. Eventually, he worked very hard at this dream and displayed insight, so that he was able to accommodate the great anxieties associated with the primitive love impulse and particularly with oral sadism. He even reached to preambivalence and the early good relationship to the mother that he had lost at three. The immediate clinical result was satisfactory and indicated a real change in the boy's personality. Incidentally, the changes in the boy produced favorable changes in the environment, and the general result was beneficial.

In this work the therapist cashes in on the child's capacity to believe in human reliability. The therapist remains a subjective object, and the work is unlike that of psychoanalysis in that it is not done in terms of nascent transference neurosis samples.

Interpretation is minimal. Interpretation is not in itself therapeutic, but it facilitates that that is therapeutic, namely, the child's reliving of frightening experiences. With the therapist's ego support, the child becomes able for the first time to assimilate these key experiences into the whole personality.

REFERENCES

1. Winnicott, D. W. "Symptom Tolerance in Pediatrics," in *Collected Papers: through Paediatrics to Psychoanalysis.* New York: Basic Books, 1958.

2. Winnicott, D. W. "Regression as Therapy Illustrated by the Case of a Boy Whose Pathological Dependence Was Adequately Met by the Parents," *British Journal of Medical Psychology*, 36 (1963), 1.
3. Winnicott, D. W. "A Clinical Study of the Effect of a Failure of the Average Expectable Environment on a Child's Mental Functioning," *International Journal of Psycho-Analysis*, 46 (1965), 1.
4. Winnicott, D. W. "Child Therapy: A Case of Antisocial Behaviour," in J. G. Howells (ed.), *Perspectives in Child Psychiatry*. London: Oliver & Boyd, 1965.
5. Winnicott, D. W. "String: A Technique of Communication," in *The Maturational Processes and the Facilitating Environment*. London: Hogarth Press, 1965.
6. Winnicott, D. W. "A Child Psychiatry Case Illustrating Delayed Reaction to Loss," in M. Schur (ed.), *Drives, Affects, Behavior*. New York: International Universities Press, 1965. Vol. 2.
7. Winnicott, D. W. "The Antisocial Tendency," in R. Slovenko (ed.), *Crime, Law, and Corrections*. Springfield: Charles C Thomas, 1966.
8. Winnicott, D. W. "The Value of the Therapeutic Consultation," in E. Miller (ed.), *Foundations of Child Psychiatry*. New York: Pergamon Press, 1968.
9. Winnicott, D. W. "The Squiggle Game," *Voices*, Spring 1968.
10. Winnicott, D. W. *Therapeutic Consultations in Child Psychiatry*. London: Hogarth Press, 1970. No. 87.

[[[18]]]

INFANTILE AUTISM

Bruno Bettelheim

A quarter of a century has passed since Kanner[28] first described eleven children whose combination of symptoms differentiated them from other children suffering from childhood psychosis. He called their syndrome "infantile autism."

Such children had been known before Kanner gave a name to their disease. In 1809, Haslam described the case of an autistic boy who was admitted in 1799 to Bethlehem asylum.[50] And in 1921, Darr and Worden[11] studied a four-year-old autistic child at the same Johns Hopkins hospital from which, some twenty years later, came Kanner's first writings on infantile autism. To these may be added my own view[5,6] that the so-called feral children of past centuries may in fact have been autistic and that the same may hold true for Itard's famous case of Victor.[24]

Though one may question Kanner's conclusions as to the origin and treatability of autism, his description of the syndrome itself remains classic:

The characteristic features consist of profound withdrawal from contact with people, an obsessive desire for the preservation of sameness, a skillful relation to objects, the retention of an intelligent and pensive physiognomy, and either mutism or the kind of language that does not seem intended to serve the purpose of interpersonal communication.

Though these children do nothing much of the time, or engage in a most simple, repetitive behavior (turning pages, tearing paper, twiddling, and rotating their fingers or simple objects), quite a few suddenly break into the wildest, most destructive fury and, occasionally, into animal-like behavior.

Despite a widespread interest in the disturbance following Kanner's publications, there is still by no means any general agreement as to its etiology or treatment. As Kanner points out,[33] the diagnosis of infantile autism became quite fashionable for a time, particularly during the 1950's and early 1960's. Since then it has given way to what he correctly calls "the ever-ready rubber stamp of 'brain-damage.' " But if the diagnosis of infantile autism is less frequent than it was a few years ago, it is not, alas, being used more correctly. The disease is comparatively rare, and very few have studied it intensively, so that misdiagnosis is understandable. Thus, even today, "children who are severely retarded, children with Heller's disease, or who are aphasic, have been miscalled 'autistic'; [while] autistic children have been miscalled mentally retarded or aphasic."[33]

When it comes to treatment methods, things seem even more deplorable, both as to extreme and unwarranted optimism and pessimism. For example, "the concept of operant conditioning, in precipitous zeal, has been championed as a foregone success on the basis of what are, in fact, fragmentary attainments."[33] And although "considerable research has so far failed to produce evidence of any consistent neurological, metabolic, or chromosomal pathology which can be connected with the origin of autism,"[33] there are those "believers [who] hope to elevate their speculative philosophy to the realm of proven fact by dint of pure zeal."[33] Thus, Rimland[39] insists, with little basis in fact, that the problem of the origin of autism has been solved: it is the result of a neurological disturbance, namely, the impairment of the reticular formation of the brain stem.

Despite such uncertainty as to cause, some facts have emerged as to etiology and there are some very definite findings on the psychodynamics of infantile autism and the meaning of autistic behavior, though matters become less certain again as regards prognosis and treatment.

ETIOLOGY

Controversy over the cause of infantile autism—whether it is inborn or psychogenic (caused essentially by parental attitudes) —can be traced to Kanner's original papers, where, on the one hand, he speaks of innate inabilities and, on the other, of parental characteristics. Thus, in 1943 he wrote:

We must, then, assume that these children have come into the world with innate inability to form the usual, biologically provided affective contact with people, just as other children come into the world with innate physical or intellectual handicaps. If this assumption is correct, a further study of our children may help to furnish concrete criteria regarding the still diffuse notions about the constitutional components of emotional reactivity. For here we seem to have pure-culture examples of *inborn autistic disturbance of affective contact.*

But also, in 1948, Kanner wrote:

There is one other very interesting common denominator in the background of these children. Among the parents, grandparents, and collaterals there are many physicians, scientists, writers, journalists, and students of art. It is not easy to evaluate the fact that all of our patients have come of highly intelligent parents. This much is certain, that there is a great deal of obsessiveness in the family background.

And (with Eisenberg) in 1956: "It is difficult to escape the conclusion that this emotional configuration in the home plays a dynamic role in the genesis of autism."

Now, it is difficult to see how the "emotional configuration in the home" can play "a dynamic role in the genesis of autism" if, because of an "innate disability," the child does not respond to this emotional configuration because he does not relate to people. The only way these two statements can be reconciled is to assume that the parents' behavior does not permit or induce the child to come out of his shell. That is, the only way one can accept Kanner's thesis that the home affects the disturbance, and still hold his view that the child cannot relate, would be to assume that the parents fail to evoke any response in the child and that he therefore remains in his original autistic state.

By now, theories of etiology range from the wholly organic and congenital[39] to the wholly psychogenic. Bender[2] sees autism not as an inborn impairment of the central nervous system, but as a defensive reaction to one. Autistic children, she feels, "withdraw to protect themselves from the disorganization and anxiety arising from the basic pathology . . . in their genes, brains, perceptual organs or social relationships."

Goldstein[20] also views autism as a secondary defense against an organic deficiency. The impairment, he feels, is the autistic child's inability to engage in abstract thinking. Autistic behavior then represents "expressions of protective mechanisms, occurring passively as a means of safeguarding the patient's 'existence' in situations of unbearable distress and anxiety." Both Goldstein and Bender thus view infantile autism as a defense against unbearable anxiety. With this I concur, but unlike these authors I believe that the source of anxiety is not an organic impairment but the child's evaluation of his life conditions as being utterly destructive.

Rank[38] stressed emotional deprivation from rejecting irresponsive parents as the etiological factor. Mahler[36] has pointed out that an overpossessive mother who anticipates the child's every need deprives him of the chance to explore, differentiate, experiment with cause and effect, communicate affect, and cause response. The child gives up, withdraws interest from the world, and thus becomes autistic. Ferster,[17] using operant conditioning terms, suggests a purely psychological basis for the extinction of outgoingness in the child, attributing it to failure of parental reinforcement. Fraknoi[18] studied mothers of autistic children, found significant identification with their children's autistic position based on a disordered relationship with their own mothers, and cited these as causal factors. Ekstein[16] speaks of a bidirectional failure in communication and countertransference—such as failure to understand the child's uniquely expressed messages. Eisenberg[13] suggests that insensitive parental pressure compounds the disorder.

Bergman and Escalona[3] discuss unusual sensitivities and perceptual distortions that result from an inadequate stimulus barrier—a deficiency in primary autonomous ego functions. They suggest that ordinary stimuli may prove overwhelming to the autistic child. Spitz[49] emphasizes the damaging effects of excessive and noxious stimulation—causing "emotional overload" and psychotoxic response.

Shevrin and Toussieing[43] suggest that autistic reactions may be caused by inadequate tactile stimulation, either via a constitutionally high barrier or maternal understimulation or—at the other extreme—overstimulation either directly or via low threshold.

Given the baffling nature of the disturbance, the difficulties of treatment, the strange behavior of the parents, and the absence of neurological signs, most careful authors who have studied and worked with autistic children lean toward a psychogenic hypothesis, without entirely excluding the possibility of an organic basis. Given the wide variations in severity, in presenting symptoms, and in response to treatment, several authors tend to think of a continuum from considerable organic to essentially psychogenic causation. Such an intermediate position is reflected in the views of Ruttenberg, Wolf, and Dratman.[41]

I feel that the hesitation about discarding the organic position has to do with present difficulties in determining whether a child is congenitally defective or whether he develops ego dysfunction in the first few weeks of life owing to early environmental impact. I believe that the answer will have to come from infant observations during the first few weeks of life. As Wolf and White[53] have shown, newborn infants respond to their environment practically from birth and are extremely vulnerable to its impact during the first weeks of life. And Call[9] has shown how radically wrong things can go in an infant's relation to the world during the very first nursing experiences.

One crucial test of organic versus psychogenic etiology is provided by identical twins. Rimland[31] discusses fourteen cases of twins that came to his attention, eleven of them monozygotic and all twenty-eight children suffering from autism. This, he feels, provides "one of the strongest lines of evidence against psychogenic etiology of autism."

Yet, even both twins being autistic does not invalidate a hypothesis of environmental origin, because both may have been subject to an identical or very similar home influence. And if there were even one instance of identical twins in which one was autistic and the other not, it would throw serious doubts on any theory of inborn origin, though it would not weaken the environmental hypothesis, because parents may react differently to each twin.

Two such instances have come to light. The twins on whom Kamp[26] reported have by now been studied intensively for five years by the department of child psychiatry of the University of Utrecht. According to a private communication,[27] "The twin sister has shown no signs of maladjustment, is doing well at school, and is getting along all right." Vaillant, too,[50] has reported on a set of identical twins who were discordant for autism.

In summary, far too little is known about infantile autism to settle the question of organicity versus a psychogenic origin. As heuristic hypotheses, both have value in the sense that, by following both, no possibility is overlooked. Though I do not accept the hypothesis that autism results from an original organic defect, I do not feel I can rule out its later appearance. On the contrary, I tend to believe that far from being organic in origin, infantile autism, when persisting too long, can have irreversible effects. This applies not to the affects—because we could restore full affective functioning to nearly all the autistic children we have worked with long enough—but to the intellectual or ego functions. What are even more essential than theories about the origin of the disease are the hypotheses that have so far led to the rehabilitation of autistic children.

THE AUTISTIC ANLAGE

According to psychoanalytic theory, the newborn infant views the world as mainly need-satisfying, more or less at his command. But this seems true only if good care is at all times provided, and if his own limited activities—a reaching up of arms, a vigorous sucking, later a smile—make him feel he had a great deal to do with securing these satisfactions.

The necessary frustrations of living, though they soon shatter the infant's feeling that the world is his for the asking, also challenge him to learn to do something about it. But all his later ability to do so may be the consequence of an earlier conviction that the world is at his fingertips. It simply turns out that the pleasures he wants are not so close at hand. He must go out and capture them first.

I suggest, then, that there may be a critical time to experience the world as frustrating. If this experience hits the infant too soon, before he has had a chance to be fully convinced that the world is essentially good, it will deter him from investing vital energy in reaching out for what he wants, even when his growth developments make that possible. Such children stop trying. They see no reason to reach out to a frustrating experience, and this is all the world seems to offer. These, then, are children who suffer from infantile marasmus, are Spitz's[45] vegetating children who suffer from hospitalism. Such children do not develop socially, emotionally, or intellectually, and many soon die physically as well.

But I believe it was not directly the mechanical, impersonal care that was given them—nor the low stimulation they experienced, nor the parents' wish that the child should not exist—that accounts for the shriveling up and withering away of autistic children's relation to the world. I think it is rather their failure to become active in their own behalf. Though the detrimental experiences of early infancy were at fault in not activating them, it was their spontaneous failure to become active that led to their emotional, intellectual, and often physical death. Otherwise, the observations of Spitz[45, 46, 47, 48, 49] and others on hospitalism would still not explain why some of these children survived and others did not, though all of them were treated alike. Some, either because of endowment, prior experience, or benign accident, became more activated than others and hence put even the most mechanical care to better use. More correctly, perhaps, the care seemed less purely mechanical to them because they were more active in receiving it.

There are other children in whom their early experience created an autistic anlage, but whose later encounter with frustration, during their second year, was not their total world experience. These children's essential needs, both to receive and be active, were satisfied to at least that minimal degree that the world did not seem to them wholly destructive.

There are others who were fairly well cared for, but who were nevertheless denied the experience that what they did made much difference. To children with either experience, the world appeared to be need-satisfying, but wholly insensitive. (This latter experience they share with the first group who hardly developed at all.) Such children remain passive, the "good" quiet infants. They develop to the point where growth and maturation, as well as society, require them to begin to act on their own, at least to some degree, in shaping their lives. This task they cannot meet. But then the world that seemed only insensitive begins to seem destructive as well, because it asks of them, for their survival, to do what they are unable to do. In reaction to this experience, they assume the autistic position.

I can now be more specific about what essentially the autistic anlage consists of—the conviction that one's own efforts have no power to influence the world, because of the earlier conviction that the world is insensitive to one's reactions.

Infantile marasmus, then, and Spitz's hospitalism, result from a combination of the conviction that one can do nothing about the world and that the world is not need-satisfying at all, but only frustrating and destructive. These convictions result in utter passivity.

Infantile autism, on the other hand, stems from the original conviction that there is nothing at all one can do about a world that offers some satisfactions, though not those one desires, and only in frustrating ways. As more is expected of such a child, and as he tries to find some satisfactions on his own, he meets still greater frustration, because he neither gains satisfaction nor can he do as his parents expect. So he withdraws to the autistic position. If this happens, the world that until then seemed only insensitive now appears to be utterly destructive, as it did from the start to the child who succumbs to marasmus. But because the autistic child once had some vague image of a satisfying world, he strives for it—not through action, but only in fantasy. Or if he acts, it is not to better his lot but only to ward off further harm. The child with infantile marasmus does not even have a fantasy world.

Thus, we may perhaps think of infantile autism as coming from the infant's experience during not only two, but even three or more critical periods. The first may occur during the first six months, the time before the so-called eight-month anxiety, the time before his reaching out to friends is being powerfully reinforced by his fear of the stranger. In order for this normal separation of friend and foe to occur, the baby's prior experience must have enabled him to single some out as friends; that is, he must have had the experience that the world is essentially good. If not, then no eight-month anxiety will be experienced either, as it is absent in Spitz's children who suffered from hospitalism. Some children are recognized as autistic at about this age. These children fail to form social relations because they have been too sorely disappointed in the world.

The second time for critical experiences to account for autism may be the period from about six to nine months, the period that normally includes the eight-month anxiety. Other persons are now recognized as individuals, and the child begins to recognize himself as such, too. If, during this period, the infant tries to relate to the other but finds him unresponsive, he may give up trying to relate. But not having found the other, he cannot find the self either.

The third critical time may be the age from eighteen months to two years, when autism is most commonly recognized. It is the age when the child can approach or avoid contact with the world not just emotionally, but by walking away from it all. This, then, may be the stage when to emotional withdrawal from the mother (in the second stage) is added emotional and physical withdrawal from the world altogether.

At best, these are highly tentative suggestions and gross approximations. In each stage, different strivings of the self have been blocked or severely interfered with: in the first with the child's being active in general, in the second with his active reaching out to others, and in the third with his active efforts to master the world physically and intellectually.

Several students of infantile autism mention how often the history of autistic children showed no obvious deviation or traumatization at the earliest age, though it may have occurred. Instead, the children were reported as developing more or less normally up to about eighteen or twenty-four months. This is an age when the infant still has many needs he cannot fill by himself, but through walking and talking is beginning to try to get what he wants on his own.

Again and again in the history of mute autistic children one finds the statement, often fully verified, that they began to speak normally. Then after the rudiments of speech were acquired—that is, after they could say a few words—they slowly gave up talking or dropped it suddenly. That is, speech was developed in an effort to influence the environment, but was given up when it failed in this purpose. The child does not withdraw from all efforts at relating because his needs are not adequately met—though this too will scar the personality. He withdraws when these efforts find him less able to modify the environment than before.

Here, parental observations of their own autistic children are significant. Most of their accounts of the child's first year indicate that the autistic child was quiet, a good child, that in the second year he amused himself on his own, often with stereotyped, empty activity, such as humming to music or turning the pages of a book. But that his behavior was strange, out of the ordinary, did not catch the attention of parents or pediatrician until the second year of life.

Isn't it possible that what these children showed, during the first year of life, was only a lowered level of activity? That they only became autistic at the age when spontaneous, goal-directed activity is part of normal development, in addition to the earlier behavior that is no less spontaneous but not consciously purposeful?

The Harlows' experiments, on the other hand,[21, 22] show that activity without response can be fatal. Monkey babies raised with terrycloth mothers could do all the clinging they wished. They grew, they gained weight, seemed to be doing all right, until such time in development as they would normally have socialized and mated. This they could not or would not do.

DYNAMICS

Despite the incredible variety of presenting symptoms, the many autistic children we have worked with over the years shared one thing in common—an unremitting fear for their lives. The reason for this, in our conviction, is that they all suffer from the experience of having been subject to extreme conditions of living that convinced them that their very existence was in jeopardy every moment. Furer,[19] speaking of all types of psychotic children, writes that they suffer "from extreme panic and anxiety." And the more autistic the schizophrenic child, the more debilitating his symptoms, the greater is his mortal anxiety. Autistic children not only fear constantly for their lives, in particular they seem convinced that death is imminent, that possibly it can be postponed just for moments through their not taking cognizance of life.

Others who have studied autistic children psychoanalytically came to the same conclusions. During the year in which I presented this view, Rodrigué wrote: "I think the intensity of the autistic child's anxiety is similar to that to which imminent death gives rise."[40]

In reviewing thoughts on etiology, it was possible to be fairly objective. This becomes more difficult in regard to dynamics, because here one is so dependent on what can be gleaned from the treatment of autistic children. So long as the children are autistic, they do not convey things clearly, and when they can eventually tell us, they are no longer autistic. But by that time, their recollections are colored by everything that happened afterward. Thus, the following remarks represent largely this author's views, rather than a balanced judgment on those of others.

Seen from outside the person, all emotional disturbance is marked by some serious breakdown in communication with others. And the defensive and determined aloneness, the doing nothing of the autistic child, represent the most extreme breakdown of communication with the world.

Ordinarily, things do not happen with dramatic suddenness, neither the giving up of relating and talking, nor of the impulse to act. They happen rather in a slow, step-by-step process. In normal development, the child begins to act as his mouth seeks the nipple, as he responds to auditory and visual stimuli, as he engages in visual pursuit. And communication begins as he nurses. Even in this earliest stage of personality formation, things may go wrong and, if radically so, then autism follows.

The infant, because of pain or discomfort and the anxiety they cause, or because he misreads the mother's actions or feelings, or correctly assesses her negative feelings, may retreat from her and the world. The mother, for her part, either frustrated in her motherly feelings, or out of her own anxiety, may respond not with gentle pursuit, but with anger or injured indifference. This is apt to create new anxiety in the child, to which may now be added the feeling that the world (as represented by the mother) not only causes anxiety but is also angry or indifferent as the case may be.

Any such retreat from the world tends to weaken the baby's impulse to observe and to act on the environment, though without such an impulse personality will not develop. Retreat debilitates a young ego barely emerging from the undifferentiated stage and leads to still further psychic imbalance.

How severe the imbalance will be depends on the nature and degree of the breakdown in communications with the outside. Those parts of reality that prove too disappointing or unresponsive will be defended against or replaced by imaginary ones that seem more satisfying; inner reactions that are too powerful will be repressed—all in efforts to retain some contact with the world and to make at least some limited part of it secure. But when things go beyond this, when reality seems too destructive, then one stops trying. Efforts to master some aspects of reality, and to come to terms with others through defense, are given up. Then the mental apparatus is made to serve only one goal—to protect sheer life by doing nothing about outside reality. All energy goes into protection, and none is available for building personality. Behind it all lies the conviction that any being or doing would bring about some disastrous response. If all this happens very early in life, autism may result.

The reasons communication breaks down may be various and take a wide range of forms. A person may not respond correctly because he misinterprets the signals he receives in terms of his anxiety or hostility, or he may read them only too correctly. He may need to send out confusing signals to "get back at others" or, more likely, to avoid dangers he is sure would follow if others could know his true thoughts. Yet, whatever the initial cause, it is the degree and persistence of the person's failure to send and receive messages correctly that account for the degree and persistence of his emotional disturbance.

Viewed from inside the person—or intrapersonally—however, this breakdown in communication is caused by overwhelming anxiety. The anxious person may seek minimal security by first reducing his contact with a world that makes him too anxious. In more severe cases, he may later avoid such contact and lose all trust in his ability to deal with the world. If the retreat is not just temporary, he may be caught in a vicious circle where anxiety leads to retreat from reality, retreat to still greater anxiety, and in the end to more permanent withdrawal. Here it makes little difference whether the anxiety began because of real or imagined dangers in the world or because of some inner psychic process. Inner hostility, for example, can arouse tremendous anxiety if we are convinced that giving vent to it will cause our destruction.

Still, as long as the person views his anxiety as caused by something outside, he remains in some distorted contact with reality. It matters little whether he is anxious about the hostile intentions of others or what they may do in response to his own hostile wishes. To the degree that he connects his anxiety or hostility to the external world he is in contact with it, though his view of it and responses to it are distorted. Depending thus on the degree of anxiety, and hence of distortion, it remains possible for him to view the source of his anxiety more or less correctly.

But if anxiety increases beyond a certain degree, if it overwhelms the organism and results in panic, the contact with reality is lost. Whether anxiety reaches panic proportions depends on whether the person believes he can take action to reduce the dangers that caused it, and with it reduce the anxiety. Here again it makes little difference whether the external source of anxiety is, in fact, irreducible. What counts is whether the anxious person thinks so.

In panic anxiety, hostility is no longer felt as such. This makes matters so much worse, because, in some fashion, as long as we feel we are hostile to the world, we can see it as a reasonable consequence that the world will hit back. This, of course, makes us anxious. But though we are frightened, the world still makes sense. It is when we no longer recognize our hostility and the world remains utterly frightening that reality stops seeming reasonable. Living in such an unreasonable, unpredictable world, the best thing, the only protection, lies in doing nothing. If any action on our part is apt to bring about disaster, then not acting is the only safe course.

To protect such nonacting, the child's only safety lies in not being provoked into action. Any stimulus reaching him from the outside might provoke action, so he must make himself insensitive to whatever might reach him from the outside. And because inner hostility might also provoke him to act, he must make himself insensitive to what comes from within his own psyche. This is autism as seen from inside the person.

THE MEANING OF AUTISTIC BEHAVIOR

Those autistic children who give up speaking and remain mute seem to feel that merely hiding their thoughts behind what seems like nonsensical language is not enough guarantee of safety. Jackson[25] reports on nine cases of nonspeaking children she has treated, all of whom could be considered autistic because of their withdrawal from human contact and their repetitive and compulsive preoccupation with objects. Mutism in these children is explained as their ultimate retreat in the face of danger:

> The three primitive forms of reaction to danger are (a) flight, (b) fight and (c) assuming complete immobility or feigning death; mutism and ignoring of other human beings can be likened to (c). Silence and the absence of relationships with others are, after all, a kind of death, non-existence as a social being.

But even when autistic children are not mute, they use language mainly as a defense, not at all as communication. And the nature of this defense, and what the child is directing it against, must be understood if we are to understand the nature of the disturbance from the subject's behavior. Thus, though the children hide defensively behind their idiosyncratic use of language, we must approach what they do and say as if these were riddles to be solved if we want to understand infantile autism. These riddles are designed to test our desire to understand them, a desire that would also attest to our willingness that they should exist. Viewed in this way, it appears that whatever the child selects for endless repetition has deep meaning. This was amply demonstrated by Marcia,[6] when this nonspeaking daughter of an

English-born mother sang, day after day, the song from *My Fair Lady* called "Why Don't the English Teach Their Children How to Speak?" Thus, she posed the question of why her mother, who had not wished her to exist, had also not helped her relate to the world.

I believe that the repetition of clusters of words is thus nonsensical only to us and shows that the children understand the meaning of language very well. In this sense, they use language in its highest—namely, its symbolic—function by performing verbal feats that both symbolize their intelligence and pose the most important question of all.

One of the characteristic symptoms of autism is that those children who talk do not use the pronoun "I." Kanner[30, 32] called this phenomenon "pronominal reversal"—where the child uses the pronoun "you," but correct grammar would require the "I." He also spoke of "delayed echolalia" and "affirmation by repetition" as when, for example, the autistic child is asked "Do you want milk?" and replies "You want milk" (meaning "I want milk," or "Yes, I want milk").

In my opinion the concept of pronominal reversal is misleading because the issue is not that autistic children reverse pronouns, but that they avoid using them. And they avoid them the more, the more directly the pronoun refers to themselves.

Cunningham and Dickson[10] studied the language of one autistic boy whose development had been normal to about two years of age. He began to speak at about one year and continued to acquire and retain new words up to the age of two, at which age he began to lose the words he had learned, and by three years had stopped speaking. Residential treatment began at five. His first word was recorded after three months; after seven months he could say a number of single words. From then on, he gathered words fairly rapidly and began to put them together in short phrases or sentences.

When he was seven, his language was at about the two-year-old level. It was therefore compared with the language of normal children who were thirty months old. There was little difference in how often verbs, articles, and so forth were used, but the story was different for nouns and pronouns. He used considerably more nouns, but the differentials were most marked in regard to pronouns, where the count was 19 per cent for normals, 5 per cent for the boy. For personal pronouns alone, the difference was 4 per cent for normals, less than 1 per cent for the boy.

Arieti[1] comments that "It will be easier for George to think 'You, George, eat'; than to think 'I, George, eat' because when he says 'You, George, eat' he verbalizes an attitude of his mother's which he has not accepted and therefore has not transformed into 'I, George, eat.'" This will be so if the adults in his life are anxiety-producing or extremely rejecting, because then he "has difficulty in incorporating attributes, feelings, points of view about himself which come from others."

It is astonishing that the writers who discuss this phenomenon have not also observed that though autistic children repeat readily such statements as "You want milk" to indicate that they want it, they will never repeat such a statement as "I want milk" if they want it. If we were dealing here with no more than echolalia, it should be as simple for them to repeat "I want milk" as to repeat "You want milk." We have tried this with all our autistic children, and the result is always the same. They will readily repeat "You want such and such" but never, before they have also begun to say "I" in other contexts, do they repeat such a statement using "I."

It has also been commonly observed that these children avoid the word "yes" as much as they avoid the word "I." But the much earlier appearance of "no" in the speech of these children, compared with "yes," is often disregarded. Now the word "yes" should be no harder to learn than the word "no" if the difficulty in learning were organically caused. In my opinion, however, the readier use of "no" compared to "yes," is an indication of extreme and deliberate negativism. Kanner[29] comes close to recognizing that the affirmation is what is not available to these children.

Maybe what we are here presented with is a most obstinate determination, but also the autistic child's single affirmation: not to commit himself to anything, or to any particular existence that would inhere in statements implying an "I am" or "I want." It is a total refusal to get involved with the world. And because any use of the "I" carries the minimal implication that "I am in this world," the use of "I" must be avoided. The survival value of such a position is that if "I" do not really exist, then neither can "I" really be destroyed. This self-protective avoidance of "I," it seems to me, is more important than all other protections it offers. It wards off the disappointment always expected by never admitting to having any wants.

That autistic children use language to hide what they really think is also Loomis' opinion.[35] Kanner,[30] too, on some occasions, has mentioned the protective function of specifics in autistic language when he speaks of "the use of simple verbal negation as magic protection against unpleasant occurrences."

It is not the autistic child's reluctance to talk alone that reveals his anxiety about being himself. What he avoids most of all is any communication of feeling. So even if he says something, he says it in a most peculiar voice. Most of the time it is like the voice of a deaf person; it has the same toneless and unaccommodating-to-the-ear quality of one who cannot hear his own voice. And, indeed, he does not wish to know what he says or to have the other person hear it. This gives the voice a most bizarre quality. If it shows any feeling at all, it is that of anger at having been seduced into speaking, and then the tonelessness changes to an angry screeching screaming.

Some autistic children speak only in a whisper and enunciate very indistinctly, put the accent on a different syllable than is customary, or slur their letters. Others, when they begin to speak in more than monosyllables, run the words of a short sentence so much together that the entire sentence is pronounced as one word. This makes it extremely difficult, often impossible, to disentangle the words and hence to understand what was said. Others speak overclearly, but with such a nonusual emphasis that they, too, turn each word into a symbol of their private preoccupations. All words, in fact, have private meanings to them that tally only in part and by chance with the meanings we attach to them.

The most important European study of autism so far published is that of Bosch,[7] who concentrated on the peculiar language these children use. Though familiar with psychoanalytic thinking, Bosch is very little influenced by it. What he tried to understand was the autistic child's thinking process, not the children's unconscious. His frame of reference derives primarily from Husserl[23] and from a psychology of language based on Karl Bühler[8] and Snell.[44]

Bosch, too, finds most important the absence, or only very late appearance, of the child's saying "I." But he finds the same to be true for those language forms normally connected with the meaning of "having" or "owning" and of "influencing" and "doing." Not only is the saying of "I" delayed, but also essential verbal forms such as those connecting "I" with the future, as well as the imperative forms. Thus, any statements of intention are lacking, any anticipation of procedures, or the purposes of doing. The autistic child cannot handle these concepts.

Bosch observes, in my opinion correctly, that

the absence of saying "I" stands in a close meaningful connection with the inadequate attention these children pay to the other, and with the absence of a clear separation between the speaking, answering, encouraging or demanding person on the one hand, and the other person who hears, answers, and responds to the demand, on the other.

In considering why autistic children show such peculiar use of language, Bosch lays stress on its origin.

Language develops in the encounter with others. Language presupposes that certain developments took place in the preverbal phase [namely] a development from touching via grasping to experimental manipulation; from holding and showing the object, to pointing to it with hand or finger.

Discussing how an autistic child will say, to empty space, as it were, "He wants to eat," Bosch remarks that it is not only the absence of "I" and its replacement by "he," but the general manner in which the sentence is constructed that makes it seem as if the child does not make a direct request, certainly not one directed to another person. What seems lacking is a desire to bring something to the other person's attention, a demand that something should take place. Also missing is any direct reference to the desired object or any personalized expression of the demand or desire. What takes place here is a reduced expression of the very personal demand "I want" to a mere impersonal statement that something is wanted. The impersonal level of the appeal brings it close to the preverbal cry of the infant.

Convincing as such an analysis is, it does not explain the strange phenomenon of why our autistic children never used the assertive form, "he wants," that seems typical of their German counterparts. Our children began with a mere repetition of enough of the question "Do you want to go out?" to produce the assertive "want go out" if the reply was affirmative. I believe the explanation may have to do with an aspect of German usage that has no parallel in English. In German, the child is addressed as "thou" by adults, a form that he himself will never use with any but the most intimate adults—certainly not with persons in authority, such as a physician. Hence, to repeat verbatim the question, "Willst du essen?" ("Wilt thou eat?") would be both a social affront to the questioner and an admission of great intimacy with him, because the child would be addressing the adult familiarly as "thou." This the German child circumvents by using "he," probably more to avoid owning to an intimacy he feels toward no one. In this way, he uses neither the tabooed "I" nor the intimate or impolite "thou," while retaining the impersonal nature of the reply.

Bosch feels that, if we want to understand the strange ways in which the autistic child deals with objects, we must consider that "the objects that surround man are not there for him alone, but for his fellow men too. . . . Many objects are constructed for common use with other persons." In order to clarify such bipersonal constitution, Langeveld[34] uses the example of the seesaw, whose function would not be grasped by a person who knows only himself.

It [was] therefore enlightening to observe an autistic child on the see-saw. [He] sat on it like a dead doll, and clung to it, but could not participate actively in the movement of the see-saw. He could neither push himself up, nor appropriately react to the activity of the other child through changing his position on the see-saw. Autistic children are also at a loss to know what to do with a ball; possibly it might be rolled, or turned while it is held in the hand; but it will not be caught or thrown back to another person.

We had observed and reported exactly the same behavior in several autistic children. Because they were also receiving treatment, they did not remain arrested at this level and could eventually understand objects that involved the interaction of people. But this learning took years. Not until they were interacting more freely with others did they also seesaw with others. And this happened at the same time that they began to play ball more freely. Thus, their progress was not related to the complexity of the object, but conditioned only by their developing ability to interact with others and hence to take part in interactional play.

In the sphere of motor behavior, autistic disorders defy description in classical neurologic terms. Though they vary greatly from child to child, they are remarkably consistent, persistent, and unique to the individual child. Thus, "twiddling" is also individually unique. One child uses mainly a unique finger movement. Another child flexes and extends the wrist as well as the fingers. A third child may twiddle in a rotary finger movement with alternating pronation and supination of the forearm, with fixation of the shoulder, elbow, wrist, metacarpal metacarpal-phalangeal, and interphalangeal joints.

Nearly all autistic children tap and twiddle with their fingers, but each does it in his own way. Many will also use an object. The choice of twiddling object, too, is unique and has personal meaning. One child utilizes a rigid object of particular shape, such as a pencil. Another child uses a floppy piece of cloth or a sock. A third child rotates a ring-shaped object about the end of her finger, as Laurie[4] may have been about to do. A fourth youngster prefers a cloth or leather strap. A fifth will juggle small objects in a characteristic manner.

Twiddling as a symptom—to which should probably be added rocking, head rolling, and head banging—is highly overdetermined, has many roots, and serves many purposes. Among its uses we have little doubt that it creates a "dream screen" on which the child projects his own private reality. For example, though autistic children show an apparent inattentiveness to external sensory stimuli, some actually achieve the inattention by the excessive, unvaried self-stimulation that arises from their strange motor behavior. In this way, outer stimuli are blotted out by and "lost" in the sensations the child stirs in himself. His own behavior converts his state of "wakefulness" into an overwhelming attentiveness to himself and effectively obliterates his perception of reality.

The twiddled fingers, as they move in front of the face, blur the vision of reality. The result is that whatever the twiddling child sees, he sees as if through a self-created screen. Reality, if seen at all, flickers by in a discontinuous manner, but a discontinuity that the child himself creates. Watching his eyes, as he stares at his twiddling fingers, suggests that he is peering, so to say, through a filmy veil he has superimposed on what is actually there. On this veil he seems to project his vague and essentially empty (because unvarying) daydreams and semihallucinations. In lieu of an unbearable reality, he creates a private one whose visual appearance he controls through the speed of his twiddling. To some degree, it is thus an effort to reshape reality and make it bearable.

By the same token, it seems likely that twiddling serves to reshape the reality of the child's own body and who controls it. Clearly, twiddling is not a diffuse activity but has a special relation to one object in particular: the child hits *himself*, twiddles against *his* chin, pushes against *his* face, displaces *himself* through space, moves *his* fingers in front of *his* eyes, shakes *his* arms, and so forth. In some vague form, this allows him the pretense of a megalomanic self-sufficiency of the body and its organs. By twiddling the part object—shreds of paper, a rattle, or straps—he tries not only to gain additional body organs but ones that he controls.

Whether or not an external object is used as part of the twiddling procedure, the emphasis is always on action and influencing and manipulating the whole world. And this, by his own actions, the child has narrowed down to the twiddling arena. Because he controls the twiddling, it permits him to hallucinate absolute mastery over both the external world and his own body—though my separating the two goes far beyond the autistic child's intellectual grasp of any reality. For Marcia, when she twiddled her fingers in front of her face, this was the sum total of the world and all experience for her.

TREATMENT

It is only on the basis of such understanding of the deep meaning of autistic behavior that treatment can succeed. It has to center greatest respect on symptomatic behaviors, because they represent the autistic child's highest ego achievements from which all further ego development must flow. Given parental attitudes, and their inability to accept the autistic child's behavior, which is, indeed, often hard to take, treatment proceeds best in a total therapeutic setting. Within it, individual psychotherapy should be only one important part of a total treatment effort that must extend to the child's entire life throughout the day and for much of the night. In many respects, Kanner is right when he repeats, in his most recent statement on infantile autism,[33] that "no better results have been obtained than [through] calm, persistent, nonspectacular attempts to wean the autistic child away from his self-isolation."

It is unfortunate that pessimism about treatment is dominant in the literature. In my opinion, the pessimism is unwarranted and may be ascribed to the fact that all too few efforts at treatment were intensive enough and, more important, were sustained for the requisite number of years.

That this may indeed be the case seems borne out by data that Professor Eisenberg[14] was kind enough to furnish at my request. Because his follow-up study of autistic children[12] is the outstanding one of its kind in the literature, it was important to know how much treatment these children had received. The most intensive treatment received by any of the sixty-three children reported on was in three cases of outpatient treatment where the children were seen in once- or twice-weekly sessions for no more than two years. It is significant that whereas a fair or good outcome is reported for only seventeen out of the entire group of sixty-three, the story is very different for the three who received the most intensive treatment. Although it was by no means as concentrated as it should have been for children suffering so severe a disturbance, the outcome was rated fair or good for two of them.

The largest group—twenty—of the sixty-three reported on were placed in private institutions where care was essentially only custodial. Fair or good outcome was reported for five of these twenty. The next largest group—sixteen—was placed in training schools or state hospitals. None of these sixteen showed fair or good outcome.[14]

In order to evaluate our 1967 results at the Orthogenic School in a comparable way, I shall use here the same categories as Eisenberg, though our results, unlike those he reported, are based on the most intensive and sustained therapy we were able to provide. Altogether we have worked with forty-six autistic children, all of whom showed marked improvement. But for purposes of comparison, the following remarks will be restricted to only forty of these forty-six, because one of them was withdrawn after a year, one, unbeknown to us when we accepted her, had been subjected to a long series of electroshock treatments a year before she came to us, which precluded effectiveness in our treatment methods, and four others, at this writing, had not been with us long enough to make valid assessments.

Applying Eisenberg's categories, there were eight in our forty for whom the end results of therapy were poor, because, despite improvement, they failed to make the limited social adjustment needed for maintaining themselves in society. For fifteen, the outcome was fair, and for seventeen, good. Thus, though Eisenberg reports only 5 per cent good outcome, our experience shows that intensive treatment can raise this figure to 42 per cent. Though he reports only 22 per cent fair improvement, we can report 37 per cent. Most important, though he found 73 per cent poor outcome, we had only 20 per cent poor results. Certainly, failure in one-fifth of the cases is disappointing. But the difference between Eisenberg's findings and ours suggests that autistic children should be given the chance that is offered by intensive institutional treatment.

On the other hand, prognosis seems closely related to the child's willingness to speak. Eisenberg[12] and Eisenberg and Kanner[15] have reported much better recovery in speaking autistic children:

(The category nonspeaking includes mute children, those who exhibit only echolalia, and those who may possess in addition a few words, usually employed in a private sense. Its meaning in this context is: unable to communicate verbally with others.)
The outcome of the group of thirty-two [speaking children] can be classified as good in three, fair in thirteen, and poor in sixteen instances. Contrariwise, the outcome of the thirty-one nonspeaking children were fair in one and poor in thirty cases.

Though our results are again much more favorable, the fact remains that of our eight failures, six were once nonspeaking (in Eisenberg's terms), whereas of the thirty-two who showed fair and good outcome only eight were nonspeaking.

The seventeen children whose improvement we classified as good can for all practical purposes be considered cured. Most of them still have some quirks in their personality, but none that would prevent them from functioning on their own in society. Nine of the seventeen were gainfully employed. Because eight were still in high school or college, this means that all who were not still completing their education were currently self-supporting. As for the academic level they had reached at the time of this writing: five of the seventeen had finished college and three of these five had, in addition, earned higher degrees; four others were still in college; one dropped out of college in his third year to seek employment; three graduated from public high school; one was a senior in a prep school; the other three were still high school students. Two of the seventeen were married, and one had a child.

The fifteen classified as fair results are no longer autistic, though eight of them should now be classified as borderline or schizoid, because they have only made a fair social adjustment. The remaining seven do somewhat better and suffer mainly from more or less severe personality disorders, which limitation has not kept them from making an adequate social adjustment.

Generalizing on both our failures and successes, we are impressed that for all forty-six children the so difficult establishment of affective relations—first to significant persons and then to the world—was achieved far more readily than what we might call ego functions. In cases classified as poor, ego functioning remained at a low level, and most progress came in the emotional sphere.

Or, to put it in psychoanalytic terms, it seems much easier to achieve full recovery in the libidinal sphere than in the ego sphere. In many cases, the ego seemed to remain pegged on a much lower platform than is normal for the youngster's age.

These findings, incidentally, suggest again that in infantile autism we are not dealing with an inborn disturbance of affective contact, but rather with an inborn time schedule that cannot be delayed for too long. This is true for the children we classified as poor results and for some of those classified as fair, though the latter achieved much higher levels of ego functioning.

THE PARENTS OF AUTISTIC CHILDREN

Earlier, I spoke of Kanner's comments about high intelligence being characteristic of the parents of autistic children. Because this factor was used by Rimland and others as suggesting a hereditary factor in infantile autism, the problem has warranted investigation. Nevertheless, such reports as Van Krevelen's,[52] Bosch's,[7] the Orthogenic School's, Schain and Yannet's[42] fail to support the assertions of Kanner, Rimland, and others as regards the parents' superior intelligence.

What can account for the strange difference between these data and those of Kanner and others? One explanation may be found in recent sociological research that tries to identify those groups of the population who seek out and have access to psychiatric service. The evidence is overwhelming that it is the educated, middle, and upper classes who do and the uneducated and lower classes who do not. We have known of autistic children who were declared feeble-minded early in life and thereafter disappeared into state schools for the defective. This seems to have happened much more often when Kanner was compiling his data than might happen today. Precisely because of his pioneering studies and other publications physicians and particularly child psychiatrists have grown much more sophisticated about recognizing infantile autism. So by now, whether or not a child is recognized as being autistic or is treated as feeble-minded or brain-damaged depends largely on whether he was examined by a competent child psychiatrist.

Bender[2] arrived at similar conclusions:

It is not clear what he [Kanner] means by saying that there is evidence that autistic children have greater intellectual potentialities, unless he is referring to the family background of his colleagues, professors and intellectual sophisticates who have selected his service.

In conclusion, let me quote from O'Gorman's monograph[37] on childhood autism, because it expresses exactly my views on the importance of the work.

When all is said, we know but little about autistic children, and a lifetime of experience with them is enough to bring humility to the most arrogant. Our efforts to learn more about them must be continued in great earnestness, not only because of our feeling that many of them, with better luck, might have become very special human beings; but also because, through studying their disabilities, we may stumble upon principles of general application in the field of the development of human abilities and human personality.

REFERENCES

1. Arieti, S. *Interpretation of Schizophrenia*. New York: Brunner, 1955.
2. Bender, L. "Autism in Children with Mental Deficiency," *American Journal of Mental Deficiency*, 63 (1960), 81–86.
3. Bergman, P., and Escalona, S. K. "Unusual Sensitivities in Very Young Children," in *The Psychoanalytic Study of the Child*. New York: International Universities Press, 1949. Vols. 3–4, pp. 333–352.
4. Bettelheim, B. "Childhood Schizophrenia as a Reaction to Extreme Situations," *American Journal of Orthopsychiatry*, 26 (1956), 507–518.
5. Bettelheim, B. "Feral Children and Autistic Children," *American Journal of Sociology*, 64, no. 5 (1959), 455–467.
6. Bettelheim, B. *The Empty Fortress*. New York: The Free Press, 1967.
7. Bosch, G. *Der Frühkindliche Autismus*. Berlin: Springer, 1962.
8. Bühler, K. *Sprachtheorie*. Jena: Fischer, 1934.
9. Call, J. D. "Newborn Approach Behavior and Early Ego Development," *International Journal of Psychoanalysis*, 45 (1964), 286–295.
10. Cunningham, M. A., and Dickson, C. "A Study of the Language of an Autistic Child," *Journal of Child Psychology and Psychiatry*, 2 (1961), 193–202.
11. Darr, G. D., and Worden, F. C. "Case Report Twenty-Eight Years after an Infantile Autistic Disorder," *American Journal of Orthopsychiatry*, 21 (1951), 559–569.
12. Eisenberg, L. "The Autistic Child in Adolescence," *American Journal of Psychiatry*, 112 (1956), 607–612.
13. Eisenberg, L. "The Fathers of Autistic Children," *American Journal of Orthopsychiatry*, 27 (1957), 715–724.
14. Eisenberg, L. Private communication, 1965.
15. Eisenberg, L., and Kanner, L. "Early Infantile Autism, 1943–1955," *American Journal of Orthopsychiatry*, 26 (1956), 556–566.
16. Ekstein, R. *Children of Time and Space, of Action and Impulse*. New York: Appleton-Century-Crofts, 1966.
17. Ferster, C. Paper presented at workshop, "A Multidisciplinary Approach to the Study and Treatment of Infantile Autism: II," at the meeting of the American Orthopsychiatric Association, 1967.
18. Fraknoi, J. "Major Defense Configurations and Identity Patterns in Mothers of a

Group of Autistic Children," paper presented at workshop, "A Multidisciplinary Approach to the Study and Treatment of Infantile Autism: II," at the meeting of the American Orthopsychiatric Association, 1967.
19. Furer, M. "The Development of a Preschool Symbiotic Psychotic Boy," in P. Greenacre (ed.), *The Psychoanalytic Study of the Child*. New York: International Universities Press, 1964. Vol. 19, pp. 448–469.
20. Goldstein, K. "Abnormal Conditions in Infancy," *Journal of Nervous and Mental Diseases*, **128** (1959), 538–557.
21. Harlow, H. F. "Affectional Responses in the Infant Monkey," *Science*, **130** (1959).
22. Harlow, H. F., and Harlow, M. K. "Social Deprivation in Monkeys," *Scientific American*, **207**, no. 5 (1962), 136–146.
23. Husserl, E. *Ideen zu einer reinen Phaenomenologischen Philosophie; Jahrbuch für Philosophie und Phaenomenologische Forschung*. Halle: Niemeyer, 1913.
24. Itard, J. M. G. *The Wild Boy of Aveyron*. New York: Century, 1932.
25. Jackson, L. " 'Non-Speaking' Children," *British Journal of Medical Psychology*, **23** (1950), 87–100.
26. Kamp, L. N. J. "Autistic Syndrome in One of a Pair of Monozygotic Twins," *Psychiatria, Neurologia, Neurochirurgia*, **67** (1964), 143–147.
27. Kamp, L. N. J. Private communication, 1965.
28. Kanner, L. "Autistic Disturbances of Affective Contact," *Nervous Child*, **2** (1943), 217–250.
29. Kanner, L. "Early Infantile Autism," *Journal of Pediatrics*, **25** (1944), 211–217.
30. Kanner, L. "Irrelevant and Metaphorical Language in Early Infantile Autism," *American Journal of Psychiatry*, **103** (1946), 242–246.
31. Kanner, L. *Child Psychiatry*. 2d ed.; Springfield: Charles C Thomas, 1948.
32. Kanner, L. "The Conception of Wholes and Pairs in Early Infantile Autism," *American Journal of Psychiatry*, **108** (1951), 23–26.
33. Kanner, L. "Early Infantile Autism Revisited," *Psychiatry Digest*, February 1968, pp. 17–28.
34. Langeveld, M. J. *Studien zur Anthropologie des Kindes*. Tübingen: Niemeyer, 1956.
35. Loomis, E. A. "Autistic and Symbiotic Syndromes in Children," *Monographs of the Society for Research in Child Development*, **25**, no. 3 (1960), 39–48.
36. Mahler, M. "Thoughts about Development and Individuation," in P. Greenacre (ed.), *The Psychoanalytic Study of the Child*. New York: International Universities Press, 1963. Vol. 18, pp. 307–324.
37. O'Gorman, G. *The Nature of Childhood Autism*. New York: Appleton-Century-Crofts, 1967.
38. Rank, B. "Adaptation of the Psychoanalytic Technique for the Treatment of Young Children with a Typical Development," *American Journal of Orthopsychiatry*, **19** (1949), 130–139.
39. Rimland, B. *Infantile Autism*. New York: Appleton-Century-Crofts, 1964.
40. Rodrigué, E. "The Analysis of a Three-Year-Old Mute Schizophrenic," in M. Klein, P. Heimann, and R. E. Money-Kyrle (eds.), *New Directions in Psychoanalysis*. New York: Basic Books, 1955. Pp. 140–179.
41. Ruttenberg, B., Wolf, E., and Dratman, M. "Orienting the Speech and Language Therapy of Autistic Children to an Understanding of the Autistic Process," paper presented at the New England Speech and Hearing Association, Boston, October 1967.
42. Schain, R. J., and Yannet, H. "Infantile Autism—An Analysis of 50 Cases," *Journal of Pediatrics*, **57**, no. 4 (1960), 560–567.
43. Shevrin, H., and Toussieing, P. "Conflict over Tactile Experience in Emotionally Disturbed Children," *Journal of the American Academy of Child Psychiatry*, **1** (1962), 564–590.
44. Snell, B. *Der Aufbau der Sprache*. Hamburg: Claassen, 1952.
45. Spitz, R. A. "Hospitalism," in P. Greenacre (ed.), *The Psychoanalytic Study of the Child*. New York: International Universities Press, 1945. Vol. 1, pp. 53–74.
46. Spitz, R. A. "Anaclitic Depression," in P. Greenacre (ed.), *The Psychoanalytic Study of the Child*. New York: International Universities Press, 1946. Vol. 2. pp. 313–342.
47. Spitz, R. A. "The Psychogenic Diseases in Infancy," in P. Greenacre (ed.), *The*

Psychoanalytic Study of the Child. New York: International Universities Press, 1951. Vol. 6, pp. 255–275.
48. Spitz, R. A. "Autoeroticism Re-examined," in P. Greenacre (ed.), *The Psychoanalytic Study of the Child.* New York: International Universities Press, 1962. Vol. 17, pp. 283–315.
49. Spitz, R. A. "The Derailment of Dialogue," *Journal of the American Psychoanalytic Association,* 12 (1964), 752–775.
50. Vaillant, G. E. "John Haslam on Early Infantile Autism," *American Journal of Psychiatry,* 119 (1962), 376.
51. Vaillant, G. E. "Twins Discordant for Early Infantile Autism," *Archives of General Psychiatry,* 9 (1963), 163–167.
52. Van Krevelen, D. A. "Early Infantile Autism," *Zeitschrift für Kinderpsychiatrie,* 19 (1952), 91–97.
53. Wolff, P. H., and White, B. L. "Visual Pursuit and Attention in Young Infants," *Journal of Child Psychiatry,* 4 (1965), 473–484.

CONTEMPORARY MISUSE OF PSYCHOACTIVE DRUGS BY YOUTH

J. Robertson Unwin

> Là, tout n'est qu'ordre et beauté,
> Luxe, calme et volupté.
> —BAUDELAIRE,
> "Invitation au Voyage,"
> *Les Fleurs du Mal*

Since the beginning of the 1960's, Baudelaire's siren song—an invitation to an intriguing inner journey (a "trip," youth would say)—has attracted a new breed of Argonauts in steadily increasing numbers. Differing in socioeconomic and cultural background from the subjects of earlier reports of adolescent drug misuse,[3, 23] the current devotees of psychoactive drugs are primarily middle class, reasonably well educated, and unusually affluent.[92, 93] The substances in popular use—often described as psychedelic or hallucinogenic—are all capable of producing, in varying degree, alterations in mood, perception, cognition, and behavior. Although cannabis products, LSD, amphetamines, and, in younger adolescents, solvents are the most prominent examples, it should be appreciated that the persistent and insistent attention paid by the communications media to these latter substances has camouflaged the fact that the illegal use, and legal abuse, of alcohol remains the prime problem of drug misuse among North American youth.

Despite the unreliability of incidence figures, it should be appreciated that the hallucinogenic drugs are so freely available in all cities and most towns of North America that each young person must decide for himself whether or not he will experiment with these substances, because the chance will almost certainly come his way. Availability has spread from the center city to suburbs and country towns; distributors ("pushers") are in contact with the student population of the majority of high schools and universities and regularly scout the places of refreshment and entertainment where young people congregate. The pushers (at least those who sell to individual customers) are themselves young, tend to confine their activities to a few trusted friends, and are protected from detection by the prideful fidelity of their peers.

INCIDENCE

It is impossible to arrive at an accurate assessment of the number of young people involved in the current drug scene. Figures from law enforcement sources tend to reflect, at least partly, the increasing vigor with which they are pursuing this relatively new type of offender, and certainly encompass only a very small minority of clandestine users. Similarly, the vast majority of users do not come to the attention of physicians.[34, 91] The most practical type of investigation, admittedly limited, has been the use of questionnaires, with anonymity guaranteed.[8, 60, 62, 71] The youthful users themselves, and professionals in close contact with them, insist, with justification, that any published figures greatly underestimate the actual incidence.

Within North America, the most consistently quoted figures suggest that some 6 to 10 per cent of high school students have had at least one experience with one of these psychedelic drugs. In one Canadian study,[62] one-half of such subjects went on to further use of the drugs. Within the Montreal area, surveys of university undergraduates in 1968 revealed the following figures for at least one experience with one of these substances: McGill University, 28.5 per cent[10]; Loyola College, 15 per cent[71]; Bishop's University, 19.55 per cent.[8] Figures for university undergraduates in the United States[46] are similar to those for Canada—an average of 15 to 20 per cent for at least one experience with marijuana, with higher incidence in such cities as San Francisco, New York, and Boston. One group of researchers took two months to find nine "marijuana-naïve" subjects within the student population of Boston![97]

Figures from Canadian law enforcement sources show that cases involving marijuana rose from 54 in 1964 to 157 in 1967; during the first eleven months of 1968, there was a total of 2,244 convictions. The Canadian Dominion Bureau of Statistics, analyzing 295 convictions for possession of marijuana, found that 241 involved persons under the age of twenty-five, 141 of these between the ages of sixteen and nineteen—confirming that marijuana is essentially a youth problem. In California, there were 7,000 arrests involving marijuana in 1964, as against 37,000 in 1967.[48]

In England, white cannabis offenders apprehended by the London police rose in number from 296 in 1963 to 1,737 in 1967; corresponding figures for Negro offenders rose from 367 to 656. Estimates of cannabis use among undergraduates at London and Oxford universities correspond to North American percentages. In England, hashish is more commonly used than marijuana, whereas the use of LSD became popular some two years after it crested in the United States.[46, 72] Estimates in 1967 suggested that about 2 to 3 per cent of North American students had had at least one experience with LSD; the incidence has dropped appreciably since mid-1968.

Amphetamine abuse is considered by the World Health Organization to have reached epidemic proportions, and North American studies[33, 41] support this judgment. England has experienced a problem with this class of drugs for some twelve years.[46] Sweden has found amphetamine abuse, especially in the intravenous form, to be a major problem among youth for some time, to the extent that prescription and sale of these and similar drugs are now forbidden. Some 5 to 10 per cent of Stockholm high school students have experimented with hashish at least once[46]; LSD misuse is of recent onset.

During the panel on International Problems of Youth at the 124th Annual Meeting of the American Psychiatric Association (Boston, May 1968), Leigh Sakamaki reported that in Hawaii the misuse of marijuana and LSD was primarily a problem among Caucasian high school and university students from the upper socioeconomic levels; solvent inhalation was confined more to the socially disadvantaged youth. At the same meeting, C. P. Wijesinghe of Ceylon indicated that in his country drug abuse was not a significant problem among youth; gangs of juveniles peddle drugs to laborers without themselves indulging. Pachéco e Silva, speaking at the Fourth World Congress of Psychiatry (Madrid, September 1966), noted that the recent introduction of youth to marijuana was causing alarm in that country, particularly in view of a suspected association with criminal activity. Lambo, in his West African studies,[43] noted that teenage abuse of drugs, especially cannabis, has become prevalent and that, for patients with a history of cannabis use, more than half are under the age of twenty-five.

The remainder of this chapter will focus primarily on the issue of psychoactive drug misuse as it pertains to North America. Awareness of this circumscribed approach will hopefully discourage extrapolation from a given intoxicant, milieu, and set of experiences to other situations with superficial similarities—a phenomenon that, through its too frequent occurrence, is responsible for a good deal of the confusion and controversy surrounding the entire issue of psychedelic drug misuse, particularly as it pertains to marijuana.

DRUGS IN COMMON USE

The ingenuity, adventurousness, persistence, and disdain for potential hazards that the youthful drug user demonstrates in his search for new varieties of subjective experience continue to amaze and alarm health professionals. Every few months, another substance is added to the peculiar pseudopharmacopoeia. Legislators, to the glee of some young users, join in the interminable paper chase—as quickly as one substance is brought under legislative control, a new intoxicant attains evanescent or long-term popularity. The enthusiasm for research, were it tempered by adequate precautions and sufficient attention to scientific procedure, might evoke the envy of more responsible workers in the ethnopharmacologic field.[18]

Which particular substance is in common use at a given time depends on availability, fashion, and novelty—and on the individual user's assessment of new information concerning established substances. Many young users have a detailed knowledge of the professional literature, a fact that has embarrassed more than one authority figure trying to dissuade them from misusing drugs. Their understanding and memory, however, seem too often to be biased in favor of those parts of various studies that might be used to exonerate misuse of the drug. Marijuana and, to a lesser extent, hashish are ubiquitous and perennially popular. Until recently, LSD came next in frequency of misuse, but there has been an appreciable decline in its popularity recently, owing primarily to the widely reported possibility of chromosomal damage and chronic brain damage. (It does seem that misusers of psychedelic drugs are deterred more by the possibility of somatic damage than by the probability of psychiatric complications.) Unfortunately, the decline in LSD use has been paralleled by an increase in the misuse of amphetamines.[92, 93] STP and Asthmador had a mercifully short-lived popularity. Solvent inhalation, confined mainly to younger teenagers, seems inexplicably to be on the increase in eastern Canada, following the discovery farther west during fall 1967 that 2 to 5 per cent of the students in some Winnipeg high schools were glue sniffers.

Solvent Inhalation

Glue sniffing, the inhalation of the fumes given off by polystyrene and household cements[2, 7, 25, 101] is widespread among older children and younger adolescents in the United States and Canada. However, a wide variety of lipid-soluble organic solvents are abused by inhalation, and the term "solvent inhalation" is more appropriate. The problem has become serious enough for legislatures to place restrictions on the sale and availability of these substances to juveniles. Commercially available products capable of producing the transient intoxication and elation sought by abusers include:

1. Glues and cements are the most frequent source, especially plastic (styrene) cements, model-building cements, and household cements. The chief solvents involved are toluene and acetone.
2. Cigarette-lighter fluid, cleaning fluid, and gasoline—containing naphtha, benzene, and sometimes carbon tetrachloride.
3. Fingernail polish remover—containing mainly acetone and aliphatic acetates.
4. Lacquer and varnish thinners—containing toluene and aliphatic acetates.
5. Ethyl ether.

Other solvent-containing products, including antifreeze, may be experimented with, particularly by the beginner.

The technique of self-administration involves the tight wrapping or soaking of the substance in a piece of cloth, which is then held to the nose or mouth and sniffed. Glues may be heated to speed the process of emission of their halogenated hydrocarbon solvents. A parallel technique is to place the substance in a plastic bag, the opening of which is then closed around the face to allow inhalation of the pure fumes. The actual concentration of toluene contained in one tube of cement may be fifty times that allowed as a maximum by law in industry.[61] Chronic users may show erosion of the mucosa of the gums, lips, or nose. The odor of the solvent is usually noticeable on the breath and clothes, and the discovery of rags, handkerchiefs, or plastic bags containing dried remnants of solvent-containing products should alert parents and teachers to the probability of solvent inhalation.

The clinical picture produced by these substances varies to a certain extent with the principal solvent involved. The acute effects, the result of an acute brain syndrome, are fairly constant, however, and include, shortly after inhalation, elation, ataxia, slurred speech, sensations of dizziness and floating, and confusion; there is interference with judgment, often to the extent that delusions of increased strength and athletic ability lead to impulsivity, accidents, self-destructive behavior, or antisocial acts (which bring most abusers to the attention of adults).[7, 61] Vivid visual, and less commonly auditory, hallucinations may be experienced by particularly susceptible individuals, especially when external stimuli are reduced.[61] This phase of intoxication usually lasts forty-five to sixty minutes, depending on the concentration and amount inhaled and on the tolerance of the individual. Drowsiness of up to one hour's duration follows, although high enough concentrations may produce stupor, convulsions, and loss of consciousness. Abnormalities of the electroencephalogram are found during the phase of acute intoxication and may persist, in heavy users, for several weeks. Marked anorexia, sometimes leading to pronounced weight loss, is seen with sustained heavy abuse. Transient abnormalities of renal functioning—pyuria and hematuria—are the most constant findings on laboratory examination; reports also exist of hepatic damage and of bone marrow malfunctioning, sometimes leading to aplastic anemia. There is no established evidence of permanent brain damage, and tests of cognitive functioning show no deterioration in chronic users. Deaths are usually the outcome of suffocation from plastic bags, though other fatalities have been associated with pulmonary edema, alveolar hemorrhage, and respiratory or cardiac arrest.

Tolerance and psychological dependency are pronounced with these solvents. Physical withdrawal symptoms are uncommon. Among chronic abusers, emotional deprivation has been a regular finding,[61] as have a history of truancy and poor school performance (not related to intelligence per se), even prior to the beginning of the habit, and a subsequent history of chronic delinquency. No convincing evidence exists to link solvent inhalation with subsequent use of narcotic drugs.[61]

Amphetamines

The use of amphetamines to delay fatigue and sustain concentration has long been practiced by students before exams, long-haul truck drivers, and airline pilots. Physicians have prescribed these drugs for fatigue and mild depression, and their widespread use for control of appetite in patients possessing or anticipating obesity has led to such a problem of dependency and abuse that several countries are considering following Sweden's lead in completely banning the sale or prescription of these and allied substances.

The widespread upsurge in the misuse of amphetamines among young people in recent years is unrelated to the above factors. Used initially within the drug milieu to intensify and prolong the effects of LSD, and sometimes to reactivate the experience without further recourse to LSD, misuse tends more and more to center around the effects of amphetamines alone, particularly methedrine. Methedrine ("speed") misuse is found especially among those who were previously heavy users of LSD ("acid freaks"). Use is by mouth (to "drop") in tablet form, by ingestion or sniffing in powder form, or by intravenous injection (to "shoot").

Oral misuse, commencing with 10 to 20 mg and building up to 150 to 250 mg per day,[41] results in a sense of well-being and self-confidence, euphoria, the absence of fatigue, a sense of increased ability to concentrate, the urge to talk and move about, and reduction of appetite, together with increased alertness and irritability.[15, 33] The mouth is dry, the pulse rapid, and palpitations may occur. With sustained use, there is usually a rebound depression after the effects wear off. Sleeplessness may encourage the use of barbiturates, whose hangover effects lead to further amphetamine ingestion and thus to a vicious circle. The amphetamines are somewhat unique among CNS stimulants in their tendency to produce tolerance,[17] and with the larger doses noted above and with sustained misuse, paranoid features are almost universal.

Intravenous use, commencing with 20 to 40 mg individual doses and building up to 100 to 300 mg, produces a sudden ecstatic feeling throughout the body (a "rush"). Following the rush, there is a compulsion to talk continuously, the experiencing of strong emotions ranging from warmth and sociability to anger and fear, driven activity that gradually becomes purposeless, and no awareness of fatigue or a need to sleep. Paranoid ideas are virtually inevitable, and though initially the paranoid ideation may be more or less realistically focused on the law violations of the group,[41] the higher doses tend to produce disordered behavior, hallucinations, and a tendency to retaliate in response to paranoid delusions—amphetamine psychosis. The lapel buttons sported by youth, proclaiming that "Speed Kills," refer not to highway slaughter but to the occasional violence precipitated by repeated high doses of intravenous methedrine and to the potential complications, such as septicemia and serum hepatitis, that accompany the communal use of nonsterile needles and syringes by hippie groups. Sustained heavy use of either the oral or intravenous forms results in cachexia, abscesses, intractable ulcers. tooth grinding, and brittle fingernails.[41] Withdrawal is followed by prolonged sleep, voracious appetite, and emotional depression.

Amphetamine psychosis is a distinct clinical entity, first described by Connell in 1958.[15] Even a single therapeutic dose may, in susceptible personalities, precipitate a paranoid psychosis indistinguishable from alcoholic hallucinosis or paranoid schizophrenia. Though the psychiatric profession was initially interested in the potential of the LSD "model psychosis" for further understanding of schizophrenia, it is now realized that there are significant differences between schizophrenia and the LSD psychosis and that the psychotic state produced by amphetamines is much closer to the schizophrenic model. The clinical picture is "a paranoid psychosis with ideas of reference, delusions of persecution, auditory and visual hallucinations, in a setting of clear consciousness."[15] Gross distortions of body image are frequent.[19] Patients recover within a week of withdrawal, during which time there are periods of prolonged deep sleep, followed by marked hunger for food and by depression that might lead to suicide. Amphetamine is found in the urine for up to seven days after withdrawal, and Connell recommends the use of a modified methyl orange test whenever the question of amphetamine use arises in a patient. In the absence of psychotic symptoms, amphetamine dependency may present clinically as a chronic anxiety state.

Personality studies indicate that schizoid types are more liable to develop the amphetamine psychosis than antisocial types.[19] Reporting to the Fourth World Congress of Psychiatry in 1966, Tatsetsu judged that 96 per cent of the intravenous methedrine abusers treated by him in Japan showed signs of psychiatric disease before becoming involved with abuse of the drug.

Abuse of amphetamines leads to pronounced tolerance and is very frequently associated with psychological dependence. Though Eddy, Halbach, Isbell, and Seevers[17] contend that amphetamine abuse is not associated with physical dependence or a characteristic abstinence syndrome, Connell[15] and Kramer, Fischman, and Littlefield[41] believe that the depth and length of the sleep following cessation of the drug, and the pronounced appetite on awakening, are strongly suggestive of abstinence effects. Further, Oswald and Thacore[58] conclude from their electroencephalographic studies that the marked increase in REM time, noted during the withdrawal sleep and reversible by reinstituting the drug, is indicative of physiological dependency. The sleep abnormalities noted on the electroencephalogram may not disappear completely until eight weeks after withdrawal of the drug.

Following strict legal controls, the misuse of inhalers containing amphetamines is now uncommon. However, the use of the contents of such inhalers as Dristan (containing the amphetamine congener mephentermine) is seen occasionally. The inhaler plug is chewed or soaked in coffee, beer, or warm water and swallowed; ingestion leads to euphoria and other amphetamine effects. Compulsion to increase the dose, a clinical state similar to amphetamine psychosis, and a confusional state on withdrawal have been noted.[28] Rotalin (methylphenidate) misuse is less commonly met with than amphetamine abuse; its effects are more central, with fewer peripheral autonomic signs, and dependency seems to be less marked. Ephedrine misuse is occasionally encountered, particularly as a means of enhancing LSD effects; the results are similar to, but less marked than, those associated with the amphetamines.

The Original Psychedelic Drugs

Prior to 1943 the main psychedelic drug in (limited) use was mescaline. After Hoffman accidentally discovered the hallucinogenic properties of LSD in 1944, psychiatric research centered around the psychotomimetic and therapeutic properties of this new substance, until sensationalist publicity during the early 1960's led to the adoption of LSD as an almost sacrificial substance by the psychedelic movement among youth. "Psychedelic" means "mind-manifesting"; other terms applied to this class of drugs include "psychomimetic" ("copying a psychosis") and "hallucinogenic" (a relative misnomer, as the perceptual distortions are more often of the nature of illusions). "Hallucinogenic" has been applied also more broadly to encompass all "soft" (nonaddictive) drugs misused by youth—including the amphetamines and the marijuana group.

Drugs of the psychedelic category include, in order of probable increasing potency, dimethyletryptamine (DMT), lysergic acid diethylamide (LSD), and DOM (STP). Some (LSD, DMT, Psilocybin) are indole derivatives; others (mescaline, STP) are phenylethylamines. One postulated biochemical mode of action involves interference with the metabolism in the brain of the catecholamines. The primary neurophysiological impact is thought to be on the afferent impulses entering the ascending RAS through collaterals from sensory pathways.[6] There are certain neurophysiological similarities between LSD-induced hallucinations in the waking state and the "dreaming" sleep (REM's); a possible relationship has been postulated between LSD action and the neurohumoral mechanisms underlying REM's.[53]

LSD-25

Lysergic acid diethylamide ("acid") is one of the most potent psychochemicals known. A dose no smaller than 1/700 millionth the weight of an average man is sufficient to yield significant alteration of psychic functioning. One ounce of the substance could "turn on" (intoxicate) a city of 300,000 inhabitants,[50] though fears of contamination of the water supply of cities are groundless, because the LSD would be inactivated by chemical purifiers in the reservoirs. In solution, LSD is colorless, tasteless, and odorless. It is ingested as a white crystalline powder in tablets or capsules, less frequently in impregnated sugar cubes; it may also be injected. Potency and purity of samples bought on the illicit market vary widely.

As with marijuana, the effect of a given dose on a given individual is a function of the complex interaction of personality, expectation, and milieu, and, as with marijuana, suggestibility is significantly heightened.[79] Depending on individual susceptibility and the surrounding circumstances, a dose of 50 to 150 micrograms can induce a psychedelic experience. Heavy users may ingest ("drop") a single dose of several hundred (and uncommonly several thousand µg. LSD is absorbed rapidly after swallowing and has disappeared from the body fluids by the time of onset of the symptoms. Increasing the dosage tends to lead to prolongation of the experience rather than to intensification of effects; the latter is obtained by the addition of atropine-like substances—an increasingly common phenomenon[78, 87]—or of amphetamines. Substances peddled as LSD (and particularly as STP) may in fact consist of varying mixtures of amphetamines, atrophine-like substances, and mescaline.

The LSD syndrome can serve as a model for the other psychedelic substances. Effects commence about thirty minutes after ingestion and persist for the average dose (100 to 200 µg) about nine to twelve hours. Effects on the autonomic nervous system include dilation of pupils, varying photophobia, slight tachycardia, elevated blood glucose, flushed face, sweating, and limb trembling. Certain subjective phenomena are invariant[17, 50, 59, 67]: perceptual alterations including depersonalization, derealization, and visual illusions (less commonly hallucinations) involving color, distance, space, and plasticity; a dissociation of the ego to produce an observing, monitoring self and an experiencing, feeling self; disturbance of cognition with fluctuating ability to concentrate and sustain attention; pressure and vagueness of ideas; and increasingly autistic preoccupation with philosophical, ethical, and highly egocentric issues. Enough contact with reality is usually maintained to realize that the experience is initiated by the drug, but judgment can be so disturbed as to allow serious accidents.

The "tripper" may be so withdrawn into his inner experiences as to appear stuperose, but his attention can, with persistence, be obtained by intervening persons. Less commonly, disorganized hyperactive behavior may ensue. The intoxication is subsequently remembered in detail and recognized as having been a paranormal drug-induced experience.

Less common phenomena, depending very much on personality, set, and suggestion, include varieties of affective responses ranging from ecstasy to despair. There may, uncommonly, be the attainment of a transcendental state with consequent change in personality functioning in the direction of better integration and improved ego strength. Such changes are not frequent outside of a psychotherapeutic alliance. Reported successes in psychotherapy using LSD do not require the attainment of such a rarefied state. More commonly, states of intense inner preoccupation, less than transcendental, produce quasi-delusional assessments of intellectual ability, self-insight, and creativity[82]; the alleged insights are not usually applied to the ongoing personality functioning of the nonintoxicated subject following the trip. The presence of an LSD sophisticate as "guide" does not guarantee a satisfying, nontraumatic experience; several studies on the behavioral effects of LSD in animals and man[66, 88] attest to the complexity and unpredictability of the experience.

A study of the long-lasting effects of LSD on normals[47] revealed that psychological testing to validate the lasting effects reported by 58 per cent of subjects after six months could provide "only minimal supporting evidence." On the other hand, a growing list of reports has more than adequately demonstrated that LSD is a potentially dangerous drug.[13, 14, 31, 69, 73, 86, 87, 88, 89] M. M. Cohen, who had earlier assessed the risk of suicide and psychosis as less than 1 in 1,000, found in 1966 that the incidence had risen considerably, owing to the increasing illicit use of the drug. He devised a classification[14] of LSD complications as follows:

I. Psychotic Disorders
   A. Accidental LSD intoxication in children
   B. Chronic LSD intoxication
   C. Schizophrenic reactions
   D. Paranoia
   E. Acute paranoid states
   F. Prolonged or intermittent LSD-like psychoses
   G. Psychotic depressions
II. Nonpsychotic Disorders
   A. Chronic anxiety reactions
   B. Acute panic states
   C. Dissocial behavior
   D. Antisocial behavior
III. Neurological Reactions
   A. Convulsions and permanent brain damage

To this classification would now have to be added, tentatively, "Chromosomal Breakage" and, perhaps, the "Amotivational Syndrome."[48] Ungerleider, Fisher, and Fuller[87] reported on seventy psychiatric patients, with a median age of twenty-one, all of whom had used LSD (and often other drugs) illicitly. In order of incidence, the patients presented with hallucinations, anxiety states, depression, and confusion. Twenty-five required hospitalization, eleven for more than one month. The same authors, with two others, undertook a questionnaire survey of Los Angeles county[89] over an eighteen-month period prior to January 1968 and found a minimum of 2,389 adverse reactions to LSD encountered by 27 per cent of respondents, all health professionals. There was an increase of 62 per cent in the number of adverse reactions seen from the first six-month period to the third, contradicting the impression of many physicians that such reactions are decreasing in frequency. Twenty-six per cent of respondents indicated that more than half their LSD patients had experienced spontaneous recurrences ("flashbacks") of the LSD experience; as pointed out by Keeler,[36] such recurrences need not necessarily be regarded as adverse reactions, unless they precipitate anxiety or interfere with function. The significance of the Ungerleider survey is clouded by the inconsistencies in definition of "adverse reaction" by some respondents—some felt any effect of LSD was an adverse reaction and others were unable to attribute effects noted to one specific drug when several had been misused in combination or sequence —a not uncommon dilemma for clinicians.

Problems of physical dependence and abstinence symptoms do not arise with LSD. There is, however, a tolerance that develops and disappears rapidly. Cross-tolerance is exhibited with mescaline, but not with the tetrahydrocannabinols (THC). Reports of chronic brain damage, following sustained heavy use, remain to be adequately assessed in the literature. The first reports of chromosome breakage associated with LSD came from M. M. Cohen in 1967[13]; some subsequent reports confirm Cohen's findings,[31] whereas others[45, 80] have not been able to replicate them. The latter of these two dissenting reports[80] has itself been criticized on the grounds of unsatisfactory statistical methodology.[42, 100] The risks to pregnancies from pregnant women taking LSD remains an open question, despite reports in the popular press.

The value of LSD in psychiatric therapy is still not established. Though earlier reports indicated its usefulness in such conditions as alcoholism and homosexuality, other studies are more skeptical. Robinson found in a controlled study that the use of LSD for abreaction had no advantage over standard psychotherapy or abreaction with intravenous methedrine and hexabarbitone in the therapy of neuroses.[64] Two recent controlled studies found LSD of no advantage in the treatment of alcoholism.[74, 95] The recent book edited by Ungerleider[86] examines the current status of LSD as a therapeutic tool, the many unanswered questions with regard to hallucinogens, and prospects for the future. There is also here a useful up-to-date review of possible acute and chronic side effects.

STP

These letters, given by the hippies to the hallucinogen DOM, stand for serenity, tranquility, and peace. The drug is a synthetic methoxylated amphetamine with the formula 2, 5-dimethyl-4-methyl-amphetamine and is related to both mescaline and amphetamine.[63, 75] When it first appeared on the illicit market in early 1967, it was considered a highly potent and dangerous substance, at least ten times as strong as LSD, a megahallucinogen that induced a trip of from three to five days' duration.[63, 81, 91] Deaths had been reported. Toxic signs were essentially those of atropine poisoning—a classical delirium with confusion, agitation, disorientation, and visual and tactile hallucinations. The mouth was dry, the pupils widely dilated, and the skin dry and flushed. Fever and tachycardia completed the picture, along with some muscle twitching and occasional convulsions. Respiratory failure could lead to death.

Subsequent experience suggested that the substance was, more often than not, a composite of large doses of atropine-like substances, methedrine, and perhaps mescaline. The recent experiment by Snyder and his coworkers[75] suggests that genuine STP (DOM) is more than fifty times as potent as mescaline and uniformly hallucinogenic at doses exceeding 5 mg/70kg. In normal male volunteers aged twenty-one to thirty-five, controlled experiments with low doses of from 2.7 to 3.3 mg STP produced "subjective effects of mild euphoria and enhanced self-awareness in the absence of hallucinogenic or psychomimetic effects." There was enhanced performance on serial learning tasks and no interference with simple visual perception tests. The only interference at this dosage was with associative organization.

It remains doubtful as to how often the young drug misuser encounters genuine STP. The vast majority of cases physicians see will evidence atropine poisoning and should be managed as such.

DMT AND DET

DMT (dimethyltryptamine) and the closely related DET (diethyltryptamine) are substituted phenethylamines found in hallucinogenic snuffs used by South American Indians.[20] Both give only a short intoxication of thirty to forty-five minutes.[50] DMT is more commonly encountered than DET and must be inhaled—it is inactive if ingested orally. It can be sniffed as a powder or prepared as a liquid into which parsley, tobacco, or marijuana is dipped and then smoked. DMT tends to give a greater variety and proportion of visual illusions than LSD, with greater (though short-lived) autonomic effects. The very rapid onset of symptoms (especially if injected intramuscularly, which is uncommon) and the occasional feeling of loss of control can cause panic states more frequently than LSD.

PSILOCYBIN

This drug is a 4-hydroxydimethyltryptamine and is unlike other substituted tryptamines, such as DMT, in that it elicits psychedelic effects when taken orally.[20] It has been described as giving a "warm, giggly high" whose characteristics are more stable and less intense than those of the LSD experience.[59] It is not in wide illicit use.

MESCALINE

Derived from the peyote cactus, it is not in wide use because ingestion first induces nausea, tremor, and perspiration. After one to two hours, these unpleasant effects subside and a dream-like intoxicated state ensues, characterized by vivid kaleidoscopic visions. Finally, the subject falls into a deep sleep.

Marijuana, Hashish, and THC

Cannabis products, especially marijuana, have in recent years become the center of such controversy and so many contradictory reports that any author must approach yet another review of the topic with considerable reluctance. The whole issue has become embroidered with so much mythology, prejudice, and dogmatism that even for professionals in close and continuous contact with the literature, research, and illicit users, bias and confusion are difficult to avoid. The subject is, to quote Winston Churchill out of context, "a riddle wrapped in a mystery inside an enigma." Despite an abundance of studies and reports,[9, 46, 49, 52, 56, 67, 76, 91, 99] reliable facts are scant and elusive, and results of adequately conducted experiments in man are surprisingly few.[11, 20, 32, 97] Equally eminent and experienced experts give diametrically opposed and mutually contradictory views. The Advisory Committee on Drug

Dependency of the British Parliament, in its recent report on cannabis,[9] noted that "the literature is vast and contradictory International discussion and decision-making have been handicapped by inexact or inadequate information." Sir Aubrey Lewis, in constructing a bibliography for the same report, noted that, despite a literature containing 1,750 entries up to 1965, "almost every theme is beset with contradictory observations and opinions."

Some beginning to the resolution of this confusion may be possible if one considers some of the contradictory statements themselves. Thus, in two very recent reviews of the literature, though Lewis concludes[9] that "a respectable body of opinion is to the effect that . . . the majority of moderate users are within the normal range of personality" (p. 46), Schwarz concludes, on the other hand,[70] that "regular users of both marijuana and hashish so far studied tend to show basic defects of personality." Again, though the Narcotic Addiction Foundation of British Columbia in a recent policy statement,[54] outlining "what we know about the drug," found "indisputable evidence that the stronger forms of the drug (resin from the plant) are directly connected with crimes of violence and anti-social behavior," Murphy in his review of the literature[52] states that "most serious observers agree that cannabis does not, per se, induce aggressive or criminal activities, and that reduction in the work drive leads to a negative correlation with criminality rather than a positive one." According to Schwarz,[70] "depending on the complex interaction of a number of variables of which the drug is only one, Hashish and to a lesser extent Marihuana, can be associated with . . . personality deterioration and chronic physical ill-health," whereas Eddy et al.[17] are of the opinion that, for cannabis, "no unequivocal evidence is available that lasting mental changes are produced," and another assessment of current knowledge[49] concludes that "no valid conclusion about the harmfulness or harmlessness of chronic marihuana use can be drawn at present." It should be noted that all the reports and reviews quoted in this paragraph were published within the last four to five years, and all but two within the seven months preceding February 1969.

Why these apparent discrepancies—a very small sample of the total number that could be demonstrated? Detailed perusal of the above examples and of published reviews suggests that confusion and apparent contradictions are related to the following factors:

1. Many reports speak of marijuana users and cannabis users, suggesting a constancy and interchangeability of potency and frequency of use

that do not exist. Cannabis products vary enormously in their strength and effects, depending not only on the particular preparation used, but also on the age of the product and the climatic conditions and geography where the parent plant was grown.[20]

2. The use of such terms as "moderate," "casual," "heavy," "chronic," and "sustained," when describing the user, though inevitable at present, are insufficiently exact, even when the same preparation is being referred to. For adequate scientific assessment, one needs to know what individual dose of the drug was used how frequently over what period of time.

3. Even when exact dosage is measured and reported (an uncommon event), valid comparisons cannot be made if different preparations are used, for example, crude marijuana[35] vs. oily extract[11] vs. tetrahydrocannabinol.[32] Satisfactory comparisons will become possible only when all preparations used in future experiments are assayed for tetrahydrocannabinol content, should this prove to be the most significant constituent of cannabis in terms of production of clinical effects.[20, 97] There is now available for research purposes a U.N. Reference Sample of constant composition and known strength. The U.S. National Institute of Mental Health is also preparing a standard sample for research.

4. There is considerable evidence to suggest that the same dose of the same preparation has different effects, depending on whether it is inhaled or taken orally.[32, 52, 56, 97] In published studies over the years, some substances have been administered orally, others by inhalation.

5. The pronounced effects of personality, set, setting, and suggestibility are crucial[21, 79, 91, 97] in determining the effects of cannabis products on a given subject at a given time. Very few experiments or reports have taken these factors into consideration or tried to control them.[97]

6. The sample of subjects to which a given report refers must be considered. Most experiments on humans have involved as samples prisoners, exopiate users, or chronic cannabis (usually marijuana) users.[9, 32] Of recent experiments, only two[11, 97] used marijuana-naïve subjects, and even here comparison is limited by the fact that different preparations were administered by different routes and equivalent doses cannot be calculated. Only one recent study[97] has used such control techniques as placebo and the administration of comparable doses to both naïve and chronic users. The vast majority of nonexperimental reports have drawn their conclusions from psychiatric patients and heavy, chronic users,[9, 35, 43, 52] mostly from African and Asian countries. The Task Force on Narcotics and Drug Abuse of the 1967 U.S. President's Commission on Law Enforcement and the Administration of Justice reported that "no careful and detailed analysis of the American Experience seems to have been attempted." It is obvious that very few of the known findings can be extrapolated honestly to the experiences of young North American

cannabis users, most of whom smoke no more than two to four (usually mild) marijuana cigarettes per week.[48] Research is urgently needed in North America on the immediate and remote effects—physical, psychiatric, psychological, and social—of occasional, moderate use and sustained heavy use of the various cannabis preparations (if these adjectives can be defined more exactly in terms of dosage).

7. It is quite common for users to mix noncannabis drugs with their cannabis preparations. In North Africa and Asia, opium and datura seeds (containing stramonium) are frequently admixed,[22] and in other countries, combinations of drugs of other types may be found.[43, 70, 91] It thus can be difficult to determine which drug causes which effect, either immediate or remote.

8. In determining the relationship of cannabis use to various outcomes (criminal activity, psychiatric disturbance, progression to other drugs, and so forth), the effects of the drug must be weighed against the personality vulnerabilities of the subject.[48, 70, 91]

9. Marijuana use has become a lightning rod, a point of focus, toward which are projected and displaced many of the anxieties, desires, fears, and indignations of contemporary society.[48, 56, 71] To some, including what many youths call the "Establishment," it seems synonymous with all that is disturbing and disturbed about contemporary youth—the protestors, hippies, student activists, dropouts, and so forth. To others (usually called "liberal"), the marijuana issue evokes other concerns of society—the arbitrariness of over-centralized, impersonal authority, the obsolescence of tradition, and the diminishing reliability of conventional wisdom and values in a society in perennial rapid transition. The entire issue is grossly overdetermined and frequently entails a degree of emotion suggestive of reaction formation or of projective identification.

Consideration of the foregoing list of factors, which is certainly not exhaustive, requires that, having acknowledged the possible emotional bias, one must assess the various reports in the following terms: how often over what period of time was how much of what strength of which cannabis product of determined purity administered by what route under what conditions to which sample of people.

Cannabis sativa L. var. *indica* is a weed that grows wild, ideally in hot, dry climates. The resinous exudate of the tops of the female plant contains most of the active ingredients. Marijuana ("pot," "grass," "tea") consists of the dried, mature flowering tops of the (preferably unfertilized) female plant. It is usually smoked, the typical cigarette ("joint," "reefer") being thinner than a regular tobacco cigarette and containing greenish-brown, dry, crushed leaves and twigs and perhaps some small seeds. The ends of the cigarette paper are twisted or folded back to prevent spillage of the loosely packed contents, which have a slight musty smell (and which dogs can be trained to sniff out despite intervening covering material). The substance can also be smoked in a pipe. It burns with a characteristic odor, rather like that of burning hay or alfalfa grass (and the latter, which has no psychoactive properties, is often fraudulently sold mixed with or instead of marijuana, in which case the client is said to have been "burned"). Because it burns rapidly, the joint is usually smoked in company, being passed round to minimize wastage. The technique of inhalation has to be learned—deep inhalation of as much smoke as possible, with the mouth open, followed by holding the breath in the inspiratory phase for as long as possible. The unused end of the cigarette ("roach"), containing a high concentration of resin, is saved to be incorporated in a new joint or hoarded against times of famine, when it will be smoked by tucking it into the evacuated end of a tobacco cigarette.

The smoke is irritating to the pharynx, particularly when inhaled suddenly by the novice. Spasms of coughing are common after several inhalations ("tokes"). Most users use one to two cigarettes at a sitting and will commonly refuse more, preferring to maintain the moderately fluctuating plateau ("high"), which they have learned pleases them most. Less commonly, heavy intoxication (being "stoned") will be sought. Effects of one to two cigarettes reach maximum intensity after thirty minutes and have dissipated after about three hours.[97]

Pharmacological effects in animals are largely confined to the CNS, with vomiting, diarrhea, ataxia, and tremors, but no marked sedation or hypnosis.

The initiate, when first introduced to the drug, often notices no effect[91, 97] apart from some throat irritation and some nausea. It appears one must learn not only the proper technique of smoking, but also how to recognize and become sensitized to the effects.[55, 97] Guidance and further experimentation using one to two cigarettes at a time lead to the typical marijuana syndrome: a feeling of tranquility and well-being, euphoria (plus easily evoked giggling), sensations of floating, and altered awareness of time (time is expanded, with a given time interval thus seeming to pass more slowly—which is not to say that the subject necessarily moves or reacts slowly). Mild depersonalization and derealization are common—the latter particularly in the form of a broadening of space and a seeming remoteness of near objects. It is primarily the distortion of time, and even more of space, that can make driving hazardous. Colors may be perceived as more vivid, and their emotional context is more pronounced, especially with higher doses; the same holds for the senses of touch, taste, smell, and sound—individual instruments in a band or orchestra can be isolated more easily and the components of a harmony dissected (to hear music "vertically"). Hunger is invariable, but though this has usually been attributed to hypoglycemia (Goodman and Gilman[27] claim slight hyperglycemia), the important recent study by Weil, Zinberg, and Nelson[97] found no changes in blood glucose in either naïve or experienced intoxicated subjects. Another popular marijuana myth contradicted by this study is that of pupillary dilation—careful measurement showed no change in pupil size for either the naïve or experienced intoxicated subjects. There are dryness of the mouth and suffusion of the conjunctiva—but the latter cannot be used as evidence of current or recent intoxication, as the injection of transverse ciliary vessels can persist for years after cessation of the drug in chronic users.[52] Though most writers report hypomotility with incoordination, Eddy et al.[17] claim hypermotility without impairment of coordination, and another report[54] finds that subjects are not nearly so uncoordinated as with alcohol. The Weil study, on a test measuring muscular coordination and attention, found a decline in performance in the nine marijuana-naïve subjects that was dose-related, but the eight chronic users, starting from a good base line, actually improved in performance while intoxicated; the authors feel that this may have been largely a practice effect, but the point is that the performance did not decline. In the same study, a test measuring capacity for sustained attention was unaffected for both the naïve and experienced intoxicated subjects, despite the addition of a strobe light for added distraction. Practice effects are not significant in this test. A test of cognitive functioning showed gross impairment during intoxication for the naïve group, but a slight improvement for the chronic users, who all once again started from a good base line. This improvement cannot be accounted for solely by practice effect.

Other findings of the Weil study[97]—apparently "the first attempt to investigate marijuana in a formal double-blind experiment with the appropriate controls"—suggest that the effects on marijuana-naïve subjects of two cigarettes (containing in toto 18 mg THC) are only slight. The authors conclude that "marihuana appears to be a relatively mild intoxicant in our studies" and suggest that "if these results seem to differ from those of earlier experiments it must be remembered that other experiments have given marihuana orally" (which tends to produce more powerful and more unpredictable effects), "have given doses much higher than those commonly smoked by users, have administered powerful synthetics, and have not strictly controlled the laboratory setting."

With higher doses, and with sustained use, depersonalization is more pronounced and illusions more prominent. Hallucinations can occur, though less frequently than the appellation "hallucinogen" might imply. Complex reaction time is slowed, and with heavy intoxication incoordination becomes more noticeable. Effects of all cannabis products are dose-related; the resin of the tops of the plant, when collected in relatively pure state, is used to make hashish, which contains about 35 to 47 per cent resin by weight (as compared with 5 to 8 per cent by weight for marijuana).[56, 70]

Hashish is sold in small blocks of the consistency of bouillon cubes. It is gray-brown to brown in color. Small pieces are flaked off the block with a knife and placed on the glowing tip of a tobacco cigarette, from which the smoke is led to the nose or mouth through a drinking straw or hollow shell of a ballpoint pen. It may also be smoked in a small pipe or through a water pipe (to which crème de menthe is often added). It may also be eaten. The effects are similar to, but more intense, than marijuana.

The tetrahydrocannabinols (THC), which appear to be the main active ingredients of cannabis, have been isolated from the resin,[40] and the synthesis of one of these—(-)-delta 1 -trans-tetrahydrocannabinol—in 1967, has opened the door for broader research. However, it has yet to be established that THC is the sole determinant of marijuana's effects.[97] It is doubtful that much THC has found its way onto the illicit market; it is very complex and expensive to synthesize and unstable under certain conditions. Regardless of the route of administration, it produces many of the effects noted in the Weil study[97]—no significant dilation of pupils, and no change in respiratory rate, but, with high doses, increased heart rate and injection of the transverse ciliary vessels.[32] THC has been found to be two or three times as potent by inhalation as by mouth, which is the opposite of naturally occurring cannabis products.[7] Isbell, Gorodetzsky, Jasinski, Claussen, Spulak, and Korte[32] found that, with a sample of forty chronic marijuana users, synthetic THC in small doses (50 µg/kg by smoking, 100 to 120 µg/kg orally) produced marijuana-like effects; in higher doses (200 to 250 µg/kg by smoking, 300 to 400 µg/kg orally), LSD-like effects were produced.

Adverse reactions to marijuana and hashish appear to be uncommon in North America. Keeler[34] reports on eleven cases seen recently—1 panic reaction, 2 depressions, 1 case of gross confusion, 1 severe depersonalization, 4 paranoid states, and 2 major changes of life style and behavior. He also interviewed four cases who had become schizophrenic after the combined use of marijuana, amphetamine, and LSD. From his review of other reports on adverse reactions and his own experience, he concludes that "perhaps all investigators would agree that marijuana cannot produce functional psychopathology but can only precipitate it in individuals so predisposed." He confirms the impression of other North American authors[91] that most marijuana users do not come to medical attention, but the unexpected findings of the Ungerleider survey[89] that respondents had seen 1,887 adverse reactions to marijuana in eighteen months contradicts this impression and the belief in the uncommonness of untoward marijuana effects. The difficulty of interpreting the Ungerleider findings has been discussed under LSD above. Keeler, Reiflin, and Liptzin[36] have reported four cases of spontaneous recurrence of marijuana effects and suggest that such phenomena should only be classified as adverse reactions if they precipitate anxiety or interfere with function. Murphy[52] concludes from his review of the literature that "the prevalence of *major* mental disorders among cannabis users appears to be little, if any, higher than that in the general population" [emphasis added] and doubts the existence of a specific cannabis psychosis, as does Lewis,[9] who further states that "there is no unequivocal evidence that cannabis can be the major or sufficient cause of any form of psychosis."

In terms of long-term harm from the use of cannabis products, the above-quoted British committee concluded that "having reviewed all the material available to us we find ourselves in agreement ... that the long-term consumption of cannabis in *moderate* doses has no harmful effects" (p. 6) and that "in terms of *physical* harmfulness, cannabis is very much less dangerous than the opiates, amphetamines and barbiturates, and also less dangerous than alcohol" [emphasis added]. Several other authors are of the same opinion.[46, 56, 71] It should be stressed again, however, that satisfactory studies on this matter do not exist for North American samples. McGlothlin and West[48] note the occurrence of the amotivational syndrome—apathy, loss of effectiveness, poor frustration tolerance, noninvolvement in long-term plans, and so on—in some chronic marijuana users, but note that there "has been no attempt to distinguish between preexisting personality traits and the effect of the drug use" in the reports on this syndrome.

The weight of opinion indicates that cannabis products do not lead to tolerance (in fact, a type of reverse tolerance has been noted.)[91, 97] It is generally agreed also that marijuana use does not lead to physical dependence or to significant withdrawal symptoms.[17, 23, 27, 91] As with any substance that relieves anxiety or depression or permits escape from frustrating life circumstances, cannabis products can be associated with psychological dependence, but, as with most drugs, such dependence is much more a function of a preexisting personality vulnerability than inherent in the drug itself.[27]

A few other issues should be touched on briefly. Progression to other drugs, especially heroin, is the most prominent current reason given by law enforcement personnel for maintaining or increasing the penalties for marijuana possession—the fact that 80 per cent of heroin users have used marijuana in the past is repeatedly quoted. The implied causal relationship and inevitability have never been substantiated[23] and are basically illogical.[49] Those who do graduate to such narcotics as heroin are liable to be the vulnerable personalities for whom the degree of escape permitted by marijuana is inadequate.[9] The "underground" nature of the trafficking in marijuana and other "soft" drugs makes it more likely that the user will come into contact with more dangerous drugs,[91] and certainly one does encounter young people who have experimented with heroin—the marijuana user is certainly more at risk than the nonuser, but, as Eddy et al. assert,[17] "transition to such drugs would be a consequence of this association" (with social groups and subcultures involved with the more dangerous drugs) "rather than an inherent effect of cannabis." The British cannabis report[9] does not feel that risk of progression to heroin is a reason for maintaining the present penalties for cannabis offenders.

The association of cannabis with crimes of violence and with unemployment has been noted, primarily in Africa, the Middle East, and Asia,[43, 90] but it is generally agreed that such an association is neither direct nor inevitable.[9, 52, 56] In countries where alcohol use is forbidden by religion, the common practice of mixing stramonium or opium with cannabis must be taken into account.[50] Lambo states that "the relationship of cannabis to crime and antisocial behaviour is complex and elusive"[43] and that unemployment may encourage cannabis use rather than vice versa. Fort found in his studies in Asia[22] that there "opium or cannabis use has had little effect on vocational life." Most authors agree that cannabis does not in itself lead to criminal activity or violence and that this type of activity is considerably more common with alcohol use.[9, 27, 48, 52, 56]

The causes and effects of cannabis misuse involve a "concatenation of factors"[23] and high-priority research in North America must assess the various biological, psychological, and sociocultural variables and their interaction. Halo effects, owing to association through use, social circumstances, or legislative misconceptions, must be obviated.[91]

Exotica

A cursory survey illustrates the variety of miscellaneous substances that youth will experiment with in its search for thrills, as if the foregoing variety of drugs were not enough.

Nutmeg, long popular among sailors and prisoners, contains myristicin, similar to mescaline, and capable of producing a psychedelic experience if sniffed or mixed in juice or water and swallowed. There are less visual phenomena than with LSD, and usually accompanying malaise.[85, 91, 96] Morning-glory seeds contain two alkaloids of lysergic acid. The seeds have to be crushed to release the psychedelic substances, and a solution is usually prepared and swallowed. Only two varieties—Heavenly Blue and Pearly Gates—have psychedelic properties; other varieties contain highly dangerous amounts of toxic ergot derivatives.[20, 59] Symptoms for the psychedelic varieties are like those of LSD, but less intense and so variable as frequently to disappoint the user.[21, 91] Asthmador ("Witches' poison") is a curry-colored powder, intended to be burned and thus inhaled for relief of asthma. Youth discovered that the ingestion of one or two teaspoonfuls would cause intoxication of the LSD type. The powder contains 0.23 to 0.31 per cent total belladonna alkaloids and is clearly labeled with a warning against oral use! The clinical picture of even a slight overdose is of atropine poisoning, with the same signs and symptoms outlined above under STP. Urinary retention is common. The pupils remain dilated for twelve to twenty-four hours after the mental symptoms subside. Deaths are apparently less common than previously believed.[83, 84, 91] Freon gas, available in aerosol containers, is intended for the chilling of cocktail glasses when released. Inhalation in a closed space or from a plastic bag produces a silly delirium—and may freeze the larynx and trachea, which, along with pulmonary edema, has caused several deaths. Gravol (dimenhydrinate) in doses of approximately 400 mg can produce an alcohol-like intoxication. Codeine in cough medicines can be abused—orally, or even by intramuscular injection. Amyl nitrate ampuls, meant for coronary insufficiency, can be used to give a "two-minute trip"; the ampuls ("snappers" or "poppers") are crushed and inhaled; this is commonly done immediately preceding sexual orgasm.

MANAGEMENT

The clinical assessment of the intoxicated individual who obtains his supplies on the illicit market is rendered difficult by several factors: (1) it is usually impossible to know what dosage of a particular drug has been taken; the claims of the user are of dubious reliability; (2) the substance taken may have no psychoactive properties—alfalfa grass has been sold as marijuana, detergent powder and powdered sugar as LSD, bouillon cubes as hashish. Even the scrapings of banana skins enjoyed a passing vogue—the prescribed extract contained nothing apart from carboniferous material[5]; nevertheless, the subject may reproduce all the subjective experiences of the LSD or marijuana trip—evidence of the importance of set and suggestibility mentioned above; (3) the frequent practice of taking several drugs in combination.[30, 65, 77, 91] Increasingly, atropine-like substances are being added to LSD (and less commonly to hashish) to intensify the effects.[78, 87] Methedrine is often added to LSD to prolong and intensify the effects. Tincture of camphor (containing 2.2 grains of opium per fluid ounce) has been added to marijuana in the United States, but occasional reports of marijuana "cured" in opium in Canada have not been substantiated on investigation by authorities.[91] Marijuana may be soaked in DMT. It is important to realize that the user may have no knowledge that his sample of a particular drug has been contaminated ("cut") with another substance; this should add to the caution and skepticism of the examining physician, who may in fact be confronted with the effects of several unidentified drugs in combination.

Because of the above factors, it has become increasingly clear that immediate treatment of the intoxication and of adverse effects has to be on a symptomatic basis. Because of the increasing risk of atropine-like substances being mixed with LSD and other drugs, and because of reported paradoxical responses to chlorpromazine,[68, 87, 91] the drug of choice for immediate use when sedation is required would seem to be diazepam (Valium)[78] in doses of 5 to 10 mg intramuscularly or 30 to 40 mg orally, followed by oral doses of 10 mg every four hours or as needed.[78] Note that the phenothiazines must be avoided if there is any sign or suspicion of atropine poisoning.[78, 91] A stomach lavage may be of use if ingestion of the drug has been very recent. Hospitalization may be indicated if the symptoms are severe, and attention to fluid intake and output, plus monitoring of the vital signs, will be required.

Psychiatric assessment will be indicated in all but the one-time experimenter. This is not to say that the casual user of many of these drugs, especially marijuana, is necessarily an unstable personality or in need of therapy (the increasing use of marijuana by professionals, educators, and responsible public figures in the same social context within which casual indulgence in alcohol is found would challenge such a contention). Nevertheless, any young person who is involved in more than passing experimentation with drugs should be evaluated, as should his family.[91] Whatever the pros and cons of marijuana use may be, it should be obvious that free, unsupervised access to and indulgence in any intoxicant (including alcohol) can be hazardous to the younger adolescent at a time when he is going through critical intellectual, biological, personality, and social development. The judgment and sense of personal and social responsibility of the younger teenager have yet to reach full maturity, and intoxicants that interfere with these functions carry a heavy risk of personal and social disaster.

Certainly, for the habitual young user, therapy of him (and if possible of his family) will be indicated. Increasingly, it is becoming apparent that, though all types of personality disorders, neurotic conflicts, and even psychotic functioning may underlie the repeated misuse of drugs, one of the most common underlying conditions among these young people is a depressive reaction.[30, 44, 55, 92, 98] This is often allied to youthful alienation[1, 29, 37,

[38, 39, 102] and can be quite difficult to uncover and treat in psychotherapy.[29, 55] Several authors have noted the way in which youth can use these drugs to escape unwelcome feelings, and particularly how often there is a need for a fusion or merging with others.[4, 24, 44, 97] The need for interpersonal closeness, if responded to, frequently reveals a degree of dependency need suggestive of regressive states.

The pervasive paranoid attitude found within the drug milieu is so prominent as to suggest psychosis, were it not for the fact that it is a feature shared in common with the subculture and usually not accompanied (except in adverse reactions) by other psychotic symptoms. For the individual, this attitude is usually a projection of his guilt, and often of the need for attention from adults that detection would produce. Both are allied to the basic depression and respond as it is managed in psychotherapy.

Any complete discussion of the management of drug misuse must include consideration of the sociocultural factors involved. One immediate need seems to be accurate, factual education of youth regarding the consequences—personal, social, and legal—of misuse.[56, 71] Other social measures depend on an accurate assessment of the basic sociocultural issues at the center of what is in fact a mass movement among youth—just as drug misuse, if habitual, is usually symptomatic of an underlying personality disturbance, so the widespread misuse of these intoxicants by young people is symptomatic of deep-seated problems within society at large.

SOCIOCULTURAL ISSUES

Motivation for use of the hallucinogenic drugs by youth can be understood in such relatively benign terms as curiosity and need to conform to peer group values,[35] the "dare" factor,[43] an expression of rebellion against authority, and even a search for a more sensible intoxicant than alcohol[35]; there are also the less benign motives, such as a search for identity and mystical experience and escape from intolerable circumstances. These understandings, although perhaps explaining (usually in unduly simplified and superficial terms) the involvement of any one individual in drug misuse, are unsatisfactory when applied to the phenomenon as a social problem involving a small, but significant, segment of contemporary youth.

That young people with individual problems of adjustment should group together around certain causes or unconventional activities seems appropriate when one recalls the findings of such sociologists as A. K. Cohen[12] that "a subculture owes its existence to the fact that it provides a solution to certain problems of adjustment shared among a community of individuals," and this is further understandable through O'Donnell's observation[57] that "most illegal or deviant roles . . . may be and usually are associated with other roles of equal or more importance to the individual." Individual life histories and problems of coping with developmental crises augment the normal tendency of the adolescent to identify with causes related to suppression of minorities, arbitrary authoritarianism, and undue reliance on tradition. These latter issues are particularly prominent in contemporary North American society, as indeed they are in most industrialized countries. An increasingly earlier onset of puberty (by four to six months every decade) and a considerably longer time required for training and education toward adult employability in a technological society mean that the period of adolescing ("becoming adult") is being progressively stretched out, so that youth is being asked to contain its biological urges, idealism, frustrations, and impatience for a longer period than any previous generation. This, plus the accent in our society on immediate consumption and instant gratification of wants—the antithesis of the Puritan ethic that stressed the postponement of desires and the saving of money for future needs—augments the normal tendency of adolescents to live in the present and to indulge desires immediately —as exemplified in the misuse of drugs.

Youth has always had a gift for identifying and resenting the apparent hypocrisies and inconsistencies of the adult world. The present generation is the first to have had a third authority in the home virtually from birth—the television set—and television has been an essential, if nonscheduled, part of the education of the vast majority of present-day youth, offering a new source of information and authority, rich in opinion and fact, and often offering viewpoints sharply at variance with the way their parents and teachers interpret and value society and history. The totally more sophisticated education to which the present youth generation has been exposed has made it generally well informed about social and political issues, and thus more able to identify and resent the imperfections and injustices within society. The indignation and resentment against racial inequality, widespread and semisanctioned violence, and the preoccupation of some segments of adult society with material possessions and fashion are readily evident among the group of young people who are active in dissent—and frequently also in drug misuse. The present generation of adolescents and young adults has made a fine art of parodying the excesses and hypocrisies of their elders. Thus, the misuse of drugs can be looked on, from one viewpoint, as a parody—a grotesque caricature—of the widespread dependence of adult society on alcohol, tranquilizers, and stimulants.

As noted earlier when discussing the marijuana controversy, drug abuse, particularly with reference to marijuana, has become a displacement target for many of the concerns of present-day transitional society. The misuse of marijuana, in particular, challenges traditional attitudes toward the use of drugs and at the same time symbolizes much of the alienation felt by youth. They note the inconsistency of a society that sanctions the use of drugs of proven danger to health—alcohol and nicotine—but treats users of another drug (considered by youth and increasingly by professionals as at least no more dangerous than these substances if used in moderation) as criminals, to be treated in the same way as narcotic abusers. The advisability of adding yet another intoxicant to society, should marijuana become more legally accessible, is not seen by these young misusers as being pertinent to the issue. By their continued disdain for punitive legislation, they not only have caused many adult groups to reexamine the justification for such laws, but also have inspired a reconsideration of what constitutes abuse of a substance, particularly if such a substance proves to be relatively innocuous when used in moderation.[24] The basic issue then becomes one of individual rights, the morality of self-indulgence and pleasure as its own reward, and the philosophical and psychiatric consequences of self-induced alterations in the perception of reality and experimentation with new varieties of inner experience.

One result of the defiance of traditional attitudes and values, as reflected in the misuse of marijuana (misuse, that is, in terms of conventional attitudes and of the law, rather than abuse in the sense of danger to health and society), has been that increasing numbers of respectable committees and organizations, made up of respected citizens (many of them in the medical profession), have called for a reexamination of the laws and a reduction in penalties for simple possession of marijuana.[9, 71] It has become apparent that giving a criminal record to a young person for simple possession of the drug serves little useful social purpose and is out of proportion to the severity of the offense. And certainly the laws have had little influence on the spreading use of marijuana.[9, 39, 91, 92]

In terms of the future, it is instructive to note the attitude of the sociologist Davis[16] toward the way of life of the hippies, including their use of hallucinogenic drugs; he feels that the hippies are "already rehearsing in vivo a number of possible cultural solutions to central life problems" and notes that there is "an elective affinity between prominent styles and themes in the hippie subculture and certain incipient problems of identity, work, and leisure that loom ominously as Western industrial society moves into an epoch of accelerated cybernation, staggering material abundance, and historically unprecedented mass opportunities for creative leisure and enrichment of the human personality." Keniston[37] offers the ultimate challenge to critics of drug misusers:

In the long run those of us who are critical of student drug abuse must demonstrate to our students that there are better and more lasting ways to experience the fullness, the depth, the variety and the richness of life than that of ingesting psychoactive drugs . . . and we can perhaps, in our lives, and by our own examples, suggest that moral courage, a critical awareness of the defects of our society, a capacity for intense experience and the ability to relate genuinely to people are not the exclusive possession of drug users.

REFERENCES

1. Allan, J. R., and West, L. J. "Flight from Violence: Hippies and the Green Revolution," *American Journal of Psychiatry*, 125 (1968), 364.
2. Allen, S. M. "Glue-Sniffing," *International Journal of Addictions*, 1 (1966), 147.
3. Bender, L. "Drug Addiction in Adolescence," *Comprehensive Psychiatry*, 4 (1963), 181.
4. Bowers, M., Chipman, A., Schwartz, A., and Dann, O. T. "Dynamics of Psychedelic Drug Abuse," *Archives of General Psychiatry*, 16 (1967), 560.
5. Bozetti, L., Goldsmith, B., and Ungerleider, J. T. "The Great Banana Hoax," *American Journal of Psychiatry*, 124 (1967), 678.
6. Bradley, P. B., and Key, B. J. "Conditioning Experiments with LSD," in R. Crocket, R. A. Sandison, and A. Walk (eds.), *Hallucinogenic Drugs and Their Psychotherapeutic Use*. London: Lewis, 1963. P. 4.
7. Brozovsky, M., and Winkler, E. G. "Glue Sniffing in Children and Adolescents," *N.Y. Journal of Medicine*, 65 (1965), 1984.

8. Campbell, I. L. *Marijuana Use at Bishop's University: A Preliminary Report.* Lennoxville, Quebec: Bishop's University, 1969.
9. *Cannabis* Report of the Advisory Committee on Drug Dependence. London: Her Majesty's Stationery Office, 1968.
10. Caron, P. Personal communication, McGill University Faculty of Medicine.
11. Clark, L. D., and Nakashima, E. N. "Experimental Studies in Marihuana," *American Journal of Psychiatry,* **125** (1968), 379.
12. Cohen, A. K. *Delinquent Boys: The Culture of the Gang.* New York: The Free Press, 1955.
13. Cohen, M. M., Marinello, M. J., and Back, N. "Chromosomal Damage in Human Leukocytes," *Science,* **155** (1967), 1417.
14. Cohen, S. "A Classification of LSD Complications," *Psychosomatics,* **7** (1966), 182.
15. Connell, P. H. *Amphetamine Psychosis,* Maudsley Monograph No. 5. London: Chapman & Hall, 1958.
16. Davis, F. "Why All of Us May Be Hippies Someday," *Trans-Action,* **5** (1967), 10.
17. Eddy, N. B., Halbach, H., Isbell, H., and Seevers, M. H., "Drug Dependence: Its Significance and Characteristics," *Bulletin of the World Health Organization,* **32** (1965), 721.
18. Efron, D. H. (ed.). *Ethnopharmacologic Search for Psychoactive Drugs,* Public Health Service Publication No. 1645. Washington, D.C.: Government Printing Office, 1967.
19. Ellingwood, E. H. "Amphetamine Psychosis: 1. Description of the Individuals and Process," *Journal of Nervous and Mental Diseases,* **144** (1967), 273.
20. Farnsworth, N. R. "Hallucinogenic Plants," *Science,* **162** (1968), 1086.
21. Fink, P. J., Goldman, M. J., and Lyons, I. "Morning Glory Seed Psychosis," *Archives of General Psychiatry,* **15** (1966), 209.
22. Fort, J. "Giver of Delight or Liberator of Sin: Drug Use and 'Addiction' in Asia," *U.N. Bulletin of Narcotics,* **17** (1965), 13.
23. Freedman, A. M., and Wilson, E. A. "Childhood and Adolescent Addictive Disorders," *Pediatrics,* **34** (1964), 283, 425.
24. Freedman, D. X. "Perspectives on the Use and Abuse of Psychedelic Drugs," in D. H. Efron (ed.), *Ethnopharmacologic Search for Psychoactive Drugs,* Public Health Service Publication No. 1645. Washington, D.C.: Government Printing Office, 1957. P. 77.
25. Glaser, H. H., and Massengale, O. N. "Glue Sniffing in Children," *Journal of the American Medical Association,* **181** (1962), 300.
26. Glickman, L. "Psychological Determinants of 'LSD Reactions,'" *Journal of Nervous and Mental Diseases,* **145** (1967), 79.
27. Goodman, L. S., and Gilman, A. (eds.). *The Pharmacological Basis of Therapeutics.* 3d ed.; New York: Macmillan, 1965.
28. Greenberg, H. R. "Misuse of Dristan Inhalers," *N.Y. Journal of Medicine,* **66** (1966), 613.
29. Halleck, S. J. "Psychiatric Treatment of the Alienated College Student," *American Journal of Psychiatry,* **124** (1967), 642.
30. Hekimian, L. J., and Gershon, S. "Characteristics of Drug Abusers Admitted to a Psychiatric Hospital," *Journal of the American Medical Association,* **205** (1968), 125.
31. Irwin, S., and Egozcue, J. "Chromosomal Abnormalities in Leukocytes from L.S.D.-25 Users," *Science,* **157** (1967), 313.
32. Isbell, H., Gorodetzsky, C. W., Jasinski, D., Claussen, U., Spulak, F., and Korte, F. "Effects of (-) delta 9 -Trans-Tetrahydrocannabinol in Man," *Psychopharmacologica,* **11** (1967), 184.
33. Kalant, O. J. *The Amphetamines: Toxicity and Addiction.* Toronto: University of Toronto Press, 1966.
34. Keeler, M. H. "Adverse Reactions to Marihuana," *American Journal of Psychiatry,* **124** (1967), 674.
35. Keeler, M. H., "Motivation for Marihuana Use: A Correlate of Adverse Reactions," *American Journal of Psychiatry,* **125** (1968), 386.
36. Keeler, M. H., Reifler, C. B., and Luptzin, M. B. "Spontaneous Recurrences of Marihuana Effect," *American Journal of Psychiatry,* **125** (1968), 384.

37. Keniston, K. "Drug Use and Student Values," paper presented at National Student Personnel Administrators' Drug Education Conference, Washington, D.C., November 1966.
38. Keniston, K. *The Uncommitted: Alienated Youth in American Society*. New York: Dell, 1967.
39. Keniston, K. "Introduction" to H. H. Nowlis, *Drugs on the College Campus*. New York: Anchor, 1969. P. x.
40. Korte, F., Sieper, H., and Tira, S. "New Results on Hashish-Specific Constituents," *U.N. Bulletin of Narcotics*, 17 (1965), 35.
41. Kramer, J. C., Fischman, V. S., and Littlefield, D. C. "Amphetamine Abuse: Pattern and Effects of High Doses Taken Intravenously" *Journal of the American Medical Association*, 201 (1967), 305.
42. Kruskal, W. H., and Haberman, S. "Chromosomal Effects and LSD: Samples of Four," *Science*, 162 (1968), 1508.
43. Lambo, T. A. "Medical and Social Problems of Drug Addiction in West Africa," *U.N. Bulletin of Narcotics*, 17 (1965), 3.
44. Levy, N. J. "The Use of Drugs by Teenagers for Sanctuary and Illusion," *American Journal of Psychoanalysis*, 28 (1968), 48.
45. Loughman, W. D., Sargent, T. W., and Israelstam, D. M. "Leukocytes of Humans Exposed to Lysergic Acid Diethylamide: Lack of Chromosomal Damage," *Science*, 158 (1967), 508.
46. Louria, D. B. *The Drug Scene*. New York: McGraw-Hill, 1968.
47. McGlothlin, W., Cohen, S., and McGlothlin, M. S. "Long-Lasting Effects of LSD on Normals," *Archives of General Psychiatry*, 17 (1967), 521.
48. McGlothlin, W. H., and West, L. J. "The Marihuana Problem: An Overview," *American Journal of Psychiatry*, 125 (1968), 370.
49. *Marihuana and Its Effects: An Assessment of Current Knowledge*. Toronto: Addiction Research Foundation of Ontario, 1968.
50. Masters, R. E. L., and Houston, J. *The Varieties of Psychedelic Experience*. New York: Holt, Rinehart & Winston, 1966.
51. Miller, D. E. "What Every Policeman Should Know about the Marihuana Controversy," paper presented to International Narcotic Enforcement Officers Association, Louisville, Ky., October 1967.
52. Murphy, H. B. M. "The Cannabis Habit: A Review of Recent Psychiatric Literature," *U.N. Bulletin of Narcotics*, 15 (1963), 15.
53. Muzio, J. N., Roffwarg, H. P., and Kaufman, E. "Alterations in the Nocturnal Sleep Cycle Resulting from LSD," *Electroencephalic Clinical Neurophysiology*, 21 (1966), 313.
54. Narcotic Addiction Foundation of British Columbia, "Policy Statement on Marijuana," *Canada's Mental Health*, 16, no. 5 (September–October 1968), 28.
55. Nicholi, A. M. "Harvard Dropouts: Some Psychiatric Findings," *American Journal of Psychiatry*, 124 (1967), 651.
56. Nowlis, H. H. *Drugs on the College Campus*. New York: Anchor, 1969.
57. O'Donnell, J. A. "The Rise and Decline of a Subculture," *Social Problems*, 15 (1967), 73.
58. Oswald, I., and Thacore, V. R. "Amphetamine and Phenmetrazine Addiction: Physiological Abnormalities in the Abstinence Syndrome," *British Medical Journal*, 2 (1963), 427.
59. Pollard, J. C., Uhr, L., and Stern, E. *Drugs and Phantasy: The Effects of LSD, Psilocybin and Sernyl on College Students*. Boston: Little, Brown, 1965.
60. *Preliminary Reports on the Attitudes of Toronto Students in Relation to Drugs*. Toronto: Addiction Research Foundation of Ontario, 1969.
61. Press, E., and Done, A. K. "Solvent Sniffing: Physiologic Effects and Community Control Measures for Intoxication from the Intentional Inhalation of Organic Solvents," *Pediatrics*, 39 (1967), 541–611.
62. Raduco-Thomas, S., Villeneuve, A., Hudon, M., Tanguay, C., Monnier, D., Gendron, C., and Raduco-Thomas, C. "Enquête sur l'Usage des Psychodysleptics (Hallucinogenes) dans les Collèges et Universités de la Province de Québec," *Laval Médical*, 39 (1968), 817.
63. "Research," *Chemical Week*, 101 (1967), 32.

64. Robinson, J. T., Davies, L. S., Sack, E. L., and Morrissey, J. D. "A Controlled Trial of Abreaction with Lysergic Acid Diethylamide," *British Journal of Psychiatry*, **109** (1963), 46.
65. Rockwell, D. A., and Ostwald, P. "Amphetamine Use and Abuse in Psychiatric Patients," *Archives of General Psychiatry*, **18** (1968), 612.
66. Schwartzman, A. E. "LSD-25 and Behavior," paper presented to Special Meeting on Psychodysleptic Drugs of Quebec Psychopharmacological Association, Hôpital des Laurentides, l'Annonciation, Quebec, June 1968.
67. Schwarz, C. J. "LSD, Marihuana and the Law," *British Columbia Medical Journal*, **9** (1967), 274.
68. Schwarz, C. J. "Paradoxical Responses to Chlorpromazine after L.S.D.," *Psychosomatics*, **8** (1967), 210.
69. Schwarz, C. J. "The Complications of LSD: A Review of the Literature," *Journal of Nervous and Mental Diseases*, **146** (1968), 174.
70. Schwarz, C. J. "Towards a Medical Understanding of Marihuana," paper presented at Western Regional Meeting of Canadian Psychiatric Association, Vancouver, January 1969.
71. Shearer, R. C. (ed.). *Loyola Conference on Student Use & Abuse of Drugs*. Proceedings of Canadian Higher Education Conference, Canadian Student Affairs Association. Montreal: Loyola College, 1969.
72. Silberman, M. *Aspects of Drug Addiction*. London: Royal London Prisoners' Aid Society, 1967.
73. Smart, R. G., and Bateman, K. "Unfavourable Reactions to LSD: A Review and Analysis of the Available Case Reports," *Canadian Medical Association Journal*, **97** (1967), 1214.
74. Smart, R. G., Storm, T., Baker, E. F. W., and Solursh, L. *Lysergic Acid Diethylamide (LSD) in the Treatment of Alcoholism*. Toronto: University of Toronto Press, 1967.
75. Snyder, S. H., Faillace, L. A., and Weingartner, H. "DOM (STP), a New Hallucinogenic Drug, and DOET: Effects in Normal Subjects," *American Journal of Psychiatry*, **125** (1968), 357.
76. Solomon, D. (ed.). *The Marihuana Papers*. New York: Bobbs-Merrill, 1966.
77. Solursh, L. P., and Clement, W. R. "Hallucinogenic Drug Abuse: Manifestations ond Management," *Canadian Medical Association Journal*, **98** (1968), 407.
78. Solursh, L. P., and Clement, W. R. "Use of Diazepam in Hallucinogenic Drug Crises," *Journal of the American Medical Association*, **205** (1968), 644.
79. Solursh, L. P., and Rae, J. M. "LSD, Suggestion & Hypnosis," *International Journal of Neuropsychiatry*, **2** (1966), 60.
80. Sparkes, R. S., Melnyk, J., and Bozzetti, L. P. "Chromosomal Effect in Vivo of Exposure to Lysergic Acid Diethylamide," *Science*, **160** (1968), 1343.
81. "S.T.P." *British Medical Journal*, **3** (1967), 570.
82. Taylor, G. C. "An Analysis of the Problems Presented in the Use of LSD," *U.N. Bulletin of Narcotics*, **19** (1967), 7.
83. Teitelbaum, D. T. "Stramonium Poisoning in 'Teeny-Boppers,'" *Annals of Internal Medicine*, **68** (1968), 174.
84. Tramontana, J. A., and Der Marderosian, A. H. "Anti-Asthmatic Drugs as Hallucinogens," *Pennsylvania Medicine*, **70** (1967), 58.
85. Truitt, E. B. "The Pharmacology of Myristicin and Nutmeg," in D. H. Efron (ed.), *Ethnopharmacologic Search for Psychoactive Drugs*, Public Health Service Publication No. 1645. Washington, D.C.: Government Printing Office, 1967.
86. Ungerleider, J. T. (ed.). *The Problems and Prospects of LSD*. Springfield, Ill.: Charles C Thomas, 1968.
87. Ungerleider, J. T., Fisher, D. D., and Fuller, M. "The Dangers of LSD," *Journal of the American Medical Association*, **197** (1966), 389.
88. Ungerleider, J. T., Fisher, D. D., Fuller, M., and Caldwell, A. "The 'Bad Trip'—The Etiology of the Adverse LSD Reaction," *American Journal of Psychiatry*, **124** (1968), 1483.
89. Ungerleider, J. T., Fisher, D. D., Goldsmith, S. R., Fuller, M., and Forgy, E. "A Statistical Survey of Adverse Reactions to LSD in Los Angeles County," *American Journal of Psychiatry*, **125** (1968), 352.

90. U. N. Commission on Narcotic Drugs. *Report of the Twentieth Session*, November 29–December 21, 1965, E/4140 (E/CN. 7/488). New York: United Nations, 1966.
91. Unwin, J. R. "Illicit Drug Use among Canadian Youth," *Canadian Medical Association Journal*, **98** (1968), 402, 449.
92. Unwin, J. R. *An Overview of the Drug Scene.* Vancouver: Narcotics Addiction Foundation of British Columbia, 1968.
93. Unwin, J. R. "Dissident Youth: National Hazard or Loyal Opposition," *Canada's Mental Health*, **17,** no. 2 (1969).
94. Unwin, J. R. "Utilisation des Hallucinogènes chez les Jeunes: Aspects Psycho-Sociaux," *Laval Medical*, **40** (1969), 70.
95. Van Dusen, W., Wilson, W., Miners, W., and Hook H. "Treatment of Alcoholism with Lysergide, *Quarterly Journal of Studies in Alcoholism*, **534** (1966), 27.
96. Weil, A. T. "Nutmeg as a Psychoactive Drug," in D. H. Efron (ed.), *Ethnopharmacologic Search for Psychoactive Drugs*, Public Health Service Publication No. 1645. Washington, D.C.: Government Printing Office, 1967. P. 188.
97. Weil, A. T., Zinberg, N. E., and Nelson, J. M. "Clinical & Psychological Effects of Marihuana in Man," *Science*, **162** (1968), 1234.
98. Welpton, D. F. "Psychodynamics of Chronic Lysergic Acid Diethylamide Use," *Journal of Nervous and Mental Diseases*, **147** (1968), 377.
99. White House Conference on Narcotic and Drug Abuse. *Proceedings.* Washington, D.C.: Government Printing Office, 1962.
100. Whitmore, F. W. "Chromosomal Effect and LSD: Samples of Four," *Science*, **162** (1968), 1508.
101. Winick, C., and Goldstein, J. *The Glue Sniffing Problem.* New York: American Social Health Association, 1965.
102. Yolles, S. F. Testimony before U.S. Subcommittee on Juvenile Delinquency, *Canada's Mental Health*, **16,** no. 6 (November–December 1968), 29.

PART FOUR

Biological Studies

PSYCHOPHARMACOLOGY: THE ROLE OF CLINICAL RESEARCH

Pierre Deniker

It is now generally acknowledged that therapeutic testing plays a determining role in psychopharmacology; applicability to human beings alone can be our source of information on the therapeutic and secondary effects of a psychotropic compound. Here we examine the clinical stage of research, its methodological problems, and the ethical questions it eventually poses. For this study we shall refer first to the lessons that have been drawn from previous findings in research and then to the experiments and problems of present research.

THE ROLE OF THE CLINIC IN MODERN DISCOVERIES

From the viewpoint of methodology, it is useful to recall some present-day achievements in psychopharmacology, defining the role played by clinical research in connection with each one.

Neuroleptics and Tranquilizers

We know how the effect peculiar to chlorpromazine was isolated from the total effect of Laborit's "Lytic Cocktail," which included two other drugs—promethazine and pethidine. The latter two were already known to psychiatrists, and their therapeutic possibilities had already been evaluated. Interest at once centered on the new phenothiazine. The relative ineffectiveness of shock treatments and known sedatives in the treatment of psychotic states of excitation and agitation was revealed during the first therapeutic tests; thus, the treatment of manic excitation became a true test of the pharmacodynamic effectiveness of the neuroleptic drugs. The favorable action of chlorpromazine in states of mental confusion, however, soon showed that it was not only a powerful sedative, but that it also had complex antipsychotic effects. On the other hand, the relative ineffectiveness of the drug in the treatment of depressive psychoses and its limited effect vis-à-vis inert forms of schizophrenia were immediately apparent. This experimentation, conducted more than fifteen years ago, foreshadowed the pilot studies of new drugs based on the selection of compounds (in relation to the effects of already known pharmacodynamics) and on the nosological selection of patients for therapeutic tests.

The similarity of the nonhypnotic sedative effect of reserpine, already utilized in the treatment of arterial hypertension, to that of chlorpromazine determined its introduction into psychiatric therapy, in spite of test indications that the dosage had to be increased approximately tenfold. The evidence of similar extrapyramidal effects of the two compounds contributed to the delimitation of the group of neuroleptics in relation to other tranquilizers.

Pharmaceutical research, in fact, had been oriented toward the search for new nonhypnotic sedatives, different from the classical products that led to the proliferation of nonneuroleptic tranquilizers. On the other hand, research that aimed at the production of extrapyramidal effects—and of its experimental equivalent, animal catalepsy—was to lead to the discovery of ever more powerful neuroleptic compounds, such as thioproperazine and fluphemazine, in the large group of phenothiazines. It is now admitted that catalepsy, rather than the production of antiemetic hypothermizing or other activities, is the essential test for the predictive selection of neuroleptics.

It seems that the observation in animals, used in laboratory experiments, of manifestations recalling the neurological semiology of man played a definite role in the discovery of haloperidol and of neuroleptic butyrophenons.

Present investigations being conducted by pharmacologists on equivalents of human neurological syndromes in animals[1] seem to be on a fruitful path. In recent years, they have made possible the selection of new neuroleptic molecules[4] that do not belong exclusively to the aforementioned series, those derived from dibenzoazepines, thioxanthemes, piperazine, procalnamide, and so forth. Moreover, they have produced interesting studies on the reciprocal potentiating effects of neuroleptics and analgesics,[2] or neuroleptanalgesia.

Antidepressant Drugs

We know how imipramine, prototype of the tricyclical antidepressants, was first tested in connection with symptoms similar to those of chlorpromazine and exhibited little effectiveness, and how later tests in endogenous depressions demonstrated its therapeutic power. These investigations are complementary examples of pilot studies *avant la lettre*. With chlorpromazine, investigators had started out from the most logical therapeutic indices in order to explore less evident indices later. With impramine, a process of elimination led only to an inconclusive result. But, in both cases, major attention was paid to clinical semiology and nosography as the guiding elements of the research. This procedure, moreover, is common to most clinical studies originating in Europe, and it must be stressed that French and German nosologies remain relatively clear and faithful factors in scientific communication.

On the other hand, the discovery of the antidepressant activity of the inhibitors of monoamine oxidase (IMAO), of American origin, seems to have followed a very different logical course. Starting from the observation of the effect of iproniazide on reserpine-administered animals and cataleptics, and perceiving an analogy in the animal between the reserpinic akinesia and schizophrenic inertia, the first—unsuccessful—therapeutic tests were on this type of illness. Later tests focused on endogenous depressions. Here, the results were telling and, in many respects, comparable to those of imipramine, although the latter is practically without effect on MAO. It remains to be noted that, although the first tests of antidepressants in schizophrenic psychoses were viewed as failures, investigators had to return to them subsequently, utilizing the association between antidepressant drugs and neuroleptics to combat inertia and apathy in schizophrenics.

The individuation of the group of antidepressants, which, like the neuroleptics, includes different chemical structures, rests essentially on clinical criteria.[6] These can be summed up as the ability to redress the depressive mood (thymoanaleptic effect) and even the ability to invert it (reversive thymoaction). This effect makes possible the differentiation of true antidepressants from sedatives and tranquilizers that can have favorable symptomatic effects in depressive syndromes without producing a radical change of mood. The antidepressants likewise have neurological effects in common, the most typical being the dysarthria tremens syndrome, particularly clear with tricyclical compounds. But here, in contrast to the existing situation in respect to neuroleptics, we are lacking correlative pharmacological tests of the characteristic therapeutic action, inasmuch as the batteries of tests utilized are as sensitive to amphetaminic effects as to those of antidepressants. Further, the absence of truly "depressed" animals in laboratory material is clearly felt.

Hallucinogens

We know that, as regards hallucinogens, the discoveries were either accidental (for example, lysergamide) or resulted from the patient investigation of the active principle of vegetals, long known because of their hallucinatory activity (for example, mescalin, psilocybine, tetrahydrocannabinol).

Nevertheless, the clinician's role is important. LSD chemists have proven a remarkable clinical spirit in identifying the effects of the drug on their own persons. Today we possess an extensive compilation of studies on hallucinogenic compounds that clearly sets off their common action and characteristics.[8]

On the other hand, if we refer to investigations of the biochemical etiology of psychosis, doubts and contradictions abound respecting the effects of supposedly pathogenic substances, which are made the subject of tests that are not at all conclusive. Perhaps the doubt is owing either to the low potency of the components under study or to the inadequacy of the clinical material, because the psychotic subjects show fewer psychodysleptic manifestations than healthy volunteers.

General Data

Clinicians have played a major role in the classification of modern psychotropes. Thus, the major categories of activities are, in general, clinical categories: psycholeptics (sedatives), psychoanaleptics (stimulants), and psychodysleptics (alterers of mental activity).

Among these major divisions, the principal psychopharmacological types are defined simultaneously by clinical characteristics and pharmacodynamic tests; as we have seen, these are notably the neuroleptics, the tranquilizers, the antidepressants, and so forth. Each group contains subgroups, differentiated by their chemical structures, which have no significance in this context except to aid in the classification.

The clinician can play a role not only through his observations, but also through his reflections and experience. Thus, one can set neuroleptics—characterized by the ability to reduce psychic excitation, which extends to real mental depression (described in particular with reserpine, thioproperazine, and taloperidol)—against antidepressants—capable of changing the depressive mood, which can extend to euphoric subexcitation. We observe that we have at our disposal a well-stocked arsenal for the regulation of a mood, or a thymic function, which the clinical findings of psychopharmacology highlight as a functional entity of prime importance.

THE CLINICIAN IN PRESENCE OF A NEW PSYCHOTROPIC MOLECULE

It is generally agreed that three stages are to be distinguished in therapeutic tests: phase I is theoretically that of tests of tolerance, phase II that of pilot or orientation studies of the therapeutic signs, and phase III that of extensive studies aimed at determining the effects of a drug and comparing it to products already in use.

Approaching the sphere of human applications, it is useful to recall the ethical and deontological imperatives they impose: the new compounds must have a possible advantage for the patients under treatment; they must be susceptible to providing new therapeutic activities or give evidence of being more active, more specific, or more manageable than existing drugs. In psychiatry, the gravity and chronic character of some mental disorders warrant some bold approaches to which the families—and sometimes the patients themselves—readily agree. In addition, the different reactions of the same patient to similar compounds justifies, to a certain point, the multiple use of these compounds.

Pilot Studies

For us, phases I and II of the tests must go hand in hand, inasmuch as it is inconceivable for a study of tolerance to be made without a therapeutic aim or for a clinical study to be followed up if the degree of tolerance is not sufficient.

We have previously discussed the guiding rules in the initial phases of clinical research by the method of triple selection: selection of the compounds to be studied, nosological selection of the patients to be treated, and the selection of responsible and knowledgeable clinicians.

STUDY OF THE EXPERIMENTAL LITERATURE

Thus, the first step in therapeutic tests is the critical study of the toxicological and pharmacological literature. We have already noted the dialectical characteristic of this study that establishes communication between the experimenters and the clinicians. The clinician must possess a sufficient fund of information concerning pharmacological methods and, if necessary, have recourse to the advice of an experienced and independent pharmacologist.

In fact, in a study of the literature, it is important to distinguish those data that refer to tests and to known experimental models[3] from those data that constitute innovations whose weight and significance should be carefully evaluated.

The study of the literature, completed if necessary by an experiment suggested by the clinician, must provide conclusive answers to the following questions: Is it a product having new effects or effects comparable to existing compounds? In the first case, is the experiment conducive to therapeutic tests? In the second case, is it conceivable that the product will be more effective or more manageable?

Initial Phase of the Tests

Just as for the questions of tolerance, this phase must confirm or disconfirm the experimental data, at least in a first approximation. It is rare in our experience that a compound, not producing any effect in a dozen consecutive cases, could be a product of the first rank. If one is dealing with a compound whose psychotropic action is as powerful as its secondary effects, there is a definite interest in assuring that as strict control as possible is assured during the first test. The technique that combines neuropsychiatric observation with polygraphic registration of the EEG, the electrocardiogram of respiration, and so forth,[5] can provide early indications of the mode of action and the risks incurred.

Orientation Study

We have seen that it is possible to base certain pilot studies on a triple system of references: first, that of the types of psychopharmacological research to which we can relate the compound under study; second, that of the classic categories of psychiatric nosography—valid in respect to the ascertainment of symptoms—and third the observation of the neurological semiology that furnishes indications on the structures affected. Verification of the data of these three orders generally enables experienced clinicians to form a composite idea of the therapeutic and secondary effects of a given compound.

Neuroleptics. According to our experience, the clinical identification of a new neuroleptic rests on two arguments: therapeutic action in acute psychoses (test for mania) and chronic psychoses (schizophrenia) coupled with neurological effects, especially those of an extra-pyramidal character.[11] As regards therapeutic activity, we have established in advance the composition of nosologic groups to be carefully selected for the evaluation of the major indices. These diagnostic categories (see Table 1) include a minimum of cases and an optimum that already permits some statistical calculations. It would serve no useful purpose to inflate without reason one category at the expense of another.

Neurological effects require minute research by daily clinical examinations (even twice daily) following a very detailed schema of which there are now several models in specialized clinical research laboratories.

Tranquilizers and Hypnotics. The nonneuroleptic and nonhypnotic sedative action enables experimenters to individuate the tranquilizers, despite the negative and somewhat vague character

TABLE 1

Composition of Nosological Groups for the Early Evaluation of Neuroleptics

1. Mania or expansive excitations	3 to 7 cases
2. Acute psychoses (confusion, flushes of acute schizophrenia)	7 to 10 cases
3. Schizophrenias of three types evolving in fewer than five years	7 to 9 cases
4. Schizophrenias of more than five years	5 to 7 cases
5. Other chronic psychoses (interpretative and hallucinatory)	3 to 7 cases
Total	25 to 40 cases

of this definition. The clinical material of a psychiatric service can be suitable for a first evaluation of this type of action; this can be completed on a population of nonpsychiatric patients with eventual reference to a placebo.

Clinical tests of hypnotics run into serious difficulties: either they are conducted among psychiatric patients, in which case it is rare that patients are exempt from another more or less synergic therapeutic, or clinicians address themselves to normal subjects and the incidence of the placebo effect must be taken into consideration. Thus, the study of the injectable product under polygraphic control can be very useful.

Antidepressants. We have seen that the best test of the clinical action of these compounds is no doubt their effectiveness in the treatment of typical depressions, in particular melancholia: unfortunately, this type of patient is tending to disappear from psychiatric hospitals in order to be treated in general hospitals and private clinics. Also, certain authors, taking the term "depression" in the broad sense, have fancied they could conduct tests in cases of atypical depressions, symptomatic of schizophrenia, which are conducive to error. Thus, a neuroleptic can ameliorate a depressive schizophrenia without, by the same token, being a real antidepressant. On the other hand, antidepressants can produce crises of agitation or of delirium in schizophrenics, although this effect might not suffice to characterize the drug, inasmuch as amphetamines can produce the same disturbances.

As with the neuroleptics, we have established a nosological selection for the clinical tests of antidepressants (see Table 2). It will be noted that schizophrenia is represented in the table, but as an accessory category. In order objectively to determine the precise nature of each case studied, the latter is characterized by a double classification in the syndromic categories (1-D, simple; 2-D, melancholic; 3-D, serious; 4-D, hypochondria; 5-D, during the course of a psychosis) and in etiopathogenic categories (A, reactional; B, on a neurotic base; C, on a psychopathic base; D, following other D; E, following cyclical manifestations; F, with homologue heredity; G, tardy or menopausal; H, with signs of organicity; and so on), so that a menopausal depression, for example, will be classified 2-FG, and a neurophatic depression 1-AB. This coding system enables us to eliminate the depressions that generally are but mildly responsive to drugs.

Compounds Producing an Original Effect. This is the rarest and the most difficult case. As examples, we can cite two possibilities. First, the drug can have a double therapeutic action, such as with derivations of neuroleptics endowed with possible antidepressant effects. The procedure of the tests must have in view the two types of indications and answer the question: Is it a neuroleptic or an antidepressant? Until now, we have knowledge only of negative answers to one of these two questions. Second are complex activities, such as those of a product presented as an antidepressant[1] or as an analgesic,[2] but endowed with hallucinatory side effects. The analysis, in particular, must bear on the latter to determine whether further study of their therapeutic usages is warranted.

In a general way, we shall always attach a primary importance

TABLE 2

Composition of Nosological Groups for the Early Evaluation of Antidepressants

1. Simple depressions	5 to 7 cases
2. Frank melancholic depressions	7 to 10 cases
3. Serious depressions	3 to 5 cases
4. Hypochondria and depressions of psychopaths	5 to 7 cases
5. Atypical depressions	5 to 7 cases
6. Cases of schizophrenic inertia	5 to 7 cases
Total	30 to 45 cases

to the analysis of neurological semiology. These symptoms, which are easy to objectify, yield information on the neural structures involved regardless of whether these are secondary or primary symptoms.

Complete Studies and Controlled Studies

We know how long it takes and how laborious it is to obtain complete information on the therapeutic effects of a drug. Therefore, we shall limit ourselves to envisaging some methodological aspects concerning controlled and extensive studies.

Massive Studies and Collaborative Research
A first procedure that has been employed, notably by the American Federal Drug Administration (FDA), requires thousands of observations in order to judge the risks of hepatic or hematological toxicity, which could very well not appear among restricted populations or patients as we envisaged above. This procedure has been perfected by collaborative studies, which can be conducted on a national or international scale between a certain number of hospitals or specialized units that have agreed, in advance, on the general rules to be applied to each establishment. In such a way, the net result can be treated sufficiently homogeneously

Controlled Studies
It may have surprised some readers that the techniques of controlled studies did not figure in the previous section on pilot studies. In the actual state of technique, however, the type of research is still too slow and ponderous for it to figure among the methods of evaluation in earlier stages.

The controlled character of investigations can bear on the therapeutic effect as such or on the nosology of therapeutic indices.

Control of Therapeutic Action. We know that blind or double blind comparative studies made their debut with antibiotics. But curiously enough, in passing on to the field of psychotropic drugs, it became customary to compare the compound to a placebo rather than to an already known and effective drug. This procedure is justifiable only in connection with products whose effect is mild or barely perceptible.

It is evident that comparisons of the efficacy of drugs of a same type are of a great interest, but they also present almost insurmountable difficulties, not only because of the nosographic variations from one experimenter to another, but also because of the variety of reactions of mental patients according to the point in time chosen to test the drug. We shall return to this below.

Control of the Homogeneity of the Diagnostic Categories. The comparison of studies from one country to another, and especially from one continent to another, clearly reveals the great variations in nosographic appraisals, hence in the indices. Efforts to remedy this situation did not lead to the method of tests,* but to behavioral rating scales that aim at quantifying the objective elements for all observers. A comparison of recent studies[12] conducted with such techniques in France and in the United States has shown that English clinicians with a predilection for the more constant diagnostic schemes furnished findings of much more uniform character than those of their American colleagues. Hence, the clinical training of observers is of great importance, even as regards the application of new techniques.

The latter, however, enable us to entertain the prospect of interesting possibilities. Thus, the registration of electronic computers of models or diagnostic profiles could make the comparison of new profiles possible. A small number of cases studied by each member of a team could be validly processed by the machine, which would furnish more or less comprehensive results for a relatively modest expenditure of individual effort.[13]

Longitudinal Studies

Despite the considerable work and the well-kept archives that they require, longitudinal studies meet some of the objections germane to psychiatric research: in particular, that of the semiological variation, that of the variation of reaction according to the stages of development, and that of the duration of the pathological process—so important in schizophrenia.

Only a few privileged units with a stable, specialized personnel, a relatively "faithful" population of patients, and a suitable system of observation and available research records can risk such studies. Under such conditions, the study of morbid process over a period of five or ten years and the comparison of the different therapies applied could prove to be a valuable contribution. Such studies, moreover, are not limited to the clinic. The development

---

* These methods, which have a diagnostic value, lend themselves poorly to the evaluation of changes ensuing from therapy.

of test results and, in particular, of repeated EEG studies or the reaction of the tracings to the treatments represent a definite interest from the viewpoint of research.

Summing up, it can be said that what conclusively results from the different aspects of the clinical research in psychopharmacology, which we have reviewed here, is that it certainly involves highly specialized research that requires specially oriented institutes or research groups staffed with experienced personnel. Such units cannot be improvised; they must be fostered and their activity vigorously encouraged, as was done, in the United States in 1960, with the creation of Early Clinical Drug Evaluation Units within the National Institute of Mental Health and, in France, ever since the formation of a Committee for Concerted Action in Neurophysiology and Psychopharmacology within the Délégation Générale à la Recherche Scientifique. It is to be hoped that this effort will not slacken, for if the pharmaceutical industry is the almost exclusive purveyor of the raw material of research, the equitable evaluation of the effects of therapies and the prevention of accidents become the responsibility of the state, which can support the only thorough intermediary organizations specializing in clinical research.

REFERENCES

1. Boissier, J. R., and Simon, P. "Équivalences expérimentales du syndrome neurologique des neuroleptiques," *L'Encéphale*, **53**, no. 1 (1964), 109–122.
2. Boissier, J. R., Simon, P., and Viars, P. "Aspects expérimentaux de la neuroleptanalgésie. Étude de l'association dextromoramide-lévomépromazine chez la souris," *Thérapie*, **20**, no. 1 (1965), 67–76.
3. Boissier, J. R., and Simon, P. "Étude pharmacologique prévisionnelle d'une substance psychotrope," *Thérapie*, **21** (1966), 799–818.
4. Delay, J., Deniker, P., and Ginestet, D. "Sur les nouveaux médicaments neuroleptiques," paper presented at the Neuropsychopharmacological Conferences, Milan, November 1965.
5. Delay, J., Deniker, P., Verdeaux, G., Ginestet, D., and Peron-Magnan, P. "Intérêt des contrôles cliniques et polygraphiques simultanés pour l'évaluation précoce de certaines drogues chez l'homme," *Neuropsychopharmacology*, **3**, 460–466.
6. Deniker, P. "Caractéristiques psychophysiologiques des médicaments anti-dépresseurs," *Thérapie*, **20**, no. 5 (September–October 1965), 1169–1184.
7. Deniker, P. "Evaluation clinique précoce des propriétés thérapeutiques des drogues psychotropes," *Thérapie*, **21**, no. 3 (1966), 819–830.
8. Deniker, P. "Pharmacologie humaine des drogues psychodysleptiques," paper presented at the First International Symposium on Psychodysleptic or Hallucinogens, Québec, September 16–19, 1968.
9. Julou, L., Ducrot, R., and Fouche, J. "Étude de quelques relations entre la structure chimique et l'activité neuroleptique," paper presented at the Neuropsychopharmacological Conferences, Milan, November 1965.

10. "L'expertise des médicaments psychiatriques," *L'Encéphale*, **50**, no. 4 (1961), 325–434.
11. Leyrie, J. *"Contribution à l'étude discriminatoire au laboratoire et en clinique des neuroleptiques et des tranquillisants."* Paris: Thèse, 1961.
12. Overall, J., Bailly, R., and Pichot, P. "Stereotypes of Psychiatric Diagnoses of Psychoses in French Psychiatrists: A Comparison with American Stereotypes." *Neuropsychopharmacology* (March 1968), 16–26.
13. Pichot, P. La nosologie psychiatrique et le diagnostic par ordinateur," *Presse Médicale*, **75**, no. 24 (1967), 1269–1275.

NEW STUDIES ON THE GENETICS OF SCHIZOPHRENIA

Einar Kringlen

No trait is exclusively hereditary, no feature exclusively environmental in origin. Reared in isolation, a human being may fail to speak. Unless a genetic potentiality for talking exists, no man can learn to speak. Just as the genes set the biological limits for development, so the various cultures set the social boundaries for growth. A priori, it is unlikely that an environment affects all genotypes equally.

The nature-nurture controversy is becoming as obsolete in the study of schizophrenia as it is in the rest of medicine. What scientists ought to dispute is how much is owing to heredity and how much to the environment or, more precisely, the task ought to be the definition of the specific biological and psychosocial factors involved and the mechanisms by which they interact in the production and development of various forms of schizophrenic illness.[26] How much genetic variation is possible for the manifestation of certain traits or disorders? Evidently, the genes for schizophrenia are not sufficient for the development of the disorder, but are the genes always necessary? Are not adverse environmental conditions in some cases sufficient?

Personality traits and illnesses tend to run in families. To some, this is a proof of genetical transmission; to others, it is a proof of social transmission. It ought, however, to be clear that family incidence of an illness can tell us little about the etiology of a disease; this is particularly true for mental illness.

There are two principal questions that may be asked in genetics: How important is the genetic factor and what is inherited? How is the trait inherited or what is the mode of inheritance? The first question can be answered by studying twins and adopted children, the second by genealogical studies.

In this chapter I have been asked to present chiefly my own contribution in the field with a brief review of earlier and recent genetical studies in schizophrenia. The main emphasis will be on twin studies, because the results of twin studies are the most important etiological information we possess about this disorder.[36, 48]

TWIN STUDIES

The Method

Applied twin research is based on the assumption that there are two types of twins, monozygotic (mz) and dizygotic (dz). Mz twins are held to be identical in hereditary equipment, and all differences between mz twins have to be attributed to environment in the widest sense of that term. Dz twins, on the other hand, are, from a genetic point of view, sibs who were accidentally born at the same time. Dz twins have on average half their genes in common. Differences between dz twins may therefore result from both hereditary and environmental factors.

The so-called classical twin method was developed during the 1920's. One compares mz and dz pairs statistically for concordance for the trait or illness in question. Concordance is usually expressed as a rate of similar occurrence in both twins or, in the case of measurable traits, as the average intrapair difference.[8] A pair is called concordant if both have the same illness, for instance, schizophrenia, discordant if one is sick and the other is not sick, that is, if one is schizophrenic and the cotwin is not. Significantly higher concordance figures in the group of identical twins have been regarded as evidence in support of a hereditary factor of the traits concerned. If the concordance is the same in both mz and dz, the illness or the trait under discussion has been thought to be mainly determined by environmental factors. For instance, in the case of infectious diseases, where genetic differences are of no importance, one would expect clustering in families, but no marked difference between the concordance rates for mz and dz.

There are at least two principal methods of computation of concordance rates, the pairwise method and the proband method.

The pairwise method is simple: one just calculates the percentage of concordant pairs in a twin population. The proband concordance rate, on the other hand, is the proportion of affected twins who have an affected partner; in other words, it is the morbidity rate for partners of affected twins. By this method each affected pair doubly ascertained counts twice.[2, 30] In this chapter, concordance refers to pairwise concordance when not otherwise stated.

Earlier Twin Studies

By and large, previous investigations of twins have shown much higher concordance figures for mz than for dz twins with respect to schizophrenia. This difference was most conspicuous in Kallmann's[22, 23] extensive samples when he reported a concordance of 86 per cent in mz and 15 per cent in dz, but also Luxenburger,[35] Rosanoff, Handy, Plesett, and Brush[42] and Slater[52] observed a marked difference that, of course, was considered strong evidence of the importance of genetic factors in the etiology of schizophrenia.

Several authors[1, 3, 19] leveled criticism against many of these previous studies, indicating other than genetic reasons for the high concordance figures in mz twins. Rosenthal,[43, 44, 45, 46] in a series of influential papers, drew special attention to the importance of sampling in twin studies and argued convincingly that the classical studies by and large showed misleadingly high concordance figures with respect to schizophrenia.

Critical reviews of the classical twin studies have also been published by Tienari,[54] Kringlen,[27, 28] and Gottesman and Shields.[11] Most likely, the high concordance rates in mz twins as regards schizophrenia can be ascribed to shortcomings in sampling, with the disproportionately large inclusion of concordant pairs, but also the establishment of zygosity diagnosis and the statistical handling of the data are disputable in Kallmann's samples.

Recent Empirical Twin Studies

At the Third World Congress of Psychiatry Inouye[18] reported a study of seventy-two pairs of schizophrenic twins, fifty-five of whom were mz. This proportion of mz twins seems very high, but according to vital statistics corresponds rather well with expected figures for Japan. The author thought that the sampling was representative. He explicitly stated, however, that the sampling was not systematic. The twins were personally investigated by the author. Zygosity was established by the similarity method in combination with serological tests.

Concordance uncorrected for age was 36 per cent in mz twins and 6 per cent in dz twins with respect to schizophrenia when a rather strict concept of schizophrenia was employed. When a broader concept of schizophrenia was used, the author arrived at concordance figures of 60 per cent in mz and 12 per cent in dz twins.

Inouye dealt especially with diagnostic and nosological problems in his report. The majority of cotwins are to be found within the schizophrenia-schizoid category. Inouye therefore suggests that the genes seem to be directly responsible for the schizoid personality, with or without primary and undeveloped symptoms, and that schizophrenia often seems to develop from an unknown process acting on this basic disorder, which is susceptible to the schizophrenic process.

Tienari's[54] study caused considerable discussion and led to a fruitful interest in the etiology of schizophrenia because of his remarkable finding of zero concordance in sixteen mz twins. The author deals with a population of twins, all males, born in Finland between 1920 and 1929. The Finnish Foundation of Alcohol Studies had in 1957 collected from the birth registration offices the names of all male twins born in the country from 1920 to 1929. After a psychological and sociological survey of the twins who had survived as complete pairs had been undertaken, Tienari performed personal psychiatric interviews and psychological tests. Zygosity was established on the basis of a number of variables including the results of a battery of serological tests.

In Tienari's sample, there were seventeen mz twin pairs in which the index case was classified as psychotic. Of these, fifteen cases were classed as schizophrenia, one as borderline schizophrenia, and one as reactive psychosis. None of the sixteen pairs was, strictly speaking, concordant for schizophrenia, but three cotwins had borderline features; so if a wide concept of schizophrenia is employed, the concordance figures might be said to be 19 per cent. Even this concordance figure is remarkably low. Because the twins had passed most of the risk period of schizophrenia and because the follow-up time was of considerable length in most cases, the probability of development of schizophrenia in the cotwins was small. However, one of the mz cotwins (case 67) has recently developed schizophrenic symptoms.[55]

As regards the ten cotwins classified as normals, the author remarked that the majority of these have displayed signs of disturbance that were not, however, sufficient for any psychiatric diagnosis. Six of these had shown schizoid or introverted traits.

Harvald and Hauge[14] have, since 1954, performed an impressive follow-up of all twins born in Denmark from 1870 to 1910. Unfortunately, the sample was not very suitable for psychiatric investigation, because so many of the probands of the cotwins had died or their original psychiatric pattern had been changed in old age. Concordance was found to be two out of seven mz and three out of fifty-nine dz pairs.

Gottesman and Shields[12] studied twenty-four mz and thirty-three dz same-sexed pairs of twins obtained through consecutive admissions to the Maudsley and Bethlehem hospitals in London by Dr. Eliot Slater. On admission to the inpatient and outpatient departments and the children's ward, each patient has been routinely asked, since 1948, as part of the prescribed intake procedure, whether he was born a twin. Zygosity was established by a combination of blood grouping, fingerprint analysis, and resemblance in appearance. The twins were investigated by means of hospital records, tape-recorded interviews, and psychological tests.

Clear-cut concordance was reported in 42 per cent for mz and 9 per cent for dz twins with respect to schizophrenia. Because concordant pairs will have a greater chance to appear in a hospital sample, these concordance figures must be looked on as maximum figures. (If one wants to calculate the real pairwise concordance rate in the population on the basis of this study, one arrives at the figure of 33 per cent for mz twins.[30])

Concerning the cotwins of the twenty-four mz schizophrenic twins, the authors state that ten of the cotwins were also schizophrenic, whereas three others had been hospitalized for a nonschizophrenic psychosis. Six cotwins were characterized as otherwise abnormal, and five were classed as normal.

Fischer, Harvald, and Hauge[9] reported on an unselected series of sixteen mz and thirty-four dz pairs of twins born during 1870 to 1920. Only pairs of which one or both had a so-called process-schizophrenic psychosis were taken as probands. Concordance was found to be 19 per cent in mz and 6 per cent in dz twins with respect to schizophrenia when a rather strict concept of schizophrenia was employed (both twins in a pair process-schizophrenia). If a broader concept was used, including schizophreniform and reactive psychoses, the concordance figure was 56 per cent in mz and 15 per cent in dz twins.

One of the main aims of the twin studies reviewed above has been to study the relative contribution of heredity and environment in schizophrenia. Most people seem to think of twin research as solely a field for geneticists; it ought, however, to be stressed that the twin method is also one of the best milieu methods, because here the genetic factor is under control and each difference encountered in mz twins can be ascribed to environmental influences. How this opportunity is utilized is shown in *The Genain Quadruplets*, edited by Rosenthal.[48] This impressive case study of a set of quadruplets, all more or less concordant for schizophrenia, provides us with valuable information about environmental factors and the nosological aspect of schizophrenia. Rosenthal and colleagues at the U.S. National Institute of Mental Health were able to show that different life experiences were related to different clinical states and, furthermore, that severity of schizophrenia and outcome were also clearly related to premorbid personality. The girl with the best premorbid personality received intensive psychotherapy and married without any further hospitalization after leaving the clinical center of the NIMH. The girl with the most deviant premorbid personality structure never left the hospital after the schizophrenic breakdown. Rosenthal concluded that genetic factors seem to be of no importance for the outcome of the illness.

Highly intensive examinations of mz twins discordantly affected with schizophrenia have been the focus of a project carried out by Pollin and Stabenau, also at the National Institute of Mental Health. Eleven pairs of mz twins in which one twin had previously been hospitalized for schizophrenia or borderline schizophrenia were carefully investigated along with their parents at the NIMH. Pollin and coworkers[40, 41] have clearly shown that there is a consistent tendency for a number of interacting features to differentiate the life course of the schizophrenic twin from that of his partner. The most remarkable finding—at variance with most of the literature—was that each of the eleven index twins was the smaller at birth. The sampling method employed may perhaps, to some degree, explain the contrasting findings of the

Pollin study. The authors also noted that the parents, particularly the mother, had regarded the schizophrenic twin as more vulnerable in childhood than the nonschizophrenic twin. He was the recipient of more anxious care and attention. His early development was slower, he was more passive and dependent, and he performed less successfully in school. Most of the index twins showed also that even if many of the nonschizophrenic cotwins were more or less disturbed, none showed typical schizoid traits. Obsessive compulsive traits were, however, rather common.

MY OWN WORK

In my first study on schizophrenia published in 1964, I found no significant difference in concordance rates between mz and dz schizophrenic males.[27] The twins of this study had been located through a systematic search of hospital records of five psychiatric institutions. Attention was focused on the male schizophrenics. Clear-cut concordance was found in only two out of eight mz and two out of twelve dz pairs. The six discordantly affected mz pairs are described and analyzed.

Because the sample in this study was small, a more comprehensive study has been conducted. In 1967, the results of this study were published as a monograph, the case histories of the fifty-five schizophrenic mz pairs being given in a separate volume.[30] Preliminary results and parts of the study have been published elsewhere.[28, 29, 31, 32]

This study had three principal aims: (1) to obtain representative concordance figures for all types of functional psychoses; (2) to study problems pertaining to nosology; and (3) to study a larger sample of discordant pairs in order to clarify crucial environmental factors. In other words, the aim was to conduct a combined hereditary and environmental study of the functional psychoses, with the main emphasis on schizophrenia.

Methods

All twins recorded in the Norwegian birth lists from 1901 to 1930 have been checked against the central register of psychosis. This has provided a relatively large and, what is more important, an unselected sample of psychotic twins. The checking of the twin register against the register of psychosis resulted in 519 pairs of twins. After exclusion of some diagnostic categories, such as organic psychoses and severe mental deficiency, and furthermore all pairs where the cotwin had died before the age of fifteen, a sample of 342 pairs of twins was left. These twins were in the age group thirty-five to sixty-four, and one or both had at some time been hospitalized in Norway for functional psychosis, that is, schizophrenia, manic-depressive illness, or reactive psychosis.

Zygosity diagnosis was arrived at by blood and serum grouping, as well as from information about identity confusion as children. Seventy-five pairs were classified as mz and 257 pairs as dz twins, whereas ten pairs of the same sex had unknown zygosity.

As many as possible of the families of the mz pairs, including parents and siblings, were personally investigated. Personal interviews were obtained with the mz twins within the schizophrenic group in 82 per cent of the cases, the rest being twins who had died prior to follow-up, had left the country, or simply refused to see me. Forty-two pairs of dz twins of the same sex were also personally investigated, but not their families.

The Frequency of Functional Psychosis in Twins

Owing to the uniqueness of the twin relationship, particularly in mz pairs, twins face special problems during childhood and adolescence, and it would seem not unlikely that twins have a higher frequency of mental illness than the normal population.

After considering admission rates to Norwegian hospitals, I have been unable to demonstrate any difference between twins and the general population in frequency of functional psychosis. No difference was found for the functional psychosis combined or for subgroups of schizophrenia, manic-depressive illness, and reactive psychosis.

These findings have implications for theory. Higher concordance rates in mz twins cannot be explained by postulating that the twinship in itself predisposes to schizophrenia or other psychoses. The findings, furthermore, cast doubt on Jackson's[19] "confusion of ego identity theory" of schizophrenia.

In the main, it should be possible to conclude safely that the evidence available from my own material and the literature[43, 54] gives very little support to the hypothesis that functional psychosis is more frequent in twins than in nontwins. If differential rates do occur, they would seem to be of a negligible nature and of no practical importance.

Survey of the Sample by Age, Sex, and Zygosity

The ages of the twins are evenly distributed between thirty-five and sixty-four, with a mean of forty-nine years. This refers to the year 1965 when the fieldwork was completed. Table 1 summarizes the sample. As shown in Table 1, there is the same number of male and female pairs of the same sex. In most previous studies there has been an excess of female pairs, most likely owing to shortcomings in sampling.

TABLE 1
Zygosity and Sex of Sample

ZYGOSITY	FEMALE	MALE	TOTAL
mz	38	37	75
dz, same sex	66	65	131
Unknown zygosity, same sex	4	6	10
dz, opposite sex	—	—	126
Total pairs	108	108	342

Concordance Figures

Table 2 gives an over-all picture of the concordance rates with the three main diagnostic groups—schizophrenia, reactive psychosis, and manic-depressive illness—lumped together. A pair is classified as concordant in this connection if both partners have received a hospital diagnosis of functional psychosis. In other words, if one twin is schizophrenic and the other is suffering from a reactive psychosis, the pair is classified as concordant. The figures were arrived at by checking the twin register against the register of psychosis, and the figures are given without age correction.

The concordance figures for strict, that is, strictly defined, schizophrenia plus the group with schizophreniform psychoses are presented in Table 3. Table 4 shows the concordance figures when a rather wide concept of concordance is used, and it is based on personal investigation as well as hospitalization. A pair is

TABLE 2

Concordance for All Types of Functional Psychoses

	NUMBER OF PAIRS	CONCORDANT PAIRS	DISCORDANT PAIRS	PER CENT CONCORDANCE
mz	75	18	57	24
dz, same sex	131	8	123	6
Unknown zygosity, same sex	10	0	10	0
dz, opposite sex	126	8	118	6
Total pairs	342	34	308	—

NOTE: These figures have been arrived at by checking the twin register against the register of psychosis. The figures are without age correction.

TABLE 3

Concordance for Schizophrenia and Schizophreniform Psychoses, Based on Hospitalized and Registered Cases

	NUMBER OF PAIRS	CONCORDANT PAIRS	DISCORDANT PAIRS	PER CENT CONCORDANCE
mz	55	14	41	25
dz, same sex	90	6	84	7
Unknown zygosity, same sex	6	0	6	0
dz, opposite sex	82	8	74	10
Total pairs	233	28	205	12

grouped as concordant if one twin has a diagnosis of schizophrenia or schizophreniform psychosis and the cotwin has either the same diagnosis or a diagnosis of reactive psychosis or borderline. Personal knowledge was utilized for half the schizophrenic dz group of the same sex. The opposite-sexed dz twins were not personally seen at all. As Table 4 shows, even if a rather wide concept of

TABLE 4

Concordance for Schizophrenia and Schizophreniform Psychoses, Based on Further Personal Investigation

	NUMBER OF PAIRS	CONCORDANT PAIRS	DISCORDANT PAIRS	PER CENT CONCORDANCE
mz	55	21	34	38
dz, same sex	90	9	81	10
Total pairs	145	30	115	21

TABLE 5

Concordance for Schizophrenia in mz and dz Twins, According to Various Investigators

INVESTIGATOR	YEAR COUNTRY	MZ		DZ	
		NUMBER OF PAIRS	CONCORDANCE* (%)	NUMBER OF PAIRS	CONCORDANCE* (%)
Luxenburger	1928 Germany	17	59–76	33	—
Luxenburger	1934 Germany	27	33	—	—
Rosanoff et al.	1934 U.S.A.	41	61	101	10
Essen-Möller	1941 Sweden	7	0–71	24	8–17
Kallmann	1946 U.S.A.	174	69	517	10
Kallmann	1950 U.S.A.	268	—	685	—
Slater	1953 England	37	65	112	11
Inouye	1961 Japan	55	36–60	17	6–12
Tienari	1963 Finland	16	0–19	21	5–14
Kringlen	1964 Norway	8	25	12	16
Harvald & Hauge	1965 Denmark	7	29	31	6
Gottesman & Shields	1966 England	24	42	33	9
Kringlen	1967 Norway	55	25–38	172	8–12

* The concordance figures tabulated here are the original figures, uncorrected for age. In Kallmann's 1946 material[22] the age-corrected figures were 86 per cent for mz and 15 per cent for dz. The original figures in his 1950[23] material were not given; the age-corrected figures, however, were the same as in 1946. Age-corrected figures for Slater's material are 76 and 14 per cent.

concordance is used, the concordance rates are still low. There is some increase for both mz and dz twins.

Table 5 gives a summary of earlier and recent twin studies in schizophrenia.

Table 6 gives the incidence of schizophrenia in different genetic and social groups, namely, mz cotwins, dz cotwins, and siblings of mz twins. As Table 6 shows, there is first of all a clear difference in morbidity rates (concordance rates) for mz cotwins compared with the other groups. The rates for dz twins and siblings are rather similar; we observe, however, that there is a difference, rates for dz being higher. From a genetical point of view, one should expect to find the same morbidity rate in cotwins of dz twins as in siblings. It is natural to attach some importance to these observed differences, although they are not statistically significant, and to ascribe the higher morbidity figures in cotwins of dz twins, compared with the morbidity rates in siblings, to the twinship itself. Table 7 summarizes the results obtained in various studies as regards morbidity figures in twins compared with siblings.

TABLE 6
Incidence of Schizophrenia in Different Groups in Percentage

	STRICT SCHIZOPHRENIA		SCHIZOPHRENIA AND SCHIZOPHRENIFORM PSYCHOSIS	
	H.R.	P.I.	H.R.	P.I.
mz cotwins (one twin index case)	26.7	31	25.4	38
dz same-sexed cotwins (one twin index case)	4.3	—	6.7	10
dz opposite-sexed cotwins (one twin index case)	4.7	—	9.8	—
Sibs of mz twins (one twin index case)	3.4	4.8	5.2	6.8

NOTE: The combined concordance for dz of the same sex and dz of the opposite sex is 8.1 per cent with respect to schizophrenia and schizophreniform psychosis (hospital register cases).
H.R. = hospital register.
P.I. = personal investigation.

TABLE 7
Morbidity Risk in Siblings of Schizophrenics, Based on Twin Populations in Per Cent

STUDIES COMPARED		RELATION TO INDEX CASE		
		MZ COTWINS	DZ COTWINS	FULL SIBS
Luxenburger	1935 Germany	54.0	14.0	11.8
Kallmann	1946 U.S.A.	69.0	10.3	10.2
		(85.8)	(14.7)	(14.3)
Slater	1953 England	68.3	11.3	4.6
		(76.3)	(14.4)	(5.4)
Kringlen	1967 Norway	25.4	8.1	5.2
		(38.2)	(12.0)	(6.8)

NOTE: The percentages in parentheses refer to age-corrected figures with respect to Kallmann's and Slater's studies. The figures in parentheses with respect to my own study refer to percentages based on personal investigation and employment of a wide concept of concordance.

Sex and Concordance

Table 8 gives the concordance with respect to schizophrenia for the two sexes separately, based on several investigations. The literature clearly shows a trend toward higher concordance rates in

TABLE 8

Concordance with Respect to Schizophrenia in Male and Female mz and dz Twins

INVESTIGATOR		MZ		DZ SAME SEX		DZ OPPOSITE SEX
		FEMALE %	MALE %	FEMALE %	MALE %	%
Luxenburger	(1928)	88	67	—	—	—
Rosanoff et al.	(1934)	78	42	14	9	6
Slater	(1953)	73	45	16	10	5
Inouye	(1961)	62	58	—	—	—
Gottesman & Shields	(1966)	45	38	12	6	—
Kringlen	(1967)*	29	23	9	6	10
		33	42	—	—	—

NOTE: Kallmann (1946) did not break down the figures according to sex, but from his figures for same-sexed and opposite-sexed pairs one can compute that the ratio is 17.6 to 11.5.

* Schizophreniform psychoses included. First row is based on hospitalized registered cases. Second row is based on personal investigation.

females, both in mz and dz same-sexed twins. This is apparent in the studies of Luxenburger, Rosanoff et al., and Slater. Kallmann and Inouye did not give breakdowns of their concordant and discordant pairs by sex. Tienari studied only male pairs. Furthermore, there is a higher concordance rate in same-sexed dz twins than in opposite-sexed dz twins in the studies for which such figures are available. The differences, however, seem to disappear in more recent studies; this is particularly so for my own study.

It is unlikely that differential sampling techniques can explain this tendency.[45] A more plausible hypothesis seems to be that girls in former days were more strictly brought up with less opportunity for social contacts outside the home than boys had, and thus they were less able to escape a schizophrenogenic family milieu. An increasing female emancipation could offer an explanation of the disappearance of the higher female concordance rates in more recent studies. If the general impression that girls are brought up more independently and liberally in Norway than in many other countries is correct, the findings of my own study become meaningful.

Nosology and Subtype of Schizophrenia

Let us now look at the cotwins of schizophrenics. As can be seen from Table 9, the cotwins of typical chronic schizophrenics

TABLE 9

Classification of the mz Cotwins of Index Cases with Typical Schizophrenia (Schizophreniform Excluded)

TYPE OF PSYCHOPATHOLOGY	NUMBER	PER CENT
Typical schizophrenia	14	31
Reactive psychosis	1	2
Borderline	3	7
Neurosis	13	29
Normality	14	31
Total cotwins	45	100

display a broad range of psychopathological conditions. In only 31 per cent, both twins show the same psychopathology. In another 9 per cent, the cotwins of schizophrenics have either been affected with a reactive psychosis or can be described as borderline cases. Our three borderline patients have never presented a clear-cut picture of psychosis; thus none of them has ever been hospitalized. However, they show certain personality traits that are more of a psychotic than a neurotic nature. One of them, for instance, is rather suspicious and withdrawn, with slight thinking disturbances, and the two others are extremely schizoid. Some would most likely classify these borderline cases as ambulatory or pseudoneurotic schizophrenics.

In the group of neurotic cotwins, we find a broad spectrum of clinical symptoms, namely character disorders, anxiety states, depressive neuroses, somatic neuroses, and one case where alcohol was the main problem.

One might wonder if all the so-called normal or neurotic cotwins are more or less randomly paired with various subtypes of schizophrenia and the various degrees of severity this disorder presents. Would, for instance, a case of malignant schizophrenia, believed by many to be of a genetic origin, be more aptly paired with a psychotic who shows either the same type of psychosis or with a borderline type with marked schizoid traits, whereas, on the other hand, a case of benign schizophrenia—believed to be of a nongenetic type—be paired with a merely neurotic cotwin or even with a normal cotwin?

The data show that the normal cotwin may be paired with any type of schizophrenia; furthermore, the normal cotwins may be paired not only with moderately severe cases of schizophrenia but even with extremely deteriorated partners. The findings, in other words, lend no support to the idea that some subtypes of schizophrenia are considerably more genetically determined than others; furthermore, there is no clear evidence of hereditary factors influencing the course and outcome.

Premorbid Personality

In the main, the results show that birth order, birth weight, difficult birth, physical strength in early childhood, and psychomotor development during the first years of life are of practically no significance for later schizophrenic development. On the other hand, there is a clear correlation between some personality factors in childhood and later schizophrenia.

In both mz and dz groups, the schizophrenic twin has been significantly more often the more submissive, reserved and lonely, obsessive, and the more dependent. The same tendency is present with such traits as sensitivity and obedience. Furthermore, in both mz and dz twins, the schizophrenic has been significantly more often the more nervous in childhood. The schizophrenic twin had fewer friends of both sexes premorbidly and was more passive sexually than the nonschizophrenic twin, and also more frequently was unmarried. The schizophrenic twin also had a lower social status than the nonschizophrenic twin.

These differences in personality can be ascribed to environmental factors, because they are present not only in dz twins, but also in mz twins.

Conclusion

In conclusion, the concordance figures for schizophrenia are found to be 25 to 38 per cent in mz twins and 4 to 10 (12) per cent in dz twins, according to whether the concordance rates are based on registered hospitalized cases or personal investigations and whether a wide or a strict concept of schizophrenia is employed. The difference in concordance rates for mz and dz twins with respect to schizophrenia is statistically significant, thus supporting a genetic factor in the etiology of schizophrenia, but the genetic factor seems to be weaker than it is usually considered to be.

In the main, my own investigation and previous studies clearly show that the clinical picture found in the nonschizophrenic cotwins is rather variable, because it ranges from a duplication of the schizophrenic psychosis to neurosis, or even clinical normalcy. The normal cotwin may be paired with any of the Kraepelinian subtypes of schizophrenia. Furthermore, the normal cotwin may be paired not only with a milder case of schizophrenia but even with a very severely affected partner.

We have detected clear differences in discordantly affected mz and dz pairs as regards personality traits and nervous symptoms premorbidly, even in childhood. The schizophrenic prior to his illness displayed a less healthy personality structure than the nonpsychotic twin. In other words, the twin with the more deviating personality has the greater probability of falling ill with schizophrenia. These premorbid traits could be forerunners of later manifest schizophrenia; most likely, however, they are just general predispositions to mental illness. Many introverted, obsessive, and even dependent children do not develop schizophrenia. Somatic factors could not account for these premorbid differences. More likely, social factors within the family are important in creating these differences.

ADOPTIVE STUDIES

The Method

One cannot dismiss the possibility that certain similarities in mz twins may to some degree be owing to similar environment. Hence, if one encounters a remarkable concordance in mz twins, one has first to overcome the objection that the similarities result from the similar environment before one can maintain that they result from hereditary factors. Accordingly, the study of twins who have been separated in early childhood and reared apart is evidently the best way of studying the effects of genes and environment. The rare occurrence of schizophrenic mz twins separated in early childhood and reared apart makes it, however, impossible to apply this research strategy very widely. The method of studying adoptive nontwins may be used instead.

By the adoptive method, it is possible to distinguish the effects of an environment made schizophrenogenic by a schizophrenic parent from the effects of genes from such a parent. This can be done by comparing a group of adults born to schizophrenic parents and permanently separated from them from early childhood on with matched controls not born to schizophrenic parents. Or one can start with schizophrenic patients adopted in infancy and study their adoptive parents. The transmitters of heredity and social experience can in this way be separated because the biological parents are not the parents who rear the children. If schizophrenia is entirely genetically determined, one should expect that adoptive children of schizophrenic parents will be suffering from schizophrenia in as many instances as children who grow up with their schizophrenic parents. On the other hand, if schizophrenia is largely socially transmitted, one would expect the biological parents to be psychiatrically normal and the adopting parents to be disturbed.

TABLE 10

Mz Twins with Schizophrenia or Schizophreniclike Psychosis Separated in Early Childhood and Brought up Apart

DESCRIBED BY	DIAGNOSIS OF THE TWINS		AGE AT SEPARATION
	TWIN A	TWIN B	
Kallmann (1938)	schizophrenia	schizophrenia	shortly after birth
Craike and Slater (1945)	schizophrenia (par.)? "sensitiver Beziehungswahn"	reactive psychosis depr. par. (schiz.?)	nine months
Kallmann and Roth (1956)	schizophrenia	schizophrenia	?
Shields (1962)	schizophrenia (par. cat.)	schizophrenia	shortly after birth
Tienari (1963)	schizophrenia (heb.)	normal, introverted	three to six years
Kringlen (1964)	schizophrenia (cat.)	normal	one year ten months
Kringlen (1967)	schizophreniform (catatonic)	schizophreniform (paranoid-depr.)	shortly after birth

Twins Reared Apart

The literature comprises only seven descriptions of schizophrenic mz pairs separated in early childhood and brought up apart. Four of these were concordant and three discordant for schizophrenia as can be seen from Table 10. Some of the concordant pairs are to some extent subject to the same criticism as twin case histories in general, namely, that the pairs were chosen for publication just because they were concordant. Second, one observes by examining the case histories in detail that the childhood conditions were in most cases extremely miserable and stressful, and rather similar for both twins. Some crude environmental characteristics for the concordant schizophrenic pairs are shown in Table 11.

TABLE 11

Mz Twins Concordant for Schizophrenia or Schizophreniclike Psychosis, Separated in Early Childhood and Brought up Apart

DESCRIBED BY	CRUDE CHARACTERISTICS OF THE MILIEUS	
	TWIN A	TWIN B
Kallmann (1938)	maternal uncle, unhappy childhood, seduced at fifteen years	maternal uncle, unhappy childhood
Craike and Slater (1945)	father a brutal alcoholic, orphanage age eight, loss of job at forty-eight, hard of hearing	stayed with unmarried maternal aunt, conflicts with twin sister from the age of twenty-four, hard of hearing
Kallmann and Roth (1956)	no description	no description
Shields (1962)	in two nurseries until age four and a half, then some months with grandmother and foster home, together with twin B, later on with grandmother, in poor district	in three foster homes until age five and a half, then foster home till seven and a half, with grandmother a few days, inconsistent upbringing
Kringlen (1967)	paternal aunt and uncle, aunt psychotic in later years, strained economy, contradictory information	paternal aunt and uncle, economic situation better than with A, but contradictory information

Mz twins who have been brought up apart and at the same time have developed the same illness are evidently the best proof of the important part played by heredity. If, however, one looks at the case histories from the environmental point of view one clearly realizes that other interpretations of the data are possible. For a more detailed critique, see Jackson[19] and Kringlen.[27, 30]

Recent Adoptive Studies

Heston[15] has reported on an impressive study of foster-home-reared children of schizophrenic mothers. The author compared the psychosocial adjustment of forty-seven adults born to schizophrenic mothers with fifty matched controls not born to schizophrenic mothers.

The experimental group was born to schizophrenic mothers in state hospitals in Oregon between 1915 and 1945 and had been adopted shortly after birth. No attempts were made to evaluate the psychiatric status of the fathers, but none were supposed to have been hospitalized for psychosis. The forty-seven children who were included in the study had not had any contact with their natural mothers after separation in early childhood, nor had they lived with their maternal relatives. The control group consisted of children of the same foster homes as the experimental group. These children were apparently normal at birth and were matched as exactly as possible for sex, type of institution, adoptive parent, foster home, and duration of stay in institution.

The results of the study are based on a review of school, police, veterans and hospital records, plus a personal interview and MMPI. Three psychiatrists independently rated the subjects. All the investigations and interviews were carried out by the author himself in fourteen states in the United States and Canada.

The results showed that five of the forty-seven persons born to schizophrenic mothers had developed schizophrenia, but none in the control group. However, not only schizophrenic but sociopathic and neurotic disorders as well as mental deficiency were also found in excess in persons born to schizophrenic mothers. Furthermore, the so-called normal persons born to schizophrenic mothers were notably successful adults who possessed artistic talents and demonstrated imaginative adaptations to life that were uncommon in the control group. In other words, the experimental group showed considerably more variability in personality and behavior than did the control group.

A few questions may be raised in connection with this important study. First, how far are the two groups of adoptive parents comparable? Because the adoptive parents evidently received information about the child's biological parents, one might wonder who would take such a child for adoption. These questions are important also because the author did not find only schizophrenic but also neurotic and sociopathic behavior as well as cases of mental deficiency in excess in the experimental group.

Similar results to those reported by Heston have, however, also been published by Karlsson,[25] who carried out his research in Iceland, although with a somewhat different method. Karlsson evaluated the sibs of schizophrenics who had a schizophrenic parent, and unexpectedly he found that the rate of schizophrenia among the sibs reared by relatives and nonrelatives was slightly higher than the rate among sibs reared in the parental home. By comparing the biological and foster sibs of schizophrenics who had been adopted before the age of one year, he found that among the biologic sibs six of twenty-nine were schizophrenics, whereas among the foster sibs none of the twenty-eight was schizophrenic. These results are definitely in support of a genetic theory of schizophrenia.

At variance with these results is the report by Ihda,[17] who in a summary article of Japanese twin research mentioned that the twin who stayed with his family was more likely to develop schizophrenia than the twin who was adopted. (In Japan, it was previously rather common to give away one child for adoption in the case of twin birth.) Regrettably, the author did not present any further data on this matter.

Kety, Rosenthal, and Wender of the National Institute of Mental Health are at present involved in analyzing data from similar studies in collaboration with Danish psychiatrists. Starting with adoptees who are now schizophrenic, they compare the incidence of schizophrenia in their biological and adoptive families. A matched group of normal adoptees serves as controls. Another study begins with schizophrenics whose children were given up for nonfamily adoption at an early age, whereas children similarly adopted, but with normal biological parents, serve as controls. All these groups of children, now adults, have been carefully examined psychiatrically and psychologically. Results of these significant studies should add valuable information to the question of the etiology of schizophrenia.

GENEALOGICAL STUDIES

The Method

In order to arrive at a better understanding of how a trait is inherited, we have relied on family studies. By the pedigree method, an attempt is made to follow certain traits or illnesses from generation to generation, and the incidence of the traits in each generation is calculated. In other family studies, one tries to arrive at risk figures for the illness in various relatives and to compare these figures with rates for the population at large.

There are many problems inherent in such studies. It is not easy to determine the rate of schizophrenia in the normal population, nor is the rate of schizophrenia in the relatives of index cases easily established. Problems owing to sex differences, fertility, mortality, marital status, social class, and differential rates of hospitalization arise. The most reliable method would be to study a random sample of the general population by the method of psychiatric interviews, but because schizophrenia is not too common, one has to investigate large samples to get some estimates. Most such studies therefore have relied on hospital figures.

The interpretation of such risk figures is no easy matter either, because in illnesses in which environmental factors play a great role the reliability of genetic calculation is debatable. As Planansky[39] says, research adhering exclusively to genetic hypotheses may in such cases be comparable to an analysis confined to a single variable in a field in which several variables are involved.

Empirical Findings

Rather few genetically oriented epidemiological studies have been carried out in recent years, but a large body of data has been accumulated during the 1930's in Germany and later on in Scandinavia, yielding findings that have been later confirmed by Kallmann,[21] Slater,[53] and Garrone.[10]

The incidence of schizophrenia in the general population is usually given as 0.85 per cent. A closer study of the literature reveals, however, a considerable variation, ranging from 0.4 to 1.5, the figure 2.85 from a North Swedish isolate being a notable exception.[4] The morbid risk figures have been found to be for parents 5–10 per cent, for siblings 9–16 per cent, and for children 9–16 per cent, according to various investigators.[57]

Families of two schizophrenic parents have been studied by Kahn,[20] Kallmann,[21] Schulz,[49] and Elsässer,[6] and recently Rosenthal[47] summarized these studies, estimating the morbid expectancy rate to be 35 per cent in the offspring. On the basis of such studies, one has tried to fit a theory of single gene hypothesis. Is the gene dominant or recessive? Is the gene sex-linked?

GENERAL DISCUSSION AND CONCLUSION

Both theoretical critique and empirical studies have today clearly documented that earlier twin studies, owing to various sources of error, gave results in which the genetic factor was overestimated. More recent investigations that have attempted to avoid the pitfalls of unrepresentative sampling and uncertain zygosity diagnosis have arrived at considerably lower concordance rates in mz twins with respect to schizophrenia. In the investigations so far, this pattern seems rather consistent: the more accurate and careful the samplings, the lower the concordance figures for mz twins. (See Table 12.)

What then are the representative concordance figures with respect to schizophrenia? On the basis of previous studies and my own findings, it seems to me reasonable to accept rates of 30–40 per cent in mz and about 10 per cent in dz twins, the exact figures being of less importance. This difference is so marked that even if one allows for some higher concordance in mz twins because of a more similar environment and stronger identification processes in mz than in dz twins, the difference must to a large degree be ascribed to hereditary factors. The genetic hypothesis is also supported by modern adoptive studies.

TABLE 12

Concordance Figures in Relation to Some Crucial Variables.

INVESTIGATOR		CONCORDANCE IN MZ		SAMPLING		ZYGOSITY DETERMINATION	PSYCHIATRIC DIAGNOSIS
		PAIRS	PER CENT	ESTABLISH-MENT OF TWINSHIP	RESIDENT, CON-SECUTIVE	BLOOD TEST	SCHIZOPHRENIA CONCEPT
Luxenburger	(1928)	17	60	B.R.	R+C	no	strict
Rosanoff et al.	(1934)	41	61	inq.	R	no	wide
Essen-Möller	(1941)	7	0	B.R.	C	yes	strict
			(71)				(wide)
Kallmann	(1946)	174	69	inq.	R+C	no	wide
Slater	(1953)	37	65	inq.	R+C	no	strict
Inouye	(1961)	55	36	?	R+C	yes	strict
			(60)				(wide)
Tienari	(1963)	16	0	B.R.	C	yes	strict
			(19)				(wide)
Kringlen	(1964)	6–8	0	H.R.	C (+R)	yes	strict
			(25)				
Gottesman & Shields	(1966)	24	42	inq.	C	yes	strict
Kringlen	(1967)	55	25	B.R.	C	yes	strict
			(38)				(wide)

NOTE: B.R. = birth register; H.R. = hospital records; inq. = inquiries; R = resident; C = consecutive.

What Is Inherited?

It is certainly not the symptoms of schizophrenia that are inherited, nor a distinct type of personality; more likely it is certain potentials for personality development. My own investigations might be said to support the view that there is a rather nonspecific genetic predisposition to severe mental illness, a view that, I think, is also supported by the findings of Heston.[15]

If one hypothesizes that schizophrenia as such is not inherited, and even that what one conceived of as personality traits are not inherited, but that certain potentials for response patterns are—which is more likely—then our effort at a meaningful genetic classification might involve a search for basic psychological and physiological reaction patterns underlying certain clinical personality and disease syndromes. In other words, the problem might be to identify, for instance, relationships between perceptual and cognitive response parameters in the hope that these reaction patterns might have some correlations with clinical psychiatric variables. If, however, these clinical variables are entirely or basically environmentally determined, whereas the fundamental physiological and psychological response patterns are more genetically determined, this research will be a failure.

The Mode of Inheritance

The following characteristics are typical for recessivity: the patient's parents are usually healthy, and they are more likely to be related to each other than parents in the normal population; siblings are affected with the same disease, on the average up to 25 per cent or somewhat higher if ascertainment is through affected children. Generally, there is good reason to suspect recessive inheritance in families with normal parents and sick sibs or in isolated cases when the parents are consanguineous. Recessive diseases are usually rare illnesses, occurring with frequencies usually from 1/10,000 to 1/50,000, with a range from 1 per 1,000 to 1 per .5 million births.

Until recently, the majority of genetically interested psychiatrists, Kallmann being the main proponent, favored a hypothesis of recessive inheritance, mainly because most schizophrenics are the offspring of two nonschizophrenic parents and because the illness is so frequent in *Neben-Linien* and the half-siblings have approximately half the risk of the siblings for developing schizophrenia. Against this hypothesis is the fact that the incidence of schizophrenia in the children of schizophrenics is higher than in siblings of schizophrenics, as is also evident from Kallmann's own figures. On a recessive hypothesis, the opposite is to be expected. Furthermore, the offspring of two schizophrenic parents become schizophrenics in only 30–40 per cent of the cases, and moreover the risk of schizophrenia in siblings of probands with one schizophrenic parent is higher, but far from doubly as high, as in the group of siblings of probands with two nonschizophrenic parents.

The usual criteria for dominant inheritance are the following: the disease is passed on from generation to generation; hence, the diseased person has either a sick father or a sick mother and begets children 50 per cent of whom are sick, on the average, the normal children having normal offspring.

Böök[4] and Slater[52] are today the main advocates of a modified dominant theory. Slater estimated that heterozygotes constituted 97 per cent of all schizophrenics and had a manifestation rate of about 26 per cent, which would allow for significant environmental influence.

In conclusion, the hypothesis of recessive or dominant inheritance has to be made rather complicated in order to get all the data to fit the theory, and usually some ad hoc hypotheses have to be established. There is also another difficulty with the single major gene hypothesis, namely, the frequency of the disease. The frequency of an inherited disease will depend on two factors: the frequency of the actual mutation and the selective value of a mutant, that is, the speed with which the mutant is eliminated. Because schizophrenics have a biological disadvantage—they produce fewer children on the average than the general population—one would expect a considerable number of schizophrenic genes to be eliminated from one generation to the next. To keep schizophrenia at its present frequency, one would have to postulate an improbably high mutation rate. Several speculative but quite unconvincing hypotheses have been advanced to make up for this imbalance.[16]

The genetic hypothesis most widely favored by researchers today seems to be the polygenic one.[13, 30, 38] Polygenic inheritance is the genetic background of quantitative traits with normal distribution. In polygenic inheritance, many gene pairs participate relatively equally, each being of minor significance. It is not easy to put forth definite criteria of a polygenic inheritance, one of the problems being that single gene inheritance with reduced penetrance owing to environmental factors might simulate polygenic inheritance. It seems to me that a polygenic inheritance can best explain the gliding transition from normality to severe mental illness found in siblings and parents of schizophrenics. A polygenic inheritance can make intelligible the great variation of clinical pictures found in families of schizophrenics and the fact that the number of patients with so-called clinical *forme fruste* is larger than the number of manifest schizophrenics. This is just what one should expect in conditions that are the expressions of variation of normal traits. This hypothesis also explains the fact that these are rather frequent diseases. Most single gene diseases are extremely rare illnesses.

Most psychiatrists who have worked therapeutically with schizophrenics will favor the idea of grades of personality disorganization. There are degrees of suspiciousness, there are grades of withdrawal and aloofness, and there are in particular degrees of thinking disturbances.[34, 51, 56] That the boundaries between neuroses and psychoses are vanishing is also apparent from the fact that new terms trying to bridge the gap between these two types of disorders are emerging, such as pseudoneurotic schizophrenia and borderline schizophrenia. One should also remember that the extreme forms of schizophrenia may in part be the result of prolonged institutional care rather than an inevitable outcome of underlying disease processes. Furthermore, one should bear in mind that a quantitative variation may present itself to the investigator as a qualitative difference when the margin of adjustment is overstepped. A study by Ödegaard[38] might be said to support the hypothesis of polygenic inheritance. In a large sample of successive first admissions for functional psychoses, he found that the tendency to the same diagnoses in probands and psychotic first-degree relatives (parents, children, siblings) was significant. But the high degree of intrafamilial and individual variability could hardly be suggestive of a specific and simple form of inheritance.

If these ideas are correct, that the genetic factor is an unspecific polygenic disposition, allowing for a significant environmental influence, this must have implications for further research on schizophrenia. The study of schizophrenia must be linked to the study of normal personality development. Most likely, the solution of the so-called schizophrenia riddle will, generally speaking, not come from any *simple* biochemical breakthrough, because there are no simple biochemical answers to variations in intelligence, height and weight, blood pressure, and epileptic disposition. Part of the solution may well be found in the near future, possibly through meticulous research in the field of social science.

Pessimists say we are today as ignorant about the etiology of schizophrenia as we were twenty to thirty years ago. I cannot share this pessimism. I think we know a lot more, and moreover I think the scientific climate for an understanding is much better today than just a few years ago. International conferences have been recently arranged where both geneticists and environmentalists have come together and exchanged viewpoints (The First International Rochester Conference on the Origin of Schizophrenia, the FFRP Conference on the Transmission of Schizophrenia). Both adherents of a genetic and proponents of an environmentalist view of schizophrenia are today more willing to accept and discuss the other viewpoint. The study of the genetics of schizophrenia is today no longer solely a European phenomenon, nor is the dynamic family research in schizophrenia any longer confined to American centers.

It has become more and more clear to psychiatry as to medicine in general that no illness is determined entirely by either genetic or environmental factors. The issue in psychiatry, as in the rest of medicine, is not whether environmental or genetical factors are involved, but whether these factors can be identified. The gene-environment interactions in human health and disease seem to be extremely complex. We should, however, remember that a social prevention has been possible in many diseases before one has been able to unravel the entire web of causation.

REFERENCES

1. Alanen, Y. O. "The Mothers of Schizophrenic Patients," *Acta Psychiatrica Scandinavica.* Suppl. 124 (1958).
2. Allen, G., Harvald, B., and Shields, J. "Measures of Twin Concordance," *Acta Genetica,* **17** (1967), 475–481.
3. Bleuler, M. "Forschungen und Begriffswandlungen in der Schizophrenielehre, 1941–1950," *Fortschritte der Neurologie Psychiatrie,* **19** (1951).
4. Böök, J. A. "A Genetic and Neuropsychiatric Investigation of a North Swedish Population, with Special Regard to Schizophrenia and Mental Deficiency." *Acta Genetica,* **4** (1953), 1–100, 133–139, 345–414.
5. Craike, W. H., and Slater, E. "Folie à Deux in Uniovular Twins Reared Apart," *Brain,* **68** (1945), 213–221.
6. Elsässer, G. *Die Nachkommen geisteskranker Elternpaare.* Stuttgart: Thieme, 1952.

7. Essen-Möller, E. "Psychiatrische Untersuchungen an einer Serie von Zwillingen," *Acta Psychiatrica Scandinavica*, Suppl. 23 (1941).
8. Essen-Möller, E. "Twin Research and Psychiatry," *Acta Psychiatrica Scandinavica*, 39 (1963), 65–77.
9. Fischer, M., Harvald, B., and Hauge, M. "A Danish Twin Study of Schizophrenia," *British Journal of Psychiatry*, 115 (1969), 981–990. Excerpta Medica Foundation, 1968. Pp. 1093–1096.
10. Garrone, G. "Étude statistique et génétique à Genève de 1901 à 1950," *Journale de Génétique Humaine*, 11 (1962), 89–105.
11. Gottesman, I. I., and Shields, J. "Contributions of Twin Studies to Perspectives on Schizophrenia," in B. A. Maher (ed.), *Progress Exp. Personality Research*. New York: Academic Press, 1966. Pp. 1–84.
12. Gottesman, I. I., and Shields, J. "Schizophrenia in Twins: Sixteen Years' Consecutive Admissions to a Psychiatric Clinic," *British Journal of Psychiatry*, 112 (1966), 809–818.
13. Gottesman, I. I., and Shields, J. "A Polygenic Theory of Schizophrenia," *Proceedings of the National Academy of Science*, 58 (1967), 199–204.
14. Harvald, B., and Hauge, M. "Hereditary Factors Elucidated by Twin Studies," in J. V. Nee, M. W. Shaw, and W. J. Schull (eds.), *Genetics and the Epidemiology of Chronic Diseases*. Washington, D.C.: U.S. Department of Health, Education, and Welfare, 1965.
15. Heston, L. L. "Psychiatric Disorders in Foster Home Reared Children of Schizophrenic Mothers," *British Journal of Psychiatry*, 112 (1966), 819–825.
16. Huxley, J., Mayr, E., Osmond, H., and Hoffer, A. "Schizophrenia as a Genetic Morphism," *Nature*, 204 (1964), 220–221.
17. Ihda, S. "Psychiatrische Zwillingforschung in Japan." *Archiv für Psychiatrie und Nervenkrankheiten*, 3 (1965), 206–220.
18. Inouye, E. "Similarity and Dissimilarity of Schizophrenia in Twins," *Proceedings of the Third World Congress of Psychiatry*, 1 (1961), 524–530. Montreal: University of Toronto Press.
19. Jackson, D. D. "A Critique of the Literature on the Genetics of Schizophrenia," in D. D. Jackson (ed.), *The Etiology of Schizophrenia*. New York: Basic Books, 1960.
20. Kahn, E. "Studien über Vererbung und Entstehung geistiger Störungen. IV: Schizoid und Schizophrenie im Erbung," *Monographien aus dem Gesamtgebiete der Neurologie und Psychiatrie*, 36 (1923), 1–143.
21. Kallmann, F. J. *The Genetics of Schizophrenia*. New York: Augustin, 1938.
22. Kallmann, F. J. "The Genetic Theory of Schizophrenia. An Analysis of 691 Schizophrenic Twin Index Families," *American Journal of Psychiatry*, 103 (1946), 309–322.
23. Kallmann, F. J. "The Genetics of Psychoses. An Analysis of 1,232 Twin Index Families," *Congrès International de Psychiatrie. Rapport VI: Psychiatrie Sociale*. Paris: Herman, 1950.
24. Kallmann, F. J., and Roth, B. "Genetic Aspects of Preadolescent Schizophrenia," *American Journal of Psychiatry*, 112 (1956), 599–606.
25. Karlsson, J. L. *The Biological Basis of Schizophrenia*. Springfield, Ill.: Charles C Thomas, 1966.
26. Kety, S. S. "The Relevance of Biochemical Studies to the Etiology of Schizophrenia," in J. Romano (ed.), *The Origins of Schizophrenia: Proceedings of the First Rochester International Conference on Schizophrenia*, International Congress Series, no. 151. Amsterdam, N.Y.: Excerpta Medica Foundation, 1967. Pp. 35–41.
27. Kringlen, E. *Schizophrenia in Male Monozygotic Twins*. Oslo: University Press, 1964.
28. Kringlen, E. "Schizophrenia in Twins: An Epidemiological-Clinical Study," *Psychiatry*, 29 (1966), 172–184.
29. Kringlen, E. "An Epidemiological-Clinical Study on Schizophrenia," in D. Rosenthal and S. Kety (eds.), *The Transmission of Schizophrenia*. New York: Pergamon Press, 1968.
30. Kringlen, E. *Heredity and Environment in the Functional Psychoses: An Epidemiological-Clinical Twin Study*. London: Heinemann, and Oslo: University Press, 1967.

31. Kringlen, E. "Hereditary and Social Factors in Schizophrenic Twins—An Epidemiological-Clinical Study," in J. Romano (ed.), *The Origins of Schizophrenia: Proceedings of the First Rochester International Conference on Schizophrenia*, International Congress Series, no. 151. Amsterdam, N.Y.: Excerpta Medica Foundation, 1967. Pp. 2–14.
32. Kringlen, E. "Twin Study in Schizophrenia," in J. J. López Ibor (ed.), *Proceedings of the Fourth World Congress of Psychiatry*, International Congress Series, No. 150. Amsterdam, N.Y.: Excerpta Medica Foundation, 1968. Pp. 1087–1090.
33. Lewis, A. J. "The Offspring of Parents Both Mentally Ill," *Acta Genetica*, 7 (1957), 349.
34. Lidz, T., Fleck, S., and Cornelison, A. R. *Schizophrenia and the Family*. New York: International Universities Press, 1966.
35. Luxenburger, H. "Vorläufiger Bericht über psychiatrische Serienuntersuchungen an Zwillingen," *Zeitschrift für die gesamte Neurologie und Psychiatrie*, 116 (1928), 297–326.
36. Meehl, P. E. "Schizotaxia, Schizotypy, Schizophrenia," *American Psychologist*, 17 (1962), 827–838.
37. Mitsuda, H. "Klinische-erbbiologische Untersuchung der endogenen Psychosen," *Acta Genetica*, 7 (1957), 371–377.
38. Ödegaard, Ö. "The Psychiatric Disease Entities in the Light of a Genetic Investigation," *Acta Psychiatrica Scandinavica*, 169 (1963), suppl., 94–104.
39. Planansky, K. "Heredity in Schizophrenia," *Journal of Nervous and Mental Diseases*, 122 (1955), 121–142.
40. Pollin, W., Stabenau, J. R., Mosher, L., and Tupin, J. "Life History Differences in Identical Twins Discordant for Schizophrenia," *American Journal of Orthopsychiatry*, 36 (1966), 492–509.
41. Pollin, W., Stabenau, J. R., and Tupin, J. "Family Studies with Identical Twins Discordant for Schizophrenia," *Psychiatry*, 28 (1965), 60–78.
42. Rosanoff, A. J., Handy, L. M., Plesset, I. R., and Brush, S. "The Etiology of So-called Schizophrenic Psychoses: With Special Reference to Their Occurrence in Twins," *American Journal of Psychiatry*, 91 (1934), 247–286.
43. Rosenthal, D. "Confusion of Identity and the Frequency of Schizophrenia in Twins," *Archives of General Psychiatry*, 3 (1960), 297–304.
44. Rosenthal, D. "Sex Distribution and the Severity of Illness among Samples of Schizophrenic Twins," *Journal of Psychiatric Research*, 1 (1961), 26–36.
45. Rosenthal, D. "Familial Concordance by Sex with Respect to Schizophrenia," *Psychological Bulletin*, 59 (1962), 401–421.
46. Rosenthal, D. "Problems of Sampling and Diagnosis in the Major Twin Studies of Schizophrenic Twins," *Journal of Psychiatric Research*, 2 (1962), 116–134.
47. Rosenthal, D. "The Offspring of Schizophrenic Couples," *Journal of Psychiatric Research*, 4 (1966), 169–188.
48. Rosenthal, D. (ed.). *The Genain Quadruplets*. New York: Basic Books, 1963.
49. Schulz, B. "Kinder schizophrener Elternpaare," *Zeitschrift für die gesamte Neurologie und Psychiatrie*, 168 (1940), 332.
50. Shields, J. *Monozygotic Twins Brought Up Apart and Brought Up Together*. London: Oxford University Press, 1962.
51. Singer, M. T., and Wynne, L. C. "Thought Disorders and Family Relations of Schizophrenics: III–IV," *Archives of General Psychiatry*, 12 (1965), 187–212.
52. Slater, E. "The Monogenic Theory of Schizophrenia," *Acta Genetica*, 8 (1958), 50–56.
53. Slater, E., and Shields, J. *Psychotic and Neurotic Illnesses in Twins*. London: Her Majesty's Stationery Office, 1953.
54. Tienari, P. "Psychiatric Illnesses in Identical Twins," *Acta Psychiatrica Scandinavica*, 171 (1963).
55. Tienari, P. Personal communication, 1967.
56. Wynne, L. C., and Singer, M. T. "Thought Disorder and Family Relations of Schizophrenics: I–II," *Archives of General Psychiatry*, 9 (1963), 191–206.
57. Zerbin-Rüdin, E. "Endogene Psychosen," in P. E. Becker (ed.), *Humangenetik. Ein kurzes Handbuch in fünf Bänden*. Stuttgart: Thieme, 1967.

ADVANCES IN THE BIOLOGY OF SCHIZOPHRENIA

Peter G. S. Beckett and Jacques S. Gottlieb

Three difficulties in particular have hindered research on the etiology of schizophrenia: (1) the problem of diagnosis—defining the limits of the syndrome; (2) the related problem of classification—is schizophrenia one disease or many? and (3) an unnecessary polarity between psychogenic theories and biogenic ones, implying that the disease must either arise from one source or the other, but not from both. A fourth difficulty at the practical level is that drug therapy, dietary patterns, and the influence of institutional life on the patient produce unavoidable artifacts in the complicated tests.

THE BIOCHEMICAL BACKGROUND

Many years of study at the biological level had a focus in the work of Hoskins at the Worcester State Hospital during the 1930's.[34] These studies demonstrated no specific or consistent biologic abnormality by the techniques then available, but did suggest a nonspecific disturbance in homeostasis or biologic control. Since then, a number of attractive and more specific hypotheses have been proposed: Osmond and Smythies,[51] faulty epinephrine metabolism, a hypothesis based on clinical studies; Woolley and Shaw,[65] serotonin blockade, a hypothesis suggested by the finding that LSD has antiserotonin properties; Kety's[53] related hypothesis of pathological transmethylation, based on the observation that schizophrenic symptoms get worse when methyl-donor compounds are administered; the taraxein, or blood protein, factor hypothesis of Heath,[42] Bergen,[52] Frohman,[24] and others. Modifications of all four of these hypotheses continue to be useful and are being actively pursued in a number of centers.

THE NEUROPHYSIOLOGICAL BACKGROUND

The problem of schizophrenia may not be decipherable by biochemical means alone. It may well reside in incorrect or inappropriate neuronal connections within the brain. Yet, probably because of the complexity of the brain, simple scalp electroencephalograms recorded both on wakeful and on sleeping schizophrenic patients have been unrewarding. More complex techniques, such as the surgically implanted electrode studies by Heath, have claimed specific findings in the septal area,[30] and these and his blood protein findings have been developed by him into a far-reaching autoimmune theory of the disease.[32] Other workers have reported that it is possible to demonstrate electrophysiological abnormalities in the temporal lobe in a small group of patients with typical schizophrenic symptoms,[59] possibly shedding light on the matter of classification. But methodological obstacles, including the lack of an animal model, and ethical limitations on the study of the human brain have greatly impeded physiological studies.

THE EXPERIMENTAL PSYCHOLOGICAL BACKGROUND

Can possible biochemical or physiological mechanisms be investigated at other levels? One of the more exciting findings of recent research has been the production of model, or artificial, psychoses. Although the syndrome produced is not schizophrenia, these experiments allow close observation of the onset of a psychosis and require an accurate theory to explain, for example, how approximately similar syndromes can be produced by sleep deprivation,[8] by sensory deprivation,[7] by LSD or other psychotomimetic agents, and by the sensory blocking agent, Sernyl (a drug that produces general analgesia in alert patients). What do these hold in common? One explanatory theory proposes that the common disturbance in these conditions—and possibly also in schizophrenia—is a disarticulation in the transmission and processing of sensory input to the brain, particularly in the processing of internally generated (proprioceptive) input.[48]

CLINICAL AND GENETIC BACKGROUND

It is not our purpose to review this very large topic; it has been well covered by others.[40, 50] But no comprehensive study of schizophrenia can ignore the past experience and background, and the course of illness, of the schizophrenic patient and the patterns of psychiatric illness in the family. Despite the very large amount of work done, it is still not clear whether the schizophrenic patient's illness is in part a reaction to his environment (particularly to his family), whether the family's often distinctive behavior is in part a reaction to illness in the patient or, finally, whether the family members' varying hereditary predispositions to schizophrenia interact to produce the observed behavior.

A MULTIDISCIPLINARY RESEARCH PROGRAM

The above summary suggests that the problem of schizophrenia should be pursued on several levels by several disciplines simultaneously. Starting from an extension of the Worcester Foundation results showing a general failure of homeostasis, and the other work mentioned, each scientific discipline at the Lafayette Clinic was encouraged to formulate its own hypotheses and to test them experimentally. The first requirement was to gather a stable group of subjects.

Subjects

Patients with unequivocal and long-lasting schizophrenia have been the primary group of subjects.[10] They are male, between eighteen and forty-five years, and without diseases other than schizophrenia. They have been demonstrated to be free of intestinal amoebae and had not taken antipsychotic drugs for at least two years at the time of the earliest studies being reported. Their diet is enriched with vitamins and animal proteins, and the regime includes a vigorous exercise program. In order ethically to permit a prolonged withdrawal of medication, it was necessary to select patients who had failed to respond to a very thorough trial of antipsychotic drugs (a trial measured in years) and who had also failed to benefit from other treatment techniques. This resulted in the selection of a group of patients with a severe and intractable illness. At a time toward the end of the studies to be reported, their mean age was 37.4±3.14 years and the mean duration of hospitalization was 11.3 ±3.39 years. Since they were first hospitalized, the patients' mean period out of hospital was 53.2 ±7.68 weeks; obviously, their illness is an unremitting one.

The control group has been less stable. In the early studies, a group of staff volunteers were examined, found healthy, and lived on the ward for the duration of the project.[29] Later, a group of healthy prisoner volunteers lived on the ward, but the arrangement had to be abandoned when management problems proved insuperable.[10] A few institutionalized patients with problems other than classical adult schizophrenia have been used as controls; this includes five patients with childhood schizophrenia and other patients with personality disorders and chronic alcoholism.[20] For most of the studies, the controls have been working hospital staff, mean age 32.1 ±7.01 years.

Demonstration of a Plasma Factor or Factors

If the schizophrenic patient has a pervasive failure of homeostasis, that is, a general inability to adapt to environmental change involving many organ systems, then it should be possible to demonstrate this failure at the cellular level. One of our early studies examined several important intermediates of energy-producing metabolic systems (for example, adenosinetriphosphate, ATP) and found in the schizophrenic patients a failure of response of this metabolic system to exogenous insulin. Further experiments aimed at a more detailed exploration of the metabolic disturbance showed that the results were apparently produced by a substance in the blood plasma,[21] that exercise magnified the effect,[22] and that the plasma substance could also alter the metabolism of such normal animal cells as chicken erythrocytes.[20]

In these studies, the method of demonstrating the metabolic disturbance was to suspend chicken erythrocytes in the subject's plasma and, after an hour's incubation, measure the ratio of lactate to pyruvate (the L/P ratio) in the mixture.[19] A high L/P ratio was found when plasma from schizophrenic patients was used, suggesting that the plasma substance or factor interfered with the cells' use of oxygen. This L/P ratio method was simple, but it had many drawbacks. These included relative nonspecificity, a markedly skewed distribution of results, and the need for extremely careful control of numerous details, including chemical reagents, biochemical techniques, and handling of chickens.[23] Nevertheless, it permitted studies of various plasma fractions and the eventual demonstration that the above metabolic effects were produced by a labile plasma protein, probably an alpha-2-globulin of high molecular weight.[20] This protein, or a similar one, had by 1965 been identified by three research groups in the United States and one in Sweden.[12] All found it to be a high molecular weight alpha globulin and to be labile in solution. Low temperatures or an atmosphere of hydrogen were found to be stabilizing factors, but the activity of the protein was found to be destroyed by freezing. We have found it to occur consistently in the blood plasma of one half of those patients with chronic schizophrenia described above.

Table 1 gives the distribution in twenty-eight members of the group. The L/P value for each patient is the mean of ten determinations after exercise. The range is from 5.34 to 36.7. A similar table of ten determinations in each of the twelve control subjects gives a range from 2.13 to 12.3. Therefore, in Table 1, fourteen of the twenty-eight schizophrenic subjects (subjects A through N) have mean L/P ratios above the control range and fourteen (subjects O through BB) have L/P ratios in the same range as controls.

At a 1967 conference on schizophrenia in Moscow, a Russian research group presented additional data on this same protein factor, which we may call factor 1. At this conference, there was agreement by workers from several countries on the properties of the substance—that it has a high lipid content, for example. Some workers, notably those from the Worcester Foundation, reported that the protein may be a carrier of a small active molecule, but others were not able to demonstrate this.

In our laboratory, the use of the L/P ratio technique has indicated, in two studies of subjects from other institutions, the pres-

TABLE 1

Means and Standard Deviations of Ten L/P Ratios Done on Each of Twenty-eight Schizophrenic Patients (after Exercise)

SUBJECT	MEAN L/P RATIO	STANDARD DEVIATION
A	36.7	18.7
B	33.3	17.2
C	33.1	17.8
D	29.6	17.6
E	29.0	19.3
F	25.5	17.5
G	21.6	18.0
H	20.9	19.3
I	19.5	18.6
J	18.4	13.0
K	18.0	14.0
L	16.3	13.5
M	15.0	13.5
N	12.8	8.8
O	12.1	13.7
P	11.7	10.2
Q	11.7	12.7
R	11.6	10.0
S	10.7	11.1
T	10.0	4.67
U	8.64	3.03
V	8.60	10.3
W	8.34	5.01
X	8.09	4.91
Y	6.65	3.61
Z	5.91	4.01
AA	5.52	2.43
BB	5.34	3.60

ence of factor 1 in a group of unidentified blood samples. On this basis, the samples from schizophrenic patients were correctly distinguished from the samples from control subjects.[6, 25] In a third study, the method failed to identify the samples from the schizophrenic subjects, and other collaborators claimed that the observed elevation of the L/P ratio was owing merely to increased hemolysis of the chicken erythrocytes.[58] Two experiments in our laboratories have failed to confirm this suggestion[16]; in one, the complete artificial hemolysis of chicken erythrocytes produced a drop rather than a rise in the L/P ratio; in the other, splitting the plasma proteins of schizophrenic patients by electrophoresis into thirty-two fractions showed that the protein that produces hemolysis is not the same protein that affects the L/P ratio.

If a blood-borne factor has a connection with a disorder of affect, thinking, and behavior such as schizophrenia, it ought to be possible to demonstrate a relationship between the administration of this factor to an animal and some subsequent behavioral disturbance. This is the basis of the rope-climbing delay test used by Bergen and his group at the Worcester Foundation to identify factor 1. This test measures in rats the inhibition of a well-learned task by preinjection of factor 1 into the animal. It was suggested by some of our workers that factor 1 might produce an even greater inhibition in the animal's ability to learn a new task.

A task was devised in which rats were placed in a box with a grid floor and a one and one-quarter inch diameter pole descending to within three inches of the floor. A conditioned stimulus (CS), a buzzer, was paired with grid shock. The criterion of learning was nine out of ten avoidance responses—that is, during nine out of ten trials, the rat would avoid shock by jumping to the pole during the CS interval. Blood plasma from schizophrenic or control subjects was injected intraperitoneally into the rat five minutes before the task.

The results of this study were quite unexpected.[11] Plasma from control subjects and plasma from schizophrenic patients with consistently high levels of factor 1 slowed the acquisition of learning, whereas saline and plasma from schizophrenic patients with consistently low levels of factor 1 did not. This suggested two possibilities: that factor 1 was not involved in this effect (because controls and high factor 1 patients differ in respect to factor 1 but are similar in respect to slowing of learning) and that plasma from low factor 1 patients is either deficient in some nonspecific inhibitor substance or that it contains an independent amphetaminelike substance that stimulates learning.[11]

Recent work summarized by Vartanian[64] at the 1967 Moscow conference supports this indication of several factors in the blood plasma of patients with schizophrenia. Table 2 summarizes data from various sources on these postulated factors. Factor 1 is already described. As regards the other factors, it is not certain that all are distinct; factors 1 and 7 may be the same, for example. It is also possible that several, notably factors 3 and 5, result from a nonspecific tissue reaction to stress. Nevertheless, the table reflects the tentative current status of research on blood-borne factors.

TABLE 2

A Summary of Postulated Factors in the Blood Plasma of Schizophrenic Patients

FACTOR	IDENTIFYING PROPERTIES	WORKERS	REFERENCE
1	a. Delays climbing time in rats	Bergen	6
	b. Raises the L/P ratio	Frohman	22
		Krasnova	38
	c. Raises amino acid uptake by cells	Frohman	17
	d. Amine oxidase activity	Ehrensvaard	12
2	a. Inhibition of lymphocyte stress response	Vartanian	64
3	a. Hemolysis of human and/or other erythrocytes	Ryan	58
		Frohman	16
		Turner	62
		Lideman	43
4	a. Prealbumin affecting erythrocyte permeability	Usnov	63
5	a. Anti-septal antibody	Heath	32
	b. Anti-brain antibody	Kolaskina	37
6	a. Lymphoblastic transformation	Gosheva	27
7	a. Inhibition of ADP response	Hoffman	33

Source: Modified with additions from J. R. Bergen et al., "Plasma Factors in Schizophrenia: A Cooperative Study," *Archives of General Psychiatry*, 18 (1968), Table 1.

POSSIBLE ORIGINS OF FACTOR 1

Studies relating extensive clinical data to the biologic indicators of factor 1 have shown a tendency for those patients with consistently high levels of this plasma factor to have had early lives that were sheltered, monotonous, and unstimulating when compared to the early lives of equally ill schizophrenic patients with less biochemical abnormality.[5] The retrospective nature of these data was unsatisfactory, however, so a study was devised to examine animals raised in an extremely monotonous, unstimulating early environment. The hypothesis was that, if this early environment is significant, the blood plasma of these animals should show factor 1. In one study of rhesus monkeys, this hypothesis was confirmed[3]; in another, of chimpanzees, it was not confirmed,[2] although complicating influences in the early life of chimpanzees made interpretation difficult. Note that in all these studies, and in our clinical work, the level of factor 1 in schizophrenic patients or experimental animals is not related, or at least is not closely related, to the severity of the disturbed behavior.

In another study done through the courtesy of the National Institute of Mental Health (NIMH), blood from nine identical twin pairs discordant for schizophrenia was examined on a blind basis.[54] Of the nine blood samples from the twins (one blood sample from each schizophrenic twin), eight were found abnormal using the L/P ratio; of eight blood samples from the twin who did not have schizophrenia (one blood sample was lost), only two were found abnormal. Because heredity is identical in these patients, these results suggest that factor 1 is not inherited. Pollin and coworkers[54] have described that, in these same twin pairs, the twin who later became schizophrenic was in every case lighter at birth and reached the milestones of development more slowly. It would appear that, in some cases at least, a prenatal insult of some kind may lead to a chain of circumstances eventually productive of factor 1.

A survey of the families of our study group of chronic schizophrenic patients has presented rather paradoxical results.[61] There is some tendency for factor 1 to run in families, but there also tends to be a negative relationship between the distribution of schizophrenia and that of the factor in the families, that is, those family members with schizophrenia tend not to have the factor. Krasnova has also found a familial trend in her studies of factor 1,[39] but has not reported any observations on the relationship to symptoms.

IS THERE MORE THAN ONE KIND OF SCHIZOPHRENIA?

The work presented in Table 1 on the distribution of the alpha-2-globulin blood factor (factor 1) in schizophrenic patients indicates that there is no clear distinction between normal and abnormal quantity of factor 1, that is, no obvious evidence of two groups of patients, that is, one group that always has a low L/P ratio and one that always has a high ratio. Nevertheless, an entire series of studies has been done to see whether data from other fields could help answer the question of whether there is evidence of two distinct kinds of schizophrenic patients. Do other independent measures rank the patients similarly? In all cases, data were collected by individuals unaware of the high factor 1-low factor 1 distribution.

Clinical Evidence

Much data have been collected by psychiatric interviews of patients and their families and by ratings by ward staff. There are no clearly significant differences between the high factor 1 and the low factor 1 patients. Of a total of seventy-five clinical variables examined in one study, only six show significant differences at the .05 level. These variables are derived from several sources, including the Lafayette Clinic Rating Scales,[4] the IMPS of Lorr, Klett, and McNair,[44] and the scale of Farina, Arenberg, and Guskins.[13] Some trends are shown in Tables 3, 4, and 5. In Table 3, it can be seen that, if the patients with high levels of factor 1 have a more severe illness than patients with low levels of this factor, they should be rated as socially less accessible, have a higher rating of conceptual disorganization, be less socially responsive, participate less in activities, and be less neat in their dress. These are five of the more reliable measures of severity of the schizophrenic illness. In all cases, the observed results are in the predicted direction—high factor 1 patients tend to be more seriously ill. But the requirements of statistical significance are not met. In Table 4, similar data are shown with respect to high factor 1 patients having an unremitting, progressive illness. In all four measures, results indicate a tendency in this direction.

The Russian workers have concluded that factor 1 is related to

TABLE 3

If High Factor 1 Patients Have a More Severe Form of Schizophrenia, Then . . .

INTENSITY OF THESE VARIABLES	SHOULD BE IN THIS DIRECTION	OBSERVED RESULTS	SIGNIFICANCE OF DIFFERENCE
Social accessibility in interview	Low	Low	ns
Conceptual disorganization	High	High	ns
Social response to other patients	Low	Low	ns
Participation in activities	Low	Low	.05
Neatness of dress	Low	Low	ns

TABLE 4

If High Factor 1 Patients Have Had Fewer Remissions during Their Illness, Then . . .

INTENSITY OF THESE VARIABLES	SHOULD BE IN THIS DIRECTION	OBSERVED RESULTS	SIGNIFICANCE OF DIFFERENCE
Ratio of discharges to time in hospital	Low	Low	ns
Ratio of days with off-ward card to time in hospital	Low	Low	ns
Variance in social response to other patients over a one-year period	Low	Low	ns
Variance in participation in activities over a one-year period	Low	Low	ns

the rate of progression of the schizophrenic illness. Its concentration is highest during the period three to eight years after onset; after ten years or so, when a residual phase of the illness is entered, factor 1 drops to low levels. Our results show no simple relationship to duration of illness, but we have not investigated the possibility of a curvilinear relationship.

In Table 5, the data concern a monotonous, nonstimulating early home life, and again the trend is as predicted. High factor

TABLE 5

If High Factor 1 Patients Were Raised in a Monotonous Nonstimulating Childhood Environment, Then . . .

INTENSITY OF THESE VARIABLES	SHOULD BE IN THIS DIRECTION	OBSERVED RESULTS	SIGNIFICANCE OF DIFFERENCE
Disruption of rearing home (by history)	Low	Low	.05
Disruption of rearing home (by home visit)	Low	Low	ns
Parental quarreling during childhood	Low	Low	ns
Mother absent from rearing home	Low	Low	.05
Discipline by mother	Low	Low	ns
Beatings by mother	Low	Low	ns
Discipline by father	Low	High*	ns
Beatings by father	Low	Low	ns

* Not in expected direction.

1 patients tend to have this. But the relationship is a tendency only.

Psychological Evidence

To pursue the hypothesis of proprioceptive deficit in schizophrenia and to explore its possible relationship to the biochemical findings, a series of psychological studies has been done. It was shown that the ability to discriminate between different weights lifted in the hand is less in schizophrenic patients when compared to controls[57] and that this failure is more obvious with light weights (40 gms) than with heavy weights (400 gms). To explore this further, a study of forearm flexion was devised in which one of the subject's arms was passively flexed at the elbow by the experimenter to a certain angle in an apparatus that hid the arm from the subject's vision. The subject was then asked to match the flexion of this with his other arm by using only nonvisual, mostly proprioceptive cues. The schizophrenic patients were significantly less able to do this than controls, with high factor 1 patients more deficient than the low factor 1 patients.[56] This suggestion of proprioceptive deficit in the high factor 1 patients is reinforced by the finding at a clinical level that these patients are less able than the low factor 1 patients to identify body parts or to imitate body movements made by the examiner.

Neurophysiological Evidence

Three approaches have been used here, all through the intact scalp. The schizophrenic patients have been compared during wakefulness with a control group by means of frequency analysis and by means of the average visual evoked responses using a computer of average transients (CAT).[55] The results suggest differences in EEG output between schizophrenic patients and controls and between high factor 1 and low factor 1 patients, but none of the findings is specific. There is some evidence of a relationship between proprioceptive deficit (weight discrimination and forearm flexion) and the amplitude of the negative visually evoked response. Work is in progress on the possibility of recording cortical response evoked by a proprioceptive stimulus.

In the sleeping subject, electroencephalographic results have been more clearcut. Though there were no differences in stage 1 REM (activated or dreaming sleep) between control and schizophrenic subjects, there were significant differences in the amount of deep sleep, stage 4.[9] The schizophrenic group had significantly less of this stage. On detailed study of the data, it became apparent that this finding was largely owing to the fact that ten of the twenty-five schizophrenic patients studied had no scorable stage 4 sleep. When these results are related to levels of factor 1 in the blood there is a strong tendency ($p<.001$) for high factor 1 patients to have low stage 4 sleep and for patients close to normal in amount of factor 1 to be also close to normal in amount of stage 4 sleep.

It is of great interest that one of the ways of producing a model psychosis is by deprivation of sleep[47] and that one of the first priorities during nights of recovery from sleep deprivation in these studies is to make up stage 4. Four chronic schizophrenic patients studied in our laboratories were unable to accomplish this make-up following eighty-five hours of sleep deprivation.[45] Jouvet[35] has proposed that the basis of slow-wave sleep (stage 4) is a serotoninergic mechanism involving the raphe system in the brain stem. Thus, the possibility arises of bridging the gap between these neurophysiological findings and some of the biochemical theories of schizophrenia previously discussed.

Further Biochemical Evidence

It was mentioned that the L/P ratio, though useful, has many disadvantages. A series of studies has been undertaken both to investigate further metabolic effects produced by factor 1 and to try to replace the L/P ratio as an assay method. A starting place for these studies was the observation mentioned previously that hemolysis of the erythrocytes in the incubation mixture, though leaving the mitochondria intact, lowered the L/P ratio and that 100 per cent artificial hemolysis obliterated the effect of factor 1,[16] suggesting that the intact cell membrane might be the site of action of this plasma factor.

Following some negative results of the effect of factor 1 on the passage of various substances across the cell membrane,[41] the effect of this factor on the permeability of certain elements of the citric acid cycle was investigated.[17] It was concluded from this study that amino acids from outside the citric acid cycle were entering the system in unusual amounts when factor 1 was present. A series of studies has recently been initiated to test the effect of factor 1 on the rate of transport of specific amino acids across the membrane of intact chicken erythrocytes. Evidence so far suggests that after a twenty-minute incubation, glutamic acid and tryptophan accumulate more rapidly than usual within the cell in the presence of plasma from schizophrenic patients,

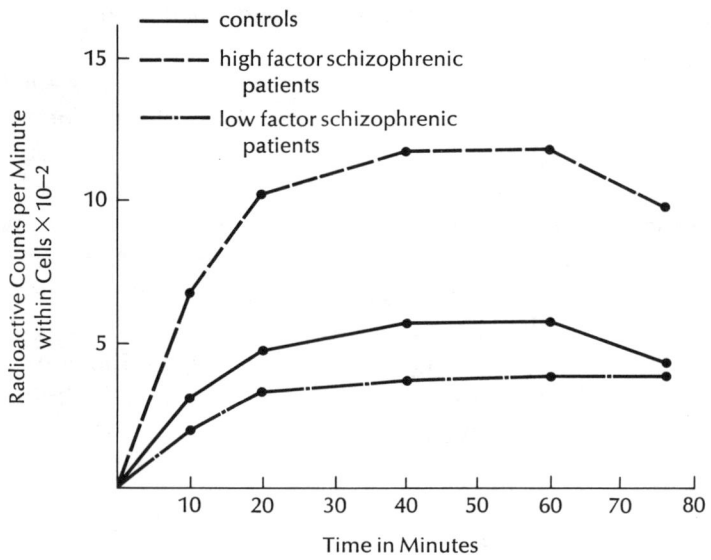

FIGURE 1
Glutamic Acid Uptake by Chicken Erythrocytes in Control Subjects and Two Groups of Schizophrenic Patients

whereas methionine, histidine, alanine, and lysine do not. This effect is much more pronounced in those patients who have consistently high levels of factor 1.

The possibility now arises that factor 1 may force the accumulation within cells, including neurones, of certain amino acids that are metabolic precursors of highly potent biogenic amines. Among the amino acids we have studied, tryptophan is a precursor of serotonin and glutamic acid is a precursor of gamma amino butyric acid (GABA).

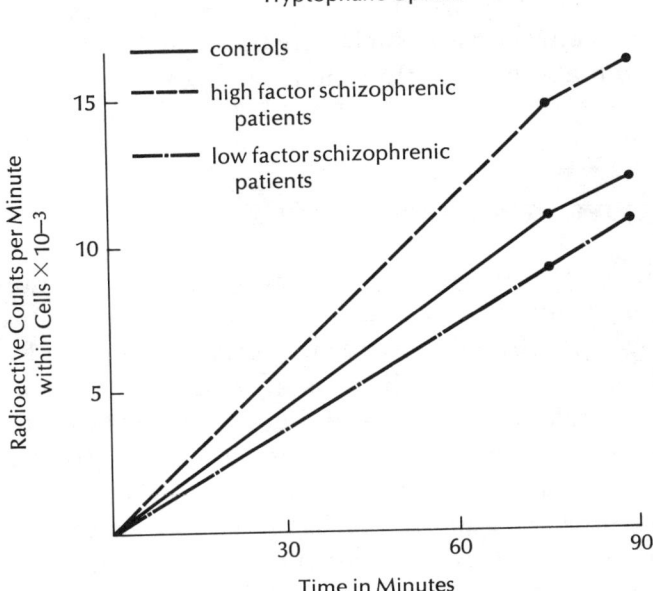

FIGURE 2
Tryptophane Uptake by Chicken Erythrocytes in Control Subjects and Two Groups of Schizophrenic Patients

Urine Findings

Although our group has not worked in this area, it is relevant at this point to bring up the disputed urine findings, the "pink spot" controversy. At least two of the substances that have been claimed as occurring in unusual amounts in the urine of schizophrenic patients are methylated products of amines. These are 3,4 dimethoxyphenylethylamine (DMPEA), reported by Friedhoff,[15] and bufotenine, reported by Fischer.[14] The first of these substances could be produced by excess methylation of dopamine and the second by the excess methylation of serotonin. Their reported occurrence in schizophrenia is in harmony both with the pathological transmethylation hypothesis of Kety[4, 36] and with our hypothesis of forced accumulation within cells and the subsequent accelerated metabolic breakdown of serotonin and of dopamine and/or the catecholamines. It is appropriate to note that Smythies has concluded that, of the phenylethylamine substitution products, only the ones methoxylated at the 4 position can produce psychotomimetic effects,[60] and such 4-methoxyphenylethylamines might arise from aberrant methylation.

A TENTATIVE REPORT OF A STATISTICAL SUMMARY

It has been indicated above that we have made a large number of measures on a group of patients with chronic schizophrenia. If all measures made by all workers are included, the total number of variables is about 900. This is on the same scale as the wide-ranging correlational studies of Gerard and his group.[26] In an attempt to bring order to this vast array, each investigator was asked to select about five of his own measures. It was suggested that the selection be made on the basis of: (1) importance to theory construction, (2) reasonably normal distribution of the data, (3) inclusion of measures independent of one another, and (4) data that were as complete as possible, that is, that had been recorded on most or all the patients. In this way, thirty-five measures from seven areas of investigation were selected. These data were close to complete on twenty-seven of the schizophrenic patients (if incomplete, group means were used).

This much-reduced number of variables is listed in the left-hand column of Table 6. The first six are psychological measures of proprioception derived from the weight discrimination study[57] (variables 1 and 2), and the arm-to-arm elbow-bending match[56] (variables 3 to 6). The next six measures (7 to 12) are derived from scalp EEG recordings of visually evoked responses over the visual and parietal areas of the brain. Variables 7 and 8 reflect the highest evoked peak, and 9 to 12 the correlation between the wave forms recorded in the areas indicated.[55] The next two measures are of the percentage of the night's sleep (second night in the sleep laboratory) spent in stage 3 and stage 4 sleep.[9] These are derived from hand-scoring of the all-night EEG.

Variable 15 is the number of trials required to acquire learning in the rat pole-jump study.[11] Variables 16 to 25 are clinical ratings of various aspects of behavior; 16 to 19 are ratings by ward staff using the Fergus Falls Scales[49] and 20 to 25 are ratings by a psychiatrist following interview, review of the record, and/or interview with parents as indicated.[4, 13, 44]

TABLE 6

Varimax Rotated Factor Loadings—by Variables: Twenty-seven Schizophrenic Patients

	1	2	3	4	5	6
1. Correct weight discrimination, heavy weights	−.083	−.763	.199	−.121	−.343	.207
2. Correct weight discrimination, light weights	.037	−.119	.138	.038	−.889	−.053
3. Proprioceptive error, arm-arm RT	.513	.645	−.122	.084	−.099	−.026
4. Proprioceptive error, arm-arm LT	.420	.623	−.331	−.132	−.251	−.039
5. Proprioceptive error, eye-arm RT	.053	.687	−.222	−.154	−.376	.063
6. Proprioceptive error, eye-arm LT	.002	.841	.061	.125	−.021	.127
7. Average VER highest peak-parietal occipital LT	.134	−.110	.223	.114	−.037	.860
8. Average VER highest peak-parietal occipital RT	.001	−.168	.249	.025	−.344	.791
9. Average VER cross-correlation occipital vs. parietal LT	−.081	−.773	−.222	.159	−.286	.220
10. Average VER cross-correlation occipital vs. parietal RT	−.044	−.591	.079	−.221	−.372	.143
11. Average VER cross-correlation LT occipital vs. RT occipital	−.233	.420	.023	−.319	−.099	.014
12. Average VER cross-correlation LT parietal vs. RT parietal	−.498	−.112	.071	−.066	−.038	.364
13. All-night EEG—per cent stage 3	−.191	−.101	−.105	.154	−.366	.119
14. All-night EEG—per cent stage 4	−.428	−.193	.062	.570	−.237	.229
15. Trials to criterion—rat learning—plasma	.407	−.448	−.554	−.271	−.016	−.193
16. Nursing rating—activity, participation	−.753	−.062	.371	.140	−.182	−.185
17. Nursing rating—ward sociability	−.460	−.170	.418	−.159	−.333	−.121
18. Nursing rating—amount of motor activity	.077	−.138	.708	.174	.115	.001
19. Nursing rating—amount of speech	−.030	−.145	.667	.213	−.108	.021
20. Psychiatric interview—muteness	.252	−.056	−.698	.239	.266	−.080
21. Psychiatric interview—inaccessibility	.334	−.115	−.111	.041	.665	−.439
22. Psychiatric interview—conceptual disorganization	.695	.036	.472	−.091	.460	.060
23. Inability to identify body parts	.423	.025	−.413	−.032	.623	−.109
24. Index of hospital discharges (by history)	−.577	−.059	−.312	.198	.048	.155
25. Mother's indulgence (by history)	−.318	.311	−.593	−.050	.287	−.354
26. Psychophysiology—GSR—reactivity	.042	.114	.024	.274	−.331	.054
27. Psychophysiology—GSR—conditioning	−.048	.051	.404	.044	−.082	.191
28. Psychophysiology—GSR—discrimination	−.250	−.124	.300	−.123	−.304	.203
29. Mean log L/P—before exercise	.193	.015	−.150	−.833	−.169	−.120
30. Mean log L/P—after exercise	.143	.060	−.245	−.867	.236	−.027
31. L/P difference—after minus before	−.034	.043	−.163	−.157	.651	.117
32. Mean log L/P—before cold pressor	.667	−.121	−.036	−.383	−.017	.113
33. Mean log L/P—after cold pressor	.713	.147	−.131	−.199	.074	−.069
34. Glutamic acid uptake	.120	−.087	−.142	−.624	.221	.221
35. Tryptophan uptake	.114	−.042	.238	−.692	.112	−.319
Per cent of variance	30%	17%	14%	13%	10%	9%

NOTE: VER = Visual Evoked Response.

TABLE 7

Summary of Factor Analysis with Tentative Titles: Twenty-seven Schizophrenic Patients, Thirty-seven Variables

30%	CLUSTER 1	DETERIORATION	VARIABLE NUMBER
	.753	Low participation in activities (O.T. and so forth)	16
	.713	High L/P peak following cold pressor test	33
	.667	High L/P before cold pressor test	32
	.695	High conceptual disorganization in interview	22
	.577	Few hospital discharges per unit time	24
	.513	Proprioceptive error—arm to arm (right)	3
	.498	Low EEG cross-correlation of VER left-right parietal	12
	.460	Low sociability on the ward	17
17%	CLUSTER 2	PROPRIOCEPTIVE FAILURE	
	.841	Proprioceptive error—eye to arm (left)	6
	.773	Low EEG cross-correlation of VER left occipital vs. parietal	9
	.763	Low accuracy at discriminating heavy weights	1
	.687	Proprioceptive error—eye to arm (right)	5
	.645	Proprioceptive error—arm to arm (right)	3
	.623	Proprioceptive error—arm to arm (left)	4
	.591	Low EEG cross-correlation of VER right occipital vs. parietal	10
14%	CLUSTER 3	AROUSAL/INDIFFERENCE	
	.708	High motor activity on the ward	18
	.698	Verbal accessibility in interview (that is, responds verbally to questions)	20
	.667	More speech on the ward	19
	.593	Rejection by mother in childhood	25
	.554	Effect of plasma is *not* to slow the acquisition of learning in the rat (control plasma does slow)	15
	.472	High conceptual disorganization in interview	22
13%	CLUSTER 4	NEUROTRANSMITTER DYSFUNCTION	
	.867	High L/P after exercise	30
	.833	High L/P before exercise	29
	.692	High tryptophan uptake	35
	.624	High glutamic acid uptake	34
	.570	Low stage 4 sleep	14

Table 7 Continued

10%	CLUSTER 5	?	
	.889	Low accuracy at discriminating light weights	2
	.665	Nonverbal inaccessibility (that is, does not respond to such social cues as shaking hands and looking at magazine)	21
	.651	High L/P difference (after minus before)—exercise study	31
	.623	High body-image disturbance by clinical rating (identifying body parts)	23
9%	CLUSTER 6	VISUAL EVOKED RESPONSE (VER)	
	.860	High peak VER right occipital-parietal	7
	.791	High peak VER left occipital-parietal	8

The three psychophysiological measures are of the GSR derived from a study of classical conditioning in which one of two tones was followed by a pain stimulus.[1] Lastly, there are seven biochemical measures of factor 1, a number of them before, or after, the stressful situations of stair-climbing (exercise) or a cold pressor test (which we had found to elevate levels of the factor).

This relatively limited data array could be encompassed at one time in the statistical technique of factor analysis. Such a procedure was done (Varimax rotation) using the thirty-five listed variables on twenty-seven schizophrenic subjects. The factors extracted will be called "clusters" to avoid confusion with blood factors.

Table 7 illustrates that six clusters containing 93 per cent of the variance were extracted; the loading on each factor by variable is presented. For simplicity, this table is arranged so that all loadings are positive, the direction of the loading being indicated by a change in the title of the variable. Thus, in Table 7, the first variable on cluster 1, number 16, is called "low participation in activities" and is given a positive loading.

These clusters are a first step toward bringing order to the mass of data available on these patients. They give an indication of which variables describe one aspect or facet of the patients. But the clusters and their titles must be considered entirely preliminary. Before firm conclusions are drawn, the same measures should be repeated on another group of chronic schizophrenic patients and the statistical procedure performed again. To the extent that the same clusters recur in a second study, firm conclusions can be drawn.

With this proviso, the clusters summarized in Table 7 present the following possibilities.

1. Something less than one third (30 per cent) of the variance seen in this group of chronic schizophrenic patients is accounted for by a group of variables summarized by "deterioration" or the "severely ill." This is cluster 1; it associates lack of socialization, disorganized thinking, and few remissions with the finding that in an unfamiliar laboratory situation, where the cold pressor test was done, plasma factor 1 is present at high levels both before and after the test. (This finding has been felt to indicate a failure of adaptation to a novel situation.[18])

2. About one sixth of the variance (17 per cent) can be summarized as "proprioceptive failure," cluster 2. In this cluster are associated psychological measures of low proprioceptive accuracy and electroencephalographic indications of low similarity of the visually evoked response (VER) in the parietal and occipital areas of the brain. No biochemical or clinical variables were found that reflect this possible failure.

3. Fourteen per cent of the variance is found to be associated with a group of variables clustering around the dimension "arousal/indifference." At one end of this hypothetical dimension, the individual is highly physically active and talks freely but with highly disorganized concepts; his plasma does not slow the acquisition of learning, and so either it contains the postulated "stimulant" substance or fails to contain a normal inhibitor substance[11]; and his history indicates a rejecting maternal relationship. At the other end of the hypothetical dimension, the individual is retarded and mute, his concepts cannot be demonstrated to be disorganized (possibly because he is mute), his plasma is either free of the "stimulant" substance or contains the normal inhibitor substance, and his maternal relationship was an indulgent nonstimulating one.[5]

4. Thirteen per cent of the variance is involved in a biological dimension tentatively entitled "neurotransmitter dysfunction." Four biochemical measures indicate high levels of plasma factor 1. As previously discussed, it has been theorized that this plasma substance promotes the entry into cells, including neurones, of precursors of neurotransmitters. Hence, it is of interest that in this same cluster of variables is found another quite independent

variable possibly dependent on the neurotransmitter serotonin; this is the percentage of the night's sleep in stage 4 sleep.[35]

The significance of the last two clusters is unclear. They account for 19 per cent of the variance between them. Cluster 5 associates a group of variables that cannot easily be conceived as a meaningful whole. Cluster 6 is entirely concerned with the maximum size of the visual evoked response.

A SUMMARY OF BIOLOGICAL WORK IN SCHIZOPHENIA

After these studies have been evaluated, the nature of schizophrenia is still not clear. There appear to be several distinct factors or substances in the blood plasma. Some of these may be specific to this illness—the evidence is best for factor 1, an alpha globulin, but even here it is not conclusive. The other blood substances may well be nonspecific. It is a reasonable speculation and there is some indirect evidence—the sleep and urine findings—that factor 1 may be interfering with the metabolism of various neurotransmitters, particularly serotonin. Possibly a psychotomimetic substance is being produced by transmethylation.

A broad look at a wide array of measures gathered at this hospital gives a tentative picture of four statistical clusters of hypothetical dimensions of the problem. One of these is deterioration, expressed both clinically and in sluggish homeostasis. A second is a failure of proprioceptive function expressed in test performance and some irregularity of electrophysiological cortical response. A third reflects the dimension of arousal to the environment vs. indifference to it; this is expressed behaviorally and may be associated with a second plasma substance. A fourth reflects the conjecture that plasma factor 1 is involved with a disturbance neurotransmitter. But in answer to the interesting question of the existence of different types of schizophrenia, it is not at all clear whether these dimensions indicate four types of illness or whether they indicate four facets of one type of illness. Studies of a new group of patients will be necessary to answer this question.

REFERENCES

1. Ax, A. F. "Psychophysiology of Schizophrenia," in J. S. Gottlieb and G. Tourney (eds.), *Lafayette Clinic Studies in Schizophrenia*, Lafayette Clinic Monograph No. 4. Detroit: Wayne State University Press, 1970.

2. Beckett, P. G. S., Frohman, C. E., Davenport, R. E., Jr., Rogers, C. M., and Gottlieb, J. S. "Biologic Effects of Infantile Restriction in Chimpanzees," *Comprehensive Psychiatry,* 4 (1963), 1–8.
3. Beckett, P. G. S., Frohman, C. E., Gottlieb, J. S., Mowbray, J. B., and Wolf, R. C. "Schizophrenic-like Mechanisms in Monkeys," *American Journal of Psychiatry,* 119 (1963), 835–842.
4. Beckett, P. G. S., Grisell, J., Crandall, R. G., and Gudobba, R. "A Method of Formalizing Psychiatric Study," *Archives of General Psychiatry,* 16 (1967), 407–415.
5. Beckett, P. G. S., Senf, R., Frohman, C. E., and Gottlieb, J. S. "Energy Production and Premorbid History in Schizophrenia," *Archives of General Psychiatry,* 8 (1963), 155–162.
6. Bergen, J. R. et al. "Plasma Factors in Schizophrenia: A Cooperative Study," *Archives of General Psychiatry,* 18 (1968), 471–476.
7. Bexton, W. H., Heron, W., and Scott, T. H. "Effects of Decreased Variation in the Sensory Environment," *Canadian Journal of Psychology,* 8 (1954), 70–76.
8. Bliss, E. L., Clark, L. D., and West, C. D. "Studies of Sleep Deprivation—Relationship to Schizophrenia," *Archives of Neurology and Psychiatry,* 81 (1959), 348–356.
9. Calwell, D. F., and Domino, E. F. "EEG and Sleep Patterns," in J. S. Gottlieb and G. Tourney (eds.), *Lafayette Clinic Studies in Schizophrenia,* Lafayette Clinic Monograph No. 4. Detroit: Wayne State University Press, 1970.
10. Crandall, R. G., Day, H., Beckett, P. G. S., Chen, C., Brosius, C., Frohman, C. E., and Gottlieb J. S. "Conflict between Treatment and Science on a Research Ward Investigating Schizophrenia," *Canadian Psychiatric Association Journal,* 2 (1966), 306–313.
11. Domino, E. F. Caldwell, D. F., Henke, J., and Henke, R. "The Differential Effects of Plasma from Two Groups of Clinically Similar Schizophrenic Patients on Learning Behavior in Rats," *Journal of Psychiatric Research,* 4 (1966), 87–94.
12. Ehrensvaard, G. "Discussion," in O. Walaas (ed.), *Molecular Basis of Some Aspects of Mental Activity.* New York: Academic Press, 1967. Vol. 2, p. 311.
13. Farina, A., Arenberg, D., and Guskins, S. "A Scale for Measuring Minimal Social Behavior," *Journal of Consulting Psychology,* 21 (1957), 265–268.
14. Fischer, E., Fernandez Lagravere, T. A., Vazquez, A. J., and Distepheno, A. O. "A Bufotenine-like Substance in the Urine of Schizophrenics," *Journal of Nervous and Mental Diseases,* 133 (1961), 441–444.
15. Friedhoff, A. J., and Van Winkle, E. "Isolation and Characterization of a Compound from the Urine of Schizophrenics," *Nature,* 194 (1962), 897–898.
16. Frohman, C. E., Latham, L. K., Beckett, P. G. S., and Gottlieb, J. S. "Biochemical Studies of a Serum Factor in Schizophrenia," in O. Walaas (ed.), *Molecular Basis of Some Aspects of Mental Activity,* New York: Academic Press, 1967. Vol. 2, pp. 241–255.
17. Frohman, C. E. "Studies on the Plasma Factor in Schizophrenia," in C. Rupp (ed.), *Mind as a Tissue,* New York: Harper & Row (1968). Pp. 181–195.
18. Frohman, C. E., Beckett, P. G. S., Grisell, J. L., Latham, L. K., and Gottlieb, J. S. "Biologic Responsiveness to Environmental Stimuli in Schizophrenia," *Comprehensive Psychiatry,* 7 (1966), 494–500.
19. Frohman, C. E., Czajkowski, N. P., Luby, E. D., Gottlieb, J. S., and Senf, R. "Further Evidence of a Plasma Factor in Schizophrenia," *Archives of General Psychiatry,* 2 (1960), 263–267.
20. Frohman, C. E., Goodman, M., Beckett, P. G. S., Latham, L. K., Senf, R., and Gottlieb, J. S. "The Isolation of an Active Factor from Serum of Schizophrenic Patients," *Annals of the N.Y. Academy of Science,* 196 (1962), 438–447.
21. Frohman, C. E., Latham, L. K., Beckett, P. G. S., and Gottlieb, J. S. "Evidence of a Plasma Factor in Schizophrenia," *Archives of General Psychiatry,* 2 (1960), 255–262.
22. Frohman, C. E., Latham, L. K., Warner, K. A., Brosius, C. O., Beckett, P. G. S., and Gottlieb, J. S. "Motor Activity in Schizophrenia: Effect on Plasma Factor," *Archives of General Psychiatry,* 9 (1963), 83–88.
23. Frohman, C. E., Latham, L. K., Warner, K. A., and Gottlieb, J. S. "The Reliability of the L/P Ratio in Measuring the Plasma Factor in Schizophrenia," in J. S. Gottlieb and G. Tourney (eds.), *Lafayette Clinic Studies in Schizophrenia,* Lafayette Clinic Monograph No. 4. Detroit: Wayne State University Press, 1970.

24. Frohman, C. E., Luby, E. D., Tourney, G., Beckett, P. G. S., and Gottlieb, J. S. "Steps toward the Isolation of a Serum Factor in Schizophrenia," *American Journal of Psychiatry*, 117 (1960), 401–408.
25. Frohman, C. E., Tourney, G., Beckett, P. G. S., Lees, H., Latham, L. K., and Gottlieb, J. S. "Biochemical Identification of Schizophrenia," *Archives of General Psychiatry*, 4 (1961), 404–412.
26. Gerard, R. W. "The Nosology of Schizophrenia: A Cooperative Study," *Behavioral Science*, 9 (1964), 311–333.
27. Gosheva, A., and Podozyonova, N. "Morphological Analysis of Human Embryo-Cerebral Cultures Affected by Schizophrenic Patients' Erythrocytes," in M. Vartanian (ed.), *Biological Research in Schizophrenia*. Moscow: Ordina Lennia, 1967. Pp. 240–243.
28. Gottlieb, J. S. "The Biologic Correlates of the Serum Factor in Schizophrenia," in O. Walaas (ed.), *Molecular Basis of Some Aspects of Mental Activity*. New York: Academic Press, 1967. Vol. 2, pp. 347–364.
29. Gottlieb, J. S., Frohman, C. E., Beckett, P. G. S., Tourney, G., and Senf, R. "Production of High-Energy Phosphate Bonds in Schizophrenia," *A.M.A. Archives of General Psychiatry*, 1 (1959), 243–249.
30. Heath, R. G. "Effect on Behavior in Humans with the Administration of Taraxein," *American Journal of Psychiatry*, 114 (1957), 14–24.
31. Heath, R. G., and Krupp, I. M. "Schizophrenia as an Immunologic Disorder: I. Demonstration of Antibrain Globulins by Fluorescent Antibody Techniques," *Archives of General Psychiatry*, 16 (1967), 1–9.
32. Heath, R. G., Krupp, I. M., Byers, L. W., and Liljekvist, J. I. "Schizophrenia as an Immunologic Disorder: III," *Archives of General Psychiatry*, 16 (1967), 24–33.
33. Hoffman, G., and Arnold, O. H. "Results of Biochemical Investigations in Schizophrenia," in O. Walaas (ed.), *Molecular Basis of Some Aspects of Mental Activity*. New York: Academic Press, 1967. Vol. 2, pp. 381–396.
34. Hoskins, R. G. *The Biology of Schizophrenia*. New York: Norton, 1946.
35. Jouvet, M. "The States of Sleep," *Scientific American*, 216 (1907), 62–72.
36. Kety, S. S. "Biochemical Theories of Schizophrenia," *International Journal of Psychiatry*, 1 (1965), 409–446.
37. Kolaskina, G., Kushner, S., and Gaskin, L. "Certain Immunological Changes in Schizophrenic Patients," in M. Vartanian (ed.), *Biological Research in Schizophrenia*. Moscow: Ordina Lennia, 1967. Pp. 238–239.
38. Krasnova, A. I. "The Influence of the Blood Serum of Patients Having Schizophrenia on Carbohydrate Metabolism in Chicken Erythrocytes," *Zh. Nevropat. i Psikh.*, 68 (1965), 1206–1211.
39. Krasnova, A. I. "The Effects of the Serum of Relatives of Schizophrenic Patients on the L/P Ratio in In Vitro Experiments," in M. Vartanian (ed.), *Biological Research in Schizophrenia*. Moscow: Ordina Lennia, 1967. Pp. 262–263.
40. Kringelen, E. "Schizophrenia in Twins: An Epidemiological-Clinical Study," *Psychiatry*, 29 (1966), 172–184.
41. Latham, L. K., Loncharich, K., Warner, K. A., Crandall, R. G., Beckett, P. G. S., Frohman, C. E., and Gottlieb, J. S. "Effects of a Protein Factor Isolated from Schizophrenic Blood on Permeability," *Vox Sang.*, 8 (1963), 491–496.
42. Leach, B. E., Byers, L. W., and Heath, R. G. "Methods of Isolating Taraxein: A Survey of Results," in R. G. Heath (ed.), *Serologic Fractions in Schizophrenia*, New York: Hoeber, 1963. Pp. 7–22.
43. Lideman, R., and Bokova, J. "The Possible Nature and Mechanism of Action of the Active Factor of the Blood Serum of Schizophrenic Patients," in M. Vartanian (ed.), *Biological Research in Schizophrenia*. Moscow: Ordina Lennia, 1967. Pp. 169–171.
44. Lorr, M., Klett, C. J., and McNair, D. M. *Syndromes of Psychosis*. New York: Macmillan, 1963.
45. Luby, E. D., and Caldwell, D. F. "Sleep Deprivation and EEG Slow Wave Activity in Chronic Schizophrenia," *Archives of General Psychiatry*, 3 (1967), 361–364.
46. Luby, E. D., Cohen, B. D., Rosenbaum, G. Gottlieb, J. S., and Kelley, R. "Study of a New Schizophrenomimetic Drug—Sernyl," *Archives of Neurology and Psychiatry*, 81 (1959), 363–369.
47. Luby, E. D., Frohman, C. E., Grisell, J. L., Lenzo, J. E., and Gottlieb, J. S. "Sleep

Deprivation: Effects on Behavior, Thinking, Motor Performance and Biological Energy Transfer Systems," *Psychosomatic Medicine*, **22** (1960), 182–192.
48. Luby, E. D., Gottlieb, J. S., Cohen, B. D., Rosenbaum, G., and Domino, E. F. "Model Psychoses and Schizophrenia," *American Journal of Psychiatry*, **119** (1962), 61–67.
49. Lucero, R. J., and Meyer, B. T. "A Behavior Scale Suitable for Use in Mental Hospitals," *Journal of Clinical Psychology*, **7** (1951), 250–254.
50. Mishler, E. G., and Waxler, N. "Family Interaction Processes and Schizophrenia: A Review of Current Theories," *International Journal of Psychiatry*, **2** (1966), 375–413.
51. Osmond, H., and Smythies, J. "Schizophrenia, A New Approach," *Journal of Mental Science*, **98** (1952), 309–315.
52. Pennell, R. B., Saravis, C. A., and Bergen, J. R. "Some Properties of a Human Plasma Protein Which Influences the Behavior of Trained Rats," in R. G. Heath (ed.), *Serologic Fractions in Schizophrenia*. New York: Hoeber, 1963. Pp. 23–32.
53. Pollin, W., Cardon, P. V., and Kety, S. S. "Effects of Amino Acid Feedings in Schizophrenic Patients Treated with Iproniazid," *Science*, **133** (1961), 104.
54. Pollin, W. Stabenau, J. R., and Tupin, J. "Family Studies with Identical Twins Discordant for Schizophrenia," *Psychiatry*, **28** (1965), 60–78.
55. Rodin, E. A. "Electroencephalographic Studies in Schizophrenic Patients," in J. S. Gottlieb and G. Tourney (eds.), *Lafayette Clinic Studies in Schizophrenia*, Lafayette Clinic Monograph No. 4. Detroit: Wayne State University Press, 1970.
56. Rosenbaum, G. "Feedback Mechanisms," in J. S. Gottlieb and G. Tourney (eds.), *Lafayette Clinic Studies in Schizophrenia*, Lafayette Clinic Monograph No. 4. Detroit: Wayne State University Press, 1970.
57. Rosenbaum, G., Flenning, F., and Rosen, H. "Effects of Weight Intensity on Discrimination Thresholds of Normals and Schizophrenics," *Journal of Abnormal Psychology*, **70** (1965), 446–450.
58. Ryan, J. W., Brown, J. D., and Durell, J. "Antibodies Affecting Metabolism of Chicken Erythrocytes: Examination of Schizophrenic and Other Subjects," *Science*, **151** (1966), 1408–1410.
59. Slater, E., and Beard, A. W. "The Schizophrenia-Like Psychoses of Epilepsy," *British Journal of Psychiatry*, **109** (1963), 95–150.
60. Smythies, J. "The Essential Hallucinogenic Molecule," in M. Vartanian (ed.), *Biological Research in Schizophrenia*. Moscow: Ordina Lennia, 1967. Pp. 215–217.
61. Sullivan, T. M., Frohman, C. E., Beckett, P. G. S., and Gottlieb, J. S. "Clinical and Biochemical Studies of Families of Schizophrenic Patients," *American Journal of Psychiatry*, **123** (1967), 947–952.
62. Turner, W. J., and Chipps, H. I. "A Heterophil Hemolysin in Human Blood: I. Distribution in Schizophrenics and Nonschizophrenics," *Archives of General Psychiatry*, **15** (1966), 373–377.
63. Usnov, G., Iordanov, B., and Doseva, I. "Cellular Membrane Permeability in Schizophrenia," in M. Vartanian (ed.), *Biological Research in Schizophrenia*. Moscow: Ordina Lennia, 1967. Pp. 163–168.
64. Vartanian, M. E. "Populational and Biological Aspects of Genetics in Schizophrenia," in M. Vartanian (ed.), *Biological Research in Schizophrenia*. Moscow: Ordina Lennia, 1967. Pp. 249–251.
65. Woolley, D. W., and Shaw, E. "A Biochemical and Pharmacological Suggestion about Certain Mental Disorders," *Science*, **119** (1954), 587–588.

[[[23]]]

PSYCHOPHYSIOLOGICAL AND RELATED APPROACHES TO PSYCHOPATHOLOGY

Heinz E. Lehmann

Psychopathology can be viewed in three different perspectives: the dynamic, the behavioral, and the functional. In the dynamic perspective, we are moving in the psychological dimension and applying theoretical methods to assess pathological conditions. In the behavioral perspective, we are moving in the social dimension and applying descriptive (phenomenological) methods for evaluation. In the functional perspective—the subject of this chapter—we are moving on a biologically oriented level, and the methodology is experimental.

To illustrate these three different perspectives, consider the example of a woman in a state of retarded depression. From the dynamic point of view, the woman may be seen as suffering from the introjection of an ambivalent libidinal object, such as her mother. From the behavioral point of view, she is depressed, retarded, and suicidal. On the functional level, this patient would show slowed reaction time, impaired learning capacity, reduced REM and stage 4 sleep, and, probably, disturbed autonomic reactions to an unconditional stimulus.

Criteria and indicators of psychopathology range widely—according to the methodologies involved—from the most objective neurophysiological (for example, evoked cortical potentials) to the completely subjective clinical (for example, empathy or the typical unstructured interview). In between there are what might be called "quasiobjective" measures, such as psychomotor, perceptual, and cognitive tests.[68]

AROUSAL

A conceptual link between various biological-functional categories and methodologies is provided by the arousal concept. Introduced by Duffy in 1934,[29] it offered a useful model for the organization of different experiential and behavioral phenomena and was later qualified and extended by Malmo,[77] who referred to it as activation. The well-known relationship between psychological arousal and behavioral performance can be graphically expressed in an inverted U-fashion. If, for instance, a drug or procedure that regularly increased arousal was applied to an individual whose basic level of arousal was known to be below the level of optimum performance, his performance could be expected to improve. But if his basic level of arousal was already beyond optimum performance, a further increase of arousal would deteriorate performance. The opposite would apply to any drug or procedure that would reduce the preexisting state of arousal.

Level of arousal can be measured objectively in at least four different ways: (1) by an electroencephalogram (EEG), which is characterized in states of high arousal by low voltage and fast, desynchronized electrical activity of the brain and in states of low arousal by increased synchronization and slowed rhythms with either low or high amplitudes; (2) by palmar galvanic skin resistance (GSR), which is inversely related to the subject's state of arousal; (3) by a subject's vigilance, measured, for instance, by his capacity to detect signals over a given period of time—the greater his vigilance, the higher his state of arousal; (4) by a subject's overt behavior—the greater his spontaneous and responsive activity, the higher his level of arousal.

It is difficult to find predictable concordance among the electrocerebral (EEG), the autonomic (GSR), the vigilance (response to stimuli), and the behavioral (motor activity) aspects of arousal. The work on rapid eye movement (REM) sleep, for instance, during the last decade has clearly brought out the fact that EEG patterns during REM sleep phases reflect a state of considerable cerebral arousal, whereas awareness, vigilance, muscle tone, and motor activity are markedly decreased.

Lacey[59] has shown that instead of cardiac acceleration in response to high arousal input, which would be expected if increased arousal were regularly associated with increased sympathomimetic tone, cardiac deceleration occurs in individuals with high cortical reactivity. This cardiac response seems to function as part of a visceral feedback system between the cerebral cortex and the cardiovascular system. Silverman[107] suggests that cardiovascular mechanisms may assume inhibitory control over thought centers of the brain and, at the same time, facilitate responsiveness to sensory stimuli, whenever stressful conditions tend to produce excessive arousal.

The majority of recent studies has revealed higher autonomic arousal in chronic schizophrenics than in normal subjects. This is a reversal of the views expressed in the literature until 1950, which almost unanimously held that chronic schizophrenics were not only behaviorally but also physiologically hyporeactive.[52]

Malmo et al.[78, 79, 80] were among the first to find higher baseline levels of electromyographic responses, heart rate, and diastolic blood pressure in chronic schizophrenics than in controls and to observe that these patients responded as much or more than the controls to experimental stress conditions. Ax,[5] reporting on recent experiments with chronic schizophrenics, has regularly found higher average base levels of palmar skin conductane (that is, lower GSR), suggesting a high level of activation. Consistently higher indices of arousal in chronic as well as acute schizophrenics, even under conditions of minimal stimulation, were also observed by Zahn.[135] In his experiments, the differences have been most pronounced in the frequency of nonspecific GSR, that is, in those changes of electrical skin resistance that occur as apparently spontaneous fluctuations. Studying these relationships, Venables and Wing[126] have found a strong positive correlation between the degree of arousal increase and the intensity of withdrawal in chronic schizophrenic patients.

Claridge[22] concludes that "the psychotic—whether acute or chronic—is not just simply either under- or over-aroused." In his formulation, a psychosis involves not only a quantitative alteration in arousal, but also a dissociation among the several components of arousal—neurophysiological, psychophysiological, psychological, and behavioral—involved in integrated central nervous activity.

Lacey[59] has recently reemphasized what he, Darrow et al.,[26] Sternbach,[113] Lazarus,[63] and others have pointed out earlier, namely, that different physiological indicators of activation or arousal do not correlate well with one another or with psychological or behavioral indicators. Taking this into account, Ax[5] points out that activation or arousal has become such a global concept that, in the light of recent experimental findings, it no longer fits the facts accurately. Nevertheless, the arousal concept still provides a useful background model for cerebrocortical processes, autonomic functions, and behavioral stimulus response contingencies. It must be clearly understood, however, that there exist few, if any, one-to-one relationships between different arousal phenomena. The arousal concept—in various forms and with many qualifications—serves better as an explanatory model or heuristic construct than as a predictive device.

NEUROPHYSIOLOGICAL PROCEDURES

Electrophysiological gauges of cerebral activity rank highest on the hierarchy of objectivity in measuring psychopathology. Their contribution to the understanding of pathogenetic mechanisms has been appreciated only in the last ten or fifteen years. Today, much lively research is carried on in at least three different aspects of electrophysiology of the central nervous system: (1) a more sophisticated evaluation of the EEG in the waking state; (2) the study of REM sleep cycles; (3) the systematic evaluation of evoked potentials.

EEG

Although the EEG does not provide a powerful means of distinguishing among various diagnostic entities in psychiatry, certain trends have been established over the years.[133] First, tension states are usually characterized by low voltage, rapid activity, and reduced alpha activity. Another frequently observed feature is the maturation defect found in the EEG patterns of many patients with personality disorders, particularly of the aggressive psychopath type. More particularly, the positive spike phenomena occurring either in bursts of slow (6 to 8 per second) or fast (14 to 16 per second) rhythms and usually appearing from both posterior temporal areas are often correlated with autonomic dysfunction, behavior disorders, and sometimes convulsive attacks. The third major EEG disorder of diagnostic significance in psychiatry is found in states of impaired consciousness and dementia occurring in organic brain disease, a condition characterized by diffuse or focal slow-wave activity as well as amplitude asymmetries and random spiking.

EEG findings of major functional psychoses, for example, schizophrenia and manic-depressive disorder, are often within the normal range, and, when they are abnormal, the pattern disturbances are not consistent or specific.

Goldman[42] has studied EEG changes in schizophrenic patients after the intravenous administration of thiopenthal and has observed bilateral, synchronic, fast and slow (theta) activity. This pattern tended to become less pronounced with improvement of the patient's condition, for instance, after treatment with antipsychotic drugs, but would appear again during a relapse.

Goldstein, Murphree, Sugerman, Pfeiffer, and Jenney[44] employed an electronic integrator to measure the coefficient of variation of the electrical energy content of the EEG and established that the EEG of schizophrenic patients is characterized by an abnormally low variability of its energy content. This feature is significantly correlated with the symptoms of retardation and apathy, motor disturbances, and conceptual disorganization. When schizophrenic patients improve symptomatically in these behavior areas, their variability coefficient increases. The authors point out that this is "perhaps the only measure on which schizophrenics show less variability than normals."

Fink[35] foresees the identification of electrophysiologically homogeneous populations based on drug-induced EEG responses that have been analyzed by means of digital computer techniques. He feels that such a system would provide a better basis for the study of the biological substrate of behavior disturbances than the present classification that relies on gross phenotypic behavior distinctions, that is, on clinical symptomatology.

REM

The discovery that periods of rapid eye movement, fast EEG rhythms, and muscular hypotonia occur in cyclic phases during normal sleep opened a new and exciting field of neurophysiological research.[2] The importance of this phenomenon for psychiatric research was strongly suggested by the fact that 80 to 90 per cent of the subjects awakened during the phases of REM would recall vivid dreams, whereas only 5 to 10 per cent of the subjects awakened during non-REM periods of sleep would report dreams.

The distinct association between REM sleep and dreaming has inspired interesting speculations. When Dement[27] observed that experimental deprivation of REM sleep produced deleterious psychological effects on the deprived subjects, several investigators hypothesized that REM pressure that had for some reason accumulated beyond a threshold limit might erupt into waking life and produce the "waking dream" of schizophrenia.[36, 109] However, in a recent critical review of all the findings, Vogel[127] concludes that there is little or no evidence that REM sleep intrusion into wakefulness provides a valid model of schizophrenia.

Because several sedative and stimulant drugs—for example, the barbiturates, phenothiazines, thioxanthenes, amphetamines,[69] and also alcohol—reduce the incidence of REM sleep, Gross et al.[46] suggested that a rebound of accumulated REM pressure might be responsible for hallucinatory psychotic states following the withdrawal of alcohol. Vogel concludes that the evidence for this hypothesis is inconclusive and is more likely negative. He points out, however, that there is laboratory evidence for the connection between an abnormal sleep cycle with a state of serious depression. Depressed patients have less REM sleep, less deep non-REM (stage 4) sleep, and also significantly less total sleep than nondepressed controls.[45, 84, 85]

Jouvet,[55] in a series of systematic experiments, studied the REM sleep cycles of cats and proposed recently that some or all aspects of REM sleep may be based on the effects of catecholamines—norepinephrine and dopamine—on the brain.

Four common sleep disorders—enuresis, somnambulism, pavor nocturnus, and nightmares—have recently been discussed by Broughton.[14] After reviewing the evidence in the work of other investigators and from his own experiments, he concludes that these classical sleep disorders are virtually never associated with the REM cycles (dreaming sleep), but occur during arousal from deep non-REM slow-wave sleep. (In view of the foregoing discussion of the changing definition of the arousal concept, it is interesting to note that Broughton questions whether the term arousal should suitably be applied to awakenings from REM sleep, because then, in contrast to awakening from non-REM sleep, the brain simply shifts from one complex pattern of intense activity to another, and on awakening some cerebral functions might even become less active than they were during REM sleep.)

Evoked Potentials

The measurement of averaged evoked potentials (AEP) in the cerebral cortex, which are recorded through scalp electrodes with electroencephalographic apparatus, has emerged as one of the most promising new psychiatric tools during the past decade. The stimuli evoking the potentials are sometimes somatosensory in nature, for example, electrical stimulation of a peripheral nerve,[100] or they might be visual[37, 111] or auditory stimuli.[18] Because the stimulus-induced changes superimposed on the basal EEG are of very small amplitude, a large number of them must be averaged by electronic (or photographic) means in order to raise them above the noise level of the ordinary EEG. It has been established that the characteristics of evoked responses change with age.[30, 101] Amplitudes tend to be higher, both in early and late life. Latencies are more prolonged in older subjects. Women tend to have higher amplitude evoked responses and recover more rapidly from the refractory period.

When two or more stimuli are given in rapid succession, the recovery function between the first and the subsequent responses differs in psychiatric patients when compared to normal controls. Shagass and Schwartz[99] demonstrated that the initial phase of recovery occurring during the first twenty milliseconds was delayed in patients with functional psychoses or personality disorders, whereas psychoneurotics or patients suffering from depression or psychosomatic disorders did not differ significantly from normal controls. However, when psychiatric patients were matched for age and sex with the control subjects, the specificity of the evoked responses related to diagnostic differences disappeared, but the patient group as a whole still showed a deficiency in the recovery process of the AEP.[98]

Callaway[17, 18]—through the use of evoked potentials provoked by auditory stimuli—showed that schizophrenic patients responded persistently to trivial differences in the pitch of two tones. Normals, when so instructed, quickly disregarded these differences and then produced very similar evoked potentials, but schizophrenics could not "avoid wasting psychological energy in attending to the physical difference between the tones." As a result, the evoked potentials to the two tones in schizophrenics were dissimilar and of a persistently low correlation.

At the same time, it appeared that clinical signs and symptoms may be related to these evoked response findings. For instance, patients with low two-tone AEP correlations tend to think in a more shifting, abstract fashion—indicating a high tolerance for incongruity of concepts. High correlations are found in paranoids with well-organized delusional systems, and low correlations are found in patients with poorly organized delusions. Callaway also found that low-correlation patients appeared to respond better to phenothiazines than those with high correlations.

Sutton, Braven, and Zubin[115, 116] observed that there are various components of the evoked potential that reflect the subject's attitudes and expectations about the nature of the stimulus. This becomes evident when two different stimulus modalities are used and the subject will attempt to predict which stimulus will come next. As an example, the amplitude of the 300 ms latency component is increased when the subject feels less certain which of the two stimuli will be used. Sutton and his team, in fact, have demonstrated four components of the evoked response related to the nature of the stimulus, the nature of the prediction, the accuracy of the prediction, and the appreciation of having been right.

Walter et al.[128] have described a slow cortical wave of negative potential that reflects a subject's awareness or expectancy of the contingency between two stimuli. Walter calls this potential the "contingent negative variation." If a subject, for example, is exposed to certain auditory signals that are invariably followed by a flash of light, the contingent negative variation will appear as soon as the auditory "warning" signal has been given. This contingent variation is distinguished in very anxious patients by low amplitude and extreme sensitivity to distraction, in obsessive-compulsive patients by high amplitude and long persistence of the wave, in schizophrenics by low amplitude, high sensitivity to distraction, and high variability. In psychopathic individuals, the contingent negative variation is absent.[129]

Chalke and Ertl[20] have investigated the possible use of the cortical evoked potential as an objective measure of intelligence. Because the latency of the evoked potential is a measure of the speed of central processing, it might be expected that intellectual processes are related to it. Although this work is still in its early stages, it seems to provide promising leads.

Though Shagass'[98] experiments have shown that the initial recovery phases of evoked potentials that seem to measure cerebral excitability "generally yield statistical differences between psychiatrically ill people and healthy ones," Callaway[17] feels that the greatest promise for clinical applications of the evoked potentials seems to be held by the long latency evoked responses "that may reflect such things as interest, expectation, the deployment of attention, and the assignment of meaning."

Implanted Electrodes

It is not likely that recordings from electrodes implanted in the human brain will ever become widely used diagnostic tools, but since the technique was first introduced more than a decade ago,[50, 94] several investigators have reported interesting results. Their subjects were mainly neurosurgical patients treated for psychosis, epilepsy, or intractable pain, and the phenomena studied were the depth electroencephalogram, depth-evoked responses, and behavior modifications resulting from electrical stimulation through implanted electrodes.[50, 76, 104] A recent observation reported by Ervin and Mark[32] is particularly intriguing: stimulation of the amygdala produces changes in mood and behavior that last much longer than the actual stimulation or its neurophysiological correlates. This suggests that neurophysiological events in the limbic system induce the release of neurochemical or neurohormonal substrates of human experience and behavior.

PSYCHOPHYSIOLOGY

Psychophysiology has been defined by Darrow[25] as "the science which concerns those physiological activities which underlie or relate to psychic functions." It is not possible sharply to demarcate neurophysiology and psychophysiology. However, there is at least one rule-of-thumb criterion: neurophysiological responses occur within a fraction of a second after the stimulus, giving emotional or other psychological factors little or no opportunity to modify the response. A second, perhaps more relevant, criterion is the requirement for the neurophysiological response to be registered directly at the level of the central nervous system rather than at peripheral target organs. Psychophysiological responses, on the other hand, are usually recorded from peripheral organs that are under autonomic control, and the interval between stimulus and response is ten to one hundred times greater than with neurophysiological responses.

Pupillography

Hakerem and Lidsky[47] showed that a sequence of light stimuli separated by variable dark periods induced a cyclic "following response" of the pupil, reflecting the information put into the retina by a train of contractile and dilatory reactions. With psychotic patients this following response, based on short-time storage of information delivered to the retina, was definitely deficient in comparison to most of the controls. Even more striking was the observation that 86 per cent of a psychotic patient sample showed a pupil contraction to light of $\leqq 1.70$ mm or less, whereas more than 80 per cent of the normals responded with a contraction >1.70 mm.

Differential Responsivity and Habituation

Several attempts have been made in recent years to distinguish schizophrenic patients who fall into two groups characterized by different autonomic responses.[41, 59, 75] Venables[122] distinguishes between schizophrenics of high and low arousal; Mednick,[82] between schizophrenics with high and low anxiety. Other studies have compared process schizophrenics vs. reactive schizophrenics. Still others use the traditional distinction of acute vs. chronic patients or differentiate between patients with a good or a poor premorbid history. For example, in response to stimuli (a loud bell or pictures depicting conflict-laden situations), process schizophrenic patients showed decreases in heart rate in contrast to reactive patients or normal controls.[28] Patients with better premorbid histories were observed to have higher resting skin potential levels than those with poorer histories.[24]

Comparing the habituation to stimuli of normals with that of schizophrenics, Zahn[135] observed that habituation of the GSR—that is, gradual disappearance of responses to stimuli—in a group of schizophrenic patients was slower than in normals. Zahn proposes that the relative difference in autonomic responsivity between schizophrenics and normals depends on the meaningfulness or demandingness of the stimulus, and he hypothesizes that schizophrenics show stronger autonomic responses to weak or irrelevant stimuli than to strong or more meaningful stimuli.

Lader[60] found significant correlations between the measures of arousal and habituation (as determined by GSR) and ratings of symptomatic improvement of neurotic patients. He was able to show that normal subjects and patients suffering from specific phobias had the highest habituation rate with agoraphobics, social phobics, patients in anxiety states, patients with anxiety and depression, and hysterical patients showing diminishing habituation, in this order. He also found that patients with frequent (nonspecific) GSR fluctuations and slow GSR habituation responded best to anxiolytic sedatives.

It should be noted here that, in spite of its many methodological and technical shortcomings, the galvanic skin resistance phenomenon has held the interest of physiologists and psychologists since it was first discovered by Féré and explained by D'Arsonval in 1888 as resulting from sweat gland activity. GSR is still the most easily recorded, continuous physical measure, which is highly correlated with different states of emotional response, autonomic arousal, or cerebral activation, whatever function one investigates—or whatever term one prefers.

Predictors

Mednick and Schulsinger,[83] in the course of a well-planned predictor study of schizophrenia conducted with a group of children known to be "at risk" because they had schizophrenic mothers, found that the subjects who broke down later had been characterized previously by more labile GSR functioning, for example, shorter latency and quicker recovery. Their GSR responses did not habituate (adapt) as well as those of the control subjects with repeated stimulation. If anything, those who broke down later manifested increasing irritability under repeated stress.

Salivary Secretion

Several investigators have demonstrated that reliable and consistent relationships prevail between salivary gland secretion and the mood changes of depressed patients. The greater the depression, the more reduced the salivary secretion.[16, 87, 90]

Sedation Threshold

Shagass and his coworkers[96] have developed the "sedation threshold" technique, which consists in the intravenous injection of a barbiturate until a certain EEG or behavioral endpoint is reached. The investigators found that sedation thresholds of a large group of psychoneurotic patients were significantly higher than those of controls. The sedation threshold seemed to correlate highly with anxious tension and allowed these workers to differentiate between neurotic and psychotic depressions.[97]

Plethysmography

The forearm rate of blood flow has been measured by plethysmography as a measure of anxiety.[56, 121] The investigators could demonstrate statistically significant differences of the forearm blood flow between groups of psychiatric patients with varying diagnoses.

CONDITIONING

In recent years the study of the conditioned response (CR) has assumed an increasingly important role as an experimental approach to psychopathology. Conditioning of the first signal system (as a response to external stimuli that are not of a verbal or symbolic nature) and of the second signal system (as a response to verbal or symbolic stimuli) or a combination and interaction of first and second signal systems all constitute paradigms of learning. Conditioning, therefore, links physiological with psychological mechanisms.

An interesting application of conditioning principles to a theory of pathogenesis of schizophrenia has been proposed by Mednick.[82] He assumes that acutely disturbed schizophrenics are highly anxious and that this anxiety—because of increased generalization and decreased discrimination potential—is induced by a wide range of everyday stimuli. The high-drive level resulting from the anxiety raises many responses, which normally would remain below the response threshold, to the point where they will become manifest. Such responses, often of an improbable and irrelevant nature, do not evoke further anxiety as more usual and relevant responses—for example, rational thoughts and actions—would evoke. Because irrelevant responses do not evoke anxiety, they are reinforced and persist, thus accounting for the strange and often absurd behavior and speech of the schizophrenic whose affect seems shallow and who does not experience overt anxiety.

Differential Diagnostic Variations

In neurotic patients with a high level of anxiety, deficient habituation to an indifferent stimulus, that is, a persistent orienting response (OR), has been observed. Neurotic patients also exhibited difficulty in extinguishing CR's and in discriminating between conditional stimuli (CS). In chronic neurotics, "protective inhibition" was often observed, that is, falling asleep under monotonous or stressful experimental conditions.[6]

Martin[81] found differential development of conditioned eyelid responses among different neurotic patients—those with animal phobias gave the highest number of CR's, social phobias, lower, and agoraphobias the lowest mean score.

It has been found that acute schizophrenics—like neurotics—do not habituate readily on the GSR to indifferent stimuli. But chronic schizophrenics often do not respond at all, that is, they show an absence of the orienting response.[3]

Ax[5] found greatly reduced mean CR's in a group of chronic schizophrenics. The statistical difference between the pathological and control groups was significant at the level of $p \geqslant .001$. He thinks that the conditioning superiority of the controls is at least partly due to significantly greater discrimination demonstrated by the control group.

In patients suffering from manic-depressive disorder, a persistent orienting response was found in manic states, whereas in depressive states the orienting response was often absent or quickly extinguished. CR formation was impaired in depressives but facilitated in manics. CS discrimination, however, was impaired in both phases.[91, 92, 119]

In organic brain disease, as in depression, the orienting response is usually absent or rapidly extinguished, and CR formation as well as CS discrimination is impaired.[6, 39]

Facilitation of Conditioning

Spence[112] and Taylor[117] demonstrated that moderate anxiety may facilitate conditioning in experimental situations. Beam[10] found that conditioning (GSR) was facilitated in real-life stress situations, for example, university examinations and stage appearances on opening nights. Welch and Kubis[131] had already shown a faster rate of conditioning and a slower rate of extinction in studies of patients who were hospitalized for anxiety.

In Mednick's previously mentioned group of children with schizophrenic mothers, those subjects who broke down psychiatrically showed more conditionability than the control groups.[83] In addition, the sick group was characterized by a tendency to higher generalization than the normal control groups.

Protective Inhibition

According to Pavlovian theory, schizophrenics are suffering from excessive "protective inhibition"—a factor that most Russian authors assume to be hereditary in nature.[4, 6, 75] This factor is thought to account for the schizophrenic's general slowness and poor conditionability. But Ax[5] proposes, as a more parsimonious concept, simply a deficit in conditionability—possibly owing to heredity or an acquired brain defect. It might also be the result of psychosomatic malfunctioning or the result of learned habit patterns.

PSYCHOPHYSICAL AND PERCEPTUAL PROCEDURES

In a recent view of perceptual performance in various schizophrenic subgroups, Silverman[107] stresses the importance of stimulus intensity control (*Reizschutz*), scanning control, and sensory input processing—ideational gating. He concludes that schizophrenics who are oversensitive to low-intensity stimulation—mainly nonparanoid, long-term schizophrenics—also show a marked disposition to reduce the intensity of strong stimuli. They appear, therefore, hypersensitive to minimal and hyposensitive to maximal stimulation. Those schizophrenics who are not hypersensitive to minimal stimulation—mainly paranoid, acute schizophrenics with good premorbid histories—are also not hyposensitive to high-intensity stimulation.

The critical flicker fusion frequency (CFF) test measures a subject's capacity to discriminate different visual stimuli on a temporal continuum by determining at which rate of flicker an intermittent light stimulus appears to become steady. This measure has been shown to be sensitive to fatigue, cerebral metabolism, age, drug effects, and differences in psychiatric diagnosis.[61, 72, 86]

Lehmann[65] has found increased CFF in acute schizophrenics and suggests that this increase is a manifestation of heightened susceptibility to perceptual bombardment because the schizophrenic cannot integrate such excess input of information. The resulting cognitive and behavioral decompensation produces anxiety, disorganization, and withdrawal. On the other hand, in chronic schizophrenics, Johannsen, Friedman, and Liccione[54] found a lowered CFF threshold. A decreased CFF is also a reliable indicator of reduced cerebral competence owing either to organic brain disease or to reversible effects of sedative and neuroleptic drugs, fatigue, or other noxious factors.[12]

Size constancy of visual objects has been the subject of many investigations. Children, for instance, because of insufficiently developed size-constancy functions, tend to judge distant objects to be smaller and close objects to be larger than they really are. Normal adults overcompensate for this and usually underestimate the size of near objects and overestimate the size of distant ones. Paranoid schizophrenics overestimate the size of distant objects even more than do normal adults. But simple or hebephrenic schizophrenics display underconstancy and base their size judgment, like children, mainly on the actual size of the retinal image.[89, 130] Underestimation of the size of objects in schizophrenics with good premorbid histories was observed by Harris.[48]

In paranoid schizophrenics there is a strong disposition to perceptual closure; in nonparanoid schizophrenics, a weak disposition.[109]

Fragmentation of visual perception in schizophrenics has been described by Arieti,[1] who noted that such patients were regressing to the phylogenetically and ontogenetically more primitive mode of part perception[51] and appeared to be incapable of organizing the parts of a percept into its appropriate whole. Bemporad[11] demonstrated this perceptual disorder by testing acute, chronic, and recovered schizophrenics and a nonschizophrenic control group with stimulus cards that could be perceived as dots or numerals. The acute schizophrenics showed almost complete fragmentation of perception (saw mostly dots), whereas chronic and recovered schizophrenics organized more percepts into wholes (saw more numerals). Nonschizophrenics perceived most wholes.

Studying autokinetic movement, Sexton[95] found high-movement (minimal scanning) responses in nonparanoid patients, whereas paranoid schizophrenics showed mainly low or no-movement responses.

Venables[123] has shown that the thresholds to light flashes and auditory clicks indicate that chronic schizophrenics are more defective in the auditory than in the visual sphere. He has recently[124] stressed the importance of experiments in which more than one stimulus is given in order to reduce the distorting influence of cultural factors, and he feels that the deficit in schizophrenia consists in an abnormally slow rate at which information in the primary channel is processed.

Silverman, Berg, and Kantor[108] observed impairment in the performance on the Titchener Illusion and the Pettigrew Category Width Test in schizophrenics, but almost identical impairment in nonpsychiatric prisoners who were equated for length of institutionalization. This finding underlines the crucial importance of considering the fact of institutionalization if one compares test performances of hospitalized patients with those of controls.

PSYCHOMOTOR PROCEDURES

King[58] points out that psychomotor function is "more complex than that of basic neuromotor integrity as the term might be used by the neurologists, yet simpler than what is called perceptuomotor by the developmental or clinical psychologist." King is convinced that psychomotor measures behave much like biological measures and are largely independent of notable social, racial, and intellectual influences.

Because many psychomotor tasks are normally performed at close to optimal speed, physical or psychological impairment will easily produce downward changes in the measured psychomotor speed, but will rarely increase speed.

A tremendous number of psychomotor measures have been used to evaluate psychiatric disorders. It is, of course, beyond the scope of this chapter to review even a significant fraction of them. However, the most frequently studied psychomotor tests are simple reaction time and tapping speed.

Working with normal volunteer subjects exposed to the action of various psychotropic drugs, Lehmann and Prescott[73] observed a negative correlation between simple auditory reaction time and latency of the GSR response. The observation was surprising because short latency and short reaction time are both considered criteria of increased arousal. This is another illustration of the fact that parameters of arousal taken from different organismic dimensions—in this case the autonomic and the behavioral—do not always lead in the same direction.

Sleep deprivation,[132] various drugs including alcohol,[33, 53] extreme cold,[118] oxygen deprivation,[120] and starvation[15] have all been shown to reduce the speed of simple psychomotor activity.

Across the field of psychopathology there is a gradient of psychomotor speed impairment most marked in the organic brain syndrome patients, less marked in the schizophrenics, still less in the manic-depressives, and least marked in the neurotics.[103]

In manic-depressive patients, slowed psychomotor responses are found in the manic as well as the depressed states, although the slowing is more marked and more consistently present in depressed patients.

Experimentally induced anxiety as well as nonexperimental anxiety, as determined by questionnaires, impairs the speed of performing several psychomotor tests.

Psychoneurotic patients do not differ much from normal controls in the speed of performing simple psychomotor tasks under ordinary conditions.[57] But their performance becomes significantly worse than that of control subjects under physiological or psychological pressure.[80]

Psychomotor slowness is thus a general factor in psychiatric patients and not clearly related to any specific diagnosis. Harris and Metcalfe[49] observed extreme slowness occurring in patients who show flattened and incongruous affect and, independently, in patients whom psychiatrists judged to have a poor prognosis.

Zahn,[135] as many investigators before him, found that most schizophrenics showed a slow reaction time. Patients diagnosed as suffering from pseudoneurotic schizophrenia show a consistent slowing on tests of tapping speed, reaction time, and finger dexterity.[58]

Venables and O'Connor[125] examined the relative speed of reaction time to auditory and visual stimuli. They found that in the most severely ill psychotic patients there was a greater slowing of auditory reaction time than of visual reaction time.

Shakow[102] discovered the now well-known "set index" disturbance from which he derived his general concept of a "segmental set" in schizophrenic patients: if normal subjects are given a warning signal prior to the stimulus to which they are instructed to react, their reaction time is shortened. If schizophrenics are given such a warning signal, they will be able to benefit from it for a shortening of their reaction time only if the interval between warning signal and stimulus does not exceed four seconds. Normals, on the other hand, are able to maintain a ready set for much longer periods of time.

When light and sound stimuli are presented in random sequence and the subject is instructed to react to either stimulus, his reaction time is affected by the sensory modality of the stimulus to which he was exposed in the preceding trial. If the sensory modality of the preceding trial was the same as in the actual trial, his reaction time is shorter than when the preceding stimulus was of another modality. The lengthening of reaction time when the modality is shifted occurs in normal and schizophrenic subjects but is considerably greater for schizophrenics. Sutton and Zubin[116] conclude from these findings that schizophrenics more than normals are at the mercy of immediately preceding stimuli.

Zahn[135] infers that high arousal, as determined by electrodermal and finger-pulse volume responses, facilitates reaction time responses for normals but inhibits them for schizophrenics.

Tapping speed is another simple, sensitive, and commonly used measure of psychomotor changes brought about by psychopathology, drug action, or other intervening factors. Wulfeck[134] found no differences in tapping speed between normals, neurotics, depressives, and schizophrenics. But most other investigators since then have found tapping speed to be slowed in depression and in many other psychiatric conditions.[13, 38, 57] A recent review of psychomotor deficits in schizophrenia can be found in an article by Lang and Buss.[62]

COGNITIVE PROCEDURES

The area of cognitive tests, among all the test categories described, employs the least instrumentation and often requires the most clinical judgment. Such tests may be aimed at evaluation of sustained attention (for example, the time-honored Bourdon Cancellation Test), at time estimation, at the coping with perceptually conflicting stimuli (for example, the Stroop Color-Word Interference Test), at short-term and long-term memory, at word association time, the learning of nonsense syllables, or a host of other often very ingeniously conceived measures. Though perceptual tests deal primarily with the mechanisms of information input, and psychomotor tests deal primarily with output of behavior, cognitive tests and also, to a considerable extent, special procedures involving neurophysiological and psychological learning (such as conditioning) probe the mechanisms of central processing of information and experience.

The schizophrenic's response to learned punishments and rewards is expressed by Garmezy[40] as follows. A normal individual, if punished, will frequently become more variable in his behavior; by contrast, the schizophrenic responds to punishment typically by becoming more stereotyped, less flexible, and, therefore, less able to cope appropriately with problems. On the other hand, learned rewards for normals tend to increase response stability, therefore leading to improved performance in learning situations. The schizophrenic is again different in that his response to rewards remains equivocal, and apparently the rewards fail to increase motivation.

The clinically recognized tendency of schizophrenics to think and speak in pathologically concrete terms has been interpreted by Goldstein,[43] who did much fundamental work on the disorders of abstract thinking as a protective mechanism, in some way akin to the schizophrenics' behavioral withdrawal. Feffer,[34] agreeing with Goldstein's position, states that "pathologically concrete thinking in schizophrenia represents an avoidant reaction to affective stimuli." Such an interpretation is, of course, along the same lines as Mednick's previously mentioned theory that the schizophrenic's bizarreness is a defense against the anxiety-provoking nature of more relevant responses to stimuli. In Mednick's predictor study of high-risk children of schizophrenic mothers, one of the significant differences between the subjects who broke down and those who did not was a marked tendency for the sick group to drift away from the stimulus word in association experiments.

The typical thought disorders of the schizophrenic, which are characterized by autistic thinking, overly concrete as well as overly abstract thinking, overinclusiveness, irrelevancy, incoherence, and loose associations, and the influence of drugs on the learning and memory disorders of schizophrenic and organic patients have been studied experimentally by many investigators.[9, 19, 21, 23, 31, 64, 74, 88, 89, 93] The classical clinical findings of flight of ideas in the manic patient and of general inhibition of intellectual processes in the depressed patient can be easily demonstrated experimentally, although they have received less attention by investigators than the perhaps more interesting thought disorders of the schizophrenic.

Silverman,[107] after discussing perceptual and psychophysiological phenomena in different types of schizophrenia, concludes that certain cognitive styles of schizophrenics serve defense and adaptation purposes that may explain some of the often observed, apparently paradoxical combinations of physiological overarousal and behavioral hyporesponsivity in schizophrenics. On the basis of experimental findings, he concluded that chronic nonparanoid schizophrenics with a poor premorbid history attend more than is normal to sensory attributes of perceptual inputs, though attending less to the meaning of the stimuli, particularly if they cannote something unpleasant or threatening.

MULTILEVEL EXPERIMENTAL APPROACHES

A Geriatric Predictor Study

At the Douglas Hospital in Montreal, a research project with geriatric patients, conducted by me in collaboration with Dr. T. Ban, has been underway for some years. Its aim is to develop methods for predicting individual therapeutic responsiveness to pharmacotherapy. In the first phase of the project, we attempted to classify geriatric patients into homogeneous groups and to predict their therapeutic responses to specific psychoactive drugs on the basis of their response profiles to a battery of psychometric tests and their immediate responses to a pharmacological load.

We also studied control groups of nonhospitalized young and aged subjects and some aged subjects living in institutions other than hospitals. In the second phase, we tested the validity of our predictions made on the basis of our first-phase findings by observing the therapeutic long-term responses of the patients to a variety of psychoactive drugs. A final evaluation of all data collected is now in process.

Our experimental population consisted of 150 aged subjects, all of them—except for four control groups—mental hospital patients. About one third of these were diagnosed as suffering from organic psychoses, one third as paranoid schizophrenics who had aged in the hospital, and one third as suffering from other functional psychoses. The average age of the patients was seventy-one years.

The following clinical psychiatric symptom clusters were evaluated on the Verdun Target Symptom Rating Scale:

1. Arousal, as measured by the symptoms irritability, excitement, and fatigue
2. Affectivity, as measured by hostility, suspiciousness, anxiety, autonomic reactivity, impulsiveness, compulsiveness, somatization, relational ability, and preoccupation with self
3. Mood, as measured by depression and elation
4. Integration, as measured by perceptual disturbance, hallucinations, thought disorder, and delusions
5. Organicity, as measured by memory disturbances, alterations of consciousness, and dementia

In addition, we used a number of psychometric tests: the critical flicker fusion frequency test to measure perception (information input); tests for word association, digit-span recall, and retention to measure cognitive processes (information storage and processing); tapping speed and reaction time tests to measure psychomotor activity (output).

The psychometric test battery was given at weekly intervals before and after each psychopharmacological load. The loads were introduced by intravenous administration of a sedative (sodium amytal, 250 mg), a stimulant (methamphetamine, 10 mg), and a placebo (normal saline). A cerebral vasodilator was administered by means of a five-minute inhalation of a mixture of 5 per cent carbon dioxide and 95 per cent oxygen.

None of the three psychotic subgroups differed significantly on the clinical rating scale or on any particular psychometric test administered before the load. However, when ranking the mean performance on each psychological test across the diagnostic groups, it became evident that patients with organic brain disease are the poorest performers on all three psychometric test groups (that is, the psychomotor, the perceptual, and the cognitive). Paranoid schizophrenics did best on five of the seven tests, mainly those of the cognitive test group, although one psychomotor test (reaction time) was included among the five. The nonparanoid functional psychotics, mainly chronic schizophrenics, had the highest flicker fusion frequency (perceptual input) of the three groups.[106]

In the postpharmacological loading tests, no significant differences in the results between methamphetamine and carbon dioxide appeared. Sodium amytal, however, produced significant decrements of performance in all three subgroups: patients with organic brain disease showed a significant impairment in both psychomotor tests; the nonparanoids showed a decrement mainly in the perceptual test, whereas the paranoids were impaired mainly in some cognitive tests, that is, the digit-forward and digit-backward recall test.

The first phase of our experiment thus provided objective procedures for assigning individual geriatric patients to particular criterion groups according to their drug responses and independent of their original clinical diagnosis. Not only were there quantitative differences, but also qualitative differences in performance between the various groups. On the other hand, an analysis of the psychiatric behavior rating scale data did not reveal significant differences among the three diagnostic groups.

In the second phase of the study, the therapeutic effects of six different drugs were tested in the same geriatric population over a period of ten weeks. The six drugs were thioridazine (a neuroleptic), nicotinic acid (an essential metabolic factor), fluoxymesterone (a steroid hormone), meprobamate (an anxiolytic sedative), methylphenidate (a psychostimulant), and amitriptyline (an antidepressant).

Using immediate pharmacological load-test performances as predictors of long-term therapeutic drug responses, indications could be obtained for choosing particular drugs for individual patients.[105] For instance, judging from the immediate postload performance, a favorable response to thioridazine is most likely to occur in geriatric patients whose psychometric test performance is impaired after pharmacological loads of methamphetamine and carbon dioxide.

Nicotinic acid, on the other hand, seems to be indicated in those patients whose test performances improve after carbon dioxide inhalation, in those who improve after sodium amytal, and in those who do poorly after methamphetamine.

Meprobamate is indicated for patients whose test performance improves following carbon dioxide inhalation, but is contraindicated in patients whose test performance deteriorates after carbon dioxide.

Fluoxymesterone appears to be indicated in patients whose test performance improves after methamphetamine and in patients whose performance becomes worse after sodium amytal.

Methylphenidate produced little long-term therapeutic improvement in our geriatric patients, but whatever improvement did occur was—somewhat surprisingly—observed in those patients who did poorly in their tests after carbon dioxide or methamphetamine.

Amitriptyline had no appreciable therapeutic effects on the patients in this study, but it was observed that those patients who did poorly after a pharmacological load of methamphetamine showed a worsening of their clinical condition with amitriptyline.

An interesting incidental finding in this study emerged from an analysis of the practice effects of the patients' test performances over the five preloading test periods.[71] The number of tests with positive practice effect increases with the presence of psychopathology, age, and institutionalization. Furthermore, unusual increases in performance of tests measuring tapping speed, reaction time, and digit-forward recall with a few weeks' practice suggest a considerable unmobilized potential in institutionalized patients and might thus serve as indicators or even measures of the secondary detrimental effects of institutionalization above and beyond the primary impairment owing to organic brain disease.

A Diagnostic Study

The data of another investigation, aimed at the diagnostic significance of a large number of different test measures on different levels of functioning, are now being evaluated by me in collaboration with Dr. Ban. Our main objective is to establish reliable, objective, or semiobjective test criteria for psychiatric diagnosis.

This study involves 120 subjects, divided into seven diagnostic groups: 20 normal paid controls, 20 hospitalized patients with personality disorder, 20 patients with neurotic depressions (10 acute and 10 chronic), 20 patients with psychotic depressions (10 acute and 10 chronic), 20 patients with schizophrenia (10 acute and 10 chronic), and 20 patients with organic brain syndromes. Diagnoses were established clinically by several staff and research psychiatrists. Acute patients were then assessed within a day or two of their admission to hospital and chronic patients after they had been withdrawn for at least two weeks from medication.

The assessment was made on the basis of seven different approaches: two clinical psychiatric rating scales, two personality inventories, three perceptual tests, one perceptual-motor test, five psychomotor tests, six cognitive tests, and a battery of eight conditioning tests.[7] These different approaches yielded a total of 144 variables.

Only the evaluation of data from the neurotic and psychotic depressed groups has been completed and reported at the time of this writing.[67]

The rank order of the ten measures with the greatest discriminatory power between depressed and normal subjects, between depression and other psychiatric conditions, between neurotic and psychotic depression, and between acute and chronic depression is as follows:

1. Unconditional stimulus response—amplitude
2. Eysenck personality inventory—neuroticism scale
3. Cancellation test—error score
4. Extinction of the conditional response
5. Critical flicker fusion frequency
6. Minnesota multiphasic personality inventory—D scale
7. Digit recall—backward
8. Orienting response—amplitude
9. Reaction time—(simple auditory)
10. Archimedes spiral—(achromatic aftereffect)

Because our aim was to render the psychiatric diagnosis more objective, we did not include results derived from behavior rating scales in this list. Behavior rating scales give results that are often far from objective—even far from the acceptable minimum of objectivity required for clinical standards of diagnostic validity.[70]

It is surprising that the best over-all test for diagnosing various aspects of depression in our sizable and varied test battery turned out to be a psychophysiological measure: the amplitude of the unconditional stimulus response, that is, the GSR response to a loud tone. This variable ranks first in discriminative power on the three parameters of screening depressed patients from normals, differentiating depressions from other psychiatric disorders, and determining the differences between acute and chronic depression.

The extinction rate of the conditional response distinguishes so well between neurotic and psychotic depression that the positions of these two diagnostic groups with this measure are on either side of the normal—the neurotic depressed extinguish slower and the psychotic depressed faster than the normal control subjects. This finding lends further strong support to the assumption that the distinction between neurotic and psychotic depression is one between two independent diagnostic entities and not simply one of increasing severity of symptoms, as has been suggested.

The unconditional stimulus response distinguishes psychotic depression from personality disorder and acute or chronic schizophrenia at the .001 level of confidence and from organic brain syndrome at the .01 level. The cancellation test, error score, discriminates between neurotic depression and personality disorder or organic brain syndrome at the .01 level of confidence and between neurotic depression and chronic schizophrenia at the .001 level of confidence. Tapping speed separates neurotic and psychotic depression from chronic schizophrenia at .001 level of confidence.

It is thus possible to construct tables that indicate the degree of probability with which one diagnostic entity may be distinguished from another in a given patient on the basis of scores obtained from psychophysiological or psychometric tests. By combining a variety of tests of which the differential diagnostic discriminatory power is known, one can conceivably construct diagnostic instruments of appreciable objectivity that may give clinically reliable and valid results.

I do not foresee that objective or semiobjective procedures will ever wholly replace the psychiatric interview and clinical observation as procedures of primary importance in the assessment of psychopathology. In fact, Dr. Ban and I deplore the fact that insufficient attention is being paid today to the teaching and further development of these classic and essential techniques of psychopathology.[66] However, we feel confident that objective indicators and experimental procedures will in the future supplement the traditional methods of making psychiatric diagnoses and of assessing change in psychopathology. Not only diagnosis based on interviewing and clinical observation could undoubtedly benefit from the additional information that would derive from more objective procedures, but also diagnosis based on the more structured yet still highly subjective evaluation by means of behavior rating scales. Metabolic and biochemical indicators and measures have long been expected to make major contributions to greater objectivity in diagnosis, but the important role of neurophysiological, psychophysiological, and psychometric tests in psychopathology is only now coming into its own and promises interesting developments for the near future.

REFERENCES

1. Arieti, S. "Contributions to Cognition from Psychoanalytic Theory," in J. H. Masserman (ed.), *Science and Psychoanalysis*. New York: Grune & Stratton, 1965.
2. Aserinsky, E., and Kleitman, N. "Regularly Occurring Periods of Eye Motility, and Concomitant Phenomena during Sleep," *Science*, 118 (1953), 273–274.
3. Astrup, C. *Schizophrenia: Conditional Reflex Studies*. Springfield, Ill.: Charles C Thomas, 1962.
4. Astrup, C. *Pavlovian Psychiatry: A New Synthesis*. Springfield, Ill.: Charles C Thomas, 1965.
5. Ax, A. F. "The Psychophysiology of Schizophrenia," paper presented at the Biometrics Research Workshop on Objective Indicators of Psychopathology, Tuxedo, New York, 1968.
6. Ban, T. A. *Conditioning and Psychiatry*. Chicago: Aldine, 1964.
7. Ban, T. A. "Annual Report of the Research Department of the Douglas Hospital," Montreal, Canada, 1966.
8. Ban, T. A., Choi, S. M., and Lee, H. "Differential Conditioning in Organic and Functional Psychoses," paper presented at the First World Congress of Social Psychiatry, London, 1964.
9. Bannister, D., and Fransella, F. "A Grid Test of Schizophrenic Thought Disorder," *British Journal of Social and Clinical Psychology*, 5 (1966), 95–102.
10. Beam, J. C. "Serial Learning and Conditioning under Real-Life Stress," *Journal of Abnormal and Social Psychology*, 51 (1955), 543–551.
11. Bemporad, J. R. "Perceptual Disorders in Schizophrenia," *American Journal of Psychiatry*, 123 (1967), 971–975.
12. Berg, O. "Study of Effect of Evipan on Flicker Fusion Intensity in Brain Injuries," *Acta Psychiatrica et Neurologia*, 58 (1949), 1–116.
13. Brooks, G., and Weaver, L. *Psychomotor Performance and Mental Disorder*, final report, U.S. Public Service Health Grant MH–01752–06. Washington, D.C.: Government Printing Office, 1963.
14. Broughton, R. G. "Sleep Disorders: Disorders of Arousal," *Science*, 159 (1968), 1070–1078.
15. Brozek, J., and Taylor, H. "Tests of Motor Functions in Investigations on Fitness," *American Journal of Psychology*, 67 (1954), 590–611.
16. Busfield, B. L., and Wechsler, H. "Salivation as an Index of High Nervous Activity in Diseases with Prominent Psychopathology," in Z. Votava (ed.), *Psychopharmacological Methods*. New York: Pergamon Press, 1963.
17. Callaway, E. "Averaged Evoked Responses in Psychiatry," *Journal of Nervous and Mental Diseases*, 143 (1966), 80–94.
18. Callaway, E., Jones, R. T., and Layne, R. S. "Evoked Responses and Segmental Set of Schizophrenia," *Archives of General Psychiatry*, 12 (1965), 83–89.
19. Cameron, N. "Reasoning, Regression and Communication in Schizophrenics," *Psychology Monograph*, 50 (1938), 1–33.
20. Chalke, F. C. R., and Ertl, J. "Evoked Potentials and Intelligence," *Life Science*, 4 (1965), 1319–1322.

21. Chapman, L. J. "Confusion of Figurative and Literal Usages of Words by Schizophrenics and Brain Damaged Patients," *Journal of Abnormal and Social Psychology*, 60 (1960), 412–416.
22. Claridge, G. S. "Psychophysiological Indicators of Neurosis and Early Psychosis," paper presented at the Biometrics Research Workshop on Objective Indicators of Psychopathology, Tuxedo, New York, 1968.
23. Craig, W. J. "Objective Measures of Thinking Integrated with Psychiatric Symptoms," *Psychology Reports*, 16 (1965), 539–546.
24. Crider, A. B., Grinspoon, L., and Maher, B. A. "Autonomic and Psychomotor Correlates of Premorbid Adjustment in Schizophrenia," *Psychosomatic Medicine*, 27 (1965), 201–206.
25. Darrow, C. W. "Psychophysiology, Yesterday, Today and Tomorrow," *Psychophysiology*, 1 (1964), 4–7.
26. Darrow, C. W., Jost, H., Solomon, A. P., and Mergener, J. C. "Autonomic Indications of Excitatory and Homeostatic Effects on the Electroencephalogram," *Journal of Psychology*, 14 (1942), 115–130.
27. Dement, W. C. "The Effect of Dream Deprivation," *Science*, 131 (1960), 1705–1707.
28. DeVault, S. "Physiological Responsiveness in Reactive and Process Schizophrenia," doctoral dissertation, Michigan State University, 1955.
29. Duffy, E. "Emotion: An Example of the Need for Reorientation in Psychology," *Psychological Review*, 41 (1934), 239–243.
30. Dustman, R. E., and Beck, E. "Visually Evoked Potentials: Amplitude Changes with Age," *Science*, 151 (1966), 1013–1015.
31. Epstein, S. "Overinclusive Thinking in a Schizophrenic and a Control Group," *Journal of Consulting*, 17 (1953), 384–388.
32. Ervin, F. R., and Mark, V. H. "Behavioral and Affective Responses to Brain Stimulation in Man," paper presented at the annual meeting of the American Psychopathological Association, New York, 1968.
33. Eysenck, H. J., and Trouton, D. "The Effect of Drugs on Behavior," in H. J. Eysenck (ed.), *Handbook of Abnormal Psychology*. New York: Basic Books, 1961. Pp. 634–696.
34. Feffer, M. H. "The Influence of Affective Factors on Conceptualization in Schizophrenia," *Journal of Abnormal and Social Psychology*, 63 (1961), 588–596.
35. Fink, M. "Clinical Neurophysiology," in D. Bente and P. B. Bradley (eds.), *Neuropsychopharmacology*. Amsterdam: Elsevier, 1965.
36. Fisher, C. "Psychoanalytic Implications of Recent Research on Sleep and Dreaming," *Journal of the American Psychoanalytic Association*, 13 (1965), 197–270.
37. Floris, V., Morocutti, C. Bernardi, G., Amabile, G., Rizzo, P. A., Sommer-Smith, J. A., and Vasconetto, C. "Cortical Recovery Cycle Modifications in Schizophrenics and Dysthymic Patients," paper presented at the symposium on the use of electronic devices in psychiatry, Fourth World Congress of Psychiatry, Madrid, 1966. Excerpta Medica Foundation. International Congress Series No. 150, January 1968. P. 1196.
38. Foulds, G. A. "Scatter of Tapping among Mental Patients," *Journal of Clinical Psychology*, 17 (1961), 168–169.
39. Gantt, W. H. "Analysis of Mental Defect in Chronic Korsakov's Psychosis by Means of Conditioned Reflex Method," *Bulletin Johns Hopkins Hospital*, 70 (1942), 467–487.
40. Garmezy, N. "The Prediction of Performance in Schizophrenia," in P. H. Hoch and J. Zubin (eds.), *Psychopathology of Schizophrenia*. New York: Grune & Stratton, 1966.
41. Gellhorn, E. *Autonomic Imbalance and the Hypothalamus*. Minneapolis: University of Minnesota Press, 1957.
42. Goldman, D. "Specific Electroencephalographic Changes with Pentothal Activation in Psychotic States," *Journal of Electroencephalography and Clinical Neurophysiology*, 11 (1959), 657–667.
43. Goldstein, K. "The Organismic Approach," in S. Arieti (ed.), *American Handbook of Psychiatry*. New York: Basic Books, 1959. Vol. 1, pp. 1333–1347.
44. Goldstein, L., Murphree, H. B., Sugerman, A. A., Pfeiffer, C. C., and Jenney, E. G.

"EEG Variability and Behavioral Change in Chronic Schizophrenics," *Clinical Pharmacology and Therapeutics*, 4 (1963), 10–21.
45. Gresham, S. C., Agnew, H. W., and Williams, R. L. "The Sleep of Depressed Patients: An EEG and Eye Movement Study," *Archives of General Psychiatry*, 13 (1965), 503–507.
46. Gross, M. M., Goodenough, D., Tobin, M., Halpert, E., Lepore, D., Perlstein, A., Sirota, M., Dibianco, J., Fuller, R., and Kishner, I. "Sleep Disturbances and Hallucinations in the Acute Alcoholic Psychosis," *Journal of Nervous and Mental Diseases*, 142 (1966), 493–514.
47. Hakerem, G., and Lidsky, A. "Characteristics of Pupillary Reactions in Psychiatric Patients and Normals," paper presented at the Biometrics Research Workshop on Objective Indicators of Psychopathology, Tuxedo, New York, 1968.
48. Harris, J. G. "Size Estimation of Pictures as a Function of Thematic Content for Schizophrenic and Normal Subjects," *Journal of Personality and Social Psychology*, 25 (1957), 651.
49. Harris A., and Metcalfe, M. "Slowness in Schizophrenia," *Journal of Neurology, Neurosurgery and Psychiatry*," 22 (1959), 239–242.
50. Heath, R. G. *Studies in Schizophrenia*. Cambridge: Harvard University Press, 1954.
51. Hebb, D. O. *The Organization of Behavior*. New York: Science Editions, 1961.
52. Hoskins, R. G. *The Biology of Schizophrenia*. New York: Wiley, 1949.
53. Jellinek, E., and McFarland, R. "Analysis of Psychological Experiments on the Effects of Alcohol," *Quarterly Journal Study of Alcohol*, 1 (1940), 272–371.
54. Johannsen, W. J., Friedman, S. H., and Liccione, J. V. "Visual Perception as a Function of Chronicity in Schizophrenia," *British Journal of Psychiatry*, 110 (1964), 651–670.
55. Jouvet, M. "Mechanisms of the States of Sleep: A Neuropharmacological Approach," in S. S. Kety, E. V. Evarts, and H. L. Williams (eds.), *Sleep and Altered States of Consciousness*. Baltimore: Williams & Wilkins Co., 1967.
56. Kelly, D. H. W. "Measurement of Anxiety by Forearm Blood Flow," *British Journal of Psychiatry*, 112 (1968), 789–798.
57. King, H. E. *Psychomotor Aspects of Mental Disease*. Cambridge: Harvard University Press, 1954.
58. King, H. E. "Psychomotor Correlates of Behavior Disorder," paper presented at the Biometrics Research Workshop on Objective Indicators of Psychopathology, Tuxedo, New York, 1968.
59. Lacey, J. I. "Somatic Response Patterning and Stress: Some Revisions of Activation Theory," in M. H. Appley and R. Trumbull (eds.), *Psychological Stress*. New York: Appleton-Century-Crofts, 1967.
60. Lader, M. H. "Arousal Measures and the Classification of Affective Disorders," paper presented at the Biometrics Research Workshop on Objective Indicators of Psychopathology, Tuxedo, New York, 1968.
61. Landis, C. *An Annotated Bibliography of Flicker-Fusion Phenomena*, publication of the Armed Forces National Research Council. Ann Arbor, Michigan, 1953.
62. Lang, B., and Buss, A. "Psychological Deficit in Schizophrenia: II. Interference and Activation," *Journal of Abnormal Psychology*, 70 (1965), 77–106.
63. Lazarus, R. L. *Psychological Stress and the Coping Process*. New York: McGraw-Hill, 1966.
64. Lehmann, H. E. "The Influence of Different Psychoactive Drugs on Cognitive and Memory Tests in Schizophrenic and Geriatric Psychotics," in *Proceedings of the Fifth International Congress of the Collegium Internationale Neuro-Psychopharmacologicum*. Washington, D.C., 1966.
65. Lehmann, H. E. "Pharmacotherapy of Schizophrenia," in P. H. Hoch and J. Zubin (eds.), *Psychopathology of Schizophrenia*. New York: Grune & Stratton, 1966.
66. Lehmann, H. E. "Empathy and Perspective or Consensus and Automation? Implications of the New Deal in Psychiatric Diagnosis," *Journal of Comprehensive Psychiatry*, 8 (1967), 265–276.
67. Lehmann, H. E. "Experimental Psychopathology of Depression," paper presented at a symposium on "Das depressive Syndrom," Berlin, 1968.

68. Lehmann, H. E. "Types and Characteristics of Objective Measures of Psychopathology," paper presented at the Biometrics Research Workshop on Objective Indicators of Psychopathology, Tuxedo, New York, 1968.
69. Lehmann, H. E., and Ban, T. A. "The Effect of Hypnotics on Rapid Eye Movement (REM)," paper presented at the Fourth Annual Meeting and Scientific Program of the Canadian Society of Chemotherapy, Montreal, 1968.
70. Lehmann, H. E., Ban, T. A., and Donald, M. "Rating the Rater," *Archives of General Psychiatry*, **13** (1965), 67–75.
71. Lehmann, H. E., Ban, T. A., and Kral, V. A. "Psychological Tests: Practice Effect in Geriatric Patients," *Geriatrics*, **23** (1968), 160–163.
72. Lehmann, H. E., and Csank, J. "Differential Screening of Phrenotropic Agents in Man: Physiologic Test Data," *Journal of Clinical and Experimental Psychopathology*, **18** (1957), 222–235.
73. Lehmann, H. E., and Lidsky, A. Unpublished research.
74. Lidz, T., Wild, C., Schafer, S., Roseman, B., and Fleck, S. "Thought Disorders in the Parents of Schizophrenic Patients: A Study Utilizing the Object Sorting Test," *Journal of Psychiatric Research*, **1** (1962), 193–200.
75. Lynn, R. "Russian Theory and Research on Schizophrenia," *Psychological Bulletin*, **60** (1963), 486–498.
76. Mahl, G. F., Rothenberg, A., Delgado, J., and Hamlin, H. "Psychological Responses in the Human to Intracerebral Electrical Stimulation," *Psychosomatic Medicine*, **26** (1964), 337–368.
77. Malmo, R. B. "Activation: A Neurophysiological Dimension," *Psychological Review*, **66** (1959), 367–386.
78. Malmo, R., and Shagass, C. "Physiologic Studies of Reaction to Stress in Anxiety and Early Schizophrenia," *Psychosomatic Medicine*, **11** (1949), 9–24.
79. Malmo, R. B., and Shagass, C. "Studies of Blood Pressure in Psychiatric Patients under Stress," *Psychosomatic Medicine*, **14** (1952), 82–93.
80. Malmo, R., Shagass, C., Bélanger, D., and Smith, A. "Motor Control in Psychiatric Patients under Experimental Stress," *Journal of Abnormal and Social Psychology*, **46** (1951), 539–547.
81. Martin, I. "Learning and Performance in Human Conditioning," paper presented at the Biometrics Research Workshop on Objective Indicators of Psychopathology, Tuxedo, New York, 1968.
82. Mednick, S. A. "A Learning Approach to Research in Schizophrenia," *Psychological Bulletin*, **55** (1958), 316–327.
83. Mednick, S. A., and Schutsinger, E. "Some Premorbid Characteristics Related to Breakdown in Children with Schizophrenic Mothers," paper presented in part at the Biometrics Research Workshop on Objective Indicators of Psychopathology, Tuxedo, New York, 1968.
84. Mendels, J., and Hawkins, D. R. "Sleep and Depression: A Controlled EEG Study," *Archives of General Psychiatry*, **16** (1967), 344–354.
85. Mendels, J., and Hawkins, D. R. "Sleep and Depression: A Follow Up Study," *Archives of General Psychiatry*, **16** (1967), 536–542.
86. Misiak, H. "Age and Sex Differences in Monocular and Binocular Critical Flicker Frequency," *Journal of Experimental Psychology*, **37** (1947), 318–332.
87. Palmai, G., Blackwell, B., Maxwell, A. E., and Morgenstern, F. "Patterns of Salivary Flow in Depressive Illness and during Treatment," *British Journal of Psychiatry*, **113** (1967), 1297–1308.
88. Payne, R. W., and Caird, W. K. "Reaction Time, Distractibility and Overinclusive Thinking in Psychotics," *Journal of Abnormal Psychology*, **72** (1967), 112–121.
89. Payne, R. W. "Attention, Arousal and Thought Disorder in Psychotic Illness," paper presented at the Biometrics Research Workshop on Objective Indicators of Psychopathology, Tuxedo, New York, 1968.
90. Peck, R. E. "Observations on Salivation and Palmar Sweating in Anxiety and Other Psychiatric Conditions," *Psychosomatics*, **7** (1966), 343–348.
91. Protopopov, V. P. "Somatic Characteristics of Manic-Depressive Psychoses," *Zhurnal Neuropatologiia Psikhiatriic*, **17** (1948), 57–64.
92. Protopopov, V. P. "Problems of the Manic-Depressive Psychosis," *Zhurnal Neuropatologiia Psikhiatriic*, **57** (1957), 1355–1362.

93. Salzinger, K., Portnoy, S., and Feldman, R. S. "Experimental Manipulation of Continuous Speech in Schizophrenic Patients," *Journal of Abnormal and Social Psychology*, **68** (1964), 508–516.
94. Sem-Jacobsen, C. W., Petersen, M. C., Lazarte, J. A., Dodge, H. W., and Holman, C. B. "Electroencephalographic Rhythms from the Depths of the Frontal Lobe in Sixty Psychotic Patients," *Journal of Electroencephalography and Clinical Neurophysiology*, **7** (1955), 193–210.
95. Sexton, M. C. "Autokinetic Test: Its Value in Psychiatric Diagnosis and Prognosis: Preliminary Report," *American Journal of Psychiatry*, **102** (1945), 399–402.
96. Shagass, C., and Naiman, J. "The Sedation Threshold as an Objective Index of Manifest Anxiety in Psychoneurosis," *Journal of Psychosomatic Research*, **1** (1956), 49–57.
97. Shagass, C., Naiman, J., and Mihalik, J. "An Objective Test Which Differentiates between Neurotic and Psychotic Depression," *Archives of Neurology and Psychiatry*, **75** (1956), 461–471.
98. Shagass, C., and Overton, D. A. "Measurement of Cerebral 'Excitability' Characteristics in Relation to Psychopathology," paper presented at the Biometrics Research Workshop on Objective Indicators of Psychopathology, Tuxedo, New York, 1968.
99. Shagass, C., and Schwartz, M. "Cortical Excitability in Psychiatric Disorder. Preliminary Results," in *Proceedings of the Third World Congress of Psychiatry*, **1** (1961), 441–446.
100. Shagass, C., and Schwartz, M. "Reactivity Cycle of Somatosensory Cortex in Humans with and without Psychiatric Disorder," *Science*, **134** (1961), 1757–1759.
101. Shagass, C., and Schwartz, M. "Age, Personality and Somatosensory Cerebral Evoked Responses," *Science*, **148** (1965), 1359–1361.
102. Shakow, D. "Psychological Deficit in Schizophrenia," *Behavioural Science*, **8** (1963), 275–305.
103. Shapiro, M., and Nelson, E. "An Investigation of the Nature of Cognitive Impairment in Cooperative Psychiatric Patients," *British Journal of Medical Psychology*, **28** (1955), 239–256.
104. Sherwood, S. L. "Electrographic Depth Recordings from the Brains of Psychotics," *Annals of the N.Y. Academy of Sciences*, **96** (1962), 375–385.
105. Silver, D., Lehmann, H. E., Kral, V. A., and Ban, T. A. "Experimental Psychiatry: III. Selection and Prediction of Therapeutic Responsiveness in Geriatric Patients," paper presented at the Canadian Psychiatric Association Annual Meeting, Quebec City, Quebec, 1967.
106. Silver, D., Lehmann, H. E., Kral, V. A., Ban, T. A., and Debow, S. L. "Experimental Psychiatry: III. The Comparative Effectiveness of Psychoactive Drugs in Hospitalized Geriatric Patients," paper presented at the Quebec Psychopharmacological Research Association Meeting, Quebec City, Quebec, 1967.
107. Silverman, J. "Variations in Cognitive Control and Psychophysiological Defense in the Schizophrenias," *Psychosomatic Medicine*, **29** (1967), 225–251.
108. Silverman, J., Berg, P. S., and Kantor, R. "Some Perceptual Correlates of Institutionalization," *Journal of Nervous and Mental Diseases*, **141** (1966), 651–657.
109. Snyder, F. "The New Biology of Dreaming," *Archives of General Psychiatry*, **8** (1963), 381–391.
110. Snyder, S. "Perceptual Closure in Acute Paranoid Schizophrenics," *Archives of General Psychiatry*, **5** (1961), 406–410.
111. Speck, L. B., Dim, B., and Mercer, M. "Visual Evoked Responses of Psychiatric Patients." *Archives of General Psychiatry*, **15** (1966), 59–63.
112. Spence, K. W. *Behavior Theory and Conditioning*. New Haven: Yale University Press, 1956.
113. Sternbach, R. A. "Two Independent Indices of Activation," *Journal of Electroencephalography and Clinical Neurophysiology*, **12** (1960), 609–611.
114. Sutton, S., Braren, M., and Zubin, J. "Evoked Potential Correlates of Stimulus Uncertainty," *Science*, **150** (1965), 1187–1188.
115. Sutton, S., Braren, M., and Zubin, J. "Sensory, Conceptual and Emotional Components of the Evoked Response to Sound Stimuli in Man," paper presented at the Psychonomic Society, Chicago, 1965.

116. Sutton, S., and Zubin, J. "Effect of Sequence on Reaction Time in Schizophrenia," in J. E. Birren and A. T. Welford (eds.), *Behavior, Aging and the Nervous System: Biological Determinants of Speed of Behavior and Its Change with Age.* Springfield, Ill.: Charles C Thomas, 1965.
117. Taylor, J. A. "Drive Theory and Manifest Anxiety," *Psychological Bulletin,* 53 (1956), 303–320.
118. Teichner, W. "Reaction Time in the Cold," *Journal of Applied Psychology,* 42 (1958), 54–59.
119. Traugott, N. N. "The Mechanisms of Affective Responses," paper presented at the First World Congress of Psychiatry, London, 1964.
120. Tufts College Institute of Applied Experimental Psychology. *Handbook of Human Engineering Data.* Part VII. *Physiological Conditions as Determinants of Efficiency.* Port Washington, N.Y.: U.S. Naval Training Service Center, 1951.
121. Vanderhoof, E., Clancy, J., and Engelhart, R. S. "Relationship of a Physiological Variable to Psychiatric Diagnoses and Personality Characteristics," *Diseases of the Nervous System,* 27 (1966), 171–177.
122. Venables, P. H. "The Effect of Auditory and Visual Stimulation on Skin Potential Response of Schizophrenia," *Brain,* 83 (1960), 77–92.
123. Venables, P. H. "Psychophysiological Aspects of Schizophrenia," *British Journal of Medical Psychology,* 39 (1966), 289–297.
124. Venables, P. H. "Signals, Noise, Refractoriness and Storage: Some Concepts of Value to Psychopathology?" paper presented at the Biometrics Research Workshop on Objective Indicators of Psychopathology, Tuxedo, New York, 1968.
125. Venables, P. H., and O'Connor, N. "Reaction Time to Auditory and Visual Stimulation in Schizophrenics and Normals," *Quarterly Journal of Experimental Psychology,* 11 (1959), 175–179.
126. Venables, P. H., and Wing, J. K. "Level of Arousal and the Subclassification of Schizophrenia," *Archives of General Psychiatry,* 7 (1962), 114–119.
127. Vogel, G. W. "REM Deprivation: III. Dreaming and Psychosis," *Archives of General Psychiatry,* 18 (1968), 312–329.
128. Walter, W. G., Cooper, R., Aldrige, V. J., McCallum, W. C., and Winter, A. L. "Contingent Negative Variation: An Electric Sign of Sensorimotor Association and Expectancy in the Human Brain," *Nature,* 203 (1964), 380–384.
129. Walter, W. G. "The Contingent Negative Variation as an Aid to Psychiatric Diagnosis," paper presented at the Biometrics Research Workshop on Objective Indicators of Psychopathology, Tuxedo, New York, 1968.
130. Weckowitz, T. E., and Blewett, D. B. "Size Constancy and Abstract Thinking in Schizophrenic Patients," *Journal of Mental Science,* 105 (1959), 909–934.
131. Welch, L., and Kubis, J. "Effect of Anxiety on Conditioning Rate and Stability of PGR," *Journal of Psychology,* 23 (1947), 83–91.
132. Williams, H., Lubin, A., and Goodnow, J. "Impaired Performance with Acute Sleep Loss," *Psychological Monograph,* 73 (1959), 1–26.
133. Wilson, W. P. *Applications of Electroencephalography in Psychiatry.* Durham, N.C.: Duke University Press, 1965.
134. Wulfeck, W. "Motor Function in the Mentally Disordered, I: A Comparative Investigation of Motor Function in Psychotics, Psychoneurotics and Normals," *Psychological Record,* 4 (1941), 271–323.
135. Zahn, T. P. "Psychophysiological Concomitants of Task Performance in Schizophrenia," paper presented at the Biometrics Research Workshop on Objective Indicators of Psychopathology, Tuxedo, New York, 1968.

EVOLUTION OF FUNDAMENTAL CNS PATHOGENIC CONCEPTS

Leon Roizin

The neuron, or the anatomical functional unit of the nervous system, in the light of present concepts, appears to be a highly organized cell "endowed and capable, within normal conditions, to assimilate, store and elaborate histometabolic, biophysical and bioelectrical energy." This complex unit,

to carry out its specific assignment, must be ready, upon reception of an appropriate stimulus, to deliver its "quantum" of energy to the synaptic field at the terminal portions of its axon. Although each cellular unit knows no function other than that of reception, conduction, and discharge, the many differences in anatomical connection, molecular organization, enzymatic and biochemical requirements and the many differences which are present in their synaptic relationships not only indicate a diversity of function of neurons, but also demonstrate the many areas where diseases, biophysical phenomena, chemical processes, and drugs may alter individual cellular function.[168]

In addition, a brief analysis of the new trends—such as phase, polarizing, ultraviolet, fluorescent, and electron microscopy; X-ray diffraction; historadioautography; and microabsorption spectrophotometry (ultraviolet, visible, and infrared)—indicates not only that they aim to obtain structural-functional correlations beyond the limitations of histologic techniques and standard microscopy, but that they also open new avenues for the localization and correlation of biochemical, biophysical, and physiological processes within nerve cells and their related subunits.

Furthermore, these relationships at the ultracellular and molecular levels of organization were (1) instrumental in the most recent discoveries, not only in genetics (particularly gene chromosomal concepts) and (2) pathogenic mechanisms of some hereditary and spontaneous metabolic diseases, but they are also very valuable in the understanding of (3) the functional interactions of neurochemical mediators as well as (4) some of the pharmacodynamic properties and the mode of action of neuropsychotropic agents.

The present review pays particular attention to the cellular organelles and membrane systems because they are considered as structural, functional, and metabolic ultracellular gradients. In this capacity, they serve also as biological tools for the exploration of functional, metabolic, and pathogenic mechanisms in the central nervous system at the ultracellular levels of organization.

NUCLEUS AND NUCLEOLAR SYSTEM

Structural (Morphobiophysicochemical) Correlates

Cytological and histochemical techniques have demonstrated that the nucleus is more or less centrally located (see Figure 1, Nuc), variable in size, and spherical or oval in shape, although at times it appears irregular, branched, or segmented. It contains chromatin arranged variously in different types of cells and according to whether the cell is in resting phase or in the phase preceding division, or mitosis. In the resting cell, the nucleus possesses principally a coarse framework; the latter is composed of strands of fibrils that may be identified with uncoiled chromosomes.[58] A sollike liquid is found between the strands of fibrils; this was called "nuclear sap," "karyolymph," or "encylema" and was considered to contain the soluble phase of the nucleus.[172]

The electron microscope has given the best results in the study of the nucleolar system (see Figure 1), which is considered[19] as a large filament formed of many granules 100–200 Å in diameter, arranged one behind the other. This filament, the nucleolonema, is surrounded by amorphous material. It is associated with chromosomes during mitosis and, thus, constitutes an element of the gene structures. The chemical nature of the nucleolonema has not been definitely determined, although it appears not to contain the DNA. Vincent[197] further suggests two types of RNA: (1) the labile fraction, which would be associated with amorphous material, and (2) the residual fraction, which might be considered a part of the nucleolonema. According to some authors,[27] the amorphous material is related to the metabolic activity of the cell, whereas the nucleolonema is more important in the maintenance of nucleoli in future generations.[116, 197]

The nuclear membrane (see Figure 1, N.m.) is a double membrane with pores, or indentations, varying from 1,200 Å in amoebae to 500 Å in many other cellular varieties.[8, 203] It is about 300 Å thick and the presence of pores (Figure 1, N.i) suggests the

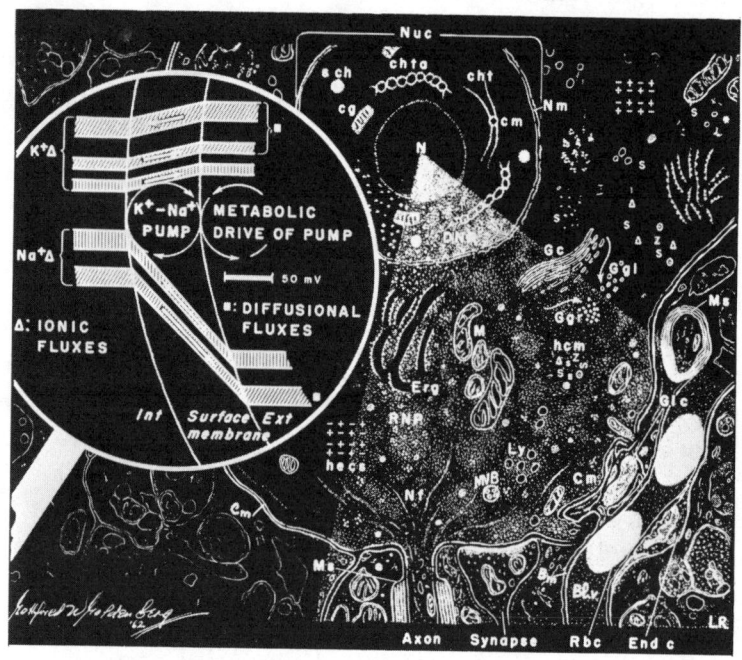

FIGURE 1

Schematic representation of a neuron as visualized on the basis of ordinary light-, phase-, and electron microscope and ultraviolet, spectroscopic, histochemical, differential, centrifugation, and microincineration studies. Reproduced with the kind permission of Prof. J. C. Eccles. Bl.v = blood vessels; Bm = basement membrane; cm, cht, chta, cg = various chromosomal constituents; Cm = cellular membrane; DNA = desoxyribonucleic acid; d.pr. = dendritic process; Erg = ergastoplasm; Glc = glia cell; Gc = Golgi complex; Ggl = Golgi globules; Ggr = Golgi granules; hcm = heterogeneous cellular material; hecs = heterogeneous electrocolloidal system; Ly = lysosomes; M = mitochondria; MVB = multivesicular body; Ms = myelin sheath; N = nucleolus; Nf = nerve fibrils; N.i. = nuclear indentation; Nm = nuclear membrane; Nuc = nucleus; Rbc = red blood cell; RNA = ribose nucleic acid; s.ch. = female sexual chromosomes.

possible passage of nuclear material into the cytoplasm.* Some authors believe that the nucleolonema granules pass into the cytoplasm to form the granules that surround the ergastoplasm saccules or appear free in its amorphous portion. The optical anisotropy of the nuclear membrane is that of a negative spherite indicating a protein lamellar texture, whereas the perinuclear layer represents a positive spherite owing to radially oriented lipid accumulation around the nucleus.[175]

The chromatic staining (with basic dyes) is owing mostly to the presence of nucleic acids. The nuclear reaction (Feulgen) points to aldehyde groups. Chemical studies have disclosed that the nuclear substances consist of nucleoproteins,[175] which can be separated into two components: proteins and phosphor containing nucleic acids; other components, such as lipids, are present in insignificant amounts. The protein components are represented by protamines, characterized by the fact that on hydrolysis they produce a striking number of basic amino acids. The polypeptide chain is not very long and would measure only 60 Å (salmine) consisting of fifteen to eighteen amino acids with molecular weight 2,000 to 25,000. The nucleic acids also possess a chain structure designated as nucleotides. On hydrolysis, they yield three components: one molecule of phosphoric acid, one molecule of sugar (from the group of pentoses), and one heterocyclic ring from pyrimidine (uracil, cytosine, thymine) or purine (guanine, adenine) types. The nucleic acids from the nucleus (DNA) differ from the nucleic acids of the cytoplasm (RNA) in that their nucleotides do not contain d-ribose but d-2-ribosedesose.

The nucleolus is composed mostly of RNA. The two types of nucleic acid contain the same purine bases, but differ with respect to one of pyrimidines. It is interesting to note that growing cells contain abundant nucleic acid and that the distribution of both kinds with the cell is such as to suggest a general pattern of the course of synthesis. These cells have dense nucleoli (RNA), which are surrounded by granules of chromosomal DNA; around the nuclear membrane is a layer of cytoplasm that contains much more RNA than is found farther out toward the boundary of the cell. Together with the evidence from the protein distribution of the proteins in the nucleus, this arrangement suggested that proteins are synthesized in the region of the nucleolus (these findings

* Densitometric tracings[97] of annular areas of nuclear membranes of mesodermal cells of the chick embryo seem to indicate that they do not represent simple openings, but are apparently more complex than previously assumed.

will be further discussed in the section on physiological and metabolic correlates). There are about 4.5 to 5 million molecules in a single nucleus (one molecule of nucleic acid links about one hundred protamine components).[53] These findings are also of particular historical interest inasmuch as they confirm Koelliker's prediction made more than a century ago—1853:

> If it be possible that the molecules which constitute cell-membranes, muscular fibrils, axile fibre of nerves, and so forth, should be discovered, and the laws of their apposition, and of the alterations which they undergo in the course of the origin, the growth, and the activity of the present so-called elementary parts, should be made out, then a new era will commence for Histology.[101]

Functional (Cytophysiological-Metabolic) Correlates

The principal functions of the nucleus are related to the hereditary concept (cell, individual, and species) and the control of metabolic functions in the normal synthetic activity of the cell. In 1854, Nageli[122] established that one plant cell is always born from the division of another. Gradually, it was demonstrated that, whenever a cell divides, either directly or by mitosis, the most outstanding phenomenon is the sequence of events developing in the nuclear substance. Subsequently, Koelliker[100] suggested that the nucleus itself might be the carrier of hereditable properties; Strasburger[187] described the chromosomes, Beneden[17] and Rabl[142] indicated their significance, and Weismann[204] proclaimed that they are the bearers of characters transmissible through heredity. In 1909, Johanssen[95] assumed that chromosomes are merely systems of genuine hereditary elements and suggested the name "genes." Subsequently, it was established that heredity consists of an always orderly transmission of structural, chemical, and physiological "features of a distinct nature in the biological sense, from which the characters of the individual and the sum total of the individual making up a species have their origin."[118]

With the application of improved cytological and cytochemical techniques, it has been established that chromosomes are not homogeneous structures. For instance, in the salivary gland chromosomes,[29] dark staining bands alternate with nonstaining interband regions. The property of stainability depends on the contents of nucleic acid, and its concentration in the band can be demonstrated with nuclear reaction (Feulgen), ultraviolet, and X-ray absorption microscopy.[52] Subsequently, the chromosomes have been conceived as a linear array of units ("the units themselves forming a hierarchy all the way from heterochromatic and euchromatic regions, some tens of thousands of mμ long to polypeptide links only a few tenths of a millimicron long"). Furthermore, it has been assumed that (1) the gene is a compound consisting of a number of identical subunits, (2) the genes are macromolecules or conglomerates thereof, (3) the immediate products that are formed under the influence of genes are also macromolecules, and (4) all primary gene products are enzymes and, therefore, proteins, which may be similar in composition to the genes themselves. From a cytogenetic point of view, the size of a gene corresponds to a cube with an edge of a few hundred Å. From the action of ionizing radiation on genetic mechanisms, it would seem that this is a sensitive target that is only 10 Å in diameter. Mutations still may occur if the effective ionization is only some ten atomic distances away from the sensitive center.[52] However, in view of the fact that genes, rather than the cells, seem to be the most ultimate functional units of living organisms, the questions of their constitution, reproduction, and function have become the most challenging research problems. In reference to the first two questions, it is considered that (1) the genes are similar to their primary product (nucleoproteins), (2) the copying goes on all the time, and (3) most of the copies are diffused into the cytoplasm, but one in each cell cycle is anchored to a chromosome.[77] They consist of a particular type of polypeptide combined with macromolecules to form a specifically orderly structural pattern that normally does not change,* and they are autoreproducible by longitudinal splitting. Distinctive features differentiate the genes from the cytoplasmic derivatives not so much on chemical as on functional and structural bases. The specific structural organization of the genes, acquired in the course of phylogenesis, is transmitted (through the chromatids) without change to daughter cells. In the latter, they remain confined to a certain location and become separated from the incessant protoplasmic activities and their metabolic turmoil. Of the inherited nucleic acids, DNA contains the genetic material (giant molecules) that directs and controls the quality and quantity of protein formation and maintains the continuity of living matter

---

* It is of interest to note that, according to Felix,[53] no metabolic reactions take place in the nuclei of fish spermatozoa because they do not contain enzymes and do not consume oxygen.

as well as the individuality of each living being. On the other hand, RNA carries the instructions from the genes to the sites of synthesis in the cytoplasm where it regulates the formation of protein molecules.[86]

The principle of progressive differentiation is also of great theoretical significance in view of the fact that each step or phase in the development is an outcome of the phase immediately preceding it and a necessary condition for those that follow it.[131] It is also of fundamental knowledge that genetic mechanisms are interrelated with environmental conditions. The essential fact is that the organism cannot reproduce itself without obtaining certain essential substances from its environment and that during development it must retain some connection with the external environment. Although the reviewed research dealt principally with the studies of mature structure and functions, their relation to the progressive dynamic aspects of development to various functional phases and to aging processes is inherently integrated as long as life functions. These conditions determine the necessity of devising mechanisms for creating, maintaining, and restoring structural-functional patterns for the atoms and molecules within the organs and cells, which are constantly changing. The available information pertains mostly to the biological synthesis and function of enzymes. Some authors[126, 127] have shown that a number of enzymes that catalyze the hydrolysis of protein themselves exist in the tissues in the form of catalytically inactive proteins. These substances—zygomoens—can be converted to enzymes by appropriate administration of enzymes. Thus, it appears that these substances are enzyme precursors, and they may represent intermediates in the biological synthesis of the enzymes to which they are converted. These findings appear to be of great significance in the study of the gene-enzyme relationship, particularly in relation to possible pathogenic mechanisms. For instance, an enzyme might not be produced because a primary gene product is not produced or because (1) substances or mechanisms controlling the orientation of the enzymes in the cell are not produced, (2) the substrate is not formed rapidly enough in relation to the functional requirements, or (3) an inhibitor for the reaction is produced.[199] Although in earlier studies the chromosome-gene concept (chromosomal gene inheritance) occupied a principal position in the study of genetics, it became possible to recognize the inheritance through extrachromosomal parts of the cell (cytoplasmic inheritance).[40, 47, 156] Two principal alternatives are considered: (1) any of the multiple intracytoplasmic components (mitochondria, microsomes, plastades, and so on) may have the continuity and stability to act as a determiner of heredity or (2) any intracellular metabolic blocks (units) may have sufficient influence within the inherited capacity of a given genome to stabilize a particular metabolic pattern. These metabolic blocks (units) have size limits extending from those of the smallest molecules (enzymes and the like) to the size of the whole cell. It appears, therefore, that a living organism consists of a coordinated system subjected to both genetic and environmental factors (adaptive extragenetic cytoplasmic system). The genetic system controls the elaboration and continuity of the adaptive system, which, in turn, ensures the survival and reproduction of the genetic system.

The recently emphasized importance of the sex-chromatin determination implies that each ovum contains among its chromosomes a specific one designated X chromosome, whereas each spermatozoon contains an X chromosome and a smaller Y chromosome. Zygotes with XX chromosomes produce females, and XY chromosomes produce males. In 1949, Barr and Bertram[10] observed characteristic "chromatin satellite bodies" in the nerve cells of mature female cats and the poorly developed nucleolar satellite in mature neurons of male cats.[11, 113] Since that time, it has been established by many investigators that the sex-chromatin body described by Barr and Bertram[12] represents the material of XX chromatin complex.*

Somatic cells, containing sex chromatin, are designated chromatin positive and are considered genetically female. Cells with invisible sex-chromatin bodies are chromatin negative and are considered genetically male. Male sex chromatin in somatic cells is presumably undetectable, rather than absent.[4, 12]

From a histometabolic point of view, it is important to mention that Alfrey and Mirsky[4] have shown (in biochemical studies of the isolated nucleus) that in the intact nucleus, the presence of DNA mediates amino acid incorporation into protein, ATP synthesis, and the uptake of purines and pyramidines into nuclear RNA. It is also important to note that different somatic cell nuclei, in a given organism, have a constant amount of DNA per nucleus.† The role of the DNA in these activities is not yet clear,

---
* Under high magnification, the chromatin body appears to consist of a pair of smaller bodies in close opposition.
† The nuclei of the germ cells contain half that amount.

but, from the DNA substitution experiments (carried out with isolated nuclei), these authors have concluded that the polyanionic nature of DNA plays a large part in its activities. The need for large negatively charged molecules as DNA substitutes, and the inhibitory action of polycationic compounds, such as polylysine, suggests a correlation between the negative electrical charge and the biochemical activity of the nucleus. Of interest are Taylor and Wood's[193] studies of polynucleotide synthesis in the nucleus and in the chromosomes with thymidine,* which was labeled with tritium. These investigations have pointed out that (1) some cells appear to have little synthesis of RNA, except perhaps in the nucleolus during DNA synthesis; (2) synthesis of RNA stops during late stages of division when chromosomes are condensed and the nucleolus disappears; (3) there is a lag of thirty minutes or more after a cell begins incorporation of an isotope before the label appears in cytoplasmic RNA; and (4) specific time curves are compatible with the hypothesis that RNA of the nucleolus and chromosomes can be transported to the cytoplasm. Thus, the nucleolus is active in RNA metabolism at all stages and incorporates labeled precursors of RNA much more rapidly than any other part of the cell.

In reviewing the structure and chemistry of nucleoli, Vincent[197] concluded that, if the nucleolus has any active function in the cell, it will play a part in the shorter term, nongenetic function of the nucleus and that it is involved in nuclear cytoplasmic interchange. In this latter instance, it will favor cell multiplication or cluster around the ergastoplasmic saccules to carry out those differentiated syntheses that enable the plasmocytes to form globulin; the epidermal cells, keratin; the erythrocytes, hemoglobin, and so on. As far as the nerve cells are concerned, it is important to note the remarkable accumulation within their cytoplasm of small granules associated with the well-developed endoplasmic reticulum. The same type of relationship is found in the ergastoplasm of glandular cells (pancreas) and liver, that is, a type of cytoplasm characterized by its intense basophil and high RNA content that is prevalent in cells maintaining intense protein production.[28, 31, 34] In the neurons, this activity is evident in the chromatolytic process that takes place in response to pronounced stimulation or injury[22, 63, 94] and certain types of generalized stress, such as colds.[130] In such circumstances, the modification of RNA metabolism is paralleled by correlated changes in the

* It is used as selective label for chromosomes.

protein metabolism of the cytoplasm. Furthermore, rapid and continuous protein synthesis in the perikaryon is noted during rapid axonal regeneration following sectioning or damage of axoplasm proximal to ligature.[205] Although the exact relationship of the components of the Nissl substances to the complex process of protein synthesis has not yet been demonstrated, the fact that its structure is of the same type as that of the ergastoplasm of the pancreas and liver cells encourages the investigation of the possibility of a similar histometabolic analogy.

Pathological Correlates

GENERAL CONSIDERATIONS

In biologically functioning organisms, dynamic systems are constantly undergoing changes related to physiological, adaptive, or reactive processes.

Within physiological conditions, the diversified, multiple, complex structural and biophysicochemical components of the cell are acting and maintaining a dynamic synergistic equilibrium determined and regulated by the intrinsic hereditary mechanisms of the individual cells. Because the intercellular materials are subject to local as well as general systemic influences and, in turn, control the cells both as substrate and by influencing exchange, they play an important role in the intracellular mechanisms. Also of particular interest are regulatory mechanisms—nucleoproteins, hormones, electrolytes, vitamins, and so forth—which do not act by forming enzyme components but by controlling the rate of enzyme reactions or by changing the orientation of these reactions.[139] Moreover, it should be kept in mind that "living cells are unique among the engines known to man, for living engines are constructed of the same kind of materials that are used for fuel. If the fires of life burned too brightly, not only the fuel, but the engines, themselves, will be consumed."[67, 68] For instance, in chromatolytic processes involving the nerve cells following physiological hyperactivity and fatigue, retrograde degeneration, vitamin B_1 and B complex deficiencies, and so forth, the Nissl substance, acid phosphatases,[22, 63] and the respiratory quotient[91] are undergoing reversible changes (histometabolic dysergia; see Table 1). Reversible alterations in growth and chromatolytic changes have also been noticed in some essential amino acid deficiencies.[54] However, if such phenomena are repeated or perpetuated for a long time and beyond the physiological endurance, then irreversible alterations with disorganization and dissolution of the integrated anatomophysiological equilibrium take place (pathergia) and degeneration may ensue (pathosis or patholysis) at cellular or subcellular levels. This concept, postulated as a working hypothesis, is summarized in Figure 2. Furthermore, in

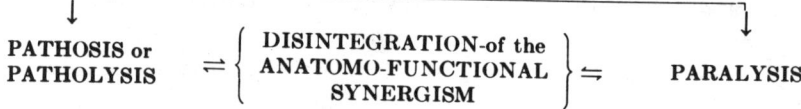

FIGURE 2

Integrated Anatomofunctional Synergism, Histometabolic Dysergia, and Related Pathogenic Mechanisms.

the living cells, enzymes may be present that are so located as to be inactive in the intact cell.[139] Physiological alterations, disorganization, or disruption of the normal cellular architecture may bring these enzymes into action. [42, 104, 129, 163]

Gene Mutations

From experiments, as well as observations in man, it has been assumed that changes in a cell or organism may come about through gene mutation or as a result of variations in environment. Neither of these factors is strictly independent of the other, in that both influence patterns of metabolism and each limits the degree to which the other may alter a given pattern. During recent years, some investigators successfully tested with Acetobacter, Escherichia coli, and Neurospora the basic premise that the biochemical processes concerned with the synthesis of essential cell constituents are gene controlled and alterable as a consequence of gene mutation.[15, 189, 190] This study was carried out in bacteria, in which many and varied naturally occurring factors required for growth were known, to see whether analogous nutritional deficiency followed exposure of bacteria to radiation. It seems[15, 106, 190] that each and every biochemical reaction in a cell of any organism from bacterium to man is theoretically alterable by gene mutation. A second consequence of the postulated relationship stems from the concept that the genetic constitution defines the potentialities of the cell, whereas the time and degree of expression of these potentialities are, to a certain extent, modifiable by the cellular environment.

Mutagenic effects also have been observed in a variety of cells following X-ray, [115, 119] ultraviolet radiation,[89] halogenated alkylamines, and mustard gas,[25] which appear to inhibit mitosis. More, Hevesy[83] found synthesis of nucleoproteins, which takes part in mitosis, is inhibited by X-ray radiation. It is of interest to note that carcinogenic substances containing a phenanthrene nucleus, when applied to tissues, caused profound alteration of cells that led to self-reproducing alterations coincidental with the assumption of neoplastic characteristics.[150] Stowell and Cooper[186] have shown that these changes are associated with alteration of nucleic acid content, and Biesele[20] has demonstrated irregular alteration of chromosome structure. The increased rate of tumor production by hybridization, like that by carcinogenic chemicals in genetically suitable material,[150] provides another example of gene mutation caused by procedures also effective in causing neoplastic disease.[207]

A variety of inherited anomalies in experimental animals[35, 112, 113] and humans have been described and considered of a mutagenic character. Of particular interest are the neural malformations arising on a genetic basis. Gluecksohn-Waelsch[66] has demonstrated that mice of different strains show distinct differences to experimental maldevelopment, thus indicating a genetic basis for their susceptibility or resistance to the effect of a pathogenic agent. On the other hand, the experimental studies of Hicks,[84] Rugh,[170] and Roizin et al.[162] on malformations in animals show that genetic factors do not always play an extensive role in the developmental anomalies of the central nervous system. Therefore, it is necessary to take into consideration the interdependence of genetic and nongenetic factors in the interpretation and evaluation of some experimental developmental anomalies.[66]

Metabolic Diseases

Gene-Enzyme-Chemical Reaction Patterns. The series of biophysical events in the supply line of nutrients to the cell is based on a long history of evolution, natural selection, and adaptation of molecular systems. These complex conditions provide multiple possibilities for alteration or dysfunction from normal metabolic processes.[75, 169] But, in many of the disorders that one may envision, the number of possibilities is multiplied enormously when one realizes that each cell is a highly individual unit with a specific function not exactly reproducible by the neighboring tissues or organs. In 1908, A. E. Garrod[60] presented his concept of inborn errors of metabolism based on four human pathologic conditions: albinism, alkaptonuria, cystinuria, and pentosuria: "They apparently result from some step or other in the series of chemical changes which we call metabolism."[61] He believed that the metabolic defect was owing to the absence or inactivity of an enzyme that, in turn, was dependent on the absence of the normal form of a specific gene. Since that time, many books, monographs, and symposia dealing with hereditary metabolic or degenerative diseases have been published.[62, 77, 140, 167, 184, 192, 199] Here, only a few selected concepts supplemented by some demonstrative examples will be mentioned in order to keep within the limit of stated aims.

Theoretically, it is possible to conceive a number of ways in which the absence or partial lack of inhibition of an enzyme could lead to a different metabolism that would eventually result in pathological processes. Recently, Snyder[182] has suggested some possibility by which mutations resulting in enzyme dysfunction may lead to genetic diseases through involvement of metabolic blocks (cerebral lipoidoses, diabetes, xanthinuria, and so on), alternative pathways (phenylketonuria and the like), and inhibitors (hereditary spherocytosis, albinism, and so on). In addition to behaving as obvious enzymes, substances controlled by genes may, in some instances, act as antigens, inhibitors, or hormones.

Environmental Effects. There are innumerable potential interactions between hereditary and environmental influences:

1. It is known that many enzymes have a coenzyme or prosthetic group as a necessary adjunct to the protein core. Although

the protein core is determined by a gene, the coenzyme is frequently vitamin in origin and, thus, is environmentally conditioned. As a result of such exogenous effects, phenocopies may be produced that mimic the genetic condition. For example, nutritional siderosis appears to be a phenocopy of genetic hemochromatosis. Incidentally, it should be indicated here that the metabolism of inorganic elements is also involved in human and some experimental diseases; this may be related to a genetic dysfunction. For instance, disorders of iron metabolism in hemochromatosis and in methemoglobinuria[65, 182]; of copper metabolism in hepatolenticular degeneration[16]; of potassium metabolism in family periodic paralysis[81]; of calcium in Fahr's syndrome[152]; and so on.

2. Although genes are normally identical in various cells of the individual, the cytoplasmic constituents of the cell need not be equivalent. The unequal distribution during mitosis of intracellular organelles and other subcellular constituents can result in the occurrence of identical genes in cytoplasmic microenvironments that differ in concentrations of enzymes, substrates, and the like from tissue to tissue. In this way, a given gene may produce an effect in one tissue and not in another.

Growth and Age Factors. Physiological and biochemical equilibrium in reversible reaction requires time to be adjusted. The achievement of equilibrium may free a substrate from a new conversion by a different enzyme. The accumulation of by-products may slowly reach a critical level at which these by-products or intermediary metabolites may act as a new substrate or inhibitor. Moreover, a biological protein is a mixed population of molecules of very different ages, with which are related dithio bonds and substitution of amino acids so that the descendant of a gene may be located in environments in the adult or old individuals, which are biochemically different from those in the embryo or young organism. Therefore, one gene may exert its influence at a certain stage of development of an individual whereas another may not be affected until another age. Ichthysosis,* Huntington's chorea,† Alzheimer's disease,‡ and so forth, are possibly demonstrative examples of these phenomena. These facts tend to suggest that genes do not exercise absolute control over the presence or absence of specific enzymes but rather determine the potential development

---

* Occurring in the embryo.
† Occurring in the adult.
‡ Occurring in the presenile stages.

of particular enzyme systems in particular environmental conditions.[1, 14, 182]

Morphogenetic Alterations. Some authors have tried to explain a number of innate structural differences as resulting from the abnormal secretion of a hormone (excess or defect). On the other hand, genes are known to alter the threshold of response of tissues to hormones. For instance, Snyder[182] has considered that such structural anomalies as polydactyly, achondroplastic dwarfism, multiple exostoses, and lobster claw may be interpreted on the basis of enzyme dysfunction as metabolic diseases. This evidence is offered by hereditary spherocytosis.[182] In this disease, the red cells develop as spherocytes lacking the expandable biconcave surfaces of the normal red cells. As a result, the erythrocytes are osmotically and mechanically fragile and rupture easily. The basic pathogenesis in this condition is a defect in glycolysis of the red cells caused by the involvement (inhibition) of enolase, which in normal glycolysis converts 2-phosphoglyceric acid to 2-phosphoenolpyruvic acid, which provides energy in the form of ATP, which in turn is essential for the maintenance of the integrity of the framework and the membrane of the cell. In some cases, it appears that genetic differences are organ specific or tissue specific as, for instance, in cases of allergic mechanisms.[159]

Before concluding this brief summary, I would also like to point out that, according to Penrose,[140] hereditary dispositions owing to metabolic errors are mainly of two kinds. The first type is almost always genetically homozygous, and the affected subject lacks an enzyme because the abnormal gene present in duplicate fails to make it. The affected people show signs of abnormality constantly throughout life or, at least, from an early age. The neurolipoidoses (amaurotic family idiocy, infantile and juvenile types; Nieman-Pick's, gargoylism) represent particular examples of this type of disease process as they are caused by rare recessive autosomal genes* and, according to Sobotka,[183] the essential feature of all these lipoidoses is the absence of specific enzymes (esterases), which normally convert one high lipid into another, whereas Thannhauser[195] suggests that coenzymes, activating enzymes that break down lipids, are faulty. In the second type, the carrier with one abnormal gene is still able to manufacture the necessary enzyme. Sometimes the inborn error only gives rise to symptoms under special conditions or stress. In this case, the irregularity in

---

* With the exception of gargoylism, which is divided into two genetic types, one owing to an autosomal recessive gene and the other to a sex-linked recessive gene.

functional or biochemical aspects is found, but not constantly—for instance, abnormal blood sugar levels,[111] which have been sometimes attributed to anti-insulin substances[117]; abnormal proportions of androgen and estrogen in the urine[90]; peculiarity in serum concentration of choline esterase.[146] Some of these abnormalities, although not necessarily harmful in the cells, may give rise to severe disturbances.

CYTOPLASM AND ITS SUBUNITS

The Cytoplasm

The cytoplasm is represented predominantly by aggregates of molecules dispersed in a colloidal system that is of a lyophilic character. Some authors consider protoplasm as being composed of granules in an amorphous matrix. Within this medium, interwoven anabolic and catabolic processes are taking place. From a physicochemical point of view, the proteins are the structural elements of the protoplasm. Their macromolecules are interlinked to form a framework whose junctions (lyophilic, hydrophilic groups, saltlike or esterlike bonds, acid and basic side groups, intramolecular and intermolecular bonds) can be disrupted by environmental[153] alternations or various physicochemical agents or technical procedures (fixation). The cytoplasm is not a homogeneous substance of uniform composition but contains structures and bodies that are considered of two main varieties[78]: organelles* and inclusions.† Among the group of intracellular organelles, we will consider those closely related to our subject of discussion and will limit our description to some fundamental features only insofar as it will be necessary to understand their specific functions.

Mitochondria

Mitochondria (mitos = thread, chondrion = granules) or PMS (pleomorphometabolosomes)[156] is unquestionably recognized as one of the most characteristic components of the cytoplasm.

---

* Specialized constituents of the cytoplasm, of various shapes and sizes, that are considered part of the living and functioning system of protoplasm.

† Aggregates or accumulations of organic or inorganic material that sometimes appear in the cells during their development and in various functional states.

Structural Correlates

The origin and morphology of mitochondria have not definitely been settled. In the past, they have been identified as pleomorphic cytoplasmic structures showing certain distinctive staining properties, but owing to difficulties in examining them in detail, they have created controversy among some investigators. However, these uncertainties have now been greatly reduced by electron microscopy.[137, 144, 156, 178, 180] Mitochondria consists of bodies surrounded by a limiting double membrane, 70 to 80 Å units thick with a system of internal ridges protruding from the inner surface of the membrane forming a relatively parallel series toward the interior called "cristae mitochondrialis" (see "M" of Figure 1). Although these structural characteristics have been observed in cells of various animals and plants, there is a certain amount of diversity among various cell types. In isolated form (by differential centrifugation in 0.25 m. sucrose), the majority appear as spherical bodies, varying in size from approximately 0.6 to 1.3μ in diameter. The double membranes consist of layers of lipoprotein molecules[178] or bimolecular lipid layers,[194] perhaps combined with other material. [57, 107, 143, 148, 171] There is, probably, sufficient lipid and protein present in the mitochondrion for the internal cristae mitochondrialis to be considered to have similar structure. The function of the membranes that divide the mitochondria may be associated with enzyme activities or/and electron transport system,[57] which will be discussed in more detail below.

Functional (Cytophysiological-Metabolic) Correlates

Cytoplasm and Its Subunits. At the level of the composite organ the cells perform not only their specific function but are also subjected to the dynamic influences of mechanical, biochemical, bioelectrical (nervous tissue) activities from one organ or tissue to another. As at a cellular level, the structures vary in relation with the specific molecular configuration, similarly their quantum of energy changes constantly in accordance with modifications of functional mechanisms, metabolic processes and environmental conditions. This over-all heterogeneous biologic dynamic organization is reciprocally interrelated with the fundamental biological processes of growth, differentiation, and function (specific, adaptive, reactive, and regressive or involutional).

The Role of Mitochondria, or PMS, in Oxidative Phosphorylation. ATP synthesis coupled with oxidative reaction has been investigated mostly in isolated mitochondria.[72] By the use of cell fractionation in the isolation of intracellular substances, according to some investigators, the mitochondria contain all of succinic dehydrogenase[76] and probably all of the cytochrome oxidase activity of the cell.[73, 107, 173, 174] The liver mitochondria contain enzymes participating in fatty acid oxidations[114] and coenzyme A. For comprehensive information concerning the known components of electron transport particle* and mitochondrial lipid the reader is referred to Green's[72] and Lehninger's[107] reviews on mitochondrial structure and function. Though, from the standpoint of chemical composition, the components of the electron transfer chain of the phosphorylating and nonphosphorylating electron transfer particles are indistinguishable, the electron microscope, however, has disclosed that the nonphosphorylating particle has a vesicular structure, whereas the phosphorylating particle has the double membrane structure of the membrane and the cristae mitochondrialis.[72] It is also highly significant that the isolated mitochondria that are morphologically intact show only a very restricted number of enzymatic activities, do not oxidize citrate or isocitrate, do not reduce externally added cytochrome C or DPN, and do not oxidize DPNH. Only when the mitochondria are damaged morphologically do these activities emerge.†

ENDOPLASMIC RETICULUM AND CORRELATED STRUCTURES

Structural Correlates. It would be inappropriate to review here the vast amount of controversial literature on the Golgi apparatus (system, complex), or smooth (a granular) reticulum. For general orientation, the reader is referred to Bourne,[29] Worley,[214] and Palay.[135] From electron microscope investigations, in particular, a general outline for the ultrastructure of the Golgi apparatus has been delineated that allows its identification in a large variety of cells (see "Gc" of Figure 1). Although its general morphologic features and distribution vary in different types of cells and under various physiological conditions, the basic cytoarchitectural organization as visualized by the electron microscope appears quite constant. In brief, the Golgi apparatus appears as a system composed of two main membranous elements[137, 161]: (1) closely packed piles of flat-

* The electron transport particle is a submitochondrial unit of variable size. Each particle may be an aggregate of many repeating units. Only a full disaggregated electron transport particle would correspond to the individual repeating unit. The particle or molecular weight of the repeating unit would be from 3.3 to 5 times 10 based on the assumption of one molecule of DPNH dehydrogenase per repeating unit.

† The pathologic correlates of the cytoplasmic organelles will be discussed as a group at the end of this chapter, because the current pathologic knowledge of the individual subunits is still limited.

tened cisternae, sometimes several micra in extent, and (2) groupings of small, spherical vesicles (approximately 250 to 650 Å in diameter) imbedded in the cytoplasmic matrix. In some cells, the cisternae branch are anastomosed with their neighbors. In places where the fenestrations are close together, the profile of the cisternae, in section, appears as a row of small circles. The packed cisternae are often arrayed in multiple curves enclosing regions of the cytoplasm that are filled with groups of the small vesicles. Groups or clusters of closely packed small vesicles may also be found outside the arrays of cisternae and even separated from the main mass of the Golgi apparatus. They are differentiated from the membranous elements of the ergastoplasm, or granular endoplasmic reticulum,[132, 133, 134] by their peculiar arrangement and the absence of ribonucleic protein granules. Because of this latter aspect, Palade and Porter have designated them as agranular, or smooth, endoplasmic reticulum.[134] On the other hand, it appears that the granular endoplasmic reticulum of the ergastoplasm continues, here and there, with the agranular reticulum of the Golgi system and that these intracellular membranes delimit a diffuse system of intracellular channels within the cell cytoplasm and the nuclear membrane into a dynamic continuity.[132, 135, 161]

Functional Correlates. More convincing than the light microscope observations of the past decades, the electron microscope revealed the close relationship between the secretory granules and the Golgi complex.[133, 135] However, its precise role still remains obscure. Although the isolated Golgi structure displays some phosphatase activity, it is doubtful whether it is capable of protein synthesis, particularly in view of the fact that recent histochemical studies indicate that protein synthesis is a function of the ergastoplasm. Therefore, some authors[135] consider the possibility that the whole cell, including the nucleus, mitochondria, and the ergastoplasm, is involved directly in the synthesis of the ultimate secretory product, which is selectively collected in the vesicles of the Golgi complex to form definite secretory droplets. Consequently, Palay[135] suggested the following hypothesis for the topographic segregation of cytoplasmic functions: The endoplasmic reticulum, which is in dynamic continuity with the plasmalema and the nuclear membrane,[132, 161] serves as a transportation system for conveying raw material from the cytoplasmic environment to the enzymatic mechanism that resides in the ergastoplasm and the mitochondria. The products of this system are released into the cavities of the endoplasmic reticulum or into the matrix of the cytoplasm whence specific substances are secreted in the Golgi complex as secretory granules to be extruded from the cells as the ultimate secretory product. Similar ideas have been expressed by some investigators and, particularly, by Worley,[215] who attempted to illustrate the possible interrelationship of the various inclusions in animals, mainly with reference to oogenesis. Further studies[128, 129, 154, 161] have complemented and extended these concepts using acid phosphatase reaction (Gomori method) as a tracer.

Multivesicular Body (MVB)—Structural and Functional Correlates

The fine organization of MVB and its distribution in the central nervous system of animals (from embryo to old age) and humans, on the basis of a review of the literature and our own studies,[161] reveals that (1) it is a round or oval organelle that is surrounded by a single membrane; (2) its matrix contains principally vesicles, although vacuoles, canalicularlike and laminated structures, as well as structureless material, may be encountered in it; (3) it shows variability of the shape, size, matrix and its contents as well as of osmiophilia; (4) it is generally located in the cytoplasm of cells and their processes including the pre- and postsynaptic terminals in the central nervous system; (5) it displays structural, probably functional, and some histochemical (acid phosphatase activity and probably that of other hydrolytic enzymes) relationship to the Golgi complex, as well as to lysosomes and possibly, through Golgi canaliculi, with the granular endoplasmic reticulum; (6) it possesses morphokinetic properties (pseudopode formations, pleomorphism); (7) it shows relationship to pinocytosis and some transport mechanisms; (8) it is capable of remarkable metamorphosis in physiological as well as in reactive and pathological processes; and (9) it spills or discharges the vesicles or matrix when the integrity of the limiting membranes (of the MVB or/and of the vesicles) is altered. In the light of these conclusions, it was suggested[161] that MVB is a component of an intracellular morphokinetic canalicular-organelle system (IMCOS) that channels and regulates the orderly transport of metabolic material from its sites of origin to the functionally interrelated ultrastructures.

The Lysosome—Structural and Functional Correlates

This group of cytoplasmic organelles was identified by De

Duve.[42] (See "Ly" of Figure 1.) It has been isolated from liver, kidney, brain, spleen, thyroid, and giant amoeba. In summary, their main structural features, in 0.25 m. sucrose, are characterized as follows: (1) spherical shape, mean diameter 0.4 μ, average density 1.15; (2) lacking several key enzymes of oxidative metabolism, but containing a number of easily soluble hydrolases (hence the name of lysosomes) and having in common an acid pH optimum; (3) surrounding membrane of lipoprotein nature that effectively prevents the enzymes from escaping from, as well as preventing their respective substrate from penetrating into, the particles; and (4) the simultaneous release of all internal enzymes in soluble and fully active form, following some injuries to the membrane as caused by various treatments.[9, 51, 56, 93, 129, 163] It is assumed[42] that the lysosome function may be involved in digestion of foreign materials, incorporated by pinocytosis; athrocytosis or phagocytosis; physiological autolysis as presumably occurs, to some extent, in all tissues and, particularly, as part of the processes of involution metamorphosis; holocrine secretion, and various pathologic processes as summarized in Table 1.[163]

TABLE 1
Structural, Metabolic, Functional, and Pathologic Correlation of Lysosomes—In Vivo and In Vitro Conditions

STRUCTURE	METABOLIC ACTIVITIES	FUNCTIONAL PROPERTIES	PATHOLOGICAL REACTIONS

In vivo	acid phosphatase
	β-glucuronidase
	ac.R.Nase,ac,D-Nase
	ac-protease(s)
	cathepsin(s)
	β-N-acetylglucose-
	  aminidase
	β-galactosidase,
	aryl sulfatase
	lysozyme (WBC)
	protein-bound
	  glycolipids
		homeokinesis
		endogenous digestion
		phagocytosis
		pinocytosis
		arthrocytosis
			metamorphosis
			abiotrophy
			autolysis
			necrobiosis
			allergic processes
			
			*

In vitro		various degrees as above	autolysis and/or necrosis (tissue culture) †

*Experimental injuries: autolysis, ischemia hypervitaminosis A, hypovitaminosis E, phagocytosis (WBC), endotoxine, traumatic shocks, IIV and X-ray irradiations.
†Experimental injuries: freezing and thawing, Waring Blender, nonionic detergents, vitamin A, U V. irradiation, hypoosmolar conditions.

Neurofibrils or Neurotubules—Structural and Functional Correlates

In nerve cells, certain of the protein molecules in the cytoplasm appear or are built up in a linear arrangement assuming the form of linear polymers.[78] (See "Nf" of Figure 1.) In some neurons, they become grouped into threadlike fibrils that are large enough to be seen with the light microscope particularly with silver impregnation techniques. With the electron microscope, they appear composed of finer structures, commonly called "neurotubules." The molecular composition of the linear polymers themselves can be studied by means of X-ray diffraction patterns. As far as the nervous system is concerned, it is assumed that they are principally related to the conductivity of the action potential current.

Cytoplasmic Inclusions, Intracytoplasmic Heterogeneous Material, and Microsomes

In nerve cells, the cytoplasmic basophile substance, Nissl bodies or Nissl material, was recently reconfirmed to preexist in the living neuron and essentially unchanged after good cytological fixation.[43, 44] Electron microscopic studies[110, 137, 156, 202] disclosed that the Nissl substance is fundamentally composed of small granules, which are either scattered at random or appear in rosettelike formation, clusters, or compact aggregations or are arranged in rows alongside or around the granular or rough endoplasmic reticulum, and variously shaped loops, spirals, or lacunarlike formations and their ramifications, which were described as cisternae and, by Garnier,[59] as ergastoplasm (see Figure 1). Irrespective of the functional specificity of the neurons, the Nissl substance always appears composed of cisternae or endoplasmic reticulum[132, 137] associated with small granules containing RNA. There are, however, noticeable differences in the degree or orientation of profiles of the ergastoplasm in various types of nerve cells. Electron microscope studies of small neurons and granule cells of the cerebellum, which do not show Nissl substance with the classical Nissl stain, disclose the presence of an endoplasmic reticulum associated with granules similar to those of larger or other neurons. Histochemically, the Nissl substance is composed principally of nucleoproteins (RNA) and contains masked iron.[33, 105, 124, 132, 151] Microincineration studies revealed that Nissl bodies represent the highest concentration of inorganic ash in the cytoplasm.[2, 176]

For many years cytologists have been aware that living cells contain a number of pleomorphic and heterogeneous structural components and have speculated about their possible physicochemical character (enzymes, organic or inorganic catalysts, and so forth) and intracellular metabolic functions (proteins, carbohydrates, lipids, and electrolytic colloidal systems). As new techniques are developed, closer cooperation between biochemists and cytologists appears necessary in order to reevaluate and reappraise the new findings, as, for instance, in the case of differential centrifugation. With this latter procedure, Claude[35] attempted to study the appearance, composition, and activity of subcellular components. As a result of such studies, the microsome fraction was isolated. Subsequent investigations have revealed that the microsomes are derived largely through fragmentation of ergastoplasm, ribonuclear protein granules,[185] and endoplasmic reticulum.[134] They also appear to be contaminated by other subcellular constituents. Therefore, extreme caution must be used in the interpretation of the biochemical results.

Microsome fractions coupled with suitable tracer techniques have revealed their role in certain mechanisms of protein metabolism and protein synthesis in the cytoplasm.[25, 87, 88, 92, 99] In addition, some authors[3, 4] have demonstrated that amino acid incorporation into microsomal proteins requires presence of ribonucleic acids.

Pathological Correlates or Interactions. The mitochondrial and PMS alterations could be summarized as qualitative (changes in shape and size, matrix, cristae, limiting membranes, and variable metamorphoses) and quantitative (topographic distribution and numerical variation) in character as well as of a histochemical nature. In order not to deviate from the main purpose of this discussion, for more detailed information the reader is referred to references 107 and 156. For similar reasons, consult references 154 and 161 for multivesicular bodies (MVB) and endoplasmic reticulum, respectively.

The pathological alteration of lysosomes is summarized in Table 2.

The study of the function and metabolic mechanisms of many subcellular structures has also reached the molecular organization.[52, 75, 85, 131, 139, 145, 210, 216, 217] In addition to previously indicated observations, recent investigations of antimetabolites, pharmacodynamic drugs affecting in particular the central nervous system and the molecular heterogeneity and evolution of enzymes are also of particular significance in the study of cytometabolic mechanism. For instance, Wooley in particular[212] has emphasized that biological functioning of diverse kinds of metabolic substances can be antagonized by the presence of other compounds closely related in chemical structure to them. These antagonistic structural analogues have been called "antimetabolites." Although they are frequently synthetic compounds (produced in the laboratory), they may at times occur naturally. For instance, if the S atom of thiamine B_1 is replaced by a venyl group (—CH:CH—), an agent, pyrithiamine, is produced that is antagonistic to thiamine. If small doses of pyrithiamine are given to mice on an adequate diet of highly purified rations of known thiamine content, symptoms resembling vitamin B_1 deficiency are produced.[213] Examples among naturally occurring compounds are indole, an antimetabolite of tryptophane, and 4-hydroxy-coumarin (sweet clover hay spoils), an antimetabolite of vitamin K.

Coenzyme analogues may also be useful for research investigations related to evolution, classification, and differentiation of enzymes. Kaplan et al.,[96] in studying the molecular heterogeneity and evolution of enzymes, observed that a group of dehydrogenases (TPNH, DPNH, or diamino DPNH) of the lactic acid type shows different substrate saturation curves with different coenzyme analogues and also shows the general property of substrate inhibition, which appears to vary quantitatively. There seems to be a distinct difference between the heart and muscle lactate dehydrogenases in the same species with regard to pyrurate saturation. The lactic dehydrogenases from the flat fish utilize the acetylpyridine analogue much better than they do the thionicotinamide analogue; this is in complete contrast to what occurs in the mammalian enzymes. These data indicate individual as well as species differentiation, which is expressed not only by morphologic and physiologic characteristics but also by their enzymatic properties. Therefore, these findings also may have significance in establishing whether changes in certain peptide chains or molecular orientation of some enzyme structures have been modified during tissue differentiation of the individual and/or as well as during species evolution.

In the course of recently used chemotherapies for treatment of mental diseases, it has been observed that they affect in various manner different functions and structures of the central nervous system.[165, 211] Similarly, some of these drugs may influence the neural metabolism[121, 166, 211] by producing a diminished supply of glucose, interfering with glycolysis, interfering with oxidation, uncoupling oxidation from phosphorylation of low-energy adenylic acid and ADP, interfering with utilization of ATP in the acetylcholine cycle or some action on the protein acceptor for the free acetylcholine in the neuronal membrane, indirect effects on the metabolism of amino acids or fats, the products of which enter the tricarboxylic acid cycle or modify the rates of turnover within it. Furthermore, recent research is aiming at separating from organs or tissue homogenates individual morphologically distinguishable components by ultracentrifugation or differential centrifugation[35, 72, 166, 172, 173, 174] in order to isolate components that are specific sites of chemical action and to establish a more specific metabolic relationship. In the evaluation of such findings, one must keep in mind the previously mentioned dependence of enzymatic functions on structural integrity. Subcellular structure obtained by differential or ultracentrifugation combined with some cytochemical and electron microscopic studies may clarify even more precisely the understanding of the cytophysiological mechanisms at the molecular level. For instance, although the ultimate site of action is the molecule itself, however, in order to establish the functional relationship of the action of the chemical substance, the molecular organization must be confined within the unit defined by the cytological structure.

CNS SYNAPSES

The gradual affirmation of the contiguity theory[32, 55, 85] over reticular,[62, 64] the assertion of the neuronal concept[201] and dynamic polarization of the neuron,[33] the demonstration of the characteristic boutons,[6, 30, 71] the studies on neural conduction and transmission,[49] and the investigations of the special properties of the reflex arc[177] lead to the development of the structural-functional concept of the synapses. The subsequent microscopic description of the neuromuscular junction of vertebrates, the various types of the synapses in the CNS, sympathetic ganglia, and neuropile in vertebrates, the giant synapses in the squid stellate ganglion, and so on, have disclosed that these organelles consist of a remarkably diversified structural organization. However, more recent electrophysiological, histochemical, and particularly electron microscope investigations indicate that these different types of synapses have a specific ultrastructural and functional uniformity that is principally correlated with the operation of the action potential of the nervous system.[48, 50] Because of space limitations, I will restrict my discussion only to a few basic aspects of the structural, functional, and pathologic aspects of the CNS synapses.

The synapses, in relation with their contacts with the neurons (see Figures 1 and 3) and their processes, have been defined as axosomatic (surface of the perikaryon), axodendritic, and axo-axonic, respectively. Furthermore, on the basis of current electron microscope observations, the fine structural organization of the synaptic organelle, or complex, consists of a presynaptic terminal, synaptic cleft, postsynaptic membrane, subsynaptic web, and, in certain regions, the synaptic spine apparatus (dendrite spines[23, 48, 50, 71]).

The presynaptic terminal (axon terminal), which corresponds to the old terms, "bouton," "bulb," or "synaptic knob," contains principally synaptic vesicles that are frequently intermixed with tubules (neurotubules), vacuoles, mitochondria (PMS), and multivesicular bodies (MVB). Among these ultrastructural compo-

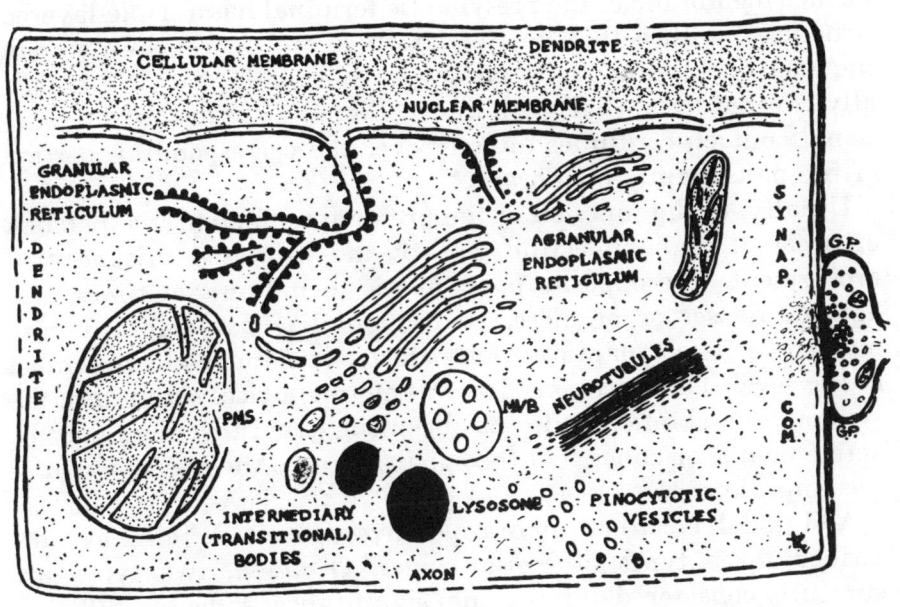

FIGURE 3

Schematic outline of various basic membrane systems of a neuron as described in the text. The location, orientation, and dimensions are arbitrary for illustrative purposes.

nents particular attention has been focused on the synaptic vesicles.[7, 23, 48, 50, 71, 123, 206, 209] They are said to contain the transmitter substances, or the neurochemical mediator. Although some finer details are still disputed, fundamentally there is common agreement that, in morphologic terms, the synaptic vesicles may vary in shape, size, concentration, and distribution within the presynaptic terminal.

In accordance with the profiles of their shape, the synaptic vesicles have been classified as circular or spheroid or S-type (Figure 4A); tubular or flattened or F-type (Figure 4B); and granular type (Figure 4C). The latter contains an electron-dense material that biochemically has been identified with catecholamines. In functional terms, it has been suggested[23] that the S-type is of an excitatory or stimulating character and the F-type inhibitory.

Furthermore, in biochemical terms, the cholinergic-containing vesicles have been named C-type, whereas the adrenergic and the catecholamine (as aforementioned) are called A-type. Because there is no space available for a thorough discussion, it should be kept in mind that, at times, two and even three types of vesicles could be encountered in the same presynaptic terminal.[157] The surface membrane of the presynaptic terminal has a triple-layered structure[48] with a thickness of 50–70 Å and in continuity with the axon membrane. This surface membrane in the CNS is usually covered by a glial membrane (Figure 3). This, at the junctional contact, continues directly over the corresponding portion of the postsynaptic membrane.*

Usually, at the junction of the presynaptic membrane, patches, or areas of higher electron density and increased thickness,[48, 7] are present. The opposite postsynaptic membrane, at times, also appears denser or of increased osmiophilia† as compared with either site. The synaptic vesicles cluster and make closer contact at this level. These are considered as morphological subunits of the synaptic membrane. It also has been suggested that they may be active points, or zones,[38] of the synapse where the transmission of the impulse occurs.

Additional electron microscope investigations[48, 50, 71] have described three types of denser zones. Of these, two types are currently considered of functional significance. Type 1 is differentiated from type 2[71] by its wider synaptic cleft (300 Å to 200 Å

---

* Small glial processes interposed between two membranes with only some partial obstruction of the direct contact have also been noted.[135]

† These electron microscope features seem to be very similar to desmonal contacts.

for type 2), thicker and denser postsynaptic membrane (this is much more extensive and occupies the greater part of the opposing synaptic membrane), and the presence in the cleft of a band of extracellular material that is nearer to the postsynaptic membrane. It is also of significance to note the selectivity in distribution and function of these two types of synapses.[48, 50, 71, 103, 138, 195]

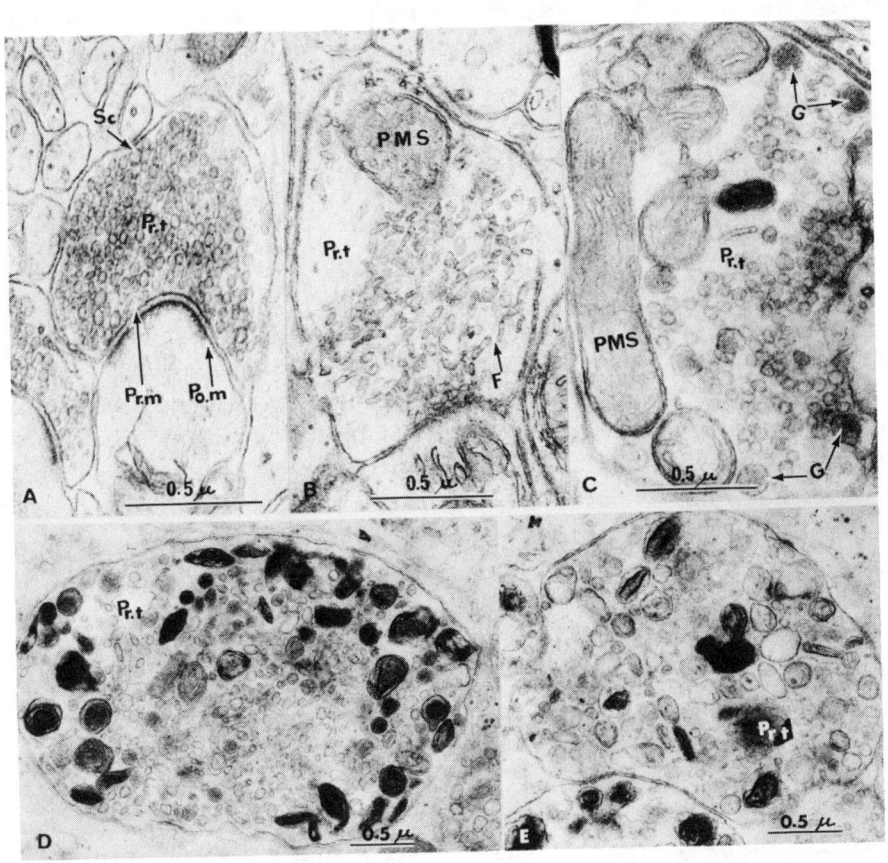

FIGURE 4
Demonstrative examples of CNS synapses as described in the text:
  A. (4, 652) *Cerebral cortex, rat, magnification 60, 200 ×;*
  B. (5, 761) *Spinal Cord, rat, magnification 54, 288 ×;*
  C. (5, 688) *Brainstem, rat, magnification 54, 288 ×;*
  D. (6, 464) *Frontal biopsy, human, magnification 28, 375;*
  E. (6, 465) *Frontal biopsy, human, magnification 36, 888.*

Abbreviations: Pr.t = presynaptic terminal; Pr.m = presynaptic membrane; Po.m = postsynaptic membrane; Sc = synaptic vesicle, circular type; F = tubular or flat-type of synaptic vesicles; G = granular type of synaptic vesicles; PMS = pleomorphometabolosomes or mitochondria.

The third type of membrane thickening is represented by a symmetrical density of the opposite membranes of an unchanged synaptic cleft. The synaptic cleft (about 120 Å–300 Å) is the interspace between the pre- and postsynaptic membranes. Recent investigations have also revealed the presence of intersynaptic filaments (about 50 Å), which form regular parallel patterns across the cleft at intervals of about 100 Å. These macromolecular structures of extracellular appearance are assumed to provide an adhesive contact or special anchorage mechanism to the opposite membranes at the synaptic junction.

The synaptic web[48] consists of a web of fine filaments, or cannaliculi, of 80Å. They extend from the postsynaptic membrane for varying distance (1500 Å or more) into the postsynaptic region.

The width of this web may vary among synapses and even at different parts of the same synapse. The significance of the subsynaptic web is still in the speculative stage. However, in view of the location in the subsynaptic region, it is suspected of being a specialized histochemical receptor zone for the transmitter substances released at the presynaptic terminal. The spine apparatus is another characteristic subsynaptic unit located in the postsynaptic[5, 71, 79, 208] depths of dentritic spines in the neocortex and hippocampus of mammalians.[103, 138] The significance of this specialized ultrastructure, as in the case of the intersynaptic filaments and subsynaptic web, is uncertain. Some investigators suggest[186] that because of its very selective location (as aforementioned), it may be related with processes of learning and memory.

Several investigators have noted glial processes beyond the synaptic junction and over the presynaptic terminal.[48, 136] This relationship is assumed to represent some kind of synaptic glial barrier, or perisynaptic barrier. According to some authors,[48] this barrier is mediated by astroglia similarly to the blood-brain-barrier (BBB) and the liquor-brain-barrier (LBB). Moreover, it is assumed that it is a protective device for the diffusion of the transmitter substance and ionic flux of the synaptic cleft as well as a shield for the underlying subsynaptic receptor from pharmacologic agents applied in the vicinity of synapses.

From a functional point of view, the electrical and chemical hypotheses of the transmission of the synaptic action across the synaptic membranes have been periodically disputed. Although the former mechanism appears to predominate, the latter has been also demonstrated for both,[45, 50, 79] the inhibitory as well as the excitatory synapses.

From a review of the current literature, it appears that the physiological operation of the synapses is mediated or regulated by its ultrastructural subunits and histochemical correlates in the following manner:

1. The nervous impulse or the action potential (bioelectrical current) induces the discharge from the synaptic vesicles of a transmitter substance, or neurochemical mediator (acetylcholine, noradrenaline, gammabutyric acid, and, possibly, 5-hydroxy tryptamine) that moves across the presynaptic membrane (active zone).

2. The quantum molecules of the transmitter substance, by coupling (anchoring) to the specific chemoreceptor of the postsynaptic membrane, causes an alteration of its polarization (depolarization or hyperpolarization).

3. The consequent increase in ionic flux (electrochemical gradients) creates the synaptic potential across the postsynaptic membrane into the subsynaptic region (web).

4. The effects of the transmitter substance is checked or terminated in the subsynaptic region (web) by the reaction of the correlated enzyme systems (acetylcholinesterase, monoaminoxydases, and so on).

Pathologic Aspects

Electron microscope alterations of the synapses and their respective subunits have been observed in some experimental conditions,[37, 39, 40, 98, 125, 164, 191, 200] and some human biopsies, for instance, in a case of psychomotor retardation[70] and a presenile psychosis.[158] Although no definite ultrastructural, electrophysiological, and histochemical correlations have been established in the aforementioned pathologic conditions, nonetheless the demonstration of qualitative and quantitative alterations of the synapses,[70, 164] the synaptic vesicles,[125, 164] the pre- and postsynaptic as well as the perisynaptic glial membranes, and the cleft[125, 164] would also imply concomitant involvement of their respective molecular patterns of organization. Furthermore, these initial pathologic observations, in the light of the previously discussed physiologic and biochemical activities of the synapses, seem to suggest that pathogenic mechanisms may occur as a result of malfunctioning of individual or combined intermediary phases of the synthesis (generation, development), storage, release, and transmission of the neurochemical mediator (transmitter substance), and/or propagation of the action potential. On this basis, the synapses, like the intracellular organelles, comply also with the principle of the integrated anatomofunctional synergism[154] in the sense that (1) each component part, through its reciprocal relationship, contributes to the same specific activity; (2) the character of each part is expressed through the chemical nature of constituent substances; (3) the specific pattern of the arrangement of the parts is of greater functional significance than the chemical nature of the individual components; and (4) the alteration of any structural component is synchronized with functional changes.

SOME BASIC STRUCTURAL-FUNCTIONAL AND PATHOGENIC ASPECTS OF MEMBRANE SYSTEMS

During recent years, the study of the structure and function of cell membranes or membranology has become one of the most debated and stimulating research topics. This is reflected in the enormous amount of cytologic, electron microscope, biophysical, biochemical or physicochemical publications.[109, 181] In brief, the elaborate membrane systems consist of "repeating units," or unit membranes.[149] Structurally, the basic patterns of the cellular membrane organization consist of single lamellae, or leaflets, which delineate the large variety of cytosomes, such as lysosomes, MVB, Golgi's intermediary or transitional structures, and pinocytotic vesicles, double lamellae, such as the nuclear membranes, the endoplasmic reticulum, and the mitochondrial, or PMS membranes (see Figure 3). The unit membrane concept proposed by J. D. Robertson[149] has evolved principally from the studies of the development of the myelin of the peripheral nerves and Davson-Danielli's model.[181] According to this concept, a unit membrane consists of a single bilayer of lipid with the nonpolar chains directed toward the center of the membrane and the polar ones outward. The latter are covered by unimolecular leaflets or films of nonlipids, or proteins. Thus, the outer surface of each membrane differs chemically from the inner and, therefore, the membrane is chemically an asymmetric structure. For details on the structure and molecular organization of the membrane systems as estimated by recent biophysical, physicochemical, and electron microscope investigations, the interested reader should refer also to references 109 and 181. Though improved or newly developed techniques and elaborate research procedures are aiming at defining the finer molecular configurations, current knowledge seems to indicate (in a simplified manner) that (1) the membrane systems enclose the cell and its organelles, compartmentalize their interior, structuralize the orderly arrangement of the enzyme assemblies, and channel the intermediary metabolites (secretory product) or histometabolic processes and (2) the properties of the membrane systems are expressed by the particular arrangement of the phospholipids (30 per cent) and protein (50 per cent) molecules. These are patterned in multiple species of repeating units (within a membrane system), and they serve as a miniaturized base for a characteristic spectrum of enzyme assemblies. Each enzyme in this membrane-bound metabolic process serves in a dual capacity as one of a group of catalysts in a sequential process and as an integral part of the membrane. Consequently, any alterations would result in concomitant changes of both the original metabolic function and the structural integrity of the membrane. A demonstrative example in support of this concept is briefly summarized in Table 2 and Figure 5, which

TABLE 2

Summary of the Structural, Chemical, and Functional Interdependence of the PMS or Mitochondrial Organelle, in Physiological Conditions

STRUCTURE	CHEMISTRY	FUNCTION
Outer and inner limiting membranes:	DPN, flavoproteins, cytochromes, E.C.E.	E.T.P., K inner membrane
Matrix:	Enzymes Krebs' and fatty ac. oxidation cycles	Oxidation Krebs' tricarboxylic ac. cycle; "respiratory assemblies", conversion of ADP in ATP; trans. H_2O and certain m.
Cristae:	Stratified proteins and phospholipid molecules	E. T. P., fatty ac. and some NH_2-ac. oxidation; oxidative phosphorylation

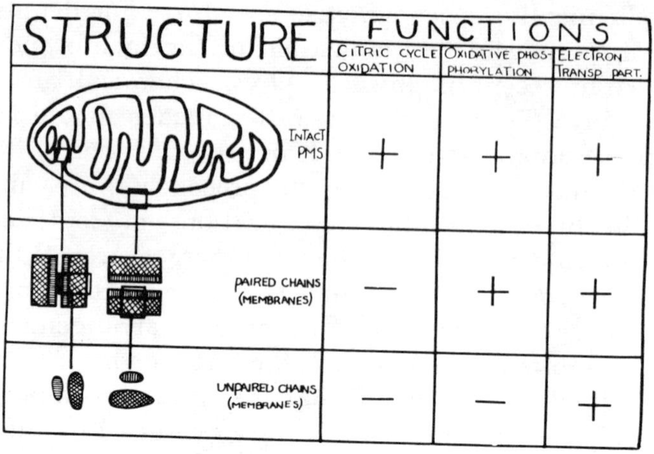

STRUCTURE	FUNCTIONS		
	CITRIC CYCLE OXIDATION	OXIDATIVE PHOSPHORYLATION	ELECTRON TRANSP. PART.
Intact PMS	+	+	+
Paired chains (membranes)	−	+	+
Unpaired chains (membranes)	−	−	+

FIGURE 5

Schematic illustration of the structural and metabolic interdependence of PMS membranes in various experimental conditions as described in the text.

illustrate the structural, functional, and histometabolic interdependency of mitochondrial subunits. It has been established that, when the mitochondria, or PMS, are damaged or disrupted,[73, 107] the enzyme assemblies of the citric cycle oxidations are apparently detached from the respective units and become water soluble. In these circumstances or when the fragmented organelles are composed principally of paired membranes, the citric cycle oxidative functions are altered or lost.

With subsequent fragmentation of the fine structural unpaired (single) membranes, the original functions of the disintegrated organelle are reduced only to the electron transport mechanisms (see Figure 4). It is also of significance that drugs may exert strong effects on organelles in situ (tissue) or in vitro[166] and on particular membrane-bound enzymes, but they may have nondemonstrable effect on the same enzyme after these have been separated or extracted from the membrane.[73] Thus, the membrane-enzyme associated systems represent the molecular basis of the histometabolism or the biological energy transformation in tissues. Their synergistic functions mediate the cybernetics* of the specialized histometabolic compartmentalized activities and regulate the flow of the living cellular energy. In association with these functions and, at times independently, some membrane varieties

* "A set of principles underlying communication information and operation of self-controlling mechanisms in either non-biological or biological systems."[108]

control the passage of electrolytic-colloidal systems and substrates, regulate the traffic of the intracellular metabolites, or direct the flux of the specialized energy transformation processes. These biological cycles involve fixation, release, transfer (translocation), and use of energy for synthesis, mechanical, digestive, secretory, bioelectrical, and similar activities. Recent investigations have also revealed that various biophysical, biochemical, and morbigenous agents can act as stabilizers or disorganizers of the membrane-bound enzyme.[21, 74, 108, 156]

CONCLUDING REMARKS

1. The organelles and the membrane units function as histochemical vectors and gradient systems at the ultracellular level of organization.

2. The diversified behavior of the cellular membranes stems not only from the structural organization of the molecular configuration but also from the interaction of their chemical components.

3. The physiological mechanisms of the organelles depend on the maintenance of the integrity of the membrane and the molecular relationship with its specialized structural architecture rather than on a particular molecule.

4. Consequently, a molecular disease or molecular pathology is not caused by a special pathologic molecule, but is the result of a mutation (genetic), disorder (biochemical and functional), or disruption (morphologic or biophysical) of a specific molecular pattern (arrangement) of the specialized structural organization.

5. The fine ultrastructural alterations of the synaptic subunits, in various experimental and pathologic conditions, demonstrate that pathogenic mechanisms in the CNS may result not only from intracellular abnormalities but also from alterations or dysfunctions of the intercellular communication systems.

REFERENCES

1. Abood, L. G., and Gerard, R. W. "A Phosphorylation Defect in the Brains of Mice Susceptible to Audiogenic Seizure," in H. Waelsch (ed.), *Biochemistry of the Developing Nervous System*. New York: Academic Press, 1955. P. 467.
2. Alexander, L., and Myerson, A. "Minerals in Normal and Pathologic Brain Tissue, Studies by Micro-incineration and Spectroscopy," *Archives of Neurology and Psychiatry*, 39 (1938), 131.

3. Alfrey, V. G., Daley, M. M., and Mirsky, A. E. "Synthesis of Protein in the Pancreas: II. The Role of Ribonucleoprotein in Protein Synthesis," *Journal of General Physiology*, 37 (1953), 157.
4. Alfrey, V. G., and Mirsky, A. E. "Biochemical Properties of the Isolated Nucleus," in T. Hayashi (ed.), *Subcellular Particles*. New York: Ronald Press, 1959. P. 186.
5. Andersen, P., Blackstad, T. W., and Lomo, T. "Location and Identification of Excitatory Synapses on Hippocampal Pyramidal Cells," *Experimental Brain Research*, 1 (1966), 236.
6. Auerbach, L. "Nachtrag zu dem Aufsatz: Nervenendigung in den Centralorganen," *Neurologisches Zentralblatt*, 17 (1898), 445.
7. Bak, I. J. "The Ultrastructure of the Substantia Nigra and Caudate Nucleus of the Mouse and the Cellular Localization of Catecholamines," *Experimental Brain Research*, 3 (1967), 40.
8. Barnes, B. G., and Davis, J. M. "The Structure of Nuclear Pores in Mammalian Tissue," *Journal of Ultrastructure Research*, 3 (1959), 131.
9. Barnum, C. P., and Huseby, R. A. "Some Quantitative Analyses of the Particulate Fractions from Mouse Liver Cell Cytoplasm," *Archives of Biochemistry*, 14 (1948), 19.
10. Barr, M. L., and Bertram, E. G. "A Morphological Distinction between Neurones of the Male and Female, and the Behavior of the Nucleolar Satellite during Accelerated Nucleoprotein Synthesis," *Nature*, 163 (1949), 676.
11. Barr, M. L., Bertram, E. G., and Lindsay, H. A. "Morphology of Nerve Cell Nucleus, According to Sex," *Anatomical Record*, 107 (1950), 283.
12. Barr, M. L., and Hobbs, G. E. "Chromosomal Sex in Transvestites," *Lancet*, 1 (1954), 1109.
13. Barron, E. S. G., Miller, Z. B., and Bartlett, G. R. "Studies on Biological Oxidations: XXI. The Metabolism of Lung as Determined by a Study of Slices and Ground Tissue," *Journal of Biological Chemistry*, 171 (1947), 791.
14. Baur, E. "Das Wesen und die Erblichkeitsverhaltnisse der Varietates albomarginate hortvon pelargonium Zonale," *Verebungs*, 1 (1909), 330.
15. Beadle, G. W. "Genes and Chemical Reactions in Neurospora. The Concepts of Biochemical Genetics Began with Garrod's 'Inborn Errors' and Have Evolved Gradually," *Science*, 129 (1959), 1715.
16. Bearn, A. G. "Wilson's Disease: An Inborn Error of Metabolism with Multiple Manifestations," *American Journal of Medicine*, 22 (1957), 747.
17. Beneden, E. van. "Recherches sur la Composition et la Signification de l'Oeuf," in *Mémoires Couronnés et Mémoires de Savants Étrangers*. Brussels: l'Académie Royale des Sciences, des Lettres et des Beaux-Arts de Belgique, 34 (1868).
18. Bennett, S. H. "The Role of Histology in Medical Education and Biological Thinking," *Anatomical Record*, 125 (1956), 327.
19. Bernhard, W., and Oberling, C. "Electron Microscopy of the Malignant Cell with Special Reference to Viruses," in *Canadian Cancer Conference*. New York: Academic Press, 1957. Vol. 2, p. 59.
20. Biesele, J. J. "Chromosome Complexity in Regenerating Rat Liver," *Cancer Research*, 4 (1944), 737.
21. Bitensky, L. "The Reversible Activation of Lysosomes in Normal Cells and Effects of Pathological Conditions," in A. V. S. de Rueck and M. P. Cameron (eds.), *Lysosomes*. Boston: Little, Brown, 1963. P. 362.
22. Bodenstein, D., and Gillette, R. "Reports of the Medical Division—Chemical Warfare Service," *Bulletin of the U.S. Army Medical Department*. Pennsylvania: Book Shop Medical Field Service School, Carlisle Barracks, 1945.
23. Bodian, D. "Synaptic Types on Spinal Motoneurons: An Electron Microscopic Study." *Bulletin of the Johns Hopkins Hospital*, 119 (July 1966), 16.
24. Bodian, D., and Mellors, R. C. "Renerative Cycle of Motoneurons, with Special Reference to Phosphatase Activity," *Journal of Experimental Medicine*, 8 (1945), 469.
25. Borsook, H., Deasy, C. L., Haagen-Smith, A. J., Keighley, G., and Lowy, P. H. "Metabolism of C^{14} Labeled Glycine, L-histidine, L-leucein and L-lycine." *Journal of Biological Chemistry*, 187 (1950), 839.
26. Borysko, E. Quoted by W. S. Vincent. "Structure and Chemistry of Nucleoli," *International Review of Cytology*, 4 (1955), 269.

27. Bourne, G. "Mitochondria and Golgi Apparatus," in G. Bourne (ed.), *Cytology and Cell Physiology*. London: Oxford University Press, 1942. P. 99.
28. Brachet, J. *Chemical Embryology*. New York: Interscience, 1950.
29. Brachet, J. "Ribonucleic Acids and the Synthesis of Cellular Proteins," *Nature*, 186 (1960), 194.
30. Cajal, S. R. "Réponse à M. Golgi à propos des fibrilles collatérales de la moelle épinière, et de la structure générale de la substance grise," *Anatomischer Anzeiger*, 5 (1890), 579.
31. Cajal, S. R. *Les nouvelles idées sur la structure du système nerveux chez l'homme et chez les vertebres*. Paris: Reinwald, 1895.
32. Cajal, S. R. "Les preuves objectives de l'unite anatomiques des cellules nerveuses," *Trabajos del Instituto Cajal de Investigaciones Biológicas* (Madrid), 29 (1934), 1.
33. Caspersson, T. "Über den chemischen Aufbau der Strikturen des Zellkerns," *Skandinavisches Archiv für Physiologie*, Suppl. 8z. 73 (1936).
34. Catcheside, D. G. "The P-locus Position Effect in Cenothera," *Journal of Genetics*, 48 (1947), 31.
35. Claude, A. "Fractionation of Mammalian Liver Cells by Differential Centrifugation: Problems, Methods, and Preparation of Extract," *Journal of Experimental Medicine*, 84 (1946), 51.
36. Colonnier, M. "Experimental Degeneration in the Cerebral Cortex," *Journal of Anatomy*, 98 (January 1964), 47.
37. Colonnier, M., and Guillery, R. W. "Synaptic Organization in the Lateral Geniculate Nucleus of the Monkey," *Zeitschrift für Zellforschung und Mikroskopische Anatomie*, 62 (1964), 333.
38. Correns, C. "Verebungsversuche mit blass (Gelb grunen und buntblattrigen Sippen bei Mirabilis, Julapa, Urtica Pilulifera und Lunaria Annua," *Zeitschrift für Vererbungslehre*, 1 (1909), 291.
39. Couteaux, R. "Morphological and Cytochemical Observations on the Post-Synaptic Membrane at Motor End-Plates and Ganglionic Synapses," *Experimental Cell Research*, 5, Suppl. (1958), 294.
40. Davidova, T. V. "Some Findings of the Synaptic Organization of the Cerebral Cortex of the Brain of the Turtle" (Russian), *Proceedings of the U.S.S.R. Academy of Sciences*, 155, no. 4 (1964), 970.
41. De Duve, C. "Lysosomes, a New Group of Cytoplasmic Particles," in T. Hayashi (ed.), *Subcellular Particles*. New York: Ronald Press, 1959. P. 128.
42. De Duve, C. "The Separation and Characterization of Subcelluar Particles," *The Harvey Lectures*, 59 (1965), 49.
43. Deitch, A. D., and Moses, M. J. "An Untraviolet Absorption Study," *Journal of Biophysical and Biochemical Cytology*, 2 (1956), 433.
44. Deitch, A. D., and Murray, M. R. "The Nissl Substance of Living and Fixed Spinal Ganglion Cells: 1. A Phase Contrast Study," *Journal of Biophysical and Biochemical Cytology*, 2 (1956), 433.
45. De Lorenzo, A. J. "Electron Microscopy: Tight Junctions in Synapses of the Chick Ciliary Ganglion," *Science*, 152 (1966), 76.
46. Denues, A. R. T. "Chromosomes: Their Constitution and Function," in S. L. Palay (ed.), *Frontiers in Cytology*. New Haven: Yale University Press, 1958. P. 42.
47. Derlin, T. M., and Lehninger, A. L. "Oxidative Phosphorylation by an Enzyme Complex from Extracts of Mitochondria: II. The Span B Hydroxybutyrate to Cytochrome C," *Journal of Biological Chemistry*, 219 (1956), 507.
48. De Robertis, E. D. P. *Histophysiology of Synapses and Neurosecretion*. New York: Macmillan, 1964.
49. Du Bois-Reymond, E. "Gesammelte Abhandlung der allgemeine," *Muskel- und Nervenphysik*, 2 (1877), 700.
50. Eccles, J. C. *The Physiology of Synapses*. New York: Academic Press, 1964.
51. Edmonds, M., and Abrams, R. "Incorporation of ATP into Polynucleotide in Extracts of Ehrlich Ascites Cells," *Biochimica et Biophysica Acta*, 26 (1957), 226.
52. Engstrom, A., and Finean, J. B. *Biological Ultrastructure*. New York: Academic Press, 1958.
53. Felix, F. In R. E. Zirkle (ed.), "Some Principles of Molecular Biology," in *A Symposium on Molecular Biology*. Chicago: The University of Chicago Press, 1959. P. 1.

54. Ferraro, A., and Roizin, L. "Essential Amino-Acid Deficiency, Clinico-pathologic Findings in Rats: II. Valine," *Journal of Neuropathology and Experimental Neurology*, **4** (1947), 383.
55. Forel, A. "Einige hirnanatomische betrachtungen und ergebnisse," *Archiv für Psychiatrie und Nervenkrankheiten vereinigt mit Zeitschrift für die Gesamte Neurologie und Psychiatrie*, **18** (1887), 162.
56. Frantz, I. D., Jr., Zamecnick, P. C., Reese, J. W., and Stephenson, M. L. "The Effect of Dinitrophenol on the Incorporation of Alanine Labeled with Radioactive Carbon into the Proteins of Slices of Normal and Malignant Rat Liver," *Journal of Biological Chemistry*, **174** (1948), 773.
57. Freeman, J. A. "The Ultrastructure of the Double Membrane System of Mitochondria," *Journal of Biophysical and Biochemical Cytology*, **2**, Suppl. 4 (1956), 337.
58. Frey, W. A. *Submicroscopic Morphology of Protoplasm*. New York: Elsvier, 1953.
59. Garnier, G. "Contribution à l'étude de la structure et du fonctionnement des cellules gladulaires, sereuses: Du role de l'ergastoplasme dans la secretion," *Journal Anatomie et Physiologie*, **36** (1900), 22.
60. Garrod, A. E. "The Croonian Lectures on Inborn Errors of Metabolism," *Lancet*, **11** (1908), 1, 73, 142, 214.
61. Garrod, A. E. *Inborn Errors in Metabolism*. 2d ed.; Oxford: Oxford University Press, 1923.
62. "Genetics and the Inheritance of Integrated Neurological and Psychiatric Patterns," *Research Publications of the Association of Nervous and Mental Diseases*. Baltimore: William & Wilkins, 1954. Vol. 33.
63. Gerch, I., and Bodian, D. "Histochemical Analysis of Changes in Rhesus Motoneurons after Root Section," *Biological Symposia*, **10** (1943), 163.
64. Gerlach, J. von. "Von dem Ruckenmarke," in S. Stricker (ed.), *Handbuch der Lehre von den Geweben des Menschen und der Thiere*. Unter Mitwirking von J. Arnold, Babuchi, [et. al.] hrsg. von . . . 2d ed.; Leipzig, 1871.
65. Gibson, Q. M. "Reduction of Methemoglobin in Red Blood Cells and Studies on the Cause of Idiopathic Methemoglobinima," *Biochemical Journal*, **42** (1948), 13.
66. Gluecksohn-Waelsch, S. "Genetic Factors and the Development of the Nervous System," in H. Waelsch (ed.), *Biochemistry of the Developing Nervous System*. New York: Academic Press. 1955. P. 375.
67. Goddard, D. R. "The Respiration of Cells and Tissues," in R. Höber, D. I. Hitchcock, J. B. Bateman, D. R. Goddard, and W. O. Fenn (eds.), *Physical Chemistry of Cells and Tissues*. Philadelphia: The Blakiston Company, 1945. P. 371.
68. Goddard, D. R. "Introduction," in J. Brachet and A. E. Mirsky (eds.), *The Cell: Biochemistry, Physiology, and Morphology*. New York: Academic Press, 1959. Vol. 1, p. xv.
69. Golgi, C. "Über den feineren bau des ruckenmarkes," *Anatomischer Anzeiger*, **5** (1890), 372.
70. Gonātas, N. K., Evangelista, I., and Walsh, G. O. "Axonic and Synaptic Changes in a Case of Psychomotor Retardation: An Electron Microscopic Study," *Journal of Neuropathology and Experimental Neurology*, **26** (1967), 179.
71. Gray, E. G., and Guillery, R. W. "Synaptic Morphology in the Normal and Degenerating Nervous System," *International Review of Cytology*, **19** (1966), 111.
72. Green, D. G. "Mitochondrial Structure and Function," in T. Hayashi (ed.), *Subcellular Particles*. New York: Ronald Press, 1959. P. 84.
73. Green, D. E., and Fleischer, S. "On the Molecular Organization of Biological Tranducing Systems," in M. Kasha and B. Pullman (eds.), *Horizons of Biochemistry*. New York: Academic Press, 1962. P. 381.
74. Green, D. E., and Goldberger, R. G. *Molecular Insights into the Living Process*. New York: Academic Press, 1967.
75. Grenell, R. G., and Mullins, L. J. (eds.). *Molecular Structure and Functional Activity of Nerve Cells*. Washington, D.C.: A.I.B.S., 1956.
76. Hogeboom, G. N., Schneider, V. C., and Palade, G. E. "Cytochemical Studies of Mammalian Tissues: I. Isolation of Intact Mitochondria from Rat Liver; Some Biochemical Properties of Mitochondria and Submicroscopic Particulate Material," *Journal of Biological Chemistry*, **172** (1948), 619.

77. Haldane, J. B. S. *The Biochemistry of Genetics.* London: Allen & Unwin, 1954.
78. Ham, A. W. *Histology.* 3d ed.; Philadelphia: Lippincott, 1957.
79. Hama, K. "Some Observations on the Fine Structure of the Synapses," in S. Seno and E. V. Cowdry (eds.), *Intracellular Membranous Structure.* Okayama, Japan: Cell Biology, 1965. P. 539.
80. Hamlyn, L. H. "The Fine Structure of the Mossy Fibre (sic) Endings in the Hippocampus of the Rabbit," *Journal of Anatomy* (London), **96** (1962), 112.
81. Harris, H. *Novant' Anni delle Leggi Mendeliane.* Rome: Instituto Gregorio Mendel, 1956. P. 206.
82. Held, H. Die Entwicklung des Nervengewebes. S. 378. Leipzig, 1909.
83. Hevesy, G. *Radioactive Indicators: Their Application in Biochemistry, Animal Physiology and Pathology.* New York: Interscience, 1948.
84. Hicks, P. S., De Harport, E. C., Johnson, L. A., and Brown, B. L. "The Neurochemical Significance of Experimentally Induced Malformations in Mammals," in H. Waelsch (ed.), *Biochemistry of the Developing Nervous System.* New York: Academic Press, 1955. P. 491.
85. His, W. "Die neuroblasten und deren entstehung im embryonalem Mark," *Abhandlungen Mathematisch-Physische, Klasse Akademie der Wissenschaften,* **15** (1889), 311.
86. Hoagland, M. B. "Nucleic Acids and Proteins," *Scientific American,* **201** (1959), 55.
87. Hoagland, M. B., Stephenson, M. L., Scott, J. F., Hecht, L. I., and Zamecnik, P. C. "A Soluble Ribonucleic Acid Intermediate in Protein Synthesis," *Journal of Biological Chemistry,* **231** (1958), 241.
88. Hoagland, M. B., Zamecnik, P. C., and Stephenson, M. L. "Intermediate Reactions in Protein Biosynthesis," *Biochimica et Biophysica Acta,* **24** (1957), 215.
89. Hollander, A., and Emmons, C. W. "Wave Length Dependence of Mutation Production in the Ultraviolet with Special Emphasis on Fungi," *Cold Spring Harbor Symposia on Quantitative Biology,* **9** (1949), 179.
90. Hoskins, R. G., and Pincus, G. "Sex-Hormone Relationships in Schizophrenic Men," *Psychosomatic Medicine,* **9** (1949), 102.
91. Howe, H. A., and Mellors, R. C. "Cytochrome Oxidase in Normal and Regenerating Neurons," *Journal of Experimental Medicine,* **81** (1945), 489.
92. Hultin, T. "Incorporation in Vivo of ^{15}N-labeled Glycine into Liver Fractions of Newly Hatched Chicks," *Experimental Cell Research,* **1** (1950), 376.
93. Hultin, T. "The Incorporation in Vitro of L-C^{14} Glycine into Liver Proteins Visualized as a Two-Step Reaction," *Experimental Cell Research,* **11** (1956), 222.
94. Hyden, H. "Protein Metabolism in the Nerve Cells during Growth and Function," *Acta Physiologica Scandinavica,* **6**, suppl. 17 (1943), 1.
95. Johanssen, W. L. Quoted by P. Suner in C. M. Stern (trans.), *Classics of Histology.* New York: Philosophical Library, 1955.
96. Kaplan, N. O., Ciott, M. M., Hamolsky, M., and Beiber, R. E. "Molecular Heterogeneity and Evolution of Enzymes," *Science,* **131** (1960), 392.
97. Kautz, J., and De Marsh, Q. B. "Fine Structure of the Nuclear Membrane in Cells from the Chick Embryo: On the Nature of the So-called 'Pores' in the Nuclear Membrane," *Experimental Cell Research,* **8** (1955), 394.
98. Kimura, R., and Wersall, J. "Termination of the Olivocochlear Bundle in Relation to the Outer Hair Cells of the Organ of Corti in Guinea Pig," *Acta Oto-Laryngologica,* **55** (1962), 11.
99. Keller, E. B., and Zamecnik, P. C. "The Effect of Guanosine Diphosphate and Triphosphate on the Incorporation of Labeled Amino Acids into Proteins," *Journal of Biological Chemistry,* **221** (1956), 45.
100. Koelliker, R. A. *Mikroskopische Anatomie und Gewebelehre der Menschen.* Leipzig: Engelman, 1852.
101. Koelliker, R. A. Quoted by S. H. Bennett, "The Role of Histology in Medical Education and Biological Thinking," *Anatomical Record,* **125** (1956), 327.
102. Koizumi, J., Roizin, L., and Pool, J. L. "Electron Microscopy of the Reactive Astrocytes and Their Vascular Walls Adjacent to Human Brain Tumors and Control Materials," *Proceedings of the Sixth International Congress of Electron Microscopists.* Kyoto, Japan, 1966. P. 479.

103. Komori, J., and Szentagothai, J. "Identification under the Electron Microscope of Climbing Fibers and Their Synaptic Contacts," *Experimental Brain Research*, 1 (1966), 65.
104. Korr, I. M. "The Relation between Cellular Metabolism and Physiological Activity," *American Journal of Physiology*, 133 (1941), 355.
105. Landstrom, H., Caspersson, T., and Wohlfast, G. "Über den Nucleotidumsatz der Nervenzelle," *Zeitschrift für Mikroskopisch-Anatomische Forschung*, 49 (1941), 534.
106. Lederberg, J. "Genes and Antibodies. Do Antibodies Bear Instructions for Antibody Specificity or Do They Select Cell Lines That Arise by Mutation?" *Science*, 129 (1959), 1649.
107. Lehninger, A. L. *The Mitochondrion: Molecular Basis of Structure and Function.* New York: Benjamin, 1964.
108. Lehninger, A. L. *Bioenergetics: The Molecular Basis of Biological Energy Transformations.* New York: Benjamin, 1965.
109. Loewry, A. G., and Siekevitz, P. *Cell Structure and Function.* New York: Holt, Rinehart & Winston, 1963.
110. Luse, S. A. "Electron Microscopic Observations of the Central Nervous System," *Journal of Biophysical and Biochemical Cytology*, 2 (1956), 531.
111. McCowan, P. K., and Quastel, J. M. "Blood-Sugar Studies in Abnormal Mental States," *Journal of Mental Science*, 77 (1931), 525.
112. McGibbon, W. H. "Cellular Antigens in Species and Species Hybrids in Ducks," *Genetics*, 29 (1944), 407.
113. MacKinney, G., and Jenkins, J. A. "Carotenoid Differences in Tomatoes," *Proceedings of the National Academy of Science*, 38 (1952), 48.
114. Mahler, H. R., Sarkar, N. K., and Vernon, L. P. "Studies on Diphosphopyridine Nucleotide Cytochrome with Reductase," *Journal of Biological Chemistry*, 199 (1952), 585.
115. March, H. C. "Leukemia in Radiologists," *Radiology*, 43 (1944), 275.
116. Mazia, D. "Nuclear Products and Nuclear Reproduction," in O. Gaebler (ed.), *Enzymes: Units of Biological Structure and Function.* New York: Academic Press, 1956. P. 261.
117. Meduna, L. J., Gerty, F. J., and Urse, V. G. "Biochemical Disturbances in Mental Disorders. 1. Anti-insulin Effect of Blood in Cases of Schizophrenia," *Archives of Neurology and Psychiatry*, 47 (1942), 38.
118. Morgan, T. H. *The Theory of the Gene.* New Haven: Yale University Press, 1928.
119. Mottram, J. C. "Abnormal Paramedia Produced by Blastogenic Agents and Their Bearing on Cancer Problems," *Cancer Research*, 1 (1941), 313.
120. Myassichtev, V. N., Goldin, L. C., and Bocova, V. V. "Electron Microscopy of Cerebral Cortex during Convulsions Induced by Electric Shock," *Zhurnal Neuropatologii i Psikhiatrii imeni S. S. Korsakova*, 59 (1959), 89.
121. Nachmanson, D. "Electrical Processes during Nerve Activity," in K. A. C. Elliot, H. Page, and J. H. Quastel (eds.), *Neurochemistry.* Springfield, Ill.: Charles C Thomas, 1955. P. 390.
122. Nageli, J. (1854) Quoted by P. Suner, in C. M. Stern (trans.), *Classics of Biology.* New York: Philosophical Library, 1955.
123. Nathaniel, E. J. H., and Nathaniel, D. R. "The Ultrastructural Features of the Synapses in the Posterior Horn of the Spinal Cord in the Rat," *Journal of Ultrastructure Research*, 14 (1966), 540.
124. Nicholson, F. M. "The Changes in Amount and Distribution of the Iron Containing Proteins of Nerve Cells Following Injury to Their Axons," *Journal of Comparative Neurology*, 36 (1923), 37.
125. Nishikawa, J., and Roizin, L., in *Proceedings of the Sixth International Congress of Electron Microscopists.* Kyoto, Japan: 1966. P. 441.
126. Northrop, J. H. "Enzymes and the Synthesis of Proteins," in A. K. Parpart (ed.), *The Chemistry and Physiology of Growth.* Princeton: Princeton University Press, 1949. P. 3.
127. Northrop, J. H., Kunitz, M., and Herriott, R. M. *Crystalline Enzymes.* 2d ed.; New York: Columbia University Press, 1952.
128. Novikoff, A. B. "Enzyme Localization and Ultrastructure of Neurons," in H. Hyden (ed.), *The Neuron.* New York: Elsevier, 1967.

129. Novikoff, A. B., Essner, E., and Quintana, N. "Golgi Apparatus and Lysosomes," *Federation Proceedings*, **23** (1964), 1010.
130. Nurnberger, J. I. "Clinical and Metabolic Effects of Exposure to Low Environmental Temperature on the C.N.S. and Related Visceral Structures. A Cytochemical Study," *Research Publications of the Association of Nervous and Mental Diseases*, **32** (1952), 132.
131. Oppenheimer, J. "Intercellular Activties in Vertebrate Development. Problems of Embryonic Organization Are Being Attacked at Subcellular, Cellular and Supracellular Levels," *Science*, **130** (1959), 686.
132. Palade, G. E. "The Endoplasmic Reticulum," *Journal of Biophysical and Biochemical Cytology*, **2** (1956), 85.
133. Palade, G. E. "Functional Changes in Structure of Cell Components," in T. Hayashi (ed.), *Subcellular Particles*. New York: Ronald Press, 1958.
134. Palade, G. E., and Porter, K. R. "The Endoplasmic Reticulum of Cells," *Anatomical Record*, **112** (1952), 370.
135. Palay, S. L. "The Morphology of Secretion," in S. L. Palay (ed.), *Frontiers of Cytology*. New Haven: Yale University Press, 1958. P. 305.
136. Palay, S. L. "The Morphology of Synapses in the Central Nervous System," *Experimental Cell Research*, **5**, suppl. (1958), 275.
137. Palay, S. L., and Palade, G. E. "The Fine Structure of Neurons," *Journal of Biophysical and Biochemical Cytology*, **1** (1955), 68.
138. Pappas, G. D., and Purpura, P. "Fine Structure of Dendrites in the Superficial Neocortical Neuropil," *Experimental Neurology*, **4** (1961), 507.
139. Pauling, L., and Itano, H. A. *Molecular Structure and Biological Specificity*. Washington, D.C.: A.I.B.S., 1957.
140. Penrose, L. L. "Inborn Errors of Metabolism in Relation to Mental Pathology," in K. A. C. Elliot, H. I. Page, and J. H. Quastel (eds.), *Neurochemistry*. Springfield. Ill.: Charles C Thomas, 1955. P. 807.
141. Porter, K. R. "The Biology of Myelin: Other Membrane Limited Structures of Cells," in S. R. Corey (ed.), *The Biology of Myelin*. New York: Hoeber, 1959.
142. Rabl, C. Quoted by P. Suner in C. M. Stern (trans.), *Classics of Biology*. New York: Philosophical Library, 1955.
143. Revel, J. P., Ito, S., and Fawcett, D. W. "Electron Micrographs of Myelin Figures of Phospholipide Simulating Intercellular Membranes," *Journal of Biophysical and Biochemical Cytology*, **4** (1958), 495.
144. Rhodin, J. *Correlation of Ultrastructural Organization and Function in Normal and Experimentally Changed Proximal Convoluted Tubule Cells of the Mouse Kidney*. Stockholm: Aktiebloget Godvil, 1954.
145. Rich, A. "The Bearing of Structural Studies on Relationships between DNA and RNA," in Zirkle, R. E. (ed.), *A Symposium on Molecular Biology*. Chicago: University Committee on publications in biology and medicine, 1959.
146. Richter, D., and Lee, M. H. "Serum Choline Esterase and Depression," *Journal of Mental Science*, **88** (1942), 435.
147. Robbins, E., Marcus, P. I., and Gonatas, N. K. "Dynamics of Acridine Orange Cell Interaction. II. Dye-induced Ultrastructural Changes in MVB Acridine Orange Particles," *Journal of Cell Biology*, **21** (1964), 49.
148. Robertson, J. D. "New Observations on the Ultrastructure of the Membranes of Frog Peripheral Nerve Fibers," *Journal of Biophysical and Biochemical Cytology*, **3** (1957), 1043.
149. Robertson, J. D. "The Membrane of the Living Cell," in D. Kennedy (ed.), *The Living Cell*. San Francisco: Freeman, 1962. P. 45.
150. Rhoads, C. P. "Neoplastic Abnormal Growth," in A. K. Parpart (ed.), *The Chemistry and Physiology of Growth*. Princeton: Princeton University Press, 1949. P. 217.
151. Roizin, L. "Comparative Morphologic and Histometabolic Studies of Nerve Cells in Brain Biopsies and Topectomies," *Journal of Neuropathology and Experimental Neurology*, **10** (1951), 177.
152. Roizin, L. "Extrapyramidal Syndrome Akin to Hallervorden-Spatz and Fahr Disease," *Transactions of the American Neurological Association*, **79** (1954), 56.
153. Roizin, L. "Neuropathology," in S. Arieti (ed.), *American Handbook of Psychiatry*. New York: Basic Books, 1959. Vol. 2, p. 1648.

154. Roizin, L. "A Review of Ultracellular Structures and Their Functions with Special Reference to Pathogenic Mechanism at a Molecular Level," *Journal of Neuropathology and Experimental Neurology*, **19** (1960), 591.
155. Roizin, L. "Mitochondria (Pleomorpho Metabolosomes) as Histometabolic Gradients (Effects of Prochlorperazine on the Rat Brain as Revealed by Electron Microscope)," *Diseases of the Nervous System*, **24** (1963), 61.
156. Roizin, L. "Some Basic Principles of 'Molecular Pathology': 3. Ultracellular Organelles as Structural-Metabolic and Pathogenetic Gradients," *Journal of Neuropathology and Experimental Neurology*, **23** (1964), 209.
157. Roizin, L., Kaufman, M. A., Caveness, W. F., and Carsten, A. L. "CNS Organellopathies: Four Fine Structural Changes of Synapses," *Journal of Neuropathology and Experimental Neurology*, **27** (1968), 150.
158. Roizin, L., Kaufman, M. A., Caveness, W. F., and Carsten, L. A. "Some Fundamental Principles of CNS Organellopathies," *Proceedings of the Second Pan American Congress of Neurology*, San Juan, Puerto Rico, 1968.
159. Roizin, L., and Kolb, L. C. "Considerations on the Neuropathologic Pleomorphism and Histogenesis of the Lesions of Experimental Allergic Encephalomyelitis in Non-human Species (Comparative Morphologic and Histochemical Studies)," in M. W. Kies and E. C. Alvold, Jr. (eds.), *Allergic Encephalomyelitis*. Springfield, Ill.: Charles C Thomas, 1959.
160. Roizin, L., and Nishikawa, K. "The Golgi Complex of the CNS: Anatomotopographic Studies Following Administration of Prochlorperazine (Compazine, SKF)," *Journal of Neuropathology and Experimental Neurology*, **24** (1965), 165.
161. Roizin, L. Nishikawa, K., and Koizumi, J. "MVB and Their Relationships to the Cellular Constituents of the CNS," *Journal of Neuropathology and Experimental Neurology*, **26** (1967), 159.
162. Roizin, L., Rugh, R., and Kaufman, M. A. "Effects of Ionizing Radiation on the Rat Embryo Central Nervous System at the Cellular and Ultra-cellular Levels," in T. J. Haley and R. S. Snider (eds.), *Response of the Nervous System to Ionizing Radiation*. Boston: Little, Brown, 1964. P. 146.
163. Roizin, L., Rugh, R., and Kaufman, M. A. "Irradiation Effects upon the Fetal Central Nervous System of Macacus Rhesus Monkeys, Effects of Lysosomes," *Acta radiologica* (Stockholm), **5** (1966), 161.
164. Roizin, L. and Schade, J. P. "V. Ultrastructural Findings," in "Pathogenesis of X-Irradiation Effects in the Monkey Cerebral Cortex," *Brain Research*, **7** (1968), 87.
165. Roizin, L., True, C., and Knight, M. "Structural Effects of Some Tranquilizing Drugs," *Research Publications of the Association of Nervous and Mental Diseases*, **37** (1959), 285.
166. Roizin, L., Wechsler-Berger, M., and Brock, D. "Ultracellular Functional and Pathogenic Mechanisms. V. In Vivo and in Vitro CNS and Liver Mitochondria, Following Administration of Phenothiazines," *Transactions of the American Neurological Association*, **89** (1964), 247.
167. "The Role of Nutritional Deficiency in Nervous and Mental Disease," *Research Publications of the Association of Nervous and Mental Diseases*. Baltimore: Williams & Wilkins, 1943. Vol. 22.
168. Rose, A. "Discussion of Metabolic and Toxic Diseases of the Nervous System," *Research Publications of the Association of Nervous and Mental Diseases*, **32** (1953), 294.
169. Rudnick, D. (ed.). *Developmental Cytology*. New York: Ronald Press, 1959.
170. Rugh, R., and Grupp, E. "Exencephalia Following X-Irradiation of the Preimplantation Mammalian Embryo," *Journal of Neuropathology and Experimental Neurology*, **18** (1958), 468.
171. Schmitt, F. O. "Ultrastructure of Nerve Myelin and Its Bearing on Fundamental Concepts of the Structure and Function of Nerve Fibers," in S. R. Korey (ed.), *The Biology of Myelin*. New York: Hoeber, 1959.
172. Schneider, W. C. "Structural Factors in Metabolic Regulations," *Proceedings of the Third International Congress of Biochemistry*. New York: Academic Press, 1956. P. 305.
173. Schneider, W. C., Claude, A., and Hogeboom, G. N. "The Distribution of Cyto-

chrome C and Succinoxidase Activity in Rat Liver Fractions," *Journal of Biological Chemistry*, **172** (1948), 451.
174. Schneider, W. C., and Hogeboom, G. M. "Intracellular Distribution of Succinoxidase and Cytochrome Oxidase Activities in Normal Mouse Liver and in Mouse Hepatoma," *Journal of the National Cancer Institute*, **10** (1950), 969.
175. Schultz, J. "Interrelation between Nucleus and Cytoplasm; Problems at the Biological Level," in "Symposium: The Chemistry and Physiology of the Nucleus," *Experimental Cell Research*, **2**, suppl. (1952), 17.
176. Scott, G. M. "The Localization of Mineral Salts in Cells of Some Mammalian Tissues by Micro-Incineration," *American Journal of Anatomy*, **53** (1933), 243.
177. Sherrington, C. S. *Integrative Action of the Nervous System*. New Haven: Yale University Press, 1906.
178. Sjostrand, F. S. "Electron Microscope of Mitochondria and Cytoplasmic Double Membranes," *Nature*, **171** (1953), 30.
179. Sjostrand, F. S. "Electron Microscopy of Cells and Tissues," in G. Oster and A. W. Pollister (eds.), *Physical Techniques in Biological Research*. New York: Academic Press, 1956. P. 241.
180. Sjostrand, F. S. "The Ultrastructure of Cells as Revealed by Electron Microscope," *International Review of Cytology*, **5** (1957), 455.
181. Snell, F., Shulman, S., Spencer, R. P., and Moos, C. *Biophysical Principles of Structure and Function*. Reading, Mass.: Addison-Wesley, 1965.
182. Snyder, L. M. "Fifty Years of Medical Genetics. The Union of Biochemistry and Genetics Offers a Rational Approach to Diagnosis, Prevention and Therapy," *Science*, **129** (1959), 7.
183. Sobotka, H. "Chemical Differentiation of Tay-Sachs Disease and Other Lipoidoses," *Journal of Mt. Sinai Hospital*, **9** (1942), 795.
184. Spillane, J. D. *Nutritional Disorders of the Nervous System*. Baltimore: Williams & Wilkins, 1947.
185. Stephenson, M. L. et al. "Intermediate Reactions in Protein Synthesis," in T. Hayashi (ed.), *Subcellular Particles*. New York: Ronald Press, 1959. P. 160.
186. Stowell, R. E., and Cooper, Z. K. "Relative Thymonucleic Acid Content of Human Normal Epidermis, Hyperplastic Epidermis and Epidermoid Carcinomas," *Cancer Research*, **4** (1944), 737.
187. Strasburger, E. A. *Das botanische Praktikum*. Jena: Fischer, 1884.
188. Tabechian, H., Altman, K. I., and Young, L. E. "Inhibition of P_{32}-Orthophosphate Exchange by Sodium Fluoride in Erythrocytes from Patients with Hereditary Spherocytosis," *Proceedings of the Society for Experimental Biology and Medicine*, **92** (1956), 712.
189. Tatum, E. L. "Induced Biochemical Mutations in Bacteria," *Cold Spring Harbor Symposia on Quantitative Biology*, **11** (1946), 278.
190. Tatum, E. L. "A Case History in Biological Research, Chance and the Exchange of Ideas Played Roles in the Discovery That Genes Control Biochemical Events," *Science*, **129** (1959), 1711.
191. Taxi, J. "Electron Microscope Study of Synaptic Areas in Various Ganglia of the Autonomic Nervous System of Some Vertebrates," in H. Jacob (ed.), *Proceedings of the Fourth International Congress of Neuropathology*. Stuttgart: George Thieme, 1962. P. 45.
192. Tayleur Stockings, G. *The Metabolic Brain Diseases and Their Treatment*. Baltimore: Williams & Wilkins, 1947.
193. Taylor, H. J., and Woods, P. S. "In Situ Studies of Polynucleotide Synthesis in Nucleolus and Chromosomes," in T. Hayashi (ed.), *Subcellular Particles*. New York: Ronald Press, 1959. P. 172.
194. Tedeschi, H. "The Structure of the Mitochondrial Membrane: Inference from Permeability Properties," *Journal of Biophysical and Biochemical Cytology*, **6** (1959), 241.
195. Thannhauser, S. J. *Lipidoses: Diseases of the Cellular Lipid Metabolism*. H. A. Christian (ed.), Oxford Looseleaf Medicine. 2nd ed.; New York: Oxford University Press, 1950.
196. Van Der Loos, H. "Fine Structure of Synapses in the Cerebral Cortex," *Zeitschrift für Zellforschung und Mikroskopische Anatomie*, **60** (1963), 815.

197. Vincent, W. S. "Structure and Chemistry of Nucleoli," *International Review of Cytology*, **4** (1955), 269.
198. Virchow, R. *Die Cellular Pathologie.* Berlin: Hirschwald, 1858.
199. Wagner, R. P., and Mitchell, M. K. *Genetics and Metabolism.* New York: Wiley, 1955.
200. Walberg, F. "An Electron Microscopic Study of Terminal Degeneration in the Inferior Olive of the Cat," *Journal of Comparative Neurology*, **125** (1965), 205.
201. Waldeyer, H. W. G. *Über einige neuere Forschungen im Gebiete der Anatomie des Central nerven systems.* Leipzig. Thieme, 1891. P. 64.
202. Walker, P. M. B., and Richards, B. M. "Quantitative Microscopical Techniques for Single Cells," in J. Brachet and A. E. Mirsky (eds.), *The Cell.* New York: Academic Press, 1959. Vol. 1, p. 91.
203. Watson, M. L. "Further Observations on the Nuclear Envelope," *Journal of Biophysical and Biochemical Cytology*, **6** (1959), 147.
204. Weismann, A. *Vortrage über Descendenz Theorie. Die Keimplasmatheorie.* Jena: Fischer, 1902.
205. Weiss, P., and Hiscoe, H. B. "Experiments on the Mechanism of Nerve Growth," *Journal of Experimental Zoology*, **107** (1948), 315.
206. Westrum, L. E. "On Origin of Synaptic Vesicles in Cerebral Cortex," *Journal of Physiology*, **179** (1965), 4.
207. Whitaker, D. M. "Physical Factors of Growth," *Growth*, **2**, suppl. (1940), 75.
208. Whittaker, V. P., and Gray, E. G. "The Synapse: Biology and Morphology," *British Medical Bulletin*, **18** (1962), 223.
209. Whittaker, V. P., Michaelson, I. A., and Kirkland, R. J. "The Separation of Synaptic Vesicles from Nerve-Ending Particles ('Synaptosomes')," *Biochemical Journal*, **90** (1964), 293.
210. Wilkins, M. H. F. "Physical Structure of Deoxyribose Acid and Nucleoprotein," *Symposia of Quantitative Biology*, **21** (1956), 75.
211. Winkler, A. *The Relation of Psychiatry to Pharmacology.* Baltimore: Williams & Wilkins, 1957.
212. Wooley, D. W. *A Study of Antimetabolites.* New York: Wiley, 1952.
213. Wooley, D. W., and White, A. G. C. "Production of Thiamine Deficiency Disease by Feeding of Pyridine Analogue of Thiamine," *Journal of Biological Chemistry*, **149** (1943), 285.
214. Worley, L. G. "The Relationship between the Golgi Apparatus and 'Droplets' in the Cell Stainable Vitally with Methylene Blue," *Proceedings of the National Academy of Science*, **29** (1943), 228.
215. Worley, L. G. "Golgi Apparatus—Interpretation of Its Structure and Significance," *Annals of the N. Y. Academy*, **47** (1946), 1.
216. Wright, S. "Genetics and the Hierarchy of Biological Sciences," *Science*, **130** (1959), 959.
217. Zirkle, R. E. (ed.). *A Symposium on Molecular Biology.* Chicago: University Committee on publications in biology and medicine, 1959.

INDEX

abandonment, fear of, 249; feelings of, 6, 249
Abraham, K., 36, 220, 222
abstract thinking, 402, 536, 547, 548
abstraction(s), 22, 23
achondroplastic dwarfism, 574
acid freaks, 432
Ackerman, N. W., 314–316, 332
acting-out, 68
adaptive extragenetic cytoplasmic system, 567
adaptive iden*ifications, 37
adoptive studies, schizophrenic, 491–496
ADP, 584
Adrian, E. D., 97
adualism, 15
adult neurosis, 69
advice-giving, 62–64
AEP (averaged evoked potentials), 535–537
affect, depression as an, 220
affective reaction, 119
affirmation by repetition, 413
agent characteristics, 119
aggression, 9; depression and, 204, 237, 241; effective, 241; internalized, 249; self-directed, 36
aggressive motivation, 22
aggressive wishes, 237
agoraphobia, 539
air pollution, 266
alanine, 518
Albert Einstein Medical School, 39
albinism, 572
alcoholic hallucinations, 433
alcoholism, 67, 225, 260, 508; folklore psychiatry and, 172–174; LSD and, 438
Alexander, F., 90, 294
Alfrey, V. G., 567
alienation, marginally asocial personality and, 258, 264, 265

alkaptonuria, 572
allergic mechanisms, 574
Alley, C., 138*n*
altruistic phobia, 299
Alzheimer's disease, 573
amaurotic family idiocy, 575
ambivalence, 67, 205, 245, 251
amenorrhea, 200
amentive disorders, 158
American Psychoanalytic Association, 40
Amiel, Henri F., 322
amino acids, 518
amitriptyline, 550, 551
amnesia, 140–141
amorphous forms of thinking, 207
amphetamine psychosis, 433–434
amphetamines, 534; misuse of, 426, 428, 430, 432–434, 447
amyl nitrate ampuls, 450
anaclitic frustration, 24
anal wishes, 125–126
analgesics, 465
analysis (*see* treatment)
analytic situation, 51, 53
anamnestic interviews, 41
anger, 14, 24; depression and, 233, 237–241; melancholia and, 220, 222
animal psychology, experimental, 39
anorexia nervosa, 197–218; differential diagnosis, 198–199; interpretation of, 199–202; interpretative conclusions, 212–213 psychogenesis of, 202–205; psychotherapeutic suggestions, 214–217; social factors in, 213–214; solvent-inhalation and, 431
anthropology, folklore psychiatry and, 165, 167–168
anthropophobia, 294
anticipation, 118; expectation and, 135
antidepressants, 465–467, 470–471, 550
antigens, 572

antimetabolites, 583
anxiety, 9, 14, 23, 123, 214; castration, 50, 52, 83–84, 142; danger and, 25, 135; depressive, 48, 61, 226, 227, 235, 239, 242; eight-month, 407; experimentally induced, 545; infantile autism and, 402, 407, 409–411; massive, 68; mortal, 409; panic, 411; paranoid, 61; plethysmography as measure of, 540; schizophrenic, 540–541; separation, 47–48, 50, 52; social, 303; symbolic, 24; theory of, 36
anxiety dreams, 83
anxiety neurosis, 293
anxiety states, 437, 539; chronic, 433
apathy, 234, 242, 448, 465–466, 533
aphasias, 76, 80, 401
Apollo astronauts, 138n
appetite, 8, 10, 14; anorexic perception of, 208
appetitive-phase behaviors, 123, 125–126
apprentice-master training model, 43
Arenberg, D., 514
Arieti, S., 3, 17, 18n, 115, 135, 136, 145, 220–223, 232, 237, 238, 298, 302, 320, 414, 543
Arlow, J. A., 34, 43, 123–125, 128, 141, 145
arousal, 530–532, 534, 538–539, 545, 546; criteria of, 545; schizophrenia and, 531, 538–539, 542–543, 546, 548
artificial hysterical paralysis, 74, 77
as-if attitude, 134, 135
as-if dualism, 96
asthenic states, 158, 159, 161
Asthmador, 430, 449–450
astronomical time, 138
ATP, 508, 567, 574, 576, 584
atropine poisoning, 439, 449–451
auditory perceptions, 7; schizophrenic, 544
authority, craving for, 323–324
autism, infantile (*see* infantile autism)
autistic thinking, 548
autoexecutive faculty, 324
automation, 181–182
autonomous gratification, fear of, 225–226, 229
averaged evoked potentials (AEP), 535–537
aversion therapy, 4
awareness, 7–8; of causality, 18, 115; motivation and, 8; repression from, 26; self- (*see* self-awareness); subjective, 16; suppression from, 26; teleological, 18; of time, discontinuity of, 124–125

Ax, A. F. 531–532, 541, 542

Baeyer, W. von, 359, 366, 371, 372
Baez, Joan, 280–281, 289
Bak, R., 34
Baldwin, J. M., 15
Ban, T., 548, 551, 553
bargain relationship, 226–228, 233, 234, 236, 238
Baros, C. P., 72
Barr, M. L., 567
Baudelaire, Charles P., 426
Beam, J. C., 542
Beatles, 259, 280, 281, 289
beatniks, 259–262, 285, 290. *See also* hippie movement
Beck, Julian, 281
Beck, L. W., 94
Beckett, P. G. S., 505
bed-wetting, 379, 534
Bemporad, J. R., 219, 544
Bender, L., 402, 422–423
Beneden, E. van, 564
Benjamin, J., 206
benzoazepines, 465
Berg, P. S., 544
Bergen, J. R., 506
Bergler, E., 133, 134
Bergman, P., 403
Berliner, B., 67, 68
Bernard, Claude, 76, 77
Bernfeld, S., 90, 98
Bertram, E. G., 567
Bettelheim, B., 400
Bibring, E., 91, 204, 220
Bieber, I., 128
Biesele, J. J., 571
Black Panthers, 290
Blitzen, N. Lionel, 62n
blushing, fear of, 293–295, 305, 308
Boado, M., 172n
bodily odor, fear of, 294, 295, 300–303, 307–310
body-cognition disturbance, 210–211
body-identity disturbance, 210–211
body image, 20, 21
body-image disturbance, 205, 210–211
body mistrust, 205, 208, 209
Bonaparte, M., 122, 144n
Bonime, W., 222, 238
Böök, J. A., 500
borderline schizophrenia, 68, 296, 303–305, 479, 481, 485, 501. *See also* schizophrenia
boredom, 127–128, 203, 258

INDEX

Bosch, G., 415–417, 422
Bourdon Cancellation Test, 547
Bourne, G., 577
Bowen, M., 312n
Brave New World, 265
Braven, M., 536
Breuer, J., 56, 74, 75, 77, 79
Brickmann, H. R., 274
brief psychotherapy, 55–71; fundamental issues of, 59–61; implications for the present, 69–70; indications and limitations, 65–69; nature of, 57–59; primary purpose of, 59; techniques, 61–64
Brill, N. Q., 68
Broughton, R. G., 534
Brown, H. Rap, 290
Brown, R., 145
Bruch, H., 199, 205, 210–211
Brücke, E. W. von, 76, 80
Bruner, J. S., 118
Brunner, E., 256
Brush, S., 478
Buber, M., 253, 254, 302
Bühler, K., 415
bulimia, 209
Burdon, A. P., 68
Burt, Cyril, 333
Buss, A., 546

Caen, Herb, 261
Call, J. D., 404
Callaway, E., 535–537
Cameron, N., 300
campus rioting, 264–265
Camus, Albert, 259
cannabis products, 426, 428–429, 440–449. *See also* marijuana, misuse of
carbon dioxide inhalation, 549, 551
cardiac transplantation, psychiatric aspects of, 336–352
Carmichael, Stokely, 290
Casper, J. V., 293
Castelnuovo-Tedesco, P., 55, 336
castration anxiety, 50, 52, 83–84, 142
CAT, 516
catatonic-oneiroid states, 157–159
catecholamines, 519, 534
cathartic method, 56, 75
cathexis, bound, 82, 84, 87–88; free, 82, 84; Freudian concept of, 79, 81, 82, 98; Helm-Ostwald intensity law and, 80
causality, 8n; awareness of, 18, 115; lack of appreciation of, 15–16
central nervous system, 560–602; cytoplasm and its subunits, 562–563, 565, 568–569, 575–584; membrane systems, 562–563, 590–593; nucleus and nucleolar system, 561–575; synapses, 584–590. *See also* specific entries
cessation, 119
CFF threshold, 543
Chalke, F. C. R., 536
character perversions, 48–50, 68
Charcot, J. M., 74, 75, 85
Chiappe, M., 169n, 172n
child psychiatry, psychotherapeutic consultation in, 377–399
chlorpromazine, 157–158, 451, 463–465
Choisy, M., 91
chromatic staining, 563, 581
chromatids, 565
chromatin, 561; sex, 567
chromosomal gene inheritance, 566
chromosomes, 564–568
Chronos, 125n
Churchill, Winston, 440
civil rights movement, hippies and, 262, 264, 267, 271, 276, 288–289
Claridge, G. S., 531
classical conditioning, 523
Claude, A., 582
Claussen, U., 446–447
Cleaver, Eldridge, 290
clinical research, 463–475; antidepressants, 465–467, 470–471; controlled studies, 472–473; general data, 467; hallucinogens, 466; hypnotics, 470; longitudinal studies, 473–474; massive studies, 472; neuroleptics, 463–465, 467, 469; orientation study, 469–472; pilot studies, 468–472; tranquilizers, 463–465, 467, 469–470
clinicopathogenetic theory, 151–152
CNS (*See* central nervous system)
codeine abuse, 450
cognition, body-, disturbance of, 210–211; cultural factors in, 26; developmental aspects, 13–17; emotions and, 23; paleologic, 17–18, 23, 25; perceptions and, 7–8; presymbolic, 9, 10; primary, 12–17, 25, 26; secondary, 12, 17–19, 22–27; *table*, 28, structural and psychodynamic role of, 3–32; symbolic, 9–13; tertiary, 12; Whorf-Sapir theory, 26
cognitive constructs, 14
cognitive tests, 529, 547, 549, 550, 552
Cohen, A. K., 453
Cohen, J., 136, 137
Cohen, M. M., 437, 438

Colby, K. M., 89
college rioting, 264-265
Colm, H., 254
communication, symbolic, 46
communications theory, 39
computer of average transients, 516
concentration-camp survivors, late symptomatology among, 353-374
concepts, emotions and, 23; reification of, 24; role of, 22-27. *See also* conceptualization
conceptual ideation, 26
conceptual thinking, 12, 22-23
conceptualization(s), 34, 35, 43; anorexic capacity for, 208, 209; utopian, 178-179
concomitance, doctrine of, 91
concrete thinking, 548
condensation, 11
conditioning, 22, 540-542, 547; classical, 523; facilitation of, 542; of first signal system, 540; operant, 401, 403; Pavlovian theory, 542; of second signal system, 540
confabulosis, 158
Connell, P. H., 433, 434
consciousness, 7, 99; clouded, 156, 158n; quantum of, 144; states of, 91
consensual validation, 11, 15
conservation of energy, Helmholtz's principle of, 79, 86
constancy, principle of, 79, 82, 88, 89, 97, 100, 105
constancy-pleasure principle, 83, 88
constructs, cognitive, 14; inferred entities and, 94
contiguity, 22, 41
contingent negative variation, 536
contrast, 41
convergence, 41
Cooper, Z. K., 571
core of man, 4
correspondence, rules of, 95
counseling, 63
counterconditioning techniques, 63
Craig, W., 123n
Craike, W. H., 492, 493
Cramond, W. A., 337
creativity, 12
crime, drug misuse and, 443, 448-449
crisis therapy, 55, 59n
critical flicker fusion frequency test, 543, 549, 550
Cromer, R. F., 118, 145
cross-cultural psychiatry, 165, 167, 305-310

culture, cognition and, 26; self-image and, 26-27
Cunningham, M. A., 413
current psychoanalytic thought, problems in, 34-54
cybercultural revolution, 182
cybernetics, 182, 592
cystinuria, 572
cytoplasm, 562-563, 565, 568-569, 575-584
cytoplasmic inclusions, 575, 581-584
cytoplasmic inheritance, 566
cytoplasmic organelles, 573, 575, 579-580, 591-593

danger(s), 25, 46; anticipation of, 135; anxiety and, 25, 135; expectancy of, 135; primitive forms of reaction to, 412; in regression, 142
Darrow, C. W., 531 537
Darwinism, 80 104
Davidenkov, S. N., 152
Davidovsky, I. V., 152
Davis, F., 455
De Duve, C., 579-580
death, fear of, 409
death instinct, 90, 97, 101
death wish, 126, 129, 141, 251
deductive processes, 12
defense(s), 37, 42, 46; anorexic, 204, 205, 209, 210, 212, 213; primary, 83, 84
delusional projection, 302
delusions, disappearance of, 157; expansive-fantastic, 158; fantastic, 157, 158; of influence, 294, 295, 299, 304; megalomanic, 157; paranoid, 135-136, 294, 299-300, 302, 303, 433, 536; reduction of, 157; of self-reference, 300, 302, 303; somatic, 303; systematized, 158
Dement, W. C., 534
dementia, 159, 161
denial, 267
Deniker, P., 463
dependency, depression and, 222-225, 227, 228, 231-233, 236, 237, 240; psychological, 434, 448
depersonalization, 141, 143, 209; drug misuse and, 436, 444, 446, 447
depression, 14-15, 17, 23-24, 219-243; as an affect, 220; aggression and, 204, 237, 241; anger and, 233, 237-241; anorexia confused with, 197; anxiety and, 48, 61, 226, 227, 235, 239, 242; bargain relationship and, 226-228, 233, 234, 236,

238; classical psychoanalytic interpretation of, 219–220, 224; craving for authority and, 323–324; deep, 204; dependency and, 222–225, 227, 228, 231–233, 236, 237, 240; distorted experience of time in, 130–132; ego and, 220; as an ego-defect neurosis, 232, 235; environmental loss and, 220–221, 232, 236, 242; family background and, 229–231; fear of autonomous gratification and, 225–226, 229; hippie feeling of, 284; hopelessness and, 221, 228–229, 237, 242; intrapsychic structure in, 231–236; motivational organization of, 130; neurotic, 553; orality and, 204; paranoid, 158; psychodynamic aspects of, 222–229; psychotic, 553; renal transplants and, 338; salivary gland secretion and, 539–540; self-esteem and, 228–229, 233, 236, 237, 241, 242
depressive-amnestic states, 158
deprivation, 24; emotional, 403, 431; oxygen, 545; sensory, 81, 338, 506; sleep, 338, 506, 517, 534, 545
derealization, 143; drug misuse and, 436, 444–445
DES, 439–440
desensitization, 63
despair, 24
desubjectivization, 29–31
DET, 439–440
determinism, psychic, 40
development, Freudian theory of, 81, 86–88
developmental psychology, 39, 46
diagnoses, future nature of, 184
diagnostic study, 551–554
diazepam, 451
Dickson, C., 413
Dietrich, H., 299, 307
differential responsivity, 538
differentiation, 207–209, 317, 320–321, 324; progressive, 566
digital computer techniques, 533
diligence, 309
Dince, P., 230
discomfort, 24
discrimination, 258–259, 289
disease(s), causes of, 152, 153; clinical pictures of, 152–153, 155, 157, 158, 161–162; clinical studies, 164; future nature of, 183–184; individual realization of, 163; internal origins, 155; laboratory studies, 164; metabolic, 572–575; nosological independence of, 154, 161;

nosological regularities in, 161–163; pathogenic mechanisms, 152–154; pathological regularities in, 156–159, 161; social etiology of, 152; stereotpyes of, 152–153, 156; symptoms in, 152, 155, 163; syndromes and, 152, 155–159, 161, 162
displacement, 11, 26
dissolution, Spencer's theory of, 80–81, 90
district general medical clinic, 189–191
DMPEA, 519
DMT, 435, 439–440, 450
DNA, 561, 563, 565, 567–568
Dobkin, Marlene, 172n.
DOM (STP), 430, 435, 439, 449–450
dominant other, 222–225, 227, 228, 231–234, 236, 237, 242
Dooley, L., 133, 140, 142
dopamine, 519, 534
Döring, G. K., 369
double-aspect theory, 91
double bind, 318
draft-card burning, 264
Dragunsky, L., 172n
Dratman, M., 403
dreams, 15, 63, 123, anorexic, 203–204; anxiety, 83; childhood, 389–396; depression and, 233–234; primary cognition and, 12, 26; psychophysiological studies of, 39–40; regression in, 90; self-image and, 31–32; self-potentiality and, 31
Dristan misuse, 434
drives, somatic, Freudian theory of, 83, 85–86, 101
drug misuse, 67, 123, 210, 426–459; abstinence effects, 434; availability and, 426–427; commonly used drugs, 429–450; convictions for, 427–428; crime and, 443, 448–449; hallucinations and, 431, 433, 435–437, 439, 446; in hippie movement, 260–263, 265, 269, 274–277, 279, 286, 289, 433, 443, 455; incidence of, 427–429; legislative control and, 429, 430, 454; management of, 450–452; pushers and, 427; sociocultural issues, 452–455; solvent inhalation, 426, 430–432. *See also* names of drugs
drug therapy, 63, 157–158, 505–506; in folklore psychiatry, 171. *See also* clinical research
dual instinct theory, 36
dualism, 91n, 96, 103, 104; as-if, 96; interactionist, 91; metaphysical parallelistic, 91; parallelistic, 91–92

dualistic theory, 96 103
Duffy, E., 530
Duhem, P., 76n
Durand, V. J., 301
dwarfism, achondroplastic, 574
Dylan, Bob, 280–281, 289
dynamic psychology, 120
dynamic psychopathology, levels of time order in, 120–125
dynamic theories, 151–152
dynamic unconscious, 40
dysarthria tremens syndrome, 466
dysmorphophobia, 293, 295, 296, 298–299, 303, 307

echolalia, 413, 414, 421
economic point of view, 88–89, 100
Eddy, N. B., 434, 441, 445, 448
EEG findings, 434, 469, 473–474, 506, 516, 517, 520, 530, 532–533, 535, 537, 540
effective aggression, 241
Efron, R., 144
ego, 5; anorexic, 201–203; binding, 84, 98, 100; depression and, 220 dissociation of, 436; impoverishment of, 220, 221; integrative capacities, 322; lateral cathexes of, 87
ego boundaries, expanding of, 287
ego boundary, lack of, 15
ego-defect neurosis, depression as, 232, 235
ego development, identifications and, 37
ego ideal, 43, 45, 84, 205
ego identity, 125, 483
ego introject, 219–222, 224, 232
ego organization, 84
ego strength, 79, 277
egoistic phobia, 299
Eisenberg, L., 402, 403, 419–421
Eissler, K. R., 134, 140
Eitinger, L., 366
Ekstein, R., 134, 403
electrodes, implanted, 506, 537
electrolytes, 569
electron microscopy, 560, 561, 576–578, 581, 586–587, 589, 590
electron transport system, 576, 577, 592
Ellenberger, H. F., 142, 166
Elsässer, G., 497
emotional catharsis, 62
emotional deprivation, 403, 431
emotional isolation, female, 244–257
emotional overload, 403
emotional tonality, 15
emotional withdrawal, 407

emotions, cognitive processes and, 23; concepts and, 23; endocepts and, 16; first-order, 8-10, 14, 15; inverted isolation of, 141; reification of, 24; third-order, 17
empathy, 37–38
empiricism, 96
encyclema, 561
endocepts, 13, 16–17, 19, 23
endoplasmic reticulum, 568, 577–579, 581, 582, 590
endopsychic structure, 4; object relations and, 6
energetic formulations, true, 78n, 79–80.
energy, conservation of, Helmholtz's principle, 79, 86; forms of, 97; free, 102, 102n; libidinal, 97, 99, 219; primary process as consumer of, 12; psychic, 73, 81, 96–98, 102–105; total, 81, 97–99
Engelmann, T. G., 116
engrams, 16
enteroceptive sensations, 10
enuresis, 379, 534
environmental loss, depression and, 220–221, 232, 236, 242
environmental manipulation, 63, 64
environmental reality, adaptation to, 3, 9, 10, 13
enzyme precursors, 566
enzymes, 565–567, 569, 570, 572–574, 582, 583
epicritic organization, 22
epilepsy, 152, 161–162
epiphenomenalism, 92–93
epistemic correlations, 95, 96
equilibrium, displacement of, 78n, 101; disturbances of, 77; dynamic, 187; factors of, 80n; reattainment of, 101; stable, 78, 101
equivalence, principle of, 89, 100
ereuthophobia, 292–311. See also fear
Erikson, E. H., 125, 132, 134
Ertl, J., 536
Ervin, F. R., 537
erythrophobia, 293
Escalona, S. K., 403
ethnopsychiatry, 166
ethology, 39
etiological equation, 85
evoked potentials, 535–537
evolutionary physicalism, 91
evolutionary theories, 40, 73, 80, 90, 91; dynamic, 93
excitation(s), neuronic, 76–79, 86; sexual, 86; tonic, 79

INDEX 609

exhibitionism, 296
exhortation, 63
exocepts, 16
expansive-fantastic delusions, 158
expectancy, anticipation and, 135; subjective or experiential feeling of, 16
experience(s), 7; endoceptual, 16–17; felt, 7, 8; fragmented, 207–210; holistic, 16; instinctual, 8; integration of, 21; preverbal, 42, 48, 116; subjective, 7, 29, 325; subliminal, 16; transformation into inner reality, 21; verbal, 42, 116–120
experimental animal psychology, 39
exploratory behavior, 81
Express Times, 283
Ey, H., 161, 293
eye-to-eye confrontation, fear of, 294–302, 304, 306–309

Fahr's syndrome, 573
Fairbairn, W. R. D., 6, 83, 89, 102
family background, depression and, 229–231; infantile autism and, 402, 422–423
family environment, schizophrenia and, 313, 316, 507, 515–516
family identity, 323
family interviews (*see* family psychotherapy)
family leadership, deficiency in, 322–324
family periodic paralysis, 573
family psychotherapy, 312–335; conjoint interviews, 328–330; definition of, 315; founder of, 315; growth of interest in, 315; individual psychotherapy and, 324–328; schizophrenic studies, 317–322; training in, 332–333
family romance, myth of, 45
fantasies, 15; depressive, 234; impregnation, 205; omnipotent, 129; phallus-stealing, 44–45; unconscious, 6, 35, 41, 43, 44, 53
fantasiophrenia, 159
fantastic delusions, 157, 158
Farina, A., 514
fatigue, 8
fear(s), 8, 9, 14; of abandonment, 249; of autonomous gratification, 225–226, 229; of being ugly, 294–296, 298–299, 303, 307; of blushing, 293–295, 305, 308; of bodily odor, 294, 295, 300–303, 307–310; of death, 409; of eye-to-eye confrontation, 294–302, 304, 306–309; of hurting others, 299; immediate danger and, 25; of pregnancy, 205; primitive, 42; of sexuality, 227; of sideglancing, 298, 309;
of social situations, 294, 301, 307–309; of stammering, 294
Federal Drug Administration, 472
Federn, P., 15
feelings, 4; inner reality and, 6–10; synonyms of, 7. *See also* sensations
Feffer, M. H., 547
Feigel, H., 91*n*
Feitelberg, S., 90, 98
Felix, F., 565*n*
felt experience, 7, 8
female isolation, emotional, 244–257
Fenichel, O., 127, 292, 294, 295, 299
Ferenzi, S., 294–296
Fergus Falls Scales, 520
Ferster, C., 403
fetishism, 48–51
Feulgen reaction, 563, 564
fighting, 327
Fink, M., 533
first signal system, conditioning of, 540
Fischer, E., 519
Fischer, F., 132–133, 142
Fischer, M., 480
Fischman, V. S., 434
Fisher, D. D., 437
Fisher, R., 143
fixation, 26, 575, 593; oral, 204
Fletcher, R., 91
Flugel, J. C., 91
fluorescent microscopy, 560
fluoxymesterone, 550, 551
fluphemazine, 464
Fogel, L. J., 144
folklore psychiatry, 165–177; anthropology and, 165, 167–168; history of, 167; importance of, 174–176; nosology of, 170; pathogenesis and, 169; plants and drugs used in, 171; sociology and, 165, 168–169; transcultural, 165, 167, 172; treatment in, 170–174
Fort, J., 449
Fougerousse, C. E., Jr., 133
Foxe, A. N., 91
fragmentation, 207–210, 249
Fraisse, P., 143
Fraknoi, J., 403
French, T. M., 144
freon-gas inhalation, 450
Freud, A., 36, 45, 51
Freud, S., 4, 5, 7, 11–12, 16, 31, 35, 36, 40, 43, 44, 55–57, 72–106, 121–122, 124, 128, 140–142, 144, 151, 219, 221, 224, 232, 240, 294, 296, 323, 324; metapsychology, 73–74, 77, 88–90, 93–94, 96,

Freud, S. *(cont'd)*
 99; psychodynamic concepts, 104–106; theory-building, steps in, 73–91
Freudianism, 106–107
Friedhoff, A. J., 519
Frohman, C. E., 506
Fromm, E., 12
Fromm-Reichmann, F., 222, 230, 235, 236, 320
frustration, 123, 214; anaclitic, 24; anal, 125–126; infantile autism and, 405–407; oedipal, 126; oral, 204; therapeutic, 239
frustration tolerance, 448
Fugs, 281
Fujinawa, A., 304
Fuller, M., 437
Furer, M., 409
fury, 237
futurology, 178, 179

galvanic skin response, 523, 530, 531, 538–539, 541, 542, 545, 552
gamma amino butyric acid, 518
gargoylism, 574
Garmezy, N., 547
Garnier, G., 581
Garrod, A. E., 572
Garrone, G., 496–497
Gebsattel, V., 295, 301
Genain Quadruplets, The, 481
gene-enzyme-chemical reaction patterns, 572
gene inheritance, chromosomal, 566
gene mutations, 565, 570–571
generalizations, 18
genes, 561, 564–566, 573, 574
genetic fallacy, 51
genetics of schizophrenia, 476–504, 507. *See also* schizophrenia
Gerard, R. W., 520
geriatric predictor study, 548–551
Gibbs free energy, 102, 102n
Gifford, S., 116
Gilbert, L., 328–329
Gill, M., 57, 64, 87, 89
Gillman, R. D., 65
Gilman, A., 445
Ginsberg, Allen, 259, 260, 265
Glick, B. S., 81
Glover, E., 314
Gluecksohn-Waelsch, S., 571
glutamic acid, 518
Goldfarb, J., 143–144
Goldfarb, W., 134
Goldman, D., 533

Goldstein, K., 402, 547
Goldstein, L., 533
Goldstone, S., 143–144
Golgi apparatus, 577–578, 590
Golgi complex, 578–579
Gomori method, 579
Goodman, L. S., 445
Gorodetzsky, C. W., 446–447
Gottesman, I. I., 478, 480
Gottlieb, J. S., 505
Gould, R. E., 258, 273
gravol, 450
Green, D. G., 577
Greenson, R., 47
Gross, M. M., 534
Group Image, 283n
group therapy, 185–186, 252–256, 315, 378
GSR, 523, 530, 531, 538–539, 541 542, 545, 552
guilt feelings, 221, 226–228, 234, 235, 238, 241, 242, 246
Guntrip, H., 5, 73, 83, 105–106
Guskins, S., 514

habituation, 538–539, 541
Haeckel, E., 91, 93
Häfner, H., 359, 366, 371, 372
Hair, 282
Hakerem, G., 538
Halbach, H., 434
hallucinations, 156–159, 163, 295, 301; alcoholic, 433; drug-induced, 431, 433, 435–437, 439, 446; schizophrenic, 303
hallucinogens, 426 435, 438–440, 455, 466. *See also* drug misuse
Handy, L. M., 478
Hansel, C. E. M., 136
Harlow, H. F., 38, 39, 408
Harlow, M. K., 408
Harris, A., 545
Harris, J. G., 543
Harrow, M., 221
Hartmann, H., 36, 50, 51
Harvald, B., 480
hashish, 428, 429, 441, 446, 450
Haslam, J., 400
hate, 17, 24
Hauge, M., 480
heart transplantation, psychiatric aspects of, 336–352
Heath, R. G., 506
hedonism, 10
Heilbrunn, G., 284
Heimann, P., 91

INDEX

Hell's Angels, 273, 290
Heller's disease, 401
Helm-Oswald intensity law, 80
Helmholtz, H. L. F. von, 79, 86
helplessness, feeling of, 203, 204, 221; therapeutic, 215
hemochromatosis, 573
Hendricks, I., 232
Henry, Matthew, 322
hepatolenticular degeneration, 573
hereditary spherocytosis, 572, 574
Hermann, K., 366
heroin, 276, 448
Heston, L. L., 494, 495, 499
Hevesy, G., 571
Hicks, P. S., 571
hierarchic integration, 207–208
hippie movement, 259–291; beginning of, 259; and civil rights, 262, 264, 267, 271, 276, 288–289; communications media, 283; dress, style of, 278–279, 289; drug misuse, 260–263, 265, 269, 274–277, 279, 286, 289, 433, 443, 455; intrafamilial psychodynamics of, 266–271; love and nonviolent ethic, 272–274, 288; mixed-media displays, 262–263, 275, 282–283; music, 262–263, 279–281, 289; psychodynamic aspects of, 272–283; social and cultural forces in, 264–266; theater, 281–282, 289; therapy and, 284–287; and Vietnam War, 262, 264, 271, 276, 289. *See also* drug misuse
histidine, 518
historadioautography, 560
historic adaptability, 187–188
historical perspective, 134
Hoagland, H., 143
hoaxer, 49
Hoch, P., 299, 303
Hoffer, A., 133
Hoffman, Abbie, 263
holistic experience, 16
Holmes, John C., 260, 261
Holt, R. R., 73, 79, 82, 97, 99–100, 103–104
homeostatic balance, 60
homilophobia, 294
homo sapiens, development of, 30
homosexuality, 49, 438
hopelessness, feelings of, 6, 221, 228–229, 237, 242
hormones, 550, 569, 572, 574
Hoskins, R. G., 505
hospitalism, 39, 405–407
hostility, 9, 237, 239–240, 411

Hudgens, R. W., 220
hunger, 7, 8, 47
Huntington's chorea, 573
Husserl, E., 415
Huxley, Aldous, 178, 259, 265
hypnosis, 40, 63, 69, 75, 143
hypnotics, 470
hypochondriasis, 10, 25, 197, 198, 204n, 302–303, 305
hysteria, 74–77; etiology of, 86; physiopathological formula for, 74; psychological mechanisms in, 75; by repression, 140
hysterical paralysis, artificial, 74, 77

I-it relationship, 302
ichthyosis, 573
id, 5, 12, 84; timelessness of, 122
ideation, conceptual, 26; repressed, 126
identification(s), 37; adaptive, 37; ego development and, 37; maladaptive, 37; oral incorporation and, 205; projective, 303
identity, body-, disturbance of, 210–211; definitive, anorexic search for, 203; ego, 125, 483; family, 323; fear of loss of, 142; reductionistic, 96–97; self-, 21, 285; similarity and, 18
identity theory, 91, 91n
Ihda, S., 495
imagery, 11, 13–15; emergence of, 25; inner reality and, 14, 19
images, body, 20, 21, 205, 210–211; kinesthetic, 83; mnemic, 83, 105; mother, 19–20; self- (*see* self-image); visual, 119
imitative learning, 224, 232
implanted electrodes, 506, 537
impregnation fantasies, 205
impulse(s), development of, 87–88; drive-energized, 85; ego-inhibited 84; instinctual, 73, 83–85; wishful, 73, 83, 84, 86–88, 102–105
impulse gratification, 241
incestuous desires, 228
inclusions, cytoplasmic, 575, 581–584
individual psychotherapy, 186, 312, 316, 317, 322; family psychotherapy and, 324–328
individual transference psychology, 43
individuality, life organization as menace to, 323
individualization, 18
individuation, 47, 230
inductive processes, 12

inertia, principle of, 81, 83, 88; schizophrenic, 465–466
infantile autism, 134, 400–425; anxiety and, 402, 407, 409–411; characteristic features, 400; diagnosis, 400–401; dynamics of, 409–412; etiology of, 401–405; family background and, 402, 422–423; frustration and, 405–407; language in, 412–417; meaning of, 412–419; motor behavior in, 417–419; treatment of, 401, 403, 419–422; withdrawal and, 400, 402, 403, 407, 408, 410
infantile marasmus, 406, 407
infantile state, reassessment of, 46–52
infantile superego, 224, 230
inferiority, sense of, 297
inferred entities, constructs and, 94
influence, delusion of 294, 295, 299, 304
influencing machine, 304
information transmission, 7
inheritance, chromosomal gene, 566; cytoplasmic, 566; schizophrenia and, 476–477, 499–502, 507, 513
inhibition, 142; depressive, 234, 240; protective, 541, 542
inhibitors, 572
inner life, 4
inner reality, 4; cognitive and affective components of, *table*, 28; feelings and, 6–10; imagery and, 14, 19; learning and, 27; phantasmic stage, 13–16, 20; presymbolic organization and, 6–10; psychoanalytic views of, 4–6; simple feelings and, 6–10; transformation of experiences into, 21
inner self, 4. *See also* inner reality
Inouye, E., 478–479
instinct(s), 73, 84, 101; death, 90, 97, 101
instinct theory, dual, 36; Freudian, 84, 86, 105–106
instinctual experiences, 8
instinctual impulse, 73, 83–85
institutional mythology, 43–45
integration, 15, 29, 30; of experiences, 21; hierarchic, 207–208
intellectualization, 142, 267
intelligence, sensorimotor, 9
intelligence test, 379
interactionist dualism, 91
internalization, 4, 6; imagery and, 13; of parental values, 224
Interpretation of Dreams, The 11, 83, 85
interpretative techniques, 63–64

intervening variables, 94–96
intrapsychic life, 4
intrapsychic self, 4
intrapsychic validation, 15
involution, Freudian theory, 90–91
iproniazide, 465
Isbell, H., 434, 446–447
isolation, 140–141, 203; female emotional, 244–257
Itard, J. M. G., 400

Jackson, D. D., 159, 161, 483
Jackson, J. H., 75, 76, 80, 91, 93
Jackson, L., 412
Jacobson, E., 222
James, W., 125
Janet, P., 292–294, 306
Jasinski, D., 446–447
Jaspers, K., 151, 221
Jenney, E. G., 533
Jewish Family Service (New York City), 315, 319, 332
Joffee, W. G., 220, 230
Johanssen, W. L., 564
Johnson, Lyndon B., 263
Jones, E., 11, 79, 91
Jouvet, M., 517, 534
joy, 17
juvenile delinquency, 132

Kaan, H., 299
Kahn, E., 497
Kallmann, F. J., 478, 488, 492, 493, 496–497, 499
Kamp, L. N. J., 404
Kandinsky-Clerambault syndrome, 157
Kanner, L., 400–402, 413–415, 419, 421–423
Kantor, R., 544
Kaplan, B., 116, 119
Kaplan, N. O., 583
Kapp, R. O., 91
Kardiner, A., 132
Karlsson, L. J., 495
karolymph, 561
Kasahara, Y., 292
Keeler, M. H., 438, 447
Kelly, G. A., 106
Kelman, H., 144
Keniston, K., 270n, 455
Kennedy, J. A., 337
Kennedy, Robert, 263, 281
Kerouac, Jack, 259, 260
Kesey, Ken, 259
Kety, S. S., 495, 505, 519

kidney transplantation, psychiatric aspects of, 336–338
Kielholz, P., 220
Kiev, A., 175n
Kind, H., 199
kinesis, 153
kinesthetic images, 83
kinesthetic sensations, 21
King, H. E., 544
King, Martin Luther, Jr., 281
Kisker, K. P., 359, 366, 371, 372
Klein, M., 37, 38, 91, 200, 203, 237, 303
Kleitman, N., 116
Klett, C. J., 514
knowledge, transmission of, 44
Koegler, R. R., 68
Koelliker, R. A., 564
Korte, F., 446–447
Kraepelin, E., 161
Kramer, J. C., 434
Krasnova, A. I., 513
Krassner, Paul, 283
Kringlen, E., 476, 478, 482, 492, 493
Kris, E., 36, 41
Kronos, 125
Kubis, J., 542

Lacey, J. I., 530–531
Lader, M. H., 539
Lafayette Clinic Rating Scale, 514
Lambo, T. A., 428–429, 449
Lang, B., 546
Langeveld, M. J., 417
language, acquisition of, 9, 17; of autistic children, 412–417; denotative functions of, 11; development of, 11; temporal reference in, 118
Lazarus, R. L., 531
Le Chatelier's principle, 78n, 80, 97, 100, 101
leadership, family, deficiency in, 322–324
learning, imitative, 224, 232; inner reality and, 27; neurophysiological, 547; paradigms of, 540; presymbolic, 10; psychological, 547; reactive, 224–225
legislation, drug misuse and, 429, 430, 454
Legninger, A. L., 577
Lehmann, H. E., 143, 144, 529, 543, 545
Leibniz, G. W. von, 92
Lennard, S., 145
Lesse, S., 178, 189
Levenson, E. A., 120–121
Levin, M., 18
Levy, D. M., 113, 123n, 131, 145

Lewin, B. D., 47, 123, 124
Lewis, Aubrey, 441, 447
Lewis, W. C., 121
Lhamon, W. O., 143–144
libidinal development, 82
libidinal drives, repression of, 235
libidinal energy, 97, 99, 219
libidinal regression, 220
libidinal tension, 79–80, 83, 100, 101
libidinous situation, 143
libido theory, 12, 36, 102–103
Lidsky, A., 538
Lidz, T., 229, 313, 317n, 318
life organization, individuality and, 323
life trajectory, 120, 122, 126, 127, 129–131, 133–134, 137, 141–142
Lifton, R., 134
Littlefield, D. C., 434
Living Theater, 281–282
lobster claw, 575
locomotion, development of, 10
logic, 12; ancient, 17
London, Jack, 178
longitudinal studies, 42, 473
long-term treatment, 57, 67–68
Loomis, E. A., 414
Lorr, M., 514
Lost Generation, 260
Lotka, A. J., 80n
love, 14, 15, 17; mature, 24
love and nonviolent ethic, hippie, 272–274, 288
LSD, 276, 279, 282, 286, 426, 429–430, 432, 434–439, 447, 450, 451, 466. See also drug misuse
LSD model psychosis, 433
LSD syndrome, 436–438
Lunde, D. T., 336n
Luxenburger, H., 478, 488
lysergamide, 466
lysine, 518
lysomes, 579–580
"Lytic Cocktail," 463

McCarthy, Eugene, 263
MacCorquodale, K., 94–95
McCulloch, W. S., 144n
McGlothlin, W. H., 448
Macnab, F. A., 244
McNair, D. M., 514
Mahler, Gustav, 56
Mahler, M., 403
maladaptive identifications, 37
Malan, D. H., 68
Malina, Judith, 281

Malmo, R. B., 530, 531
manic-depressive psychosis, 157, 161, 184, 230, 235; psychomotor speed impairment in, 545. See also depression
manic states, 156
manipulation, 238, 241, 323; environmental, 63, 64
Mannheim, K., 134
marasmus, infantile, 406, 407
marginally asocial personality (see hippie movement)
marijuana, misuse of, 265, 275–277, 286, 427–429, 435, 449–451, 454–455. See also drug misuse
marijuana syndrome, 444–445
Mark, V. H., 537
Martin, I., 541
Masserman, J. H., 261
massive anxiety, 68
master-apprentice training model, 43
materialism, French mechanistic, 92–93; metaphysical, 91, 92; methodological, 91, 92
materialistic monism, 91, 96
Matos, D., 172n
mature love, 24
Matussek, P., 353, 359, 371
Maudsley, G., 155, 163
Mayer, A., 151
Mead, G. H., 123n
Meadow, A., 172n
medical academician, 187–188
medical technical expert, 188–189
medicine, future role of, 186–193
Mednick, S. A., 538–542, 547
Meehl, P. E., 94–95
Meerlo, J. A. M., 134
megalomanic delusions, 157
melancholia, 219–222, 232, 236. See also depression
Melges, F. T., 133
membrane systems, CNS, 562–563, 590–593
memory, 9, 115, 124
memory traces, 13, 16
meprobamate, 550, 551
mescaline, 436, 438–440, 449, 466
metabolic diseases, 572–575
metaphysical materialism, 91, 92
metaphysical parallelistic dualism, 91
metapsychology, current, 89–90; Freudian, 73–74, 77, 88–90, 93–94, 96, 99
metascientific assumptions, 72, 73, 91–96
Metcalfe, M., 545
methamphetamine, 549–551

methedrine, 276, 432–434, 439, 450
methemoglobinuria, 573
methionine, 518
methodological empirical parallelism, 91–93
methodological materialism, 91, 92
methyl-donor compounds, 505-506
methylphenidate, 550, 551
microabsorption spectrophotometry, 560
microgenetic process, 12
micropsychosis, 299
microsomes, 567
Mill, J. S., 75
Millet, J., 145
mind-body problem, 29, 73, 91–93, 95–96
Minkowski, E., 142, 221
Mirsky, A. E., 567
Mishler, E. G., 317n
mitochondria, 567, 575–584, 592
mitosis, 561, 564, 573
mixed-media displays, 262–263, 275, 282–283
mnemic images, 83, 105
Money-Kyrle, R. E., 91
monism, 91n; materialistic, 91, 96
monoamine oxidase, 465
moralistic rationalizations, 235
More, Thomas, 178
Morita, S., 293–294, 309
morning-glory seeds, psychedelic properties of, 449
mortal anxiety, 409
mother image, 19–20
motivation, aggressive, 22; awareness and, 8; at conceptual level of development, 25; imagery and, 14; physiologic-protoemotional, 9; self-gratification and, 25; at sensorimotor level of development, 25; sexual, 22; unconscious, 11–12
motor engrams, 16
multilevel experimental approaches, 548–554
multiple exostoses, 574
Murakami, M., 294–295, 299
Murphree, H. B., 533
Murphy, H. B. M., 441, 447
Muses, C., 145
music, hippie movement and, 262–263, 279–281, 289
mutations, gene, 565, 570–571
mutism, 400, 408, 412–413, 421
mutuality, 255
myristicin, 449
mythology, institutional, 43–45

INDEX

Nageli, J., 564
narcissism, 36
narcissistic function, 314
nature-nurture controversy, 476
need tension, 123
Nelson, J. M., 445–446
neurasthenia, 293
neuroleptanalgesia, 465
neuroleptics, 463–465, 467, 469, 550
neuromotor integrity, 544
neuronic excitation, 76–79, 86
neurophysiological hypothesis, basic, 76–80
neurophysiological learning, 547
neurophysiological research, 532–537
New Radical Left, 290
nicotinic acid, 550, 551
nightmares, 534
Nissl stain, 581
Nissl substance, 569, 581
nonviolent and love ethic, hippie, 272–274, 288
norepinephrine, 534
nosographic approach, 74
Novey, S., 144
nuclear sap, 561
nucleoproteins, 563, 565, 569
nucleus and nucleolar system, CNS, 561–575
Nunberg, H., 49
nutmeg, psychedelic properties of, 449
nutritional siderosis, 573

Oberndorf, C. P., 141
object relationships, 60, 219; endopsychic structure and, 6; principle of, 84, 88
obsessive-compulsive neurosis, 68, 536
obsessive-compulsive syndromes, 26
obsessive neurosis, 305
oceanic feeling, 16
O'Connor, N., 546
Ödegaard, Ö., 501
O'Donnell, J. A., 453
oedipal conflict, 224
oedipal frustration, 126
oedipal wishes, 47, 125, 126
O'Gorman, G., 423
olfaction, 7
oligon, 144
omnipotence, feeling of, 20
omnipotent fantasies, 129
oneiroid-catatonic disorders, 157–159
ongoingness, 119
operant conditioning, 401, 403
opium, 443, 449

oral fixation, 204
oral frustration, 204
oral incorporation, 205
oral wishes, 47
orality, 38, 204, 233
organelles, cytoplasmic, 573, 575, 579–580, 591–593
orienting response, 541–542
Orr, D. W., 62n, 91
Orwell, George, 178
Osmond, H., 133, 505
Oswald, I., 434
oxygen deprivation, 545

pain, 7, 9, 83, 124
Palade, G. E., 578
Palay, S. L., 577, 578
Palazzoli, M. S., 197
paleologic cognition, 17–18, 23, 25
paleologic thinking, 17, 18, 26
paleosymbols, 14n
pallium psi neuronic system, 82–84, 87, 98, 102, 105
panic anxiety, 411
Paradise Now, 282
parallelism, methodological empirical, 91–93
parallelistic dualism, 91–92
paralysis, artificial hysterical, 74, 77; family periodic, 573
paranoia, 25, 286
paranoid anxiety, 61
paranoid delusions, 135–136, 294, 299–300, 302, 303, 433, 536
paranoid depression, 158
paranoid schizophrenia, 157, 543, 544, 549, 550. *See also* schizophrenia
paraphrenia, 157, 161
parental values, internalization of, 224
pathergia, 570
pathogenesis, 153, 154, 158, 161; folklore psychiatry and, 169
pathokinesis, 153, 155
pathological transmethylation, 505–506, 519
patholysis, 570
pathosis, 570
Pavlovian theory, 542
pavor nocturnus, 534
Pcs (Cs), 87, 88, 96
Peace Corps, 290
pedigree method, 496
Penrose, L. L., 574
Penrose, L. S., 91
pentosuria, 572

perception(s), 4, 7–8; anorexic capacity for, 208–210; auditory, 7, 544; cognition and, 7–8; schizophrenic, 543–544; sensory, 7, 10; visual, 7, 543–544
perceptumotor function, 544
periodic paralysis, family, 573
personality assessment, 379
personality organization, identifications and, 37
pethidine, 463–464
Pettigrew Category Width Test, 544
petty liar, 48–49
petty swindler, 48–50
peyote, misuse of, 279, 440
Pfeiffer, C. C., 533
phallus-stealing fantasies, 44–45
pharmacological load-test performances, 548–550
pharmacotherapy, 548–551
phenomenological theories, 151–152
phenothiazines, 451, 464, 534, 536
phenylketonuria, 572
phi neuronic system, 81–82
phobias, 26, 47–48, 63, 292–311, 539; altruistic, 299; egoistic, 299; social, 539. *See also* fear
photophobia, 436
physicalism, evolutionary, 91
physiodynamics, 187
physiological-protoemotional motivation, 9
physiopathological formula, 74, 76
physiosensations, 8
Piaget, J., 9, 13, 114–116, 118, 135, 138
Pick's disease, 162
piperazine, 465
Pitres, A., 293
placebo, 442, 549
Plague, The, 282
Planansky, K., 496
plastades, 567
Plato, 178
play therapy, 378, 381–389
pleasure principle, 79, 83, 88, 89
Plesett, I. R., 478
plethysmography, 540
Pollin, W., 481–482, 513
polydactyly, 574
population expansion, 181, 182
Porter, K. R., 578
possessiveness, leadership and, 323
postulational concepts, Freudian, 93–94
potentiality, self-; 29–31
practical joker, 48, 49
preconceptual thinking, 13, 17–19

predictor study, geriatric, 548–551; schizophrenic, 539, 547–548
pregnancy, fear of, 205; LSD and, 438
prelogical thinking, 17
premonition, 141
Presley, Elvis, 280
presymbolic cognition, 9, 10
presymbolic learning, 10
presymbolic organization, 6–10; *table*, 28
preverbal experience, 42, 48, 116
Pribram, K., 82
primary autonomous ego functions, deficiency in, 403
primary cognition, 12–17, 25, 26
primary defense, 83, 84
primary process, 11–12, 15, 22
primitive fears, 42
procalnamide, 465
progressive differentiation, 566
projection, anorexic, 212, 213; delusional, 302
projective identification, 303
promethazine, 463–464
Prometheus, 44–45
pronominal reversal, 413
proprioceptive sensations, 10
proprium, 4
protective inhibition, 541, 542
Protestant Ethic, 265
protoemotions, 8–10
protopathic organization, 22
protoplasm, 575
pseudoanorexia nervosa, 198, 204*n*
pseudodualism, 96
pseudomutuality, 318
pseudoneurotic schizophrenia, 303, 501, 546. *See also* schizophrenia
psi neuronic system, 80–82, 98, 103–105; pallium, 82–84, 87, 98, 102, 105
psilocybine, 440, 466
psychedelic drugs (*see* drug misuse)
Psychiatric News, 319
psychiatric nosology, 154
psychiatric theories, 151–152
psychiatrist, future role of, 184–186
psychic analysis, techniques of, 75
psychic apparatus, 81, 96–101, 103, 104
psychic automatisms, 158, 159
psychic determinism, 40
psychic energy, 73, 81, 96–98, 102–105
psychic mechanisms, physiopathology of, 75–76
psychic reality, 4, 5, 13–15. *See also* inner reality
psychoanaleptics, 467

INDEX 617

psychoanalytic investigation, dissatisfaction with method of, 41–42
psychoanalytic knowledge, state of development of, 35–38
psychoanalytic literature, 35–36; cultural lag in, 36
psychoanalytic movement, leaders in, 42–45
psychoanalytic situation, 35, 40, 46
psychoanalytic theories, 106–107, 151
psychoanalytic thought, current, problems in, 34–54
psychoanalytic training, 332–333, 377, 378
psychobiological theories, 105–106, 151
psychodynamic concepts, Freudian, 104–106
psychodynamics, 187
psychodysleptics, 467
psychointegration, 317
psycholeptics, 467
psychological dependency, 434, 448
psychological learning, 547
psychometric tests, 548–550
psychomotor measures, 529, 544–546, 549–552
psychopathology, cognitive measures, 529, 547–550, 552; criteria and indicators of, 529; diagnostic study, 551–554; dynamic, levels of time order in, 120–125; experimental approach, 540–542; geriatric predictor study, 548; multilevel experimental approaches, 548–554; neurophysiological approaches, 532–537; perceptual approaches, 543–544; perspectives in, 529; psychomotor measures, 529, 544–546, 549–552; psychophysical approaches, 542–543; psychophysiological approaches, 537–540. *See also* schizophrenia
psychopharmacology, 463–475. *See also* clinical research
psychophysiological approaches, 537–540
psychosomatic illnesses, 67
psychotemporal field, restriction of, 135, 136
psychotherapist, future role of, 184–186
psychotoxic response, 403
psychotropic drugs, 157–158
pupillography, 538
Puritan ethic, 453

quantal concept, 144
quantitative factors, 36
quantitative formulations, 77–79
quasienergetic formulation, 78, 80

Rabl, C., 564
Radical Theater Repertory, 281
Rado, S., 123, 130, 220, 222
rage, 8, 9, 14, 24; hypothalamic functions of, 5
Rank, B., 403
Rapaport, D., 89, 128
Rat, 283
rationalization(s), 267; moralistic, 235
reaction-formation, 30
reaction-time measures, 545-546, 549, 551
reactive learning, 224–225
Realist, The, 283
reality: environmental, adaptation to, 3, 9, 10, 13; functions mirroring aspects of, 7; inner (*see* inner reality); psychic, 4, 5, 13–15; subjective, 29; wishes and, 20
reality principle, 83, 88, 100
reassurance, 63
recall, 9
reductionistic identity, 96–97
reflexive validation, 15
regional specialty center, 191–192
Régis, E., 293
regression, 26, 68, 90, 139, 140, 159; dangers appearing in, 142; in dreams, 90; libidinal, 220; schizophrenic, 204
reification, of concepts, 24; of emotions, 24
REM sleep, 39–40, 434, 435, 517, 529, 530, 533–534
remission, 157, 158
renal transplantation, psychiatric aspects of, 336–338
repetition, 22, 41; affirmation by, 413
repressed ideation, 126
repression, 26, 31, 83, 123, 124; from awareness, 26; hysteria by, 140; of libidinal drives, 235
repulsion, 83
resperine, 464, 467
resperinic akinesia, 465
responsivity, differential, 538
reversive thymoaction, 466
Rimland, B., 401, 404, 422
RNA, 563, 566, 567, 581
RNA metabolism, 568–569
RNA synthesis, 568
Robertson, J. D., 590
Robinson, J. T., 438
Rodrigué, E., 409
Róheim, G., 133, 134
Roizin, L., 560, 571
Rolling Stones, 281

Rorschach test, 199, 206–211, 302
Rosanoff, A. J., 478, 488
Rosenthal, D., 478, 481, 495, 497
Rotalin misuse, 434
Roth, B., 492, 493
rubber fence, 318
Rubin, Jerry, 263
Rubinstein, B. B., 73, 95–96, 104
Rugh, R., 571
Russell, B., 94
Ruttenberg, B., 403

Sadock, B., 273
Saint-Exupery, Antoine de, 256
Sakamaki, Leigh, 428
Sakamoto, K., 292
salivary gland secretion, 539–540
Samiatin, J., 178
Sandler, J., 220, 230
satisfaction, 8, 14
Schacter, J., 145
Schain, R. J., 422
Schaltenbrand, G., 144*n*
Schapiro, D., 145
Schilder, P., 133, 141
schizoaffective psychosis, 157
schizoid personality, 305
schizophrenia, 12, 23, 26, 152; acute, 531, 538, 541, 543, 544; adoptive studies in, 491–496; anxiety and, 540–541; arousal and, 531, 538–539, 542–543, 546, 548; auditory perception in, 544; autoimmune theory of, 506; autokinetic movement in, 544; biochemical background, 505–506, 517–518; biology of, advances in, 505–528; borderline, 68, 296, 303–305, 479, 481, 485, 501; CFF threshold in, 543; chronic, 520, 531, 538, 543, 544, 548, 550, 553; classification, problem of, 505, 506, 513–520, 525; clinical background, 507; diagnosis, problem of, 505; drug therapy and, 505–506; EEG findings, 506, 516, 517, 520, 533; ego identity theory of, 483; etiology of, 313, 319, 476, 478, 479, 502, 505; evoked potentials and, 535, 536; factor analysis, *table*, 522–523; family environment and, 313, 316, 507, 515–516; family studies in, 317–322; finger dexterity in, 546; genealogical studies, 496–497; genetics of, 476–504, 507; GSR in, 523, 531, 538–539, 541; hyporesponsivity in, 548; incidence of, 497; inheritance factor, 476–477, 499–502, 507, 513; Kraepelinian subtypes, 491; learned punishments and rewards and, 547; metabolic disturbance in, 508–509; morbid expectancy rate, 497; morphological brain changes in, 162; multidisciplinary research program, 507–513; neurophysiological background, 506, 516–517; paranoid, 157, 543, 544, 549, 550; predictor study in, 539, 547–548; proprioceptive deficit in, 516, 525; protective inhibition and, 542; pseudoneurotic, 303, 501, 546; psychomotor deficit in, 545–546; reaction-time measures, 545–546; segmental set in, 546; size distortions in, 543; sleep studies, 517, 520, 534; statistical study, tentative report of, 520–525; tapping-speed measures, 546, 553; temporal orientation in, 132–135, 143–144; twin studies, 477–494, 513; urine findings, 519–520; visual perception in, fragmentation of, 543–544; waking dream of, 534; withdrawal in, 531
schizophrenic inertia, 465–466
schizophrenic regression, 204
schizophrenic thinking, 207, 524, 547–548
Schmideberg, M., 293*n*
Schüle, G., 155
Schulsinger, E., 539
Schulz, B., 497
Schur, M., 12
Schwartz, M., 535
Schwarz, C. J., 441
scopophilia, 296
scopophobia, 295, 296
Scott, W. C. M., 129
second signal system, conditioning of, 540
secondary cognition, 12, 17–19, 22–27; *table*, 28
secondary process, 11, 15, 18, 19, 22, 41–42
secondary-process thinking, 338
security, 14, 15, 23; lack of, 26
sedation-threshold technique, 540
Seevers, M. H., 434
Segal, H., 91
Seguin, C. A., 165
self, general aspects of, 29–32
self-abasement, 220, 221
self-affirmation, 254–256
self-aggrandizement, 251
self-alienation, 258
self-assertion, 126
self-awareness, 124, 125, 202, 249, 284; enhanced, 439; increasing of, 287
self-blame, 231, 236–239, 242, 302
self-concept, 20–21. *See also* self-image

self-confirmation, 254-256
self-consciousness, 295–298
self-directed aggression, 36
self-disclosure, 253–254
self-esteem, 21, 26, 284; depression and, 228–229, 233, 236, 237, 241, 242; fear of obtaining, 225; hippie search for, 285; reduction of, 220
self-evaluation, 21
self-fulfillment, 278
self-gratification, motivation and, 25
self-identity, 21; hippie search for, 285
self-image, 10, 20–22, 24–27, 208–209, 224, 228; culture and, 26–27; depression and, 228; dreams and, 31–32
self-indulgence, 240, 454
self-mortification, 27
self-potentiality, 29–31
self-preoccupation, 251, 344
self-preservation, 252
self-realization, 251–253
self-recriminations, 221, 233
self-reference, delusions of, 300, 302, 303
self-sacrifice, 225–227, 237, 238
self-ugliness, fear of, 294–296, 298–299, 303, 307
Selye's stress theory, 366
sensations, 7–9; enteroceptive, 10; kinesthetic, 21; proprioceptive, 10; tactile, 21; visual, 21. See also feelings
sensoriomotor intelligence, 9
sensoriomotor period, motivation in, 25; time orders in, 114–116
sensory deprivation, 80, 338, 506
sensory perceptions, 7, 10
separation anxiety, 47–48, 50, 52
Sernyl, 506
serotonin, 518, 519
serotonin blockade, 505
set-index disturbance, 546
sex, hypothalamic functions of, 5
sex-chromatin determination, 567
Sexton, M. C., 544
sexual excitations, 86
sexual intercourse, shame associated with, 245, 247
sexual life, etiological equation for neuroses and physiology of, 85
sexual motivation, 22
sexual revolution, 318
sexual urges, 8
sexuality, depressive disinterest in, 235; fear of, 227
Shagass, C., 535–537, 540
Shakow, D., 546

shame, sexual intercourse and, 245, 247
Shaw, E., 505
Sheehan's disease, 198
Shevrin, H., 403
Shields, J., 478, 480, 492, 493
shock treatments, 464
short-term psychotherapy (see brief psychotherapy)
sibling rivalry, 380–381, 394, 397
sideglancing, fear of, 298, 309
Silverberg, W., 241
Silverman, J., 531, 542, 548
similarity, 41; identity and, 18
Simmonds' disease, 198
size distortions, schizophrenic, 543
Slater, E., 478, 480, 488, 492, 493, 496–497, 500
sleep, psychophysiological studies of, 39–40, 434, 517, 520, 533–534
sleep deprivation, 338, 506, 517, 534, 545
sleep disorders, 534
sleep-wakefulness cycle, 47
Smith, M. W., 134
Smythies, J., 505, 519–520
Snell, B., 415
Snezhnevsky, A. V., 151
Snyder, L. M., 572, 574
Sobotka, H., 574
social anxiety, 303
social phobics, 539
social psychiatry, 165, 166
social situations, fear of, 294, 301, 307–309
social workers, 379
sociodynamics, 187
socioeconomic forces, 180–181
sociology, folklore psychiatry and, 165, 168–169
sociopolitical forces, 180–181
sodium amytal, 549, 551
solvent inhalation, 426, 430–432
somatic delusion, 303
somatic drives, Freudian theory, 83, 85–86, 101
somnambulism, 534
Soviet psychiatry, 151–152
Spence, L. W., 542
Spencer, Herbert, 80–81, 90
Spengler, O., 134
spherocytosis, hereditary, 572, 574
sphincter control, 126
Spiegel, J. P., 134
Spiegel, R., 226, 231
Spielrein, S., 116
spiritualistic monism, 91n
Spitz, R. A., 403, 405–407

spontaneous organization, 22
Spulak, F., 446-447
Stabenau, J. R., 481-482
stable equilibrium, 78, 101
stage fright, 295-297
stammering, fear of, 294
stationary-state formulations, 77-78, 89, 101
Stein, M. H., 141
Stekel, W., 61, 62n
Sterba, R., 91
Sternbach, R. A., 531
Sterne, L., 312
stoichiometric formulation, 78
Stone, L., 63-64
Stowell, R. E., 571
STP (DOM), 430, 435, 439, 449-450
Strachey, J., 95
Strasburger, E. A., 564
Straus, E., 130, 142, 145
stress theory, Selye's, 366
Stroop Color-Word Interference Test, 547
Stubbeline, J. M., 262
Stunkard, A. J., 197
subjective awareness, 16
subjective experiences, 7, 29, 325
subjective reality, 29
subjectivity, 3, 7, 29
sublimations, 37
subliminal experiences, 16
Sugerman, A. A., 533
suicidal risks, 67, 437
Sullivan, H. S., 15, 20-21, 220-221
superego, 5, 105; infantile, 224, 230; strict, 232
superego approval, fear of loss of, 142
suppression, 26, 31
Sutton, S., 536, 546
Sylvester, J. D., 136
symbolic anxiety, 24
symbolic cognition, 9-13
symbolic communication, 46
symbolic organization, *table*, 28
symbolism, 13; of time, 125-126, 133; unconscious, 220
symbolization, verbal, 11, 17
symptoms, 152, 155, 163
synapses, CNS, 584-590
syndromes, 152, 155-159, 161, 162; complex, 159; simple, 158-159
syphilis, 299
systematized delusions, 158
Szalita, A. B., 312, 319
Szasz, T. S., 91

tachycardia, 436, 439
tactile sensations, 21
Takaki, M., 145
Taketomo, Y., 112, 137
Talland, G. A., 143
taloperidol, 467
tapping-speed measures, 546, 549, 551, 553
taste, 7
Tausk, V., 304
Taylor, H. J., 568
Taylor, J. A., 542
teleological awareness, 18
Tellenbach, H., 295, 301
temperature perception, 7
temporality, 112-150; behavioral context of, *table*, 114; depression and, 130-132; disintegration of levels of, 137-142; in dynamic psychopathology, 120-125; orality-sleep, 116; schizophrenia and, 132-135, 143-144; during sensoriomotor period, 114-116; studies of in introspective and inspective frames of reference, 142-145; in verbalized experiences, 116-120. *See also* time
tension, 8, 10, 14; libidinal, 79-80, 83, 100, 101; need, 123
termination of treatment, considerations concerning, 52-53
tertiary cognition, 12
Thacore, V. R., 434
Thaler Singer, M., 206, 209
Thannhauser, S. J., 574
THC, 438, 445-447
theater, hippie movement and, 281-282, 289
theory-building, Freudian, steps in, 73-91
therapeutic alliance, 52-53, 233, 249
therapeutic frustration, 239
thermodynamic concepts, 73, 90, 96-97
thermodynamic constructs, 82
thermodynamic homologies, 96-97
thermodynamic regulative principle, 88
thermodynamic system, 80, 97-99
thinking, abstract, 402, 536, 547, 548; amorphous forms of, 207; autistic, 548; conceptual, 12, 22-23; concrete, 548; fragmented, 207-210; paleologic, 17, 18, 26; preconceptual, 13, 17-19; prelogical 17; schizophrenic, 207, 524, 547-548; secondary-process, 338
thioproperazine, 464, 467
thioridazine, 550
thioxanthemes, 465, 534
thirst, 7-9
Thoreau, Henry David, 259

INDEX

Thygesen, P., 366
thymoanaleptic effect, 466
Tienari, P., 478, 479
time, awareness of, discontinuity of, 124–125; passage of, distortion of speed in, 126–130; symbolism of, 125–126, 133
time orders (see temporality)
timelessness, 121–124
Tinbergen, N., 17, 123n
Titchener Illusion Test, 544
tofranil, 158
tonic excitation, 79
total energy, 81, 97–99
Toussieing, P., 403
training, psychoanalytic, 332–333, 377, 378
tranquilizers, 463–465, 467, 469–470
transcultural psychiatry, 165, 167, 172
transference, 45, 51, 56, 287; dependent, 68; latency-type, 66. See also transference reactions
transference neurosis, 58, 61
transference psychology, individual, 43
transference reactions, 58, 325; negative, 60–61; positive, 61, 62
transient maladaptation, 305
transmethylation, pathological, 505–506, 519
transvestism, 49–51
treatment, in folklore psychiatry, 170–174; long-term, 57, 67–68; shortening of (see brief psychotherapy); termination of, considerations in, 52–53
Trüb, H., 250
true energetic formulations, 78n, 79–80
truncated psychotherapy, 58
trytophan, 518
"Twenty-Minute Hour, The," 58, 63
twin studies, 404, 477–494, 513
two-clock theory, 92

Ucs, 87, 88, 121–122
ultraviolet microscopy, 560, 564
unconscious, dynamic, 40; timelessness of, 121–124
unconscious fantasies, 6, 35, 41, 43, 44, 53
unconscious motivation, 11–12
unconscious symbolism, 220
unconscious wishes, 220
undoing, 141
Ungerleider, J. T., 437, 438, 447
unrealistic character, 48
Unwin, J. R., 426
urge, Freudian concept of, 101–103, 105
urine findings, schizophrenic, 519–520
utopian conceptualizations, 178–179

Vaillant, G. E., 400, 404
validation, consensual, 11, 15; intrapsychic, 15; reflexive, 15
Valium, 451
values, parental, internalization of, 224
Van Krevelen, D. A., 422
Varimax rotation, 523; table, 521
Vartanyan, M. E., 162
Venables, P. H., 531, 538, 544, 546
ventilation, 62
Venzlaff, U., 372
verbal experience(s), 42; time orders in, 116–120
verbal symbolization, 11, 17
Verdun Target Symptom Rating Scale, 549
Vietnam War, protest movement against, 262, 264, 271, 276, 289
Villaret's encyclopedia, 77
Vincent, W. S., 561, 568
Vista volunteers, 290
visual images, 119
visual perceptions, 7; schizophrenic, 543–544
visual sensations, 21
vitamins, 569, 572–573
Vogel, G. W., 534
Von Bertalanffy, L., 29, 89
Von Daramus, E., 17, 18n, 135
Von Gebsattel, W. E., 142
Vygotsky, L. S., 22–23

Waelder, R., 45, 91
Walker, N., 91
Walter, Bruno, 56
Walter, K., 295, 301
Walter, W. G., 536
water pollution, 266
Watts, Alan, 259
Waxler, N. E., 317n
Weigert, E., 142
Weil, A. T., 445–446
Weismann, A., 564
Weiss, E., 221
Welch, L., 542
Werner, H., 12, 29, 116, 119, 134, 137, 207
West, L. J., 448
Westophal, C., 296
Wheeler, D. R., 144
White, B. L., 404
Who's Afraid of Virginia Woolf?, 327
Whorf, B. L., 26, 134
Wijesinghe, C. P., 428
Wing, J. K., 531
Winnicott, D. W., 377

wish(es), 14, 46; aggressive, 237; anal, 125–126; death, 126, 129, 141, 251; Freudian concept of, 102–103; incestuous, 228; oedipal, 47, 125, 126; oral, 47; preconscious, 87; reality value of, 20; unconscious, 220
wish-fulfillment, 25, 83, 84, 88, 93, 123
wishful impulses, 73, 83, 84, 86–88, 102–105
"Witches' poison", 449–450
withdrawal, drug-induced, 433; emotional, 407; infantile autistic, 400, 402, 403, 407, 408, 410; schizophrenic, 531
Wolberg, L. R., 68
Wolf, E., 403
Wolf, W., 180, 189
Wolf-man, 56
Wolfe, Tom, 262n
Wolff, P. H., 404
Woods, P. S., 568
Wooley, D. W., 505, 583

Worden, F. C., 400
working alliance, 52
working through, 58, 61, 63, 285, 287, 357, 366
Worley, L. G., 577, 579
Wulfeck, W., 546
Wynne, L. C., 206, 209, 317n

Yamamura, M., 294, 295
Yannet, H., 422
Yippies, 263–264, 268
You Are What You Eat, 281
Youth International Party, 263–264

Zahn, T. P., 538–539, 545–546
Zinberg, N. E., 445–446
zone specialty hospital, 192–193
Zubin, J., 536, 546
zygomoens, 566
zygotes, 567